MANAGEMENT
GUIDELINES
FOR NURSE
PRACTITIONERS
WORKING IN
FAMILY PRACTICE

MANAGEMENT GUIDELINES FOR NURSE PRACTITIONERS WORKING IN FAMILY PRACTICE

Alice F. Running, RN, PhD, FNP, ANP

Associate Professor
Coordinator, Family Nurse Practitioner Program
Orvis School of Nursing
University of Nevada, Reno
Reno, Nevada

Amy E. Berndt, RN, MSN, FNP

Assistant Professor
Orvis School of Nursing
University of Nevada, Reno
Reno, Nevada

 F. A. DAVIS COMPANY | Philadelphia

F. A. Davis Company
1915 Arch Street
Philadelphia, PA 19103
www.fadavis.com

Printed in Canada

Last digit indicates print number: 10 9 8 7 6 5 4 3 2 1

Publisher: Joanne P. DaCunha, RN, MSN
Developmental Editor: Diane Schweisguth, RN, BSN
Production Editor: Hearthside Publishing Services
Cover Designer: Louis P. Forgione

As new scientific information becomes available through basic and clinical research, recommended treatments and drug therapies undergo changes. The author(s) and publisher have done everything possible to make this book accurate, up to date, and in accord with accepted standards at the time of publication. The author(s), editors, and publisher are not responsible for errors or omissions or for consequences from application of the book, and make no warranty, expressed or implied, in regard to the contents of the book. Any practice described in this book should be applied by the reader in accordance with professional standards of care used in regard to the unique circumstances that may apply in each situation. The reader is advised always to check product information (package inserts) for changes and new information regarding dose and contraindications before administering any drug. Caution is especially urged when using new or infrequently ordered drugs.

Library of Congress Cataloging-in-Publication Data

Management guidelines for nurse practitioners working in family practice / [edited by] Alice F. Running, Amy E. Berndt.
    p. ; cm.
  Includes bibliographical references and index.
  ISBN 0-8036-0810-1 (alk. paper)
    1. Family nursing. 2. Nurse practitioners. I. Running, Alice F. II. Berndt, Amy E.
    [DNLM: 1. Nurse Practitioners. 2. Family Practice—Nurses' Instruction. 3. Nursing Care—methods. 4. Practice Management, Medical. WY 128 M266 2002]
RT120.F34 M36 2002
610.73—dc21

2002067312

We would like to dedicate this book to the past, present and future Family Nurse Practitioner students at the Orvis School of Nursing—University of Nevada, Reno. You continue to inspire us, and to make us proud.

AFR and AEB

I dedicate this book to the memory of my parents Fern and Ardean, and to my children Mary and Ross; "I'm the luckiest Mommy in the whole wide world."

AFR

PREFACE

Management Guidelines for Nurse Practitioners Working in Family Practice serves as a reference book for advanced practice nurses and students and is useful in both clinical and classroom environments. Contributors for each chapter were selected for their expertise in their knowledge in specific content areas. Each disorder follows a consistent format to make finding needed information easy. The headings include:

Signal Symptoms (to help quickly locate a potential diagnosis)
ICD – Codes
Definition
Epidemiology
Etiology
Physiology/Pathophysiology
Clinical Manifestations (subjective and objective)
Differential Diagnosis (with pertinent findings for each differential
    diagnosis listed to assist with targeting the appropriate diagnosis)
Diagnostic Tests (rationale for the test, expected outcomes)
Management/Treatment (pharmacological and non-pharmacological,
    complementary/alternative therapies, client education, and follow-up)
Referral
Notes—Medical information changes so rapidly that any reference
    source, even the content found on the Internet, may not be the most
    current thinking. This section is provided to allow the user to annotate
    pertinent changes and note what works best in his/her individual
    practice making this book truly his/her own personal and reputable
    reference resource.

Color photographs for common skin diagnoses are included because identifying rashes are often the most challenging diagnoses the provider must make. And to validate the content, references and resources for each chapter.

Health and its promotion have always been a central concept in the practice of nursing. Even as the role of the advanced practice nurse emerges, its clear that assessing for health and being a partner with the client in obtaining the information about health promotion and disease prevention they need remains a central component of practice. Chapter One, Health Promotion, is just the reference needed to ensure that health promotion needs are being addressed.

ACKNOWLEDGMENTS

I would like to acknowledge:

My husband, Mark, for his constant encouragement and love.

The faculty and staff at the Orvis School of Nursing.

Diane Schweisguth and Joanne DaCunha—you two were always there to answer questions, to set things up right, and to give encouragement.

Each of the contributors for their time and willingness to help with this project.

Kitty Kelly, RN, MS, FNP, your help made the last revisions possible—thank you!

AFR

To my parents, for their never-ending support and encouragement.

To DSB, for your ability to always make me laugh and your wonderful love.

AEB

CONTRIBUTORS

Sherri Aikin, RN, MS, CFNP
Nurse Practitioner
Digestive Health Associates
Reno, Nevada
Chapter 7 Gastrointestinal System

Christine Aramburu-Drury, RN, MSN, CS, FNP
Assistant Professor
Orvis School of Nursing
University of Nevada, Reno
Reno, Nevada
Chapter 2 Skin (co-author)

Amy E. Berndt, RN, MSN, CFNP
Assistant Professor
Orvis School of Nursing
University of Nevada, Reno
Reno, Nevada
Chapter 2 Skin (co-author)
Chapter 4 Ear, Nose and Throat
Chapter 6 Cardiovascular System (co-author)
Chapter 8 Renal and Genitourinary Systems
Chapter 12 Nervous System

Peggie A. Black, RN, MS, CFNP, CACNP
Nurse Practitioner
Reno Heart Physicians
Reno, Nevada
Chapter 6 Cardiovascular System (co-author)

Mary Burman, RN, PhD, FNP, CNS
Associate Professor
School of Nursing
University of Wyoming
Laramie, WY
  Chapter 5 Respiratory System

Paul DeBaldo, MSN, RN, CS
Mental Health Nurse Practitioner
Mount Hood Community Mental Health Center
Portland, Oregon
  Chapter 13 Mental Health

Kathryn Eckert, MD
Assistant Professor, Pediatrics
School of Medicine
University of Nevada, Reno
Reno, NV
  Chapter 10 Endocrine System (co-author)

Janice Hausauer, RN, MS, FNP
College of Nursing
Montana State University
Bozeman, Montana
  Chapter 3 Eye

Mari Holt, RN, PNP
Assistant Professor
School of Medicine
University of Nevada, Reno
Reno, Nevada
  Chapter 10 Endocrine System (co-author)

Margaret K. Knapp, BA, BSN, MS, CFNP
Nurse Practitioner
Washoe Health System
Reno, Nevada
  Chapter 9 Reproductive System (co-author)

Beverly Mustain, MS, RN, CS, FNP
Nurse Practitioner
Specialty Health Nevada
Reno, Nevada
  Chapter 9 Reproductive System (co-author)

Demetrius Porche RN, DNS, FNP, CS
Associate Professor
School of Nursing/Community Health Department
Louisiana State University Health Sciences Center
New Orleans, Louisiana
  Chapter 14 Infectious Diseases

Alice F. Running, RN, PhD, FNP, ANP

Associate Professor
Coordinator, Family Nurse Practitioner Program
Orvis School of Nursing
University of Nevada, Reno
Reno, Nevada
  Chapter 1 Health Promotion
  Chapter 7 Gastrointestinal System (co-author)
  Chapter 9 Reproductive System (co-author)
  Chapter 10 Endocrine System (co-author)

Sue Yarbrough, RN, MSN, CS, FNP

Assistant Professor
Southwest Missouri State University
College of Health and Human Services
Springfield, Missouri
  Chapter 11 Musculoskeletal System

Joseph Zelk, MS, RN, CS, FNP

Nurse Practitioner
Reno Heart Physicians
Reno, Nevada
  Chapter 2 Skin (co-author)

CONSULTANTS

Kimberly Ann Devine, RN, MSN, CRNP, ACNP-CS, CCRN
Cardiovascular Nurse Practitioner
St. Mary Medical Center
Langhorne, PA

Rosanne Iacono, RNCS, MSN, ARNP
Nurse Practitioner
Philadelphia, PA

Pamela McDonald, RNFA-C, WHCNP, ACNP
Nurse Practitioner
Blackhawk Medical Center
Blackhawk, CA

Alice S. Poyss, RN, PhD, CRNP
Associate Professor
MCP Hahnemann University
Philadelphia, PA

CONTENTS

Chapter *1*
HEALTH PROMOTION

Health and its promotion have always been a central concept in the practice of nursing. Today the role of advanced practice nurses is emerging, but it still contains at its core the continued provision of valuable information and advanced assessment related to health promotion and disease prevention for clients throughout their lives. This is even more compelling when we reflect on the most commonly identified causes of death:

Leading Causes of Death, 1997 (Healthy People 2010)

Heart disease
Cancer
Stroke
Chronic obstructive lung disease
Unintentional injuries
Pneumonia and influenza
Diabetes
Suicide
Kidney disease
Chronic liver disease/cirrhosis

When we are able to understand what the actual causes of these deaths are, our roles as disease preventer and health promoter are even more apparent:

Actual Causes of Death

Tobacco use
Diet and inactivity patterns
Alcohol abuse
Infections
Toxic agents
Firearms
Sexual behavior
Motor vehicles
Drugs

This chapter provides the practitioner with tools for assessing and then promoting health, thereby reducing disease.

IMMUNIZATION SCHEDULE

See Table 1–1 for childhood, adolescent, and adult immunization recommendations.

Table 1–1 Recommended Childhood Immunization Schedule United States, 2002

Legend: Range of recommended ages · Catch-up vaccination · Preadolescent assessment

Age Vaccine	Birth	1 mo	2 mos	4 mos	6 mos	12 mos	15 mos	18 mos	24 mos	4-6 yrs	11-12 yrs	13-18 yrs
Hepatitis B[1]	Hep B #1	only if mother HBsAg(-) Hep B #2			Hep B #3						Hep B series	
Diphtheria, Tetanus, Pertussis[2]			DTaP	DTaP	DTaP		DTaP			DTaP	Td	
Haemophilus influenzae type b[3]			Hib	Hib	Hib	Hib						
Inactivated Polio[4]			IPV	IPV	IPV					IPV		
Measles, Mumps, Rubella[5]						MMR #1				MMR #2	MMR #2	
Varicella[6]						Varicella					Varicella	
Pneumococcal[7]			PCV	PCV	PCV	PCV			PCV	PCV	PPV	
Hepatitis A[8]									Hepatitis A series			
Influenza[9]					Influenza (yearly)							

Vaccines below this line are for selected populations

This schedule indicates the recommended ages for routine administration of currently licensed childhood vaccines, as of December 1, 2001, for children through age 18 years. Any dose not given at the recommended age should be given at any subsequent visit when indicated and feasible. ▮ Indicates age groups that warrant special effort to administer those vaccines not previously given. Additional vaccines may be licensed and recommended during the year. Licensed combination vaccines may be used whenever any components of the combination are indicated and the vaccine's other components are not contraindicated. Providers should consult the manufacturers' package inserts for detailed recommendations.

Approved by the Advisory Committee on Immunization Practices (www.cdc.gov/nip/acip), the American Academy of Pediatrics (www.aap.org), and the American Academy of Family Physicians (www.aafp.org).

1. **Hepatitis B vaccine (Hep B).** All infants should receive the first dose of hepatitis B vaccine soon after birth and before hospital discharge; the first dose may also be given by age 2 months if the infant's mother is HBsAg-negative. Only monovalent hepatitis B vaccine can be used for the birth dose. Monovalent or combination vaccine containing Hep B may be used to complete the series; four doses of vaccine may be administered if combination vaccine is used. The second dose should be given at least 4 weeks after the first dose, except for Hib-containing vaccine which cannot be administered before age 6 weeks. The third dose should be given at least 16 weeks after the first dose and at least 8 weeks after the second dose. The last dose in the vaccination series (third or fourth dose) should not be administered before age 6 months.

   Infants born to HBsAg-positive mothers should receive hepatitis B vaccine and 0.5 mL hepatitis B immune globulin (HBIG) within 12 hours of birth at separate sites. The second dose is recommended at age 1–2 months and the vaccination series should be completed (third or fourth dose) at age 6 months.

   Infants born to mothers whose HBsAg status is unknown should receive the first dose of the hepatitis B vaccine series within 12 hours of birth. Maternal blood should be drawn at the time of delivery to determine the mother's HBsAg status; if the HBsAg test is positive, the infant should receive HBIG as soon as possible (no later than age 1 week).

2. **Diphtheria and tetanus toxoids and acellular pertussis vaccine (DTaP).** The fourth dose of DTaP may be administered as early as age 12 months, provided 6 months have elapsed since the third dose and the child is unlikely to return at age 15–18 months. **Tetanus and diphtheria toxoids (Td)** is recommended at age 11–12 years if at least 5 years have elapsed since the last dose of tetanus and diphtheria toxoid-containing vaccine. Subsequent routine Td boosters are recommended every 10 years.

3. **Haemophilus influenzae type b (Hib) conjugate vaccine.** Three Hib conjugate vaccines are licensed for infant use. If PRP-OMP (PedvaxHIB® or ComVax® (Merck)) is administered at ages 2 and 4 months, a dose at age 6 months is not required. DTaP/Hib combination products should not be used for primary immunization in infants at ages 2, 4 or 6 months, but can be used as boosters following any Hib vaccine.

4. **Inactivated polio vaccine (IPV).** An all-IPV schedule is recommended for routine childhood polio vaccination in the United States. All children should receive four doses of IPV at ages 2 months, 4 months, 6–18 months, and 4–6 years.

5. **Measles, mumps, and rubella vaccine (MMR).** The second dose of MMR is recommended routinely at age 4–6 years but may be administered during any visit, provided at least 4 weeks have elapsed since the first dose and that both doses are administered beginning at or after age 12 months. Those who have not previously received the second dose should complete the schedule by the 11–12 year old visit.

6. **Varicella vaccine.** Varicella vaccine is recommended at any visit at or after age 12 months for susceptible children, i.e. those who lack a reliable history of chickenpox. Susceptible persons aged >13 years should receive two doses, given at least 4 weeks apart.

7. **Pneumococcal vaccine.** The heptavalent pneumococcal conjugate vaccine (PCV) is recommended for all children age 2–23 months. It is also recommended for certain children age 24–59 months. **Pneumococcal polysaccharide vaccine (PPV)** is recommended in addition to PCV for certain high-risk groups. See MMWR. 2000;49(RR-9):1–35.

8. **Hepatitis A vaccine.** Hepatitis A vaccine is recommended for use in selected states and regions, and for certain high-risk groups; consult your local public health authority. See MMWR. 1999;48(RR-12):1–37.

9. **Influenza vaccine.** Influenza vaccine is recommended annually for children age > 6 months with certain risk factors (including but not limited to asthma, cardiac disease, sickle cell disease, HIV, diabetes; see MMWR. 2001;50(RR-4):1–44), and can be administered to all others wishing to obtain immunity. Children aged ≤12 years should receive vaccine in a dosage appropriate for their age (0.25 mL if age 6–35 months or 0.5 mL if age ≥3 years). Children aged ≤8 years who are receiving influenza vaccine for the first time should receive two doses separated by at least 4 weeks.

For additional information about vaccines, vaccine supply, and contraindications for immunization, please visit the National Immunization Program Web site at www.cdc.gov/nip or call the National Immunization Hotline at (800) 232-2522 (English) or (800) 232-0233 (Spanish).

GROWTH

Weight

Between 5 and 6 mo of age, the infant should double his/her weight; by 1 year the birth weight should triple.

Toddler (1–3) average yearly gain: 4.4–6.6 lb
Preschool child (3–6) average yearly gain: 4–6 lb
School-age child (6–12) average yearly gain: 4–6 lb
Preadolescent girl (10–14) average total gain: 38.5 lb
Preadolescent boy (12–16) average total gain: 52.1 lb

Length

Increases about 1 inch/month, with an average yearly increase in height between 10 and 12 inches.

Toddler (1–3) average yearly gain: 1–2 years, 12 cm; 2–3 years, 6–8 cm;
    height at 2 years, approximately half of adult height
Preschool child (3–6) average yearly gain: 6–8 cm
School age child (6–12) average yearly gain: 5 cm
Preadolescent girl (10–14) average yearly gain: 6–8.3 cm; 95% of adult
    height achieved by menarche
Preadolescent boy (12–16) average yearly gain: 6–9.5 cm; 95% of adult
    height achieved by 15 years

Fontanels

The anterior fontanel closes between 9 and 12 mo; the posterior fontanel closes by 4 mo (see Table 1–2).

Table 1–2

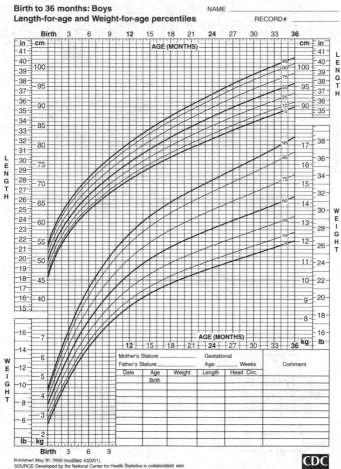

Birth to 36 months: Boys
Length-for-age and Weight-for-age percentiles

NAME _____

RECORD# _____

Published May 30, 2000 (modified 4/20/01).
SOURCE: Developed by the National Center for Health Statistics in collaboration with
the National Center for Chronic Disease Prevention and Health Promotion (2000).
http://www.cdc.gov/growthcharts

CDC

SAFER · HEALTHIER · PEOPLE™

Birth to 36 months: Girls
Length-for-age and Weight-for-age percentiles

NAME _____

RECORD # _____

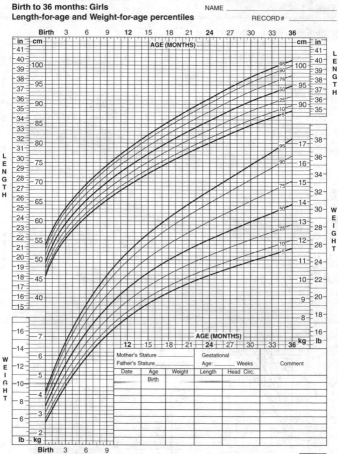

Published May 30, 2000 (modified 4/20/01).
SOURCE Developed by the National Center for Health Statistics in collaboration with
the National Center for Chronic Disease Prevention and Health Promotion (2000).
http://www.cdc.gov/growthcharts

SAFER · HEALTHIER · PEOPLE™

Birth to 36 months: Boys
Head circumference-for-age and
Weight-for-length percentiles

NAME _____

RECORD# _____

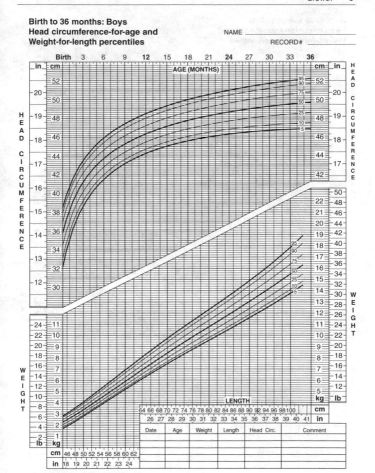

Published May 30, 2000 (modified 10/16/00).
SOURCE: Developed by the National Center for Health Statistics in collaboration with
the National Center for Chronic Disease Prevention and Health Promotion (2000).
http://www.cdc.gov/growthcharts

CDC

SAFER·HEALTHIER·PEOPLE™

Birth to 36 months: Girls
Head circumference-for-age and
Weight-for-length percentiles

NAME _____

RECORD# _____

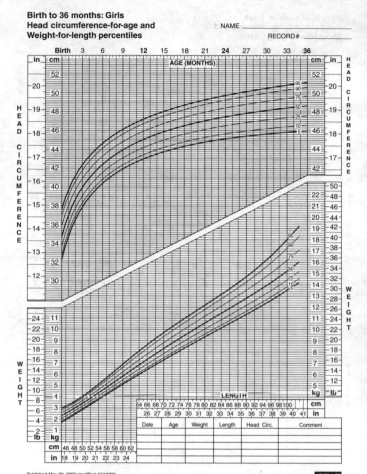

Published May 30, 2000 (modified 10/16/00).
SOURCE: Developed by the National Center for Health Statistics in collaboration with
the National Center for Chronic Disease Prevention and Health Promotion (2000).
http://www.cdc.gov/growthcharts

2 to 20 years: Boys
Stature-for-age and Weight-for-age percentiles

NAME _____

RECORD# _____

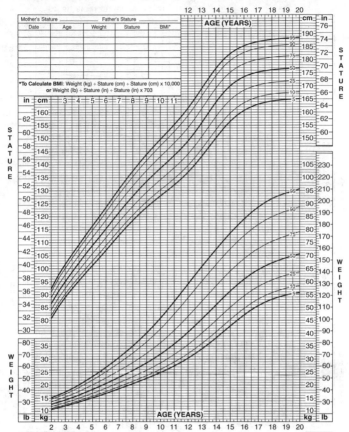

Published May 30, 2000 (modified 11/21/00).
SOURCE: Developed by the National Center for Health Statistics in collaboration with
the National Center for Chronic Disease Prevention and Health Promotion (2000).
http://www.cdc.gov/growthcharts

CDC
SAFER · HEALTHIER · PEOPLE™

2 to 20 years: Girls
Stature-for-age and Weight-for-age percentiles

NAME _____

RECORD# _____

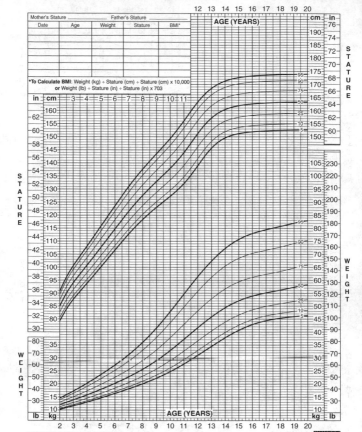

Published May 30, 2000 (modified 11/21/00).
SOURCE: Developed by the National Center for Health Statistics in collaboration with the National Center for Chronic Disease Prevention and Health Promotion (2000).
http://www.cdc.gov/growthcharts

CDC
SAFER · HEALTHIER · PEOPLE™

2 to 20 years: Boys
Body mass index-for-age percentiles

NAME _____

RECORD # _____

Date	Age	Weight	Stature	BMI*	Comments

*To Calculate BMI: Weight (kg) ÷ Stature (cm) ÷ Stature (cm) x 10,000
or Weight (lb) ÷ Stature (in) ÷ Stature (in) x 703

BMI values shown on chart: 35, 34, 33, 32, 31, 30, 29, 28, 27, 26, 25, 24, 23, 22, 21, 20, 19, 18, 17, 16, 15, 14, 13, 12

Percentile curves: 95, 90, 85, 75, 50, 25, 10, 5

AGE (YEARS): 2 3 4 5 6 7 8 9 10 11 12 13 14 15 16 17 18 19 20

kg/m²

Published May 30, 2000 (modified 10/16/00).
SOURCE: Developed by the National Center for Health Statistics in collaboration with
the National Center for Chronic Disease Prevention and Health Promotion (2000).
http://www.cdc.gov/growthcharts

CDC

SAFER · HEALTHIER · PEOPLE™

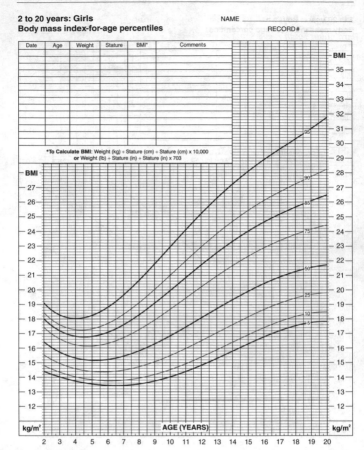

2 to 20 years: Girls
Body mass index-for-age percentiles

NAME _____

RECORD# _____

*To Calculate BMI: Weight (kg) ÷ Stature (cm) ÷ Stature (cm) x 10,000
or Weight (lb) ÷ Stature (in) ÷ Stature (in) x 703*

Published May 30, 2000 (modified 10/16/00).
SOURCE: Developed by the National Center for Health Statistics in collaboration with
the National Center for Chronic Disease Prevention and Health Promotion (2000).
http://www.cdc.gov/growthcharts

CDC
SAFER • HEALTHIER • PEOPLE™

Normal Pattern of Development

See Tables 1–3, 1–4, and 1–5.

Table 1–3   Eruption of Teeth

Primary Teeth	Age of Eruption in Months
Central incisor	6–7.5
Lateral incisor	7–9
Cuspid	16–18
First molar	12–14
Second molar	20–24

Table continued on following page.

Table 1–3   Eruption of Teeth (*Continued*)

Permanent Teeth	Age of Eruption in Years
Central incisor	6–8
Lateral incisor	7–9
Cuspid	9–12
First bicuspid	10–12
Second bicuspid	10–12
First molar	6–7
Second molar	11–13

Table 1–4   Milestones of Development—A Summary*

Newborn	When prone, pelvis is high, knees are under abdomen
2–4 wk	Watches mother intently as she speaks to him
1 mo	Ventral suspension (held prone, hand under abdomen)—head up momentarily, elbows flexed, hips partly extended, knees flexed
4–6 wk	*Smiles at mother in response to overtures*
6 wk	*Ventral suspension—head held up momentarily in same plane as rest of body; some extension of hips and flexion of knees and elbows* *When prone, pelvis is largely flat, hips mostly extended* (but when sleeping, the baby lies with pelvis high, and knees are under abdomen, like a newborn) Pulls to sit from supine position—much head lag, but not complete; hands often open When supine, follows object 90 cm away over angle of 90°
2 mo	Ventral suspension—maintains head in same plane as rest of body Hands are largely open When prone, chin is off couch; plane of face is 45° to flat surface (e.g., bed or floor) Smiles and vocalizes when talked to Eyes follow a moving person
3 mo	Ventral suspension—holds head up long time beyond plane of rest of body When prone, plane of face is 45–90° from flat surface When pulled to sit, there is only a slight head lag Hands loosely open *Holds rattle placed in hand* Vocalizes a great deal when talked to Follows object for 180° (lying supine) *Turns head to sound (3–4 months) on a level with the ear*
4 mo	When prone, plane of face is 90° to flat surface Hands come together Pulls dress or shirt over face Laughs aloud
5 mo	When prone, weight is on forearms When pulled to sit, there is no head lag When supine, feet come to mouth; plays with toes *Able to go for object and get it*
6 mo	When prone, weight is on hands; extended arms When pulled to sit, there is no head lag *When supine, lifts head spontaneously* Sits on floor, hand forward for support When held in standing position, full weight is on legs Rolls, prone to supine Begins to imitate (e.g., a cough) *Chews* Transfers cube from one hand to another
7 mo	*Sits on floor seconds, no support* Roll, supine to prone When held standing, bounces

Table continued on following page.

Table 1–4 Milestones of Development—A Summary* (Continued)

	Feeds self with biscuit Attracts attention by cough or other methods Turns head to sound below level of ear
8 mo	Sits unsupported; leans forward to reach objects Turns head to sound above level of ear
9 mo	Stands, holding on; pulls to stand or sitting position Crawls on abdomen
9–10 mo	*Uses index finger approach* *Uses finger-thumb apposition*—picks up pellet between tip of thumb and tip of forefinger
10 mo	Creeps on hands and knees; abdomen off flat surface Can change from sitting to prone and back Pulls self to sitting position *Waves goodbye* *Plays pat-a-cake* *Helps to dress*—holding arms out for coat, foot for shoe, or transferring object from one hand to another for sleeve
11 mo	Offers object to mother, but will not release it Utters one word with meaning When sitting, pivots around without overbalancing Walks, holding on to furniture; walks with two hands held
12 mo	Utters two to three words with meaning When prone, walks on hands and feet like a bear Walks, one hand held Casting objects, one after another, begins *Gives object to mother*
13 mo	*Walks, no support* Mouthing of objects stopped Slobbering largely stopped
15 mo	Creep up stairs; kneels Makes tower of two cubes Takes off shoes *Feeds self, picking up an ordinary cup, drinking, putting it down* Imitates parent in domestic work ("domestic mimicry") Jargon
18 mo	*No more casting* Gets up and down stairs, holding rail Jumps, both feet Seats self in chair Makes tower of three to four cubes Throws ball without falling Takes off gloves and socks; unzips Manages spoon well Points to three parts of body on request Turns pages of books, two or three at a time Points to some objects on request Toilet control—tells parent that he wants to go potty; largely dry by day
21–24 mo	*Spontaneously joins two or three words together to make sentence*
24 mo	Picks up object from floor without falling Runs Kicks ball Turns doorknob Makes tower of six or seven cubes Puts on shoes, socks, pants; takes off shoes and socks Points to four parts of body on request Imitates vertical and circular strokes with a pencil

Table continued on following page.

Table 1–4   Milestones of Development—A Summary* *(Continued)*

Turns pages of a book singly
Is mainly dry at night
Climbs stairs, two feet per step
Motor
   Gross: Runs well, no falling
   Walks up and down stairs alone
   Kicks large ball on request
   Fine: Turns pages of book singly
Adaptive
Builds tower of six to seven cubes
Aligns cubes for train
Imitates vertical and circular strokes with pencil
Language
Uses pronouns
Uses three-word sentences; jargon discarded
Carries out four directions with ball ("on the table", "to mother," "to me," "on the
    chair")
Personal-social
Verbalizes toilet needs consistently
Pulls on simple garments
Inhibits turning of spoon in feeding
Exhibits domestic mimicry

30 mo *Motor*
   Gross: Jumps up and down
   Walks backward
   Fine: Holds crayons in fist
Adaptive
Copies crude circle, closed figure
Names some drawings: house, shoe, ball, dog
Language
Refers to self as "I"
Knows full name
Personal-social
Helps put things away
Unbuttons large buttons

3 yr *Motor*
   Gross: Alternates feet going upstairs
   Jumps from bottom step
   Rides tricycle, using pedals
   Fine: Holds crayon with fingers
   Pincer grasp
Adaptive
Builds tower of 9–10 cubes
Imitates three-cube building
Names own drawing
Copies circle and imitates cross
Language
Uses plurals
Names action in picture book
Gives sex and full name
Obeys two prepositional commands (e.g., "on" and "under")
Personal-social
Feeds self well
Puts on shoes

4 yr *Motor*
Walks downstairs alternating feet
Does broad jump
Throws ball overhand
Hops on one foot

Table continued on following page.

Table 1–4 Milestones of Development—A Summary* *(Continued)*

Adaptive
Draws person with two parts
Copies cross
Counts three objects with correct pointing
Imitates five-cube gate
Pick longer of two lines
Language
Names one or more colors correctly
Obeys five prepositional commands (e.g., "on," "under," "in back," in front," "beside")
Personal-social
Washes and dries face and hands; brushes teeth
Distinguishes front from back of clothes
Laces shoes
Goes on errands outside of home

5 yr   *Motor*
Skips, alternating feet
Stands on one foot more than 8 sec
Catches, bounces ball
Adaptive
Builds two steps with cubes
Draws unmistakable person with body, head, etc
Copies triangle
Counts 10 objects correctly
Language
Knows four colors
Names penny, nickel, dime
Gives descriptive comment on pictures
Carries out three commands (e.g., "go under the table, get the penny, and give it to me.")
Personal-social
Dresses and undresses without assistance
Asks meaning of words
Prints a few letters

6 yr   *Motor*
Has advanced throwing
Stands on each foot alternatively, eyes closed
Walks line backward, heel-toe
Adaptive
Builds three steps with blocks
Draws person with neck, hands, and clothes
Adds and subtracts within 5
Copies drawing of diamond
Language
Uses Stanford-Binet items (vocabulary)
Defines words by function or composition (e.g., "house is to live in")
Personal-social
Ties shoelaces
Differentiates AM from PM
Knows right from left
Counts to 30

*Most important milestones in italics.
Source: Adapted from Palmer, FB: Streams of development. In Oski, FA, et al (eds): Principles and Practice of Pediatrics. JB Lippincott, Philadelphia, 1990, pp. 606–615.

Table 1–5   Normal Reflexes in Infants and Children

Response	Age at Time of Appearance	Age at Time of Disappearance
Reflexes of Position and Movement		
Moro reflex	Birth	1–3 mo
Tonic neck reflex (unsustained)	Birth	5–6 mo (partial up to 2–4 yr)
Neck righting reflex	4–6 mo	1–2 yr
Landau response	3 mo	1–2 yr
Palmar grasp reflex	Birth	4 mo
Adductor spread of knee jerk	Birth	7 mo
Plantar grasp reflex	Birth	8–15 mo
Babinski response	Birth	Variable
Parachute reaction	8–9 mo	Variable
Reflexes to Sound		
Blinking response	Birth	
Turning response	Birth	
Reflexes to Vision		
Blinking to threat	6–7 mo	
Horizontal following	4–6 wk	
Vertical following	2–3 mo	
Optokinetic nystagmus	Birth	
Postrotational nystagmus	Birth	
Lid closure to light	Birth	
Macular light reflex	4–8 mo	
Food Reflexes		
Rooting response—awake	Birth	3–4 mo
Rooting response—asleep	Birth	7–8 mo
Sucking response	Birth	12 mo
Handedness	2–3 yr	
Spontaneous Stepping	Birth	
Straight Line Walking	5–6 yr	

EVALUATION OF PHYSICAL ABUSE (adapted from Burns et al., 2000)

Pattern of the injuries

Skin and soft tissue:

Shape of bruise: imprints from hanger, jewelry, finger/hand, paddle

Colorations:

Red/purple/blue: 0–5 days old

Green: 5–7 days old

Yellow: 7–10 days old

Brown: 10–14 days old

Locations: look for multiple bruising on buttocks, trunk, back, genitals, ears and face

Burns:

Location:

Accidental if on hand, arm, or leg

Intentional if on both palms, both soles, flexor surfaces of thighs, or perineum

Scalding:
>Hot liquid most common intentional injury
>>Young children: immersion most common
>>Older children usually have hot liquid thrown at them or poured on them
>Burn pattern:
>>Sharply demarcated or circumferential burns when children are held in hot water (sock or glove burns)
>>Donut-shaped burn on buttock of child who is forcibly held in tub of hot water so that center part of buttock is spared from burning
>>Zebra stripe effect: typical pattern when child is held by the hands and legs under a faucet of hot water and the creases in the abdomen and upper legs fold up and are spared from burning
>>Cigarette burns: often multiple; found on soles and palms

Common Sites for Unintentional Injuries

Shins, elbows, knees
Skin:
>Scrapes
>Scars
>Scabs
Splash marks, such as may occur when a child tries to escape hot liquid

Common Sites for Intentional Injuries

Eyes: black
Earlobe: pinched and/or pulled
Cheek: slapped/squeezed
Upper lip: lacerations/bruises
Scalp: bare spots on scalp and broken hair, bruises
Neck: choke marks
Chest: bite marks, burns
Buttocks lower back: paddling and strap marks, burns
Genitals: pinch marks, bruises, bladder/vaginal infections
Extremities (upper): grab marks, friction burns (rope), burns (cigarettes), fractures
Extremities (lower): razor, tattoo marks, burns, fractures
Abdomen: bruises, scars, burns
(Adapted from Burns et al. Pediatric Primary Care, pgs 444–447)

EVALUATION OF PSYCHOLOGICAL ABUSE/MALTREATMENT OF CHILD

In your evaluation of the child, be alert for the following behavioral signs associated with abuse:

Overly compliant or exhibits exaggerated fearfulness

Clingy and indiscriminate attachment

Extremes in behavior (aggressive/passive)

Apprehensive when other children cry

Wary of physical contact with adults

Frightened of parents or of going home, or both

Exhibits drastic behavioral changes in and out of parental or caregiver presence

Depressed, hypervigilant, withdrawn, apathetic, antisocial, exhibits destructive behavior, suicidal (suicide attempts and/or plans) and/or engages in self-mutilation

Overprotective of parents or caregivers

Displays sleep or eating disorders

Dirty, malnourished, poor hygiene, inadequately dressed for weather

Inadequate medical and dental care (multiple caries)

Always sleepy (chronic fatigue) or hungry

(Adapted from Burns et al. Pediatric Primary Care, pg 444)

SCREENING RECOMMENDATIONS (birth–18 mo)

See Table 1–6

Leading causes of death:

    Conditions that originate in the perinatal period

    Congenital anomalies

    Heart disease

    Injuries (non-motor-vehicle)

    Pneumonia/influenza

Table 1–6 Screening Recommendations (Birth–18 mo)

Screening	Parent Counseling	Immunizations	Watch for
Height at birth: boys, 19–21 in.; girls, 20 in. Weight at birth: boys, 7.5 lb; girls, 7 lb Head circumference: 12.4–14.8 in. Schedule of visits: 2 weeks (ask about Apgar scores); 2 mo, 4 mo, 6 mo, 1 yr, 15–18 mo	Breast-feeding (teach parents about drugs that cross into the breast milk) Encourage parents to place infant on his/her back while sleeping	See Table 1–1	Ocular misalignment
Hemoglobin: at 6 mo evaluate for iron deficiency and anemia; by 18 mo should be normal adult range (12–18 gms)	Nutrient intake: Stomach capacity: Newborn: 10–20 ml 1 wk: 30–90 ml 2–3 wk: 75–100 ml 1 mo: 90–150 ml 3 mo: 150–200 ml 1 yr: 210–360 ml (Murray and Zentner, 2001, p 352)	Influenza (6–18 mo) if receiving ongoing aspirin therapy because of risk of Reye's syndrome after influenza	Tooth decay (tooth buds begin to appear at 4–6 mo; most teeth should be in by 18–20 mo) Encourage dental visit at 2 yr of age
Hearing (can be tested at birth but must be checked 18 mo)	Child safety seats Recommend five-point restraint safety seat and rear-facing car seat		Abuse/neglect (watch for shaken-baby syndrome, failure to thrive, neglect)
Fontanels: Anterior closes at 8–18 mo; posterior closes at 2–3 mo Vital signs: 1–3 mo: Respirations, 50–80/min Temperature, 97–100°F Heart rate 100–160 beats/min Blood pressure, 80–40 mm Hg 6–9 mo: Respirations, 32/min Heart rate 115 beats/min Blood pressure, 90/60 mm Hg 9–12 mo: Respirations, 20–30/min Temperature, 99.7°F Heart rate, 100–110 beats/min Blood pressure, 96/66 mm Hg (Murray and Zentner, 2001, p 349)	Smoke detector Hot-water-heater temperature—most are set at 140–150, which will cause serious burns in 2–3 seconds. **Set at 120°F or below** (National Safe Kids Campaign and Burn Foundation)		

Table continued on following page.

Table 1–6 Screening Recommendations (Birth–18 mo) (*Continued*)

Screening	Parent Counseling	Immunizations	Watch for

Vision:
  Should be tracking
    1 day after birth;
    accommodation
    at 8 in. by 1 mo
	Use gates across stairways, window guards, and fences around swimming pools		

Feeding schedule:
  1 wk, 2–3 oz Q2–4 H
  1 mo, 3–4 oz Q4–5H
  2–3 mo, 4–6 oz,
    5 feedings QD;
    may add rice
    cereal
  4–5 mo, 5–7 oz, 5–6
    feedings QD; may
    add iron-fortified
    cereals, strained
    vegetables)
  6–7 mo, 6–8 oz, 4–5
    feedings QD; can
    add solids and
    finger foods at this
    time
  8–9 mo, 8 oz, 3–4
    feedings QD;
    regular foods
    mashed or
    chopped
  9–12 mo, 3 feedings
    QD; add whole
    milk at 12 mo and
    encourage parents
    to have child drink
    from a cup
  (Murray and Zentner,
    2001, p 354)
  Breast-feeding, if possible, is recommended for the first 10 to 14 mo
	Storage of medications/drugs and toxic chemicals (i.e., paints)
	Teach parents that some of the glossy pages used in magazines and/or books actually contain lead and should be kept from children.
	Day-care checklist:
	  Ask these questions to help assess a potential day-care center for a child:
	  How long has the center been in operation?
	  How long have current staff members been working there?
	  What credentials do the caregivers have?
	  What is the average teacher salary?
	  How big are classes?
	  What is the staff: child ratio?
	  How do children spend their days?
	  Is the schedule flexible?
	  How are children disciplined?
	  Are parents free to visit the center at any time?
	  Poison control center (1-888-252-7751); have ipecac syrup on hand		

	Sunscreen (avoid PABA if under 6 mo):
	  Use at least 15 SPF and reapply Q2H
	  Avoid sun exposure between the hours of 10 AM and 2 PM
	(www.epa.gov)		

Source: http://kidshealth.org/

SCREENING RECOMMENDATIONS (2–6 years)

See Table 1–7.
Leading Causes of Death:
Injuries (non-motor-vehicle)
Motor-vehicle accidents
Congenital anomalies
Homicide
Heart disease

Table 1–7 Screening Recommendations (2–6 yr)

Screening	Parent Counseling	Immunizations	Watch for
Height/Weight—Girls 2 yr: 35 in./29 lb 3 yr: 38½ in./33¾ lb 4 yr: 41¾ in./38¾ lb 5 yr: 44 in./42½ lb 6 yr: 46 in./47½ lb Height/Weight—Boys 2 yr: 36″/30½ lb 3 yr: 39 in./34¾ lb 4 yr: 42 in./39¾ lb 5 yr: 44 in./44½ lb 6 yr: 46¾ in./48½ lb (www.babybag.com)	Limit sweets and between-meal snacks	See Table 1–1	Vision disorders (strabismus, amblyopia)
Blood Pressure: Screen annually beginning at age 3 80–100 systolic/64 diastolic (hypertension for this age group is a diastolic pressure greater than 90 mm Hg, usually measured on three occasions) (Murray and Zentner, 2001, p 389)	Iron-enriched foods, sodium restriction	Fluoride supplements Begin fluoride supplements as soon as first teeth arrive If not in the water supply (6 mo–3 years 0.25 mg NaCl PO QD, 3–6 years 0.5 mg PO QD 6–16 years 0.5–1 mg PO QD) (epocrates.com)	Dental decay, malalignment, premature loss of teeth, mouth breathing. Ask parents about use of pacifier and begin to discourage use. Discuss dental consultation for protective coating on molars. Continue with fluoride treatments if not in water supply.
Eye examination (amblyopia and strabismus to the age of 3–4 yr—if asymptomatic no need for further eye examinations until school (Gonzales & Kutner, 2000, p 56)	Calorie balance (children 2–6 yr old need about 1600 cal/day) (Dietary Guidelines, 2000, p 6)	Pneumococcal vaccine (for those with chronic cardiovascular, pulmonary disease [except asthma], diabetes, alcoholism, chronic liver disease or cerebrospinal leaks; those who are immunocompromised, or at	Child abuse or neglect

Table continued on following page.

Table 1–7　Screening Recommendations (2–6 yr) (*Continued*)

Screening	Parent Counseling	Immunizations	Watch for
		high risk because of social or environmental conditions (Alaskan natives or certain American Indian populations)	
Urinalysis	Appropriate exercise program		Abnormal bereavement
TB skin test (high risk)	Safety belts Car seat with five-point restraint until 40 lb, then may convert to booster seat		
Hearing Testing at ages 3, 4, 5, 10, 12, and 15 years (Burns, 2000, pg 783)	Smoke detector Replace battery 2 times per year (when clocks change) and test for working order monthly. Replace detector every 7–10 years (U.S. Department of Housing and Urban Development, 2000)		
TB screening recommended related to likelihood of exposure—must be screened at the preschool level prior to entering kindergarden	Hot-water temperature (see Table 1-6)		
	Use stairway gates, window guards, and fences around swimming pools (Safety Barrier Guidelines for Home Pools and How to Plan for the Unexpected at (www.acpm.org) Storage of medications/drugs and toxic chemicals (i.e., paints) Poison center control telephone, ipecac syrup Sunscreen at least SPF 15 (preferably 35 or more) reapply every 2 hr if perspiring or sweating Avoid sun exposure between the hours of 10 A.M. and 2 P.M. (www.epa.gov) (use sunglasses, hat, and protective clothing.		

SCREENING RECOMMENDATIONS (7–12 years)

See Table 1–8

Leading Causes of Death:

Motor vehicle accident

Injuries (non-motor-vehicle)

Congenital anomalies

Leukemia

Homicide

Heart disease

Table 1–8   Screening Recommendations 7–12 Years

Screening	Parent Counseling	Immunizations	Watch for
Height: Average schoolchild grows 2–2½ in. per year to gain 1–2 ft by age 12. By age 12 child has reached 90% of adult height (Murray and Zentner, 2001, p 472)	Fat (especially saturated fats) cholesterol, sweets and between meal snacks, sodium	Fluoride supplements (see Table 1–7)	Vision disorders
Weight: Gain of 4–7 lb per year	Caloric balance (teen girls need about 2200 cal/day; teen boys need about 2800) (Dietary Guidelines, 2000, p 6)	Pneumococcal vaccine (for those with chronic cardiovascular, pulmonary disease [except asthma], diabetes, alcoholism, chronic liver disease or cerebrospinal leaks; or who are immunocompromised or at high risk because of social or environmental conditions (Alaskan natives or certain American Indian populations)	Decreased hearing

Table continued on following page.

Table 1–8   Screening Recommendations 7–12 Years (*Continued*)

Screening	Parent Counseling	Immunizations	Watch for
Blood Pressure: Average systolic blood pressure, 94–112 mm Hg; average diastolic, 56–60 (Murray and Zentner, 2001, p 473)	Selection of exercise program (60 min daily)		Dental decay, mal-alignment, mouth breathing (first permanent teeth erupt [6-yr molars] by age 7—Don't evaluate for braces until until all 6-yr molars are in place.
TB	Safety belts		Signs of abuse or neglect
Scoliosis: Screen all children beyond 8 yr, especially girls at age 12, and boys at ages 13–14 (www.aaos.org)	Smoke detector		Abnormal bereavement
Vision: Should be 20/20 by age 8	Storage of firearms, drugs, toxic chemicals, matches		Depression
	Bicycle/scooter/skate board/roller blade safety helmets and protective padding Regular tooth brushing and flossing and dental visits (6-mo checkups) Evaluation of television viewing (content, time), computer time, Sunscreen		

SCREENING RECOMMENDATIONS (13–18 years)

See Table 1–9
Leading Causes of Death:
    Motor-vehicle accidents
    Homicide
    Suicide
    Injuries (non-motor-vehicle)
    Heart disease

Table 1–9 Screening Recommendations (13–18 yr)

Screening	Parent Counseling	Immunizations	Watch for
Dietary intake: Total fat, <30% saturated fat Protein, 15% of total caloric intake NA, no more than 2400 mg/day	Fat (especially saturated), cholesterol, sodium, iron, calcium (especially if on Depo Provera) Calcium 1200 mg/day for both boys and girls; pregnant teens, 1200–1800 mg/day	Tetanus-diphtheria booster (every 10 yr) Evaluate immunization schedule—may want to do titer for hepatitis B if had as child TB—evaluate if high risk	Depressive symptoms (see Beck Depression scale) CLUES: 1) Change in weight or eating habits (more or less intake) 2) Insomnia/hypersomnia 3) Loss of energy or fatigue 4) Change in motor activity such as from inactivity to constant motion 5) Loss of interest in usual activities 6) Out of proportion feelings of self-reproach or guilt 7) Drop in school performance 8) Preoccupation with death
Physical activity	Caloric balance (teen girls need about 2200 cal/day; teen boys, about 2800) (Dietary Guidelines, 2000, p 6) Food pyramid (Murray and Zentner, 2001, p 1616)	Pneumococcal vaccine (for those with chronic cardiovascular, pulmonary disease [except asthma], diabetes, alcoholism, chronic liver disease or cerebrospinal leaks; or who are immunocompromised or at high risk because of social or environmental conditions (Alaskan natives or certain American Indian populations) Meningococcal vaccine recommended prior to college admission (www.cdc.org)	Suicide risk factors CLUES: 1) Delinquency, aggressiveness, sexual promiscuity, running away, drug or alcohol use, headaches, abdominal pain, accident-proneness, fatigue, slow speech, anorexia, sloppiness and preoccupation with death. 2) Statements like: "The world would be better off without me" or "I wouldn't be around anymore" 3) Resigning from organizations, giving away cherished belongings, writing suicide notes, exhibiting sudden changes in usual

Table continued on following page.

Table 1–9   Screening Recommendations (13–18 yr) (*Continued*)

Screening	Parent Counseling	Immunizations	Watch for
			patterns of behavior (the good student who begins to fail, the quiet student who becomes aggressive)
Tobacco/alcohol/ drug use	Exercise program (60 min aerobic exercise daily)		Abnormal bereavement
Sexual practices (evaluate for unsupervised periods of time—e.g., home alone after school)	Tobacco/alcohol/ drug cessation/ prevention Ask annually		Tooth decay, malalignment, gingivitis
Height and weight: Girls: Growth spurt, age 8–17; peak at 12 Menarche, 10–16 Breast development, 8–18 Pubic and underarm hair, 11–14 Boys: Growth spurt, age 10–20; peak at 14 Penile development, 10–16 Testicular development; 9–17 Pubic, facial, underarm, and chest hair, 12–16 (for females full height is attained by 17 yr, for males full height is attained by 20 yr (Murray and Zentner, 2001, pp 531, 601)	Driving/other dangerous activities while under influence of alcohol or other drugs		Abuse or neglect National Committee for Prevention of Child Abuse (312-663-3520) National Center on Child Abuse and Neglect (202-205-8586)
Blood pressure: Boys, 116–120/ 74–80 Girls, 118–120/ 76–80 Pulse, 60–80 (www.brightfutures. com)	Sharing/using unsterilized needles and syringes Helpful books for parents of adolescents: *Reviving Ophelia, Saving the Selves of Adolescent Girls* by Mary Pipher, Ph.D.; *Raising Cain: Protecting the Emo-*		Eating Disorders: Anorexia, bulimia Warning signs of anorexia: 1) Deliberate self-starvation with weight loss 2) Fear of gaining weight 3) Refusal to eat 4) Denial of hunger 5) Constant exercising

Table continued on following page.

Table 1–9   Screening Recommendations (13–18 yr) (Continued)

Screening	Parent Counseling	Immunizations	Watch for
	tions of Boys, by Daniel J. Kindlon and Michael Thompson; *Our Last Best Shot: Guiding Our Children through Early Adolescence* by Laura Sessions Step; *Get out of My Life, but First Could You Drive Me and Cheryl to the Mall,* by Anthony E. Wolf; *Venus in Blue Jeans: Why Mothers and Daughters Need to Talk about Sex,* by Nathalie Bartle		6) Greater amounts of hair on the body or the face 7) Sensitivity to cold 8) Absent or irregular periods 9) Loss of scalp hair 10) A self-perception of being fat when the person is really too thin (Patient Information Handouts, American Family Physician, 1996, 54(4)
Skin examination: Screen for cancers and acne	Protected sex and sexually transmitted infections		
Testicular examination	Contraceptive and unintended pregnancy options		
Pap examination if sexually active (along with evaluation for sexually transmitted diseases and human immunodeficiency virus infections). Encourage Pap with every new partner	Injury prevention (seat belts, helmets) helmet should be snug on head and allow conversation (www.cpsc.gov) excellent resource for bicycle/scooter safety information		
Clinical breast examination, monthly breast self-examination	Firearms (Physician Firearm Safety Guide may be obtained from the AMA by calling 312-464-5066)		
Hearing	Smoke detectors		
Vision	Violent behaviors		
Rubella	Dental health (brushing, flossing, dental visits every 6 mo)		
Scoliosis Annually for females	Sunscreen (as above), sunglasses, hats		

SCREENING RECOMMENDATIONS (19–39 years)

See Table 1–10

Leading Causes of Death:
  Motor vehicle accidents
  Homicide
  Suicide
  Injuries (non-motor-vehicle)
  Heart disease

Table 1–10   Screening Recommendations (19–39 yr)

Screening	Counseling	Immunizations	Watch for
Females are at full height by 17 or 18, Males are at full height by 21 (though some grow another inch before 25)	Fat (especially satu-raturated), choles-terol, complex carbohydrates, fiber, sodium, iron, calcium (1000 mg/day)	Tetanus-diphtheria booster	Depressive symp-toms
Blood Pressure: 110–120 systolic/ 60–18 mm Hg diastolic	Caloric balance (active women and most men need about 2200 cal/ day) (Dietary Guidelines, 2000, p 6)		
Physical activity	Moderate physical activity (uninter-rupted) (30–45 min every day)	Hepatitis B vaccine	Suicide risk factors
Tobacco/alcohol/ drug use	Tobacco/drug/ alcohol cessation/ prevention (CAGE screening tool)	Pneumococcal vac-cine (for those who have chronic car-diovascular, pul-monary disease [except asthma], diabetes, alco-holism, chronic liver disease or cerebrospinal; or who are immuno-compromised or at high risk be-cause of social or environmental conditions (Alaskan natives or certain Ameri-can Indian popula-tions)	Abnormal bereave-ment
Sexual practices Family planning	Sharing syringes/ needles	Influenza vaccine (residents of nurs-	Malignant skin lesions

Table continued on following page.

Table 1–10   Screening Recommendations (19–39 yr) (Continued)

Screening	Counseling	Immunizations	Watch for
Infertility evaluation if necessary	Sexually transmitted infections, condoms, anal intercourse, partner selection	ing homes, who have chronic diseases, women in their 2nd or 3rd trimester of pregnancy during season, healthcare providers) Measles/mumps/ rubella vaccine	Tooth decay, gingivitis
	Unintended pregnancy and contraception options		Signs of abuse
Testicular examination (clinical, and monthly self-examination) and breast (breast self-examination monthly and annual clinical)	Safety belts, helmets		
Complete skin examination	Violent behavior		
Cholesterol ≤200 mg/dl; HDL, >35; LDL, <150 Lipid profile every 5 yr (more frequently if strong family history	Firearms (Physician Firearm Safety Guide may be obtained from the AMA by calling 312-464-5066)		
Pap smear (every year for 2 yr; if 2 normal examinations and no change in partner may lengthen screening interval to 3 yr at practitioner's discretion) (Gonzales and Kutner, 2000, p 9)	Smoke detectors		
Fasting plasma glucose, urinalysis (include microalbuminemia eval), sexually trasmitted diseases, human immunodeficiency virus, and tuberculosis	Back-conditioning exercises		
Vision	Regular tooth brushing and flossing and dental visits every 6 mo		
Rest and sleep patterns (evaluate for stress, relaxation etc)	Sunscreen (see Table 1–6)		

SCREENING RECOMMENDATIONS (40–64 years)

See Table 1–11
Leading Causes of Death:
  Heart disease
  Lung cancer
  Cerebrovascular disease
  Breast cancer
  Colorectal cancer
  Obstructive lung disease

Table 1–11   Screening Recommendations (40–64 yr)

Screening	Counseling	Immunizations	Watch for
Dietary history Encourage no more than 2 cups/day of caffeinated beverages Encourage water intake (½ weight converted to ounces) (i.e., 100-lb woman would need to drink 50 oz of water/day)	Fat (especially saturated <30% total) cholesterol, complex carbohydrates, fiber, sodium, calcium	TD booster	Depression
Physical activity	Caloric balance (active women and most men need about 2200 cal/day) (Dietary Guidelines, 2000, p 6)	Hepatitis B Hepatitis A if traveling out of country	Suicide risk factors
Tobacco/alcohol/drug use Evaluate for sleep apnea	Moderate physical activity (uninterrupted) (30–45 min every day)	Pneumococcal vaccine Pneumococcal vaccine (for those with chronic cardiovascular, pulmonary disease [except asthma], diabetes, alcoholism, chronic liver disease or cerebrospinal; or those who are immunocompromised or at high risk because of social or environmental conditions (Alaskan natives or certain American Indian populations)	Abnormal bereavement (ask about parental responsibilities and family responsibilities)

Table continued on following page.

Table 1–11 Screening Recommendations (40–64 yr) *(Continued)*

Screening	Counseling	Immunizations	Watch for
Sexual practices and concerns	Tobacco cessation	Influenza vaccine	Abuse or neglect
Height and weight	Alcohol/drugs—limit consumption, driving under the influence, treatment for abuse		Malignant skin lesions
Blood pressure 95–130 systolic/ 60–85 mm Hg diastolic (Jarvis, 2000, p 211)	Sharing/using unsterilized needles		Peripheral vascular disease
Clinical breast examination, breast self-examination, base-line mammography and every 1–2 yr thereafter; Pap smear (every year for 2 yr; if two normal examinations and no change in partner may lengthen screening interval to 3 yr at practitioner's discretion) (Gonzales and Kutner, 2000, p 9) Prostate examination (also appropriate checks for sexually transmitted diseases and human immunodeficiency virus)	Unintended pregnancy and contraceptive options Hormone-replacement therapy Menopause evaluation (emotional changes, physical changes, empty nest syndrome, depression, sexual dysfunction)		Tooth decay, gingivitis, loose teeth
Skin examination	Sexually transmitted diseases, partner selection, condoms		
Oral cavity examination	Safety belts, helmets, padding		
Palpation for thyroid nodules Thyroid screening annually over age 50 (Murray and Zentner, 2001, p 715)	Smoke detector, smoking near bedding or upholstery		
Auscultation for carotid bruits	Back-conditioning exercises, falls		
Fasting lipids, glucose and cholesterol	Regular tooth brushing/flossing and dental visits		

Table continued on following page.

Table 1–11   Screening Recommendations (40–64 yr) *(Continued)*

Screening	Counseling	Immunizations	Watch for
Cholesterol ≤200 mg/dl; HDL >35; LDL <150			
Fecal occult blood (yearly digital rectal examination and fecal occult blood test) and flexible sigmoi-doscopy every 3–5 yr after 50 (Gonzales and Kutner, 2000, p 10)	Sunscreen		
Bone mineral content evaluation for chronic steroid use, repeated fractures, early menopause, family history (Gonzales & Kutner, 2000, p 50)			
TB test Yearly if risk of exposure high			
Vision Examination every 2 yr for ages 41–60, then every year thereafter (American Academy of Opthamology, www.eyenet.org)			
Electrocardiography			
Urinalysis (include microalbuminemia evaluation), complete blood count, chemistry panel			

SCREENING RECOMMENDATIONS (65 years and over)

See Table 11–12
Leading Causes of Death:
    Heart disease
    Cerebrovascular disease
    Obstructive lung disease

Pneumonia/influenza
Lung cancer
Colorectal cancer

Table 1–12   Screening Recommendations (65 yr and over)

Screening	Counseling	Immunizations	Watch for
Symptoms of transient ischemic attack (cardiac risk factors: high cholesterol, hypertension, cigarette smoking, diabetes mellitus, family history of coronary artery disease)	Fat (especially saturated) cholesterol, complex carbohydrates, fiber, sodium, calcium (1500 mg for postmenopausal women)	Tetanus-diphtheria booster	Depression symptoms
Dietary intake	Caloric balance	Influenza vaccine (yearly)	Suicide risk factors
Physical activity	Moderate physical activity (30–45 min, uninterrupted, every day)	Pneumococcal vaccine (if received first dose more than 5 yr previously)	Abnormal bereavement
Tobacco/alcohol/drug use	Tobacco cessation	Hepatitis B (evaluate records)	Changes in cognitive function (Mini-Mental evaluation)
Functional status	Limiting alcohol consumption (1 oz for women and 2 oz for men/day), treatment for abuse, driving while under the influence		Medications that increase risk of falls
Height and weight	Prevention of falls		Signs of physical abuse or neglect (Murray and Zentner, 2000, p 762)
Blood pressure: 95–130 systolic/ 60–85 mm Hg diastolic	Safety belts, helmets		Malignant skin lesions
Visual acuity Most elderly will have presbyopia, which causes them to take longer to focus on near objects Color vision is altered after age 60 Evaluate for cataracts and macular degeneration	Smoke detectors		Peripheral vascular disease

Table continued on following page.

Table 1–12   Screening Recommendations (65 yr and over)
(Continued)

Screening	Counseling	Immunizations	Watch for
Hearing (loss and aids): about 75% of people over the age of 75 have hearing loss	Smoking near bedding or upholstery		Tooth decay, gingivitis, loose teeth, denture evaluation
Clinical breast examination, breast self-examination, mammography (every 1–2 yr); Pap smear (discontinue screening if on regular screening there have been two satisfactory smears, and no abnormal smear within the previous 9 yr. If no previous screening, three normal smears before discontinuation) (Gonzales and Kutner, 2000, p 9), and prostate examination	Hot-water-heater temperature		
Auscultation for carotid bruits	Regular dental visits, brushing/flossing		
Complete skin examination	Glaucoma examination		
Oral cavity examination	Discussion of aspirin therapy, hormone-replacement therapy		
Palpation of thyroid	Sunscreen		
Fasting cholesterol, lipids, and glucose Cholesterol ≤200 mg/dl; HDL >35; LDL <150 If history of coronary artery disease, may want to have lower levels: LDL <100; HDL >35 (Dunphy & Winland-Brown, 2001, p 517)			

Table continued on following page.

Table 1–12 Screening Recommendations (65 yr and over)
(Continued)

Screening	Counseling	Immunizations	Watch for
Urinalysis (include microalbuminemia evaluation), chemistry panel, complete blood count Evaluate for urinary continence and/ or incontinence			
Fecal occult blood test every 1–2 yr and flexible sigmoidoscopy every 5 yr (some sources say every 10 yr) (Gonzales and Kutner, 2000, p 11)			
Electrocardiogram			

SCREENING TOOLS

Apgar Scoring

SIGN:	0	1	2
Heart rate	Absent	<100 beats/min	>100 beats/min
Respirations	Absent	Slow, irregular	Cry; regular tone
Muscle tone	Flaccid	Some flexion of extremities	Active movements
Reflex irritability	None	Grimace	Cry
Color	Cyanotic or pale	Body pink; extremities cyanotic	Body pink; overall

Baby evaluated at 1 minute and 5 minutes after birth. Scores range from 0 to 10. Score <7—having difficulty, may need life-saving intervention. Score >7—doing well

CAGE (screening tool for problem drinking)

Have you ever felt the need to **C**ut down on drinking?
Have you ever felt **A**nnoyed by criticism of your drinking?
Have you ever felt **G**uilty about your drinking?
Have you ever taken a morning **E**ye opener?

Interpretation: Two yes answers are considered a positive screen. One yes answer should make you suspicious of alcohol abuse.

Differentiation of Substances and Treatment of Withdrawal (Figure 1–1)

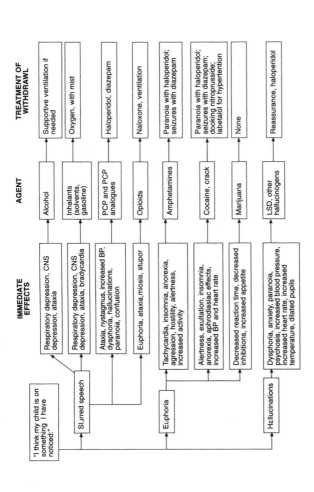

FIGURE 1–1 Differentiation of substances and treatment of withdrawal. (BP = blood pressure; CNS = central nervous system; LSD = lysergic acid diethylamide; PCP = phencyclidine hydrochloride.)

Assessment Tool for Eating Disorders

Yes   **No**

1. Do you spend most of your time thinking about food?
2. Do you panic if you gain a pound or two?
3. Do you ever eat uncontrollably?
4. Do you feel guilt and remorse after eating?
5. Do you ever fast or restrict your diet?
6. Do you vomit or use laxatives to control your weight?
7. Are your periods irregular, or have you stopped menstruating?
8. Do you have a strict exercise program?
9. Do you panic if you are unable to exercise as much as you would like?

Source: Decker, S.D. (1993). Eating disorders: Anorexia and bulimia. In B.S. Johnson (Ed.), *Psychiatric-mental health nursing: Adaptation and growth* (4th ed.) (p 706). Philadelphia: Lippincott Williams & Wilkins. Used with permission.

Mini Mental State (screening test for cognitive impairment)

Suspect dementia if score is less than or equal to 24

NAME:_____   AGE:_____

NAME OF EXAMINER:_____   YEARS OF SCHOOL COMPLETED:_____

DATE OF EXAMINATION:_____

Approach the patient with respect and encouragement.

SCORE   **ITEM**

    5 ( )   TIME ORIENTATION

Ask:

What is the year _____ (1), season _____ (1),
month of the year _____ (1), date _____ (1),
day of the week _____ (1)?

    5 ( )   PLACE ORIENTATION

Ask:

Where are we now? What is the state _____ (1), city _____ (1),
part of the city _____ (1), building _____ (1),
floor of the building _____ (1)?

    3 ( )   REGISTRATION OF THREE WORDS

Say: Listen carefully, I am going to say three words. You say them back after I stop. Ready? Here they are. . . . **Pony** (wait 1 second), **Quarter** (wait 1 second), **Orange** (wait one second). What were those words?

_____ (1)
_____ (1)
_____ (1)

Give one point for each correct answer, then repeat them until the patient learns all three.

5 (   )　　　　　　　　SERIAL 7s AS A TEST OF
　　　　　　　　　　ATTENTION AND CALCULATION

Ask: Subtract 7 from 100 and continue to subtract 7 from each
subsequent number until I tell you to stop. What is 100 minus 7?
_____ (1)

Say:

Keep going _____ (1), _____ (1), _____ (1), _____ (1)

3 (   )　　　　　　　　RECALL OF THREE WORDS

Ask:

What were those three words I asked you to remember?
Give 1 point for each correct answer _____ (1), _____ (1),
_____ (1)

2 (   )　　　　　　　　NAMING

Ask:

What is this? (show pencil) _____ (1)
What is this? (show watch) _____ (1)

1 (   )　　　　　　　　REPETITION

Say:

Now I am going to ask you to repeat what I say. Ready? "No ifs, ands
or buts." Now you say that _____ (1)

3 (   )　　　　　　　　COMPREHENSION

Say:

Listen carefully because I am going to ask you to do something.
Take this paper in your left hand (1), fold it in half (1), and put it on
the floor (1).

1 (   )　　　　　　　　READING

Say:

Please read the following and do what it says, but do not say it aloud
(1)

　　　　　　　　　　CLOSE YOUR EYES

1 (   )　　　　　　　　WRITING

Say:

Please write a sentence. If the patient does not respond, say: Write about
the weather (1)

1 (   )　　　　　　　　DRAWING

Say: Please copy this design

TOTAL SCORE _____

Assess level of consciousness along a continuum from alert to drowsy to stupor to coma.

Record yes or no answers to the following:

Cooperative: _____	Deterioration from previous level of
Depressed: _____	functioning: _____
Anxious: _____	Family history of dememtia: _____
Poor vision: _____	Head trauma: _____
Poor hearing: _____	Stroke: _____
Native language:	Thyroid disease due to alcohol abuse: _____

FUNCTION BY PROXY

Record the date when the patient was last able to perform the following tasks. Ask caregiver if patient independently handles:

	YES	**NO**	**DATE**
Money/Bills			
Medication:			
Transportation			
Telephone			

Source: Reproduced with permission from Folstein, MF, Folstein, SE, McHugh, PR: "Mini Mental State: A Practical Method for Grading the Cognitive State of Patients for the Clinician" (1975). *Journal of Psychiatric Research, 12,* 189.

Beck Depression Inventory, Short Form

Instructions: This is a questionnaire. On the questionnaire are groups of statements. Please read the entire group of statements in each category. Then pick the one statement in the group that best describes the way you feel today, that is *right now.* Circle the number beside the statement you have chosen. If several statements in the group seem to apply equally well, circle each one. Sum all numbers to calculate a score.

Scoring: 0–4, no or minimal depression

5–7, mild depression

8–15, moderate depression

>15, severe depression

Be sure to read all the statements in each group before making your choice

A. Sadness	B. Pessimism
3. I am so sad or unhappy that I can't stand it	3. I feel that the future is hopeless and that things cannot improve
2. I am blue or sad all the time and I can't snap out of it	2. I feel I have nothing to look forward to people and have little feeling for them
1. I feel sad or blue	1. I feel discouraged about the future
0. I do not feel sad	0. I am not particularly pessimistic or discouraged about the future
C. Sense of Failure	**D. Dissatisfaction**
3. I feel I am a complete failure as a person (parent, husband, wife, daughter, son . . .)	3. I am dissatisfied with everything
2. As I look back on my life, all I can see is a lot of failures	2. I don't get satisfaction out of anything anymore
1. I feel I have failed more than the average person	1. I don't enjoy things the way I used to
0. I do not feel like a failure	0. I am not particularly dissatisfied

E. Guilt
3. I feel as though I am very bad or worthless
2. I feel guilty
1. I feel bad or unworthy a good part of the time
0. I don't feel particularly guilty

F. Self-Dislike
3. I hate myself
2. I am disgusted with myself
1. I am disappointed in myself
0. I don't feel disappointed in myself

G. Self-Harm
3. I would kill myself if I had the chance
2. I have definite plans about committing suicide
1. I feel I would be better off dead
0. I don't have any thoughts of harming myself

H. Social Withdrawl
3. I have lost all of my interest in other people and don't care about them at all
2. I have lost most of my interest in other people and have little feeling for them
1. I am less interested in other people than I used to be
0. I have not lost interest in other people

I. Indecisiveness
3. I can't make any decisions at all anymore
2. I have great difficulty in making decisions
1. I try to put off making decisions
0. I make decisions about as well as ever

J. Self Image Change
3. I feel that I am ugly or repulsive-looking
2. I feel that there are permanent changes in my appearance and they make me look unattractive
1. I am worried that I am looking old or unattractive
0. I don't feel that I look any worse than I used to

K. Work Difficulty
3. I can't do any work at all
2. I have to push myself very hard to do anything
1. It takes extra effort to get started at doing something
0. I can work about as well as before

L. Fatigability
3. I get too tired to do anything
2. I get tired from doing anything
1. I get tired more easily than I used to
0. I don't get any more tired than usual

M. Anorexia
3. I have no appetite at all anymore
2. My appetite is much worse now
1. My appetite is not as good as it used to be
0. My appetite is no worse than usual

Source: Beck, A.T., & Back, R.W. (1972). Screening depressed patients in family practice: A rapid technique. *Postgrauate Medicine, 52,* 81.

INTERNET RESOURCES FOR NURSING (ACADEMIES, ASSOCIATIONS, ETC.)

http://www.library.unisa.edu.au/internet/pathfind/nursing.htm#proforg

Association/Government Web Sites

http://www.cdc.gov/nip/ (Immunizations)

http://www.cdc.gov/nip/recs/adult-schedule.pdf (adolescent/adult immunization schedule)

http://wonder.cdc.gov (wonderful assortment of CDC reports/databases)

http://www.aafp.org (American Academy of Family Physicians)

http://www.nursingworld.org (American Nurses Association)

http://www.nih.gov/ninr/ (American Academy of Nurse Practitioners)

http://www.acponline.org (American College of Physicians)

http://www.aap.org (American Academy of Pediatricians)

http://www..aad.org (American Academy of Dermatologists)

http://www.acpm.org (American Academy of Preventive Medicine)

http://www.cancer.org (American Cancer Society)

http://www.acsm.org (American College of Sports Medicine)

http://diabetes.org (American Diabetes Association)

http://www.americangeriatrics.org (American Geriatrics Society)

http://nccam.nih.gov (National Center for Complementary and Integrative Medicine)

http://www.ahcpr.gov/clinic/uspsfact.htm (United States Preventive Services Task Force)

http://www.cdc.gov (Centers for Disease Control and Prevention)

http://www.nih.gov/ninr/ (National Institute for Nursing Research)

http://www.nih.gov/ninr/ (Health Finder—United States Government)

http://www.nonpf.com/ (National Organization of Nurse Practitioner Faculty)

http://www.usda.gov/cnpp/Pubs/DG2000/DietGuidBrochure.pdf (food pyramid guidelines)

http://www.usda.gov/cnpp/Pubs/DG2000/Full%20Report.pdf (Report of the Dietary Guidelines Advisory Committee on the Dietary Guidelines for Americans, 2000)

http://web.health.gov/healthypeople/ (Healthy People 2010 Document)

Journals (online)

Postgraduate Medicine—Choose patient notes and have access to patient teaching hand outs.-http://postgradmed.com

Family Medicine Med Plus—http://members.aol.com/suzannehj/naed.htm (online nursing editor with connection to 150 nursing journals)

Herbal/Integrative Medicine Sites

http://www.sbherbals.com (Snow Ball Herbals)

http://www.hergalgram.org (American Botanical Council)

http://www.herbs.org (Herb Research Foundation)

http://onemedicine.com (Integrative Medicine Communications)

http://wholehealthmd.com (Whole Health MD)

REFERENCES

Bradey, M. (2000). Role relationships. In C.E. Burns, M.A. Brady, A.M. Dunn, & N.B. Starr (Eds.), *Pediatric primary care: A handbook for nurse practitioners* (2nd ed.) (pp 444–447). Philadelphia: Saunders.

Burns, C.E., Brady, M.A., Dunn, A.M., Starr, N.B. (Eds.) (2000). *Pediatric primary care: A handbook for nurse practitioners* (2nd ed.). Philadelphia: Saunders.

Dunphy, L.M., & Winland-Brown, J.E. (2001). *Primary care: The art and science of advanced practice nursing.* Philadelphia: F.A. Davis.

Edelman, C.L., & Mandle, C.L. (1998). Health promotion throughout the lifespan (4th ed.). St. Louis: Mosby.

Facts about anorexia nervosa, *American Family Physician, 54*. Available at http://www.aafp.org/afp/091596/960915c.html.

Gonzales, R., & Kutner, J. (2000). *Practice guidelines in primary care.* New York, Lang Medical Books/McGraw Hill.

Healthy People 2010. Available at http://web.health.gov/healthypeople/.

Hill, N.L., & Sullivan, L. (1999). *Management guidelines for pediatric nurse practitioners.* Philadelphia, F.A. Davis.

Jarvis, C. (2000) Physical examination and health assessment. (3rd ed.) Philadelphia, W.B. Saunders Company.

Murray, R.B., & Zentner, P. (2001). *Health promotion strategies through the life span.* 7th ed. Upper Saddle River, NJ: Prentice-Hall.

Report of Dietary Guidelines. Available at http://www.usda.gov/cnpp/Pubs/DG2000/Full%20Report.pdf.

U.S. Department of Health and Human Services (1990). *Healthy people 2000: National health promotion and disease prevention objectives for the year 2000.* Washington, DC: Government Printing Office.

U.S. Department of Health and Human Services (1998). *Healthy people 2010: National health promotion and disease prevention objectives for the year 2010.* Washington, DC: Government Printing Office.

ACNE

SIGNAL SYMPTOM ► inflamed papules/pustules

ICD-9 Codes	706.1	Acne NOS [not otherwise specified]
	706.1	Acne vulgaris
	704.8	Folliculitis

Acne (acne vulgaris) consists of two types:

Inflammatory: The follicle becomes blocked by sebum and bacteria proliferate in the canal. The follicle bursts and contents are released into the dermis, causing inflammation.

Noninflammatory: The follicle does not burst but remains dilated. Sebum either moves to skin, an open comedone (blackhead) or the canal remains blocked, a closed comedone (whitehead).

Epidemiology

Acne is the most common of all skin diseases. It affects 80% of all people at some point in their lives; most commonly between ages 11 and 30 years.

Up to 85% of adolescents will be affected.

Severe disease affects males 10 times more often than females.

Sites most commonly affected are face, upper neck, back and chest (areas with most numerous sebaceous glands).

Commonly appears at onset of puberty. Affects all ages, especially teens, young adults, and perimenopausal women.

Etiology

Acne is a disease of a sebaceous gland associated with a hair follicle; this is called a pilosebaceous unit. Excess sebum accumulates in the follicle, causing it to swell.

The mechanism is caused by abnormal desquamation of follicular epithelium that results in obstruction.

Physiology and Pathophysiology

Multifactorial causes. Sebaceous glands are sensitive to androgen. They are present at birth and react to maternal hormones, which can lead to milia and infantile acne. These glands atrophy until puberty, when they reappear under the influence of androgen.

The primary cause is obstruction of a pilosebaceous canal, due to a variety of factors.

First—sebum overproduction.

Second—increased epithelial cell turnover.

Third—*Propionibacterium acnes* (inflammatory acne) converts sebum to free fatty acid (FFA) and stimulates an immune response.

Clinical Manifestations

Subjective

Age of onset
Description of problem
Aggravating factors
Cleansers or lubricants used on face
Previous treatment
Oral contraceptive use, cyclic changes
Medical history
Family history of acne
Medication list

Objective

Detailed skin examination reveals:

Comedonal acne is the earliest clinical expression of acne (preteen and teen).

Characteristic lesions are noninflammatory comedones located on the central forehead, chin, nose, and paranasal area.

Comedones are open or closed.

Colonization with *P. acnes* has not yet occurred (noninflammatory lesions present at this stage).

Mild inflammatory acne usually occurs in teens and young adult women.

Characterized by scattered small papules or pustules with a minimum of comedones.

Inflammatory acne is the final phase in the evolution of acne.

Acne consists of comedones, papules, and pustules on the face and trunk.

In a minority of clients large, deep nodules (cysts) develop, which represent a destructive inflammatory condition.

Cystic acne requires prompt attention (to avoid scarring)

Differential Diagnosis

Mild or severe folliculitis (inflamed papules, pustules occurring anywhere on the body)

Rosacea (papules, pustules, and hyperplasia of soft tissue around the nose, usually in adults) (See Table 2–1.)

Table 2–1 Acne Rosacea

ICD-9 Codes	695.3
Definition	Acne rosacea is a chronic facial dermatitis, usually found in older adults.
Epidemiology	Affects over 10 million Americans Women affected more often than men Lighter skinned persons more affected than darker skinned persons
Etiology	Unknown, but currently believed to have a vascular component, that is precepted by continuous sun damage. Other triggers include: Spicy/hot foods, Exercising, Cold weather, Alcohol, Stress
Physiology and Pathophysiology	Sun damage causes blood vessels to dilate, creating a bluish tint in the skin. There is also accumulation of extracellular fluid within this area, which results in erythema, swelling and tenderness of the skin.
Clinical Manifestations	<u>Subjective</u> Redness, usually around the nose, mouth and/or cheeks, Swelling, Burning, Stinging, Sensitive skin, Eye redness, Irritation
	<u>Objective</u> Red papules, pustules, Telangiectasia, Edema, Flushing, Nodular lesions, Blepharitis, Rhinophyma (in advanced cases)
Differential Diagnosis	Acne vulgaris (papules, pustules, usually found all over the face, and possibly on the neck and back) Seborrheic dermatitis (white to yellow scaly, greasy plaques) Contact dermatitis (red, itchy, scaly papules/plaques) Lupus erythematosus (red, flushing malar rash; other systemic symptoms)
Diagnostic Tests	Usually none
Management/ Treatment	<u>Pharmacologic Management</u> Topical: Metronidazole (MetroGel) 0.75% cream/gel–Apply topically BID Systemic: Tetracycline 500mg BID for 2 weeks. Then decrease to 500mg QD Minocycline (Minocin) 50mg BID for 2 weeks, then 100mg BID Accutane can be used in severe cases (non-FDA use) [NOTE: This is prescribed under the care of a dermatologist] *must* use contraception Beta blockers may be helpful with flushing/blushing
	<u>Non-Pharmacologic Management</u> Use gentle cleansers, such as Cetaphil or Aquanil Use sunblock at all times
	<u>Client Education</u> Disease process and treatment, Avoiding triggers, Be gentle with skin, Reduce stress, Limit alcohol intake
Referral	Dermatologist if patient does not respond to topical or systemic treatment.

Molluscum contagiosum (small, waxy, umbilicated globular epithelial papules)

Steroid rosacea (rosacea caused by steroid use)

Diagnostic Tests

None indicated.

Management/Treatment

Pharmacologic Management

COMEDONAL ACNE

Goal: Reduce abnormal desquamation of follicular epithelium.

Topical comedolytic: Azelaic acid (both comedolytic and antibacterial effects), available as cream (30 g). This medication can bleach clothing. Apply BID, in morning and evening to clean dry skin. Causes less irritation than tretinoin. Treatment should continue until there are no new lesions. Gels are preferable in hot/humid weather, creams in cold/dry. Increased photosensitivity.

Topical tretinoin (Retin-A): Topical comedolytic agents are the treatment of choice.

Cream: 0.025, 0.05, and 0.1% (20, 45 g); gel: 0.01, 0.025% (15, 45 g)

Liquid: 0.05% (28 ml); apply QD QHS, beginning with a lower concentration of cream, gel, or liquid and increasing if local irritation does not occur. *Note:* Advise client to apply thin layer of the topical agent to the entire face, not just the individual lesions. Warn about increased photosensitivity. Client must apply sunscreen daily for any sun exposure. It may take several months to achieve good results. Treatment should continue until no new lesions are developing.

PO Isotretinoin: Indicated for acne resistant to antibiotic therapy and severe acne; dosage is 0.5–1 mg/kg/day; duration of therapy is generally 20 wk, for a cumulative dose > 120 mg/kg for severe cystic acne. (*Note:* This is generally administered under the care of a dermatologist must be on contraceptives!)

MILD INFLAMMATORY ACNE

Same goal as comedonal, but also prevent *P. acnes* proliferation.

Topical therapy: comedolytic and antibiotic

Benzoyl peroxide gel 5–10% (60 g), apply QD to skin in morning. Erythromycin 2% (30 g), apply QD QHS.

Most clients respond to treatment after 2–4 weeks

INFLAMMATORY ACNE

Goal is the same as previously stated, with a focus on preventing inflammation produced by the *P. acnes* organism.

Topical comedolytic mentioned before with oral antibiotic: Doxycycline 100 mg BID for 1 day, then 50 mg BID; maintenance, 50 mg QD. Do not use Tetracycline derivatives in pregnant client. Protection from the sun is very important during treatment.

Decision about topical or oral antibiotics: extent of involvement and severity.

Topical antibiotics may be used once then tapered to maintenance oral antibiotics.

Nonpharmacologic Management

Explain mechanism of acne and treatment plan.

Explain that little improvement is possible for 2–3 months.

Counsel on general measures of therapy.

Wash areas with mild soap gently, 2–3 times a day.

Avoid oil-based cosmetics, mousse, and creams and avoid picking at lesions.

Use cleaners like cetaphil lotion, nonacnegenic moisturizes, like Moisturel and cosmetics like Clinique Pore Minimizer makeup.

Complementary/Alternative Therapies

Hormonal treatment: Oral contraceptive pills (OCPs) (Ortho Tri-Cyclen has been approved for the treatment of acne by the FDA).

Lavender essential oils, burdock, echinacea, bergamot, geranium, and sandalwood, tea tree oil.

Alternatives: Spironolactone (antiandrogenic).

Metronidazole gel.

Laser peels.

Ultraviolet light therapy (contraindicated with topical tretinoin and tetracycline).

Client Education

Eat well-balanced diet and avoid foods you associate with exacerbations of acne.

Avoid excessive or abrasive cleaning.

Stress management.

Heavy sweating may exacerbate.

Mechanical trauma may exacerbate.

Oily makeup and pollution may exacerbate.

Vigilance for hepatotoxicity with medications (Retin A); avoid vitamin A.

Explain pathophysiology to dispel myths.

Warn client that acne may initially look worse before it improves.

Explain any medications and side effects.

Be supportive and encouraging.

Follow-up

Schedule at least 3 visits over 8–10 weeks in order to establish a successful treatment program; adjust strength and frequency of medications depending on irritation and effectiveness.

Referral

Refer to dermatologist for initial use of isotretinoin and for clients not responsive to therapy after 10–12 weeks of treatment.

BITES (Animal and Human)

SIGNAL SYMPTOMS ▶ teeth marks on skin, redness

ICD-9 Codes	879.8	Animal bites
	879.8	Open wound or laceration NOS

Bites (animal and human) are a disruption of the integrity of the skin by an animal or human.

Epidemiology

Between 1 and 2 million animal bite wounds occur yearly in the United States.

Pet dogs and cats inflict most of these wounds; the majority of dog bites involve children aged 2 to 19.

Etiology

Most bites do not require medical care; however, serious effects can occur, including infection or damage to a tendon sheath, joint capsule, bone, or nerve.

Human bites can cause more serious infections than dog or cat bites. Approximately 15% to 20% of dog bites become infected, and more than 50% of cat and human bites become infected.

Aerobes and anaerobes have been cultured from dog-bite wounds. The most common aerobes are *Pasteurella multocida, Staphyloccus* species, alpha-hemolytic streptococci, and *Capnocytophaga canimorsus.* Anaerobes include *Actinomyces, Fusobacterium, Prevotella,* and *Porphyromonas* species.

Cat bites harbor *P. multocida. Afipia felis,* and *Bartonella benselae* can cause infection that is usually self-limiting.

Common infectious organisms found in human bites include *Streptococcus viridans, Staphlococcus aureus, Eikenella corrodens, Haemophilus influenzae,* and beta-lactamase–producing bacteria.

Physiology and Pathophysiology

The infection originates from the oropharyngeal flora of the biting animal or human and the victim's skin, which causes an inflammatory reaction. The severity of infection can vary from cellulitis to osteomyelitis or septic arthritis.

Human bites are categorized as either occlusal injuries or clenched-fist injuries. Occlusal injuries occur when the teeth sink into the skin. The clenched-fist injury occurs when a tooth penetrates the skin. The clenched-fist injury is the more serious of the two and initially can appear to be a minor wound, until infection develops.

Clinical Manifestations

Subjective

History of bite, injury—when, where, and how it occurred.

Whether animal has been vaccinated for rabies.

Client may report signs of infection such as fever, erythema, drainage, and swelling.

Joint and/or bone pain.

Inquire about tetanus status.

Objective

Signs of infection in cat bites are evident 12 hours after the bite occurs.

Signs of infection in dog bites are evident 24 hours after the bite occurs.

Signs of infection in human bites are usually evident in less than 24 hours.
Wound such as laceration, puncture, crush injury.
Erythema.
Drainage.
Fever.
Adenopathy.
Impaired neurovascular status of affected area.
Impaired range of motion.

Differential Diagnosis

Generally none

Diagnostic Tests

Generally, none needed, but may consider:

X-ray examination (if hand is affected or if injury is over bone)
Anaerobic and aerobic cultures and Gram stain (if sign of infection is present to determine specific pathogen)
Complete blood count (CBC; to rule out infection)
Consider HIV testing (if human bite)

Management/Treatment

Pharmacologic Management

GENERAL

Tetanus toxoid is given to patients who require a booster.
Rabies prophylaxis is indicated for bites by carnivorous wild animals (skunks, raccoons) and unvaccinated domestic cats and dogs.
Prophylactic antibiotics are not indicated in low-risk bites and nonimmunocomprised clients, but they are recommended in high-risk wounds such as deep puncture, those needing surgical repair, human bites, and bites involving the hand. Antibiotics should be given to clients with diabetes, vascular disorders, prosthetic heart valves, history of splenectomy, and other immunocompromising conditions.

DOG BITES

Adults: Amoxicillin/clavulanic acid (Augmentin), 875/125 mg BID or 500/125 mg TID PO.
If allergic to penicillin: Clindamycin (Cleocin), 300 mg QID PO **and** a fluoroquinolone.
Children: Amoxicillin/clavulanic acid (Augmentin), 45 mg/kg BID. If allergic to penicillin: Clindamycin (Cleocin), 16–20 mg/kg/day divided QID **and** trimethoprim/sulfamethoxazole (TMP/SMX; Bactrim), 8 mg/40 mg/kg/day BID.

CAT BITES

Adults and children: Amoxicillin/clavulanic acid (Augmentin), 875/125 mg BID or 500/125 mg TID PO. If allergic to penicillin: Doxycycline (Monodox), 100 mg BID PO.

HUMAN BITES (ADULTS)

Prophylactic: Amoxicillin/clavulanic acid (Augmentin), 875/125 mg BID PO for 5 days.

Therapeutic: Ampicillin/sulbactam (Unasyn), 1.5 g Q6H IV or cefoxitin (Mefoxin), 2 g Q8H IV or ticarcillin/clavulanate potassium (Timentin), 3.1 g Q6H IV. If allergic to penicillin: clindamycin (Cleocin) **and** either ciprofloxacin (Cipro) or TMP/SMX (Bactrim).

Nonpharmacologic Management

Copious irrigation of the wound with saline

Wound closure in select cases

Complementary/Alternative Therapies

Topical witch hazel may be used as an astringent.

Topical arnica gel or ointment may be helpful with insect bites.

Client Education

Signs of developing or deteriorating infection

Adverse drug reactions

Follow-up

24 to 48 hours after initiating antibiotic treatment

Referral

Refer to plastic surgeon for face wounds.

BURNS

SIGNAL SYMPTOMS ▶ damage to skin, blisters

ICD-9 Codes	949.0	Burn NOS
	949.1	Burn, first-degree
	949.2	Burn, second-degree
	949.3	Burn, third-degree

Burns are thermal injuries to the skin that can be classified as:

First-degree

Second-degree (partial-thickness)

Third-degree (full-thickness)

Epidemiology

Burns are the third leading cause of accidental deaths in United States (after motor vehicle accidents and firearms accidents).

Annually, more than 1 million persons seek medical care for burns.

95% of burns can be managed in ambulatory setting.

Etiology

Tissue damage can be caused by agents such as heat, chemicals, mechanical abrasion, sunlight, electricity, nuclear radiation, or any other source of heat. The degree of damage depends on the duration of exposure and the source of heat.

Physiology and Pathophysiology

The epidermis is the thin outer layer of skin; it is made up of epithelial cells. The dermis is a thicker layer that contains nerve endings, blood vessels, collagen, elastin fibers, and the epidermal appendages. Two important functions of the skin are keeping microorganisms out of and moisture and electrolytes in the body. These functions are lost with significant burns

Clinical Manifestations

Subjective

First- and second-degree burns: hypersensitive and painful

Third-degree burns: destroy nerves, resulting in anesthesia

History of injury and source of heat

Assess pain on a pain scale

Assess for other injuries, especially if patient had fallen and/or smoke inhalation

Objective

First-degree burns: erythema, edema, and involves just the superficial layers of epidermis.

Second-degree burns: erythema, blistering, edema, possible weeping, and involves dermis and epidermis (may by superficial or deep).

Third-degree burns: total skin necrosis, charred appearance; involves all layers of dermis, epidermis, and penetrates to underlying fat and muscle.

Physical examination

Determine burn severity and whether inpatient or outpatient treatment is indicated.

Assess for signs of secondary bacterial infection.

Determine total percentage of body-surface area (TBSA) of burn and grade it according to the American Burn Association's grading system for burn severity. (See Table 2–2.)

Consider pulmonary insufficiency if patient has been exposed to smoke.

Differential Diagnosis

Consider abuse or neglect in pediatric age group and in the elderly (see Chapter 1 for signs and symptoms).

Diagnostic Tests

Usually none needed

ECG (to rule out cardiac dysfunction in patient with high-voltage electrical injury)

Management/Treatment

Triage

Minor burn: Outpatient treatment

Second-degree burns, <15 percent of TBSA

Table 2–2 Grading System for Burns

Minor: Manage as an outpatient
  <10 percent total percentage of body surface area (TBSA) in adult (age 10–50 years)
  <5 percent TBSA in young client (<10 years old) or older client (>age 50 years)
  <2 percent full-thickness burn

Moderate: Manage as an inpatient
  10–20 percent TBSA burn in adult
  5–10 percent TBSA burn in young or older client
  2–5 percent full-thickness burn
  High-voltage injury
  Suspected inhalation injury
  Circumferential burn
  Concomitant medical problem predisposing client to infection

Major: Refer to burn center
  >20 percent TBSA burn in adult
  >10 percent TBSA burn in young or older client
  >5 percent full-thickness burn
  High-voltage burn
  Know inhalation injury
  Any significant burn to face, eyes, ears, genitalia, or joints
  Significant associated injuries

Adapted from: American Family Physician, Volume 62, Number 9, November 1, 2000.

Third-degree burns, <2 percent of TBSA
Burns that spare face, hands, feet, and perineum
Moderate/major burns: Inpatient treatment
  More extensive burns
  Chemical or electrical burns
  Associated inhalation injury or major trauma
  Clients with significant medical problems

Pharmacologic and Nonpharmacologic Management

First-degree burns
  Immerse in cold water. (Do not induce hypothermia.)
  No dressings are necessary.
  Avoid sun exposure.

Second-degree burns
  Leave blisters intact.
  Gently clean with mild soap and water.
  Apply silver sulfadiazine (Silvadene) 1% cream topically to burned
    area.
  Use nonadherent gauze and bulky dry sterile dressing.
  Tetanus prophylaxis.
  Avoid sun exposure.

Third-degree burns
  Refer to physician/plastic surgeon in all cases; usually requires skin
    grafting.
  Antibiotics may be needed if there are signs and symptoms of infection.

Complementary/Alternative Therapies
Topical St. John's wort oil extract may be helpful in first-degree burns only.

Client Education
If burn overlies a joint, encourage full range-of-motion (ROM) exercises TID.

Elevate burned part as often as possible to limit edema.

Follow-up
First-degree burn: PRN.

Second-degree burn: Have client return in 2 days for dressing change and every 1–2 days thereafter until epithelialization occurs without infection.

Referral
All third-degree burns, facial burns and extensive second-degree burns should be referred to a plastic surgeon.

Circumferential burns, all burns to hands, eyes, ears, or perineum should be referred to a burn center.

If there is suspicion of child abuse or neglect, report to social services.

Patients with concurrent medical conditions such as diabetes or immunosuppression may need hospitalization even for minor burns.

CELLULITIS

SIGNAL SYMPTOMS ▶ redness, warmth, streaking

ICD Codes	682.9	Cellulitis

Cellulitis is an acute inflammation of the skin and subcutaneous tissues, characterized by hyperemia, edema, and leukocyte infiltration.

Epidemiology
Common skin infection that may occur at any age.

May be seen more often in diabetes or immunocompromised patients.

Etiology
Bacteria enters through a disruption in the integrity of the skin, through extension from a contiguous source such as an abscess, or as a complication of bacteremia. The majority of cases are caused by Group A beta-hemolytic *Streptococcus* and *Staphlococcus aureus. Streptococcus pyogenes* and other organisms are occasionally causal as well. In children, *Haemophilus influenzae* is the most common infecting organism.

Physiology and Pathophysiology
The pathogen invades the compromised area, overwhelming the immune response. As the cellulitis progresses, surrounding tissue is affected.

Clinical Manifestations

Subjective

Fever, chills, malaise

Pain, tenderness, swelling, warmth at affected site

Precipitating trauma/injury

Any recent break in integrity of skin (scrape, laceration, insect bite)

Possible immunocompromised state

Objective

Erythema, swelling, warmth.

Lymphadenopathy.

Tenderness with palpation.

Pitting edema may be present.

Preexisting lesion.

Fever.

Differential Diagnosis

Erysipelas (superficial cellulitis involving skin but not soft tissue; streaking is prominent).

Deep-vein thrombosis (common in elderly clients with cellulitis; symptoms of pain and cordlike structures on palpation; skin is usually normal and cool).

Inflammatory carcinoma of the breast and cutaneous neoplasms may look like cellulitis.

Diagnostic Tests

CBC with differential (to rule out infection; may reveal left shift)

Sedimentation rate (may be slightly elevated due to inflammation)

Blood cultures and skin-site cultures (to determine specific pathogen)

Management/Treatment

Pharmacologic Management

Treatment is generally empiric

If cellulitis is limited and client is not seriously ill:

Dicloxacillin, 500 mg PO QID for 10 days, or

Cephalexin (Keflex), 500 mg PO QID for 10 days, or

Erythromycin (PCE), 500 mg PO QID for 10 days if allergic to penicillin.

For more severe infections or in immunocompromised clients, IV antibiotics and/or inpatient treatment may be required.

If open wound, consider tetanus toxoid booster if no booster in 5 years.

Nonpharmacologic Management

Elevation of the affected area

ROM exercises to affected limb

Complementary/Alternative Therapies

Warm Epsom salt soaks of the site may help localize the infection.

Client Education

Disease process

Importance of taking entire course of antibiotics

Prevention of recurrences through good skin hygiene, foot care, and support stockings

Follow-up

Follow-up is a must to ensure eradication.

Every 1–2 days in severe infections.

Every 4–7 days in less severe infections.

Referral

Refer to infectious disease specialist or dermatologist:

Recurrent cases

Cases that fail to respond to treatment

When serious comorbidities are present (i.e., diabetes, alcoholism, IV drug abuse, immunocompromise)

Facial cellulitis

Periorbital/orbital cellulitis

CORNS AND CALLUSES

SIGNAL SYMPTOM soft or hard thickening of skin

ICD-9 Codes	700	Calluses and corns

Corns and calluses arise from hyperkeratosis, a normal physiological response to chronic excessive pressure or friction. Calluses are not well circumscribed and lack the central core that is found in corns. Corns (helomas) may be classified into two types: soft (heloma molle) spongy hyperkeratosis in the interdigital areas of the toes and hard (heloma durum) cone-shaped keratin.

Epidemiology

Population at risk includes all age groups.

Worldwide occurrence.

Behaviors associated with calluses include manual labor, weight-lifting, sports (e.g., jogging), increased activity with bare feet, and repetitive activities; those associated with corns include ill-fitting shoes (e.g., history of wearing high heels and footwear with a tight-fitting frontal portion) and anatomical abnormalities of the foot.

Etiology

Corns and calluses can be a painful reaction to pressure or friction on the underlying dermis covering the digital and plantar surfaces of the feet and hands (callus).

Areas of excessive pressure or friction lead to hyperkeratotic, thickened skin that forms a padded area of protection for the underlying skin structure.

Pressure on the skin over the heads and bases of the condyles of the metatarsals and phalanges results from extrinsic factors, including tight-fitting shoes, stiff soles, and improperly fitting toe boxes, or from intrinsic factors, such as arthritic changes, fractures, or congenital foot deformities.

Physiology and Pathophysiology

Corns may be hard or soft. Hard corns are usually found on the lateral surface of the toes or the plantar surface of distal metatarsal heads, typically with surrounding callus. Horny thickening of the stratum corneum forms a conical, deep central core pointing toward the dermis. Soft corns are usually found between the fourth and fifth digits and may appear grayish white and soft to palpation, with accompanying odor caused by maceration. Corns are tender to direct pressure.

Calluses are formed by increased cell cohesion, reduced shedding and thickening of the outer epidermal layer of dead skin. They are generally found over bony prominences and have accentuated normal skin lines. Calluses are usually not painful and serve a protective purpose to maintain integument.

Clinical Manifestations

Subjective

Thickening, hardening of skin.

Pain in localized area.

Pain on weight-bearing.

Interference with the performance of daily activities.

Obtain a good occupational history.

Inspect the style and fit of the shoes.

Inability to move the toes in the toe box or wearing pointed-toe or high-heeled shoes are commonly reported.

Assess self-treatment (e.g., cutting or using over-the-counter plasters to remove tissue).

Inquire into evidence of maceration, inflammation, oozing, and severe pain.

Question about previous trauma, hobbies, and sport participation.

Objective

Skin exam:

Hard, dry, soft, or wet.

Diameter and location.

May be translucent.

Pain or point tenderness on palpation.

Corns should appear well circumscribed, and translucent. Both corns and calluses are located in areas of trauma. Dorsolateral aspect of the fifth toe or the dorsal surface of the distal interphalangeal (DIP) joints of the second, third, and fourth toes are most common.

Seed corns are small, localized lesions anywhere on the plantar surface. "Pump bumps" in adolescents, located on the posterior aspect of the calcaneus caused by wearing short shoes.

Differential Diagnosis

Warts (circumscribed skin elevations, may have black dots)
Foreign-body granuloma (chronic inflammation around a foreign body)
Porokeratosis plantaris discreta (thickening of the stratum corneum, often linear)
Plantar fasciitis (pain in heel or arch of foot, often worse in the morning)
Calcaneal spur (a exostotic growth on the calcaneus bone)

Diagnostic Tests

Usually none necessary
X-ray if differentiating etiology or anatomical anomaly

Management/Treatment

Pharmacologic Management

Salicylic acid preparation (available over-the-counter) may be helpful in treating calluses:

Compound W
Duofilm
Mediplast
Salacid

Nonpharmacologic Management

Provide pain relief.
Correct the etiology for increased mechanical stress
Recommend appropriate footwear or orthotic devices.
Corns and calluses: Can be scraped or pared by provider: Pare down the callus with concentric strokes of a number 15-blade scalpel. No anesthetic usually needed. Leave a depression in center of callus.
Soft corn infections: warm soaks BID and topical antibiotic such as mupirocin.
  After healing, the client should be instructed to wear lamb's wool between the affected toes.
Calluses: Regular sanding with a pumice stone after softening with warm soaks.
Hammer toes: Shoe pads and toe crests.

Complementary/Alternative Therapies

Topical comfrey root may help healing

Client Education

Educate about the etiology of corns and calluses; encourage prevention.
Promote properly fitting shoes (e.g., adequate toe box) and proper posture.
Shoes should provide shock absorption and sufficient toe space for even weight distribution.

Instruct about use of pumice stone

Follow-up
Recheck in 4–6 weeks.

Referral
Refer to podiatrist if client has diabetes.

Refer to orthopedic surgeon or podiatrist if conservative measures are ineffective.

DERMATITIS (Atopic, Seborrheic, Contact)

SIGNAL SYMPTOM ▶ itchy, flaky skin

ICD-9 Codes	691.8	Atopic dermatitis
	690.11	Seborrhea capitis/cradle cap
	690.18	Dandruff
	692.9	Contact dermatitis
	693	Dermatitis, drug-related

Dermatitis is a general term for inflammation of the skin characterized by redness, itching, and various skin lesions. Types of dermatitis include:

Atopic dermatitis (AD) (commonly called eczema) is an eczematous eruption that is pruritic, symmetric, and associated with a personal family history of allergic manifestations (atopy).

Seborrheic dermatitis is a chronic inflammatory disease with a characteristic pattern for different age groups. It can be found on the head, forehead, eyebrows/eyelashes, nasolabial folds, or sternal or diaper region.

Contact dermatitis is inflammation and irritation of the skin due to contact with an irritating substance.

Epidemiology

Atopic Dermatitis
Common disease affecting 7–24 people per 1000; more common in infancy and childhood (5%) than in adulthood.

Some individuals are affected throughout life; the incidence in women is equal to that in men.

Heredity is thought to be the single most important predisposing factor.

Onset of disease before age 5 years in 85% of clients.

9%–12% of children have AD.

Asthma and allergic rhinitis develop in over 50% of children with generalized atopic dermatitis by age 13 years.

Annual estimated cost of treating AD in the United States is over $300 million.

Seborrheic Dermatitis
Familial—genetic predisposition.

Most common in adult males.

Common self-limiting condition of infancy usually seen within the first 3 months after birth.

Typically worsens in cool seasons.

Shows an association with diabetes mellitus, sprue, Parkinson's disease, and epilepsy.

Peak incidence is in adults 20–50 or older.

Affects 3% of general population, but 85% of people infected with HIV.

Contact Dermatitis

Often due to contact with poison ivy, poison oak, or poison sumac.

Latex contact dermatitis is becoming more common.

Etiology

Atopic Dermatitis

Atopic dermatitis is caused by overstimulation of T lymphocytes and mast cells.

Histamine from mast cells cause pruritus.

Unknown; may be due to T-lymphocyte activation.

Defective cell immunity.

B-cell IgE overproduction may play a significant role.

Seborrheic Dermatitis

Etiology unknown. May be due to a T-lymphocyte deficit, *Pityrosporum ovale* density and nutritional factors.

Persons with central nervous system disorders (Parkinson's disease, cranial-nerve palsies, or major truncal paralysis) are prone to dermatitis.

Possibly related to increased sebum pooling caused by immobility, which permits growth of *P. ovale*.

Contact Dermatitis

May be due to any irritating substance, including soaps, lotions, detergents, clothing, latex, plants, or other noxious chemicals.

Physiology and Pathophysiology

Atopic Dermatitis

AD is intercellular edema that eventually separates the epidermal cells and forms vesicles and bullae. Rupture of numerous thin blisters can lead to crusting. The final stage is lichenification. Some speculate that a deficiency in cell-mediated deficiency and possibly an IgE deficiency early in life makes it possible to ingest an allergen that enters the bloodstream, producing immune responses that would not be there otherwise. Established lesions show edema and variable infiltration with polymorphonuclear (PMN) cells and eosinophils.

There are two clinical forms of type 1 hypersensitivity, infantile and adult.

Seborrheic Dermatitis

Presents with no diagnostic microscopic changes and may be described as a skin condition rather than a disease. Neutrophils are sometimes seen in the stratum corneum with focal spongiosis. The yeast *P. ovale* may play a role in the etiology. Both genetic and environmental factors seem to influence onset and course.

Contact Dermatitis
When the skin comes in contact with an irritating substance or chemical, hypersensitivity to the specific antigen may occur, causing acute or chronic inflammation.

Clinical Manifestations

Subjective
See Table 2–3.

Objective
See Table 2–3.

Differential Diagnosis

Atopic Dermatitis
Contact dermatitis (see above)
Irritant or allergic dermatitis
Seborrheic dermatitis (see above)
Nummular dermatitis (chronic, well-defined pruritic, round scales and plaques)
Scabies (pruritic papules and burrows on hands, waist, genitalia; very pruritic)
Tinea corporis (red, scaling annular lesions)
Psoriasis (silvery, scaly plaques; can be generalized all over body)

Seborrheic Dermatitis
Tinea capitis (round or oval lesions on the scalp that scale; may include hair loss)
Psoriasis (silvery, scaly plaques, can be generalized all over body)
Atopic dermatitis (see above)
Impetigo (honey colored, crusting vesicles)
Acne rosacea (papules, pustules, and hyperplasia of soft tissue around the nose, usually in adults)

Contact Dermatitis
Atopic dermatitis (see above)
Impetigo (honey color, crusting vesicles)

Diagnostic Tests
Diagnostic tests usually not necessary
Serum IgE (elevated in 80%–90% of clients with atopic dermatitis)

Management/Treatment

Pharmacologic Management
See Table 2–3.

Table 2–3 Clinical Manifestations and Management/Treatment of Dermatitis

Type of Dermatitis	Atopic Dermatitis	Seborrheic Dermatitis	Contact Dermatitis
Clinical Manifestations: *History: Questions to Ak*	Onset (infantile, adult) Areas affected; neck, face, upper trunk, and flexural areas of elbows and knees, adults may have hand itching Recurrent flares, worse at any one time Triggers including food and temperature changes Family history of eczema and/or allergic rhinitis Aggravating factors—changes in humidity, wool intolerance, and emotional stress. Relieving factors If eruption occur in paroxysms, especially in evening Routine of skin care at home, e.g. frequency of baths and products used	Onset, duration, and location of lesions Personal or family history of seborrheic dermatitis Immuno-suppressed status of treatments tried and results	Recent exposure to new soaps, lotions, detergents, chemicals and latex. Employment and possible chemical exposure
Subjective	Redness Itching (often very intense) Crusting of lesions	Typically affects areas of the skin where sebaceous glands appear in high numbers. Usually distributed symmetrically and in designated sites. One characteristic is dandruff, characterized by a fine, powdery white scale on the scalp; associated pruritus is typical.	Acute itching, flaking, burning of the skin Usually localized to a specific area of the body

Table continued on following page.

Table 2–3 Clinical Manifestations and Management/Treatment of Dermatitis (*Continued*)

Type of Dermatitis	Atopic Dermatitis	Seborrheic Dermatitis	Contact Dermatitis
		An extremely common condition which waxes and wanes and may be aggravated by stress. Occurrence in infants: scalp (cradle cap) and diaper area Adults: scalp, eyebrow, paranasal, nasolabial fold, external ear canals, posterior auricular old, and pre-sternal areas	
Objective	Characterized by vesicle formation, oozing, and crusting with excoriation. Begins in the cheeks and may progress to include the scalp, arms, trunk, and legs. Adolescents and adults generally have dry leathery and hypopigmented lesions located in the antecubital and popliteal areas. May spread to neck, hands, feet, eyelids and behind the ears. Examine skin methodically; determine extent of the eruption, its distribution. Examine flexural areas for erythema and scaling, also look for lichenification. Examine hands, look for erythema on dorsal aspects of hands and dry, fissured fingertip pads.	Examine skin for characteristic lesion: Fine, dry, white or yellow scale on inflamed base or dull, red plaques with thick white or yellow greasy appearing scale. Mild seborrheic dermatitis presents as fine, dry, white or yellow scale, on an inflamed base. More severe eruptions appear as dull, red plaques with thick, white or yellow scale in a diffuse distribution. Determine distribution	Erythematous plaques in localized area (area of contact) Scaling Excoriation Lichenification may be seen, if chronic

Table continued on following page.

Table 2–3   Clinical Manifestations and Management/Treatment of Dermatitis (*Continued*)

Type of Dermatitis	Atopic Dermatitis	Seborrheic Dermatitis	Contact Dermatitis
	Blood eosinophilia correlates with severity of disease Several patterns of lesions: Erythematous papular lesions that become confluent. Diffuse erythema and scaling. Lichenification. Allergic triad: Asthma, Allergic rhinitis and Atopic dermatitis		
Management/ Treatment: *Pharmacologic Management*	Identify triggers and exacerbating factors Systemic lubrication of the skin daily If inflammation topical corticosteroids applied thinly 2 times/day until well-controlled. Hydrocortisone ointment 2.5% (1% on face and intertriginous areas) Triamcinolone acetonide ointment 0.1% Apply lubricant to inflamed area 3–4 ×/day Moisturizing lotions: Dermasil, Eucerin lotion, Lubriderm, Cetaphil Moisturing creams: Keri, Cetaphil, Eucerin, Neutrogena creams Moisturing ointments: Vaseline pure petroleum jelly, Aquaphor natural healing ointment	Cradle cap: Bland shampoo left on 5–10 min then rinse 2–3/week Apply topical steroid lotion– hydrocortisone 1% BID × 2/wks Face and diaper area: 1% hydrocortisone cream QD or QOD no longer than 2 weeks; leave diaper area open to air as much as possible. Scalp: Selenium sulfide (Selsun Blue), coal tar: Leave these shampoos on a minimum of 5–10 min before rinsing. Ketoconazole (Nizoral) 2–3 ×/week × 1 month/ can use once a week for maintenance Moderate to severe: Topical corticosteroid lotions/solutions can be used if shampoos fail after 2–3 weeks.	Do not use "very high potency steroids" on the face or groin area or with occlussive dressings. Application of BID dosing is most useful and economical. More frequent dosing does not speed improvement. Start BID and decrease as improvement occurs. High potency topical steroids should not be used longer than maximum two-week periods. The duration of use time limitation is related to increased side effects like dermal atrophy, striae, rebound flare of lesions and HPA axis depression. For an infant younger than 6 months, nothing

Table continued on following page.

Table 2–3 Clinical Manifestations and Management/Treatment of Dermatitis (*Continued*)

Type of Dermatitis	Atopic Dermatitis	Seborrheic Dermatitis	Contact Dermatitis
		Betamethasone valerate (Luxiq) 0.1% lotion BID × 2 weeks; no improvement then use hydrocortisone 1–2.5% lotion QD or taper QOD, D/C over the next 2 weeks. Antipruritics: See atopic dermatitis; antihistamines/ anti-pruritus lotions Refractory Seborrhea: Try different combinations, for example a dandruff shampoo, an anti-fungal agent and a topical steroid. If this fails, use "pulse steriod treatment" e.g.: Elocon, temovate or Lidex. Apply once or twice per day stop after 2 weeks	stronger than 1% hydrocortisone should be used. For a child older than 6 months but younger than 12 years, medium potency steroids can be used for short periods of time like 7–10 days.
	Pruritis Oral antihistamines Infants: hydroxyzine (Atarax) 0.5mg/kg/ dose TID, prn, Adults: diphenhy-dramine (Benadryl) 25–50 mg po q 4–6 hours Pruritus control: A single dose QHS is freq all that is necessary. Adults: loratadine (Claritin) 10 mg QD po, fexofenadine (Allegra) 60 mg po BID, Child >6 yr: loratadine (Claritin) 10 mg QOD then 10 mg Q day		

Table continued on following page.

CP2–1 **Clinical Pearl:** Because of the vast number of topical steroid creams, ointments, and gels, it is advised to pick/memorize one or two in each potency category (low, intermediate, high, and super high)

Nonpharmacologic Management
See Table 2–3.

Table 2–3 Clinical Manifestations and Management/Treatment of Dermatitis (*Continued*)

Type of Dermatitis	Atopic Dermatitis	Seborrheic Dermatitis	Contact Dermatitis
	It is important to prescribe non-sedating medications for clients who attend school or have daytime responsibilities. Topical agents: Sarna lotion, OTC antipruritics, Cetaphil with menthol 0.25% and phenol 0.25% Doxepin HCL cream 5% on adults ($<$ 8 days). Apply QID, prn in addition to topical steroid Severe: Oral prednisone, IM triamcinolone Goekman regimen, PUVA		
Non-Pharmacologic Management	Avoid sudden temp changes, excessive sweating, and low humidity in the winter. Avoid irritating substances (e.g. wool, cosmetics, some soaps and detergents, tobacco) Avoid foods that provoke exacerbations (e.g. eggs, peanuts, fish, soy, wheat, milk) Avoid stressful situations, allergens, dust, and excessive handwashing.	Hygiene plays a key role in controlling seborrheic dermatitis. Frequent cleansing with soap removes oils from affected areas and improves seborrhea. Clients should be counseled that good hygiene must be a lifelong commitment. Outdoor recreation can improve seborrhea; UV-A and UV-B inhibit the growth of P. ovale.	

Complementary/Alternative Therapies

Chamomile (topical) is helpful with itching.

Essential oils.

Biofeedback.

Hypnosis.

Client Education

Causes, triggers, signs, symptoms, and management

Chronic nature of condition with course characterized by remissions and intermittent flare-ups

Follow-up

ATOPIC DERMATITIS

2–4 weeks after initial therapy, then as needed

SEBORRHEIC DERMATITIS

Not indicated unless client does not respond to treatment

CONTACT DERMATITIS

Not indicated unless client does not respond to treatment

Referral

Refer to dermatologist clients who are not responsive to conservative therapy or those who require isotretinoin therapy.

HERPES SIMPLEX INFECTION/HERPES ZOSTER INFECTION

SIGNAL SYMPTOMS vesicles, redness, pain

ICD-9 Codes	053.9	Herpes zoster
	054.2	Herpes simplex, oral
	054.1	Herpes simplex, genital

Herpes simplex is a viral infection caused by the herpes simplex virus (HSV). Herpes zoster virus (HZV), also known as shingles, is an acute dermatomal infection associated with reactivation of varicella–zoster-virus. There are six strains of human herpes: herpes simplex type 1, herpes simplex type 2, cytomegalovirus, varicella–zoster virus (VZV), Epstein–Barr virus, and herpesvirus type 6.

Epidemiology

Approximately 100 million persons have HSV-1 and 60 million have HSV-2.

Herpes is most commonly found in young adults; range—infancy to senescence.

Incidence is equal in men and women (zoster). The prevalence in blacks is one-fourth that of whites.

Immunocompromised clients are especially at risk for contracting the herpesvirus (and for recurrence).

HZV incidence is >66% in the cohort over 50 years of age; 5% of cases occur in children <15 years; cumulative lifetime incidence is 10% to 20%.

Approximately one-third of persons with herpes labialis will experience a recurrence; half will have at least two recurrences annually. Postherpetic neuralgia develops in 20% of persons with HZV.

Etiology

Labialis: HSV-1, 80–90%; HSV-2, 10–20%
Urogenital: HSV-2, 70–90%; HSV-1, 10–30%
Neonatal: HSV-2, 70%; HSV-1, 30%
HSV is a double-stranded DNA virus that enters the host through abraded skin or intact mucous membranes. Epithelial cells are the initial target.

Physiology and Pathophysiology

HSV is transmitted by direct contact with active lesions or with secretions containing the virus. HSV-1 and HSV-2 share approximately 50% of their DNA; infection with one form affords some protection against the other. The virus attaches itself to epithelial cells, enters the cells, and replicates, exploiting cellular components. During the infection process, the virus gains access to and infects the regional sensory or autonomic nerves. The virus travels via nerve axon to the ganglion, where it becomes a latent infection. The virus can reactivate and cause recurrent infection in the cutaneous area innervated by the affected root.

HSV-VZV is a related virus that remains dormant in the dorsal-root ganglia. Reactivation may result from stress, trauma, re-exposure to varicella, radiation therapy, or immunosuppressive therapy. This causes the release of the virus along the nerve to the skin (dermatome).

The three distinct phases of HSV infection are:

Primary: Lesions appear 1–26 days after inoculation. Prodrome of burning or tenderness at eruption site may occur. Associated symptoms are fever, dysuria, vaginal discharge, or malaise. May last 2–6 weeks.

Latent: Virus remains dormant in the ganglion of the nerve that serves the affected dermatome.

Recurrent: Virus reactivation and the reappearance of lesions in the dermatome affected during the primary outbreak. Triggers are menses, sunburn, or illness. Duration is typically 4–6 days. It is less severe than primary symptoms.

Clinical Manifestations

Subjective

Incubation period is 2–20 days (average, 6 days) for the primary infection.

At-risk populations are those with multiple partners, increasing age, female gender, low socioeconomic status, HIV infection, long-term steroid therapy, and atopic dermatitis.

Primary HSV may be asymptomatic or have only trivial symptoms.

Symptomatic primary HSV: associated with regional lymphadenopathy, fever, headache, malaise, myalgia.

Recurrent: prodrome of tingling, itching, or burning sensation usually precedes visible skin changes by 24 hours. Systemic symptoms are usually absent.

Precipitating factors: Skin/mucosal irritation (UV radiation), altered hormonal milieu (menstruation), fever, the common cold, altered immune states, site of infection, intimate contact.

HZV: Prodrome presents with hyperesthesia, paresthesias, burning dysesthesias, or pruritus along the affected dermatome (duration, 1–2 days).

History

    Inquire about burning, tingling, nausea, fatigue, or even fever.

    Ask about any generalized symptoms.

    Are there any tender inguinal lymphadenopathies or possible deep pelvic pain?

    Any past HSV infection? Sexual history? Exposure to someone with overt HSV?

Objective

HSV-1 nongenital herpes is characterized clinically by grouped vesicles arising on an erythematous base on keratinized skin or mucous membrane.

HSV-2 genital herpes is a sexually transmitted viral infection, characterized by primary infection with grouped vesicles at the site of inoculation and regional lymphadenopathy and recurring outbreaks.

Erythemas are often noted initially. Followed by grouped often umbilicated vesicles. Become eroded. Erosions may enlarge to ulcerations.

Epithelial cells sloughs within 2–4 weeks.

Mucous membrane: Vermilion border of lip, rarely in the mouth. Vesicular fluid is contagious.

HZV: Begins as a maculopapular rash that follows a dermatomal distribution, commonly referred to as a "beltlike pattern". This evolves into vesicles with an erythematous base. Vesicles are often painful and associated with flulike symptoms or anxiety. T5 and T6 are most affected. Cranial nerve most frequently involved is the ophthalmic division of the trigeminal nerve.

Generalized viremia is characterized by 20 lesions outside the affected dermatome (1 in 7 may die).

HZV—Vesicles eventually become hemorrhagic or turbid and crust over within 7–10 days. Scarring and pigmentary changes may occur after the crust falls off.

Differential Diagnosis

Erythema multiforme (macular eruption with dark red papules and tubercles)

Excoriated scabies (papules, vesicles, pustules and burrows; intense itching)

Chancroid (open pustule or ulcer that may have exudate ; often found on genitalia)

Candidiasis (red, macerated lesions on skin ; white adherent plaques on
   tongue)

Granuloma inguinale (granulomatous painless nodule, usually in genital
   area)

HZV (vesicular lesions on red base, usually confined to dermatome)

Ulcerative balanitis (open sores and inflammation of the skin of the glans
   penis).

Aphthous stomatitis (painful, open, ulcerlike lesions usually found on the
   buccal mucosa, gums and palate)

Herpangina (a benign infectious disease of oral vesicles)

Syphilis (small red papules that change into a painless ulcer or chancre)

Neoplasia (abnormal tissue growth; can vary greatly)

Lymphogranuloma venereum (infectious vesicular venereal disease; as lesions
   heal, lymph nodes become enlarged and may block lymph channels)

Stevens–Johnson syndrome (nonpruritic, painless dark red maculopapular
   eruption, usually on extremities)

Mechanical ulceration caused by trauma (inquire during history-taking)

Diagnostic Tests

Tzanck smear (if able to unroof vesicle and obtain fluid)

Viral culture (to rule out specific herpes infection)

Antigen detection or direct fluorescence antibody test (DFA) (for crusted
   lesions)

Polymerase chain reaction (PCR) test (to rule out encephalitis)

Management/Treatment

Pharmacologic Management

HSV

Primary infection: Antiviral therapy is recommended. The drug of choice is
   oral acyclovir (Zovirax), 200 mg, PO, five times a day for 10 days

 CP 2–2   Clinical Pearl: Topical treatment of acyclovir reduces the
duration of viral shedding and the length of time before all lesions become
crusted, but this treatment is much less effective than oral or intravenous acyclovir.

Recurrent outbreaks: Acyclovir (Zovirax), 200 mg PO 5 times/day **or** 400
   mg PO TID **or** 800 mg PO BID until lesions are crusted or for approximately 5 days.

Topical penciclovir cream applied Q2H (while awake) for 4 days has been
   successful in treating recurrent episodes, reducing pain, and expediting
   the healing of lesions.

One time immediate dose of acyclovir (800 mg) at the onset of prodrome
   may prevent recurrent outbreaks.

Alternative:

   Recurrent: famciclovir (Famvir), 250 mg PO BID; valacyclovir (Valtrex),
   500 mg PO BID.

Primary: Valacyclovir (Valtrex), 1g PO BID.

Suppressive Therapy: Traditionally reserved for patients who have >6 recurrences a year. It is intended to decrease the frequency and severity of symptoms, decrease transmission of HSV to sexual partners and infants of infected mothers, and decrease the transmission of associated viral diseases (HIV). Only the first goal has proved to be attainable.

Therapy should be discontinued once a year to assess whether its continuation is necessary.

HZV

Treat acute viral infection

Treat acute pain associated with HZV

Prevention of postherpetic neuralgia

Antiviral agents, oral corticosteroids, and adjunctive individualized pain management methods are used. Regardless of agent, instituting antiviral therapy within 48 to 72 hours is crucial to avoid chronic pain.

Oral or IV corticosteroid therapy—i.e., prednisone, 30 mg PO BID (days 1–7); 15 mg BID (days, 8–14); then 7.5 mg BID (days 15–21)

Tricyclic Antidepressant (Amitryptyline 10–25 mg nightly in conjunction with antiviral reduces incidence of pain)

Lidocaine patches

Capsaicin

Topical corticosteroids

Transcutaneous electrical nerve stimulation (TENS) or nerve blocks

 CP 2–3   Clinical Pearl: Mild cutaneous episodes in younger immunocompetent clients can be adequately treated in an expectant manner with topical soaks and locally applied drying salves.

Treat complications such as secondary bacterial infections.

POSTHERPETIC NEURALGIA

The most common long-term complication of HZV is postherpetic neuralgia. Pain that persists for longer than 1–3 months after resolution of the rash is generally accepted as the sign of postherpetic neuralgia. It is characterized by constant burning, hyperesthesia, or lancinating pain that may be radicular in nature.

Capsaicin cream (Zostrix)—Apply to affected area 3–5 times a day.

Lidocaine patch—Apply to affected area Q4–12H PRN.

Amitriptyline (Elavil), 10–25 mg PO QHS; increase by 25 mg Q2–4 weeks until adequate response (maximum, 150 mg/day); imipramine (Tofranil) and desipramine (Norpramin) both have same dosing schedule as amitriptyline (maximum, 150 mg/day).

Phenytoin (Dilantin), 100–300 mg PO QHS; increase until adequate response or blood level is 10–20 μg/ml.

Carbamazepine (Tegretol), 100 mg PO QHS; increase by 100 mg Q3D until dose is 200 mg TID, response is adequate, or blood level is 6–12 μg/ml.

Gabapentin (Neurontin), 100–300 mg PO QHS; increase by 100–300 mg Q3D until dose is 300–900 mg TID or response is adequate.

Client Education

Transmission of virus, including neonatal transmission during pregnancy. Safe sex practices, including use of condoms.

Lifelong condition with no cure, but suppressive treatment is available. In most people, the frequency and severity decreases with time.

Use of sunscreen-containing lip protectants prior to sun exposure.

Follow-up

As needed for support and evaluation of recurrence

Referral

Refer to infectious disease specialist:

Clients in whom HSV is suspected who are on immunosuppressive therapy or have HIV infection.

Clients whose disease fails to respond to routine therapy.

Clients who require large amounts of pain medication or who have severe disseminated infections, have severe superimposed bacterial infection, are unable to void, or are unable to take medications PO.

PEDICULOSIS

SIGNAL SYMPTOMS ▶ itching, infestation

ICD-9 Codes	132	Pediculosis capitis
	132.2	Pediculosis pubis
	132.1	Pediculosis corporis

Pediculosis is a parasitic infestation. There are three types of pediculosis, more commonly known as lice: *Pediculosis humanus capitis* (head lice), *P. humanus corpora* (body lice), and *Phthirus pubis* (pubic lice).

Epidemiology

10–12 million persons are affected annually in the United States.

Head lice are most common among children aged 3 to 12 years.

Etiology

Lice are obligate human parasites and feed on human blood. No free-living lice live in the environment. Transmission occurs through close personal contact and through the sharing of hats, combs, and other personal items. Lice cannot jump or fly.

Physiology and Pathophysiology

The life span of the female louse is approximately 1 month. During that time she will lay approximately 5 to 10 eggs per day. The eggs are within a casing (nit) that attaches to the human hair shaft. The nit is brown in color prior to hatching and white after it hatches. Pruritus is a common symptom, and secondary infection from excoriation is common.

Clinical Manifestations

Subjective

Pruritus

Scaling of skin

Fatigue and low-grade fever if secondary infection is present

Objective

Obvious adult lice and/or nits in pruritic area

Nits attached to hair shaft

Lymphadenopathy

Excoriation

Differential Diagnosis

Dandruff and seborrheic scale (these can be slid along the hair shaft)

Scabies (generally involves the hands and feet, areas that are spared by body lice)

Diagnostic Tests

Usually none needed

Management/Treatment

Pharmacologic Management

HEAD AND PUBIC LICE

Permethrin (Nix), 1% (OTC); application needs to be repeated for pubic lice.

Malathion (Ovide), 0.05% (prescription); application needs to be repeated for pubic lice.

BODY LICE

Malathion (Ovide), 0.05%

Permethrin (Nix), 5% (prescription)

Nonpharmacologic Management

Infested clothing should be discarded.

Home should be cleaned thoroughly.

Vacuuming of rugs, furniture, and mattresses and hot-water laundering of personal items is necessary.

Items such as stuffed toys should be placed in a plastic bag for 10 days, and the lice will die from lack of food.

Nits must be meticulously removed: a solution of 50% vinegar and 50% water may be helpful.

Insecticidal sprays should be avoided.

Client Education

Stress prevention of transmission.

Emphasize nit removal.

Check child's head weekly, especially if classmates have recently had lice.

Lice are not a sign of poor hygiene.
Lice cannot jump or fly.

Follow-up
Follow up if secondary infection occurs.

Referral
Usually not necessary

PRESSURE ULCERS (Decubitus Ulcers)

SIGNAL SYMPTOMS▶ red, painful lesions

ICD-9 Codes	707.0	Decubitus ulcer

Pressure ulcers (decubitus ulcers) are areas of cellular necrosis of the skin and subcutaneous tissue that occur most commonly over bony prominences. Pressure ulcers are categorized by four stages of severity:

Stage 1: Erythema. Epidermis intact.
Stage 2: Partial-thickness skin loss. Extends into but not through dermis.
Stage 3: Full thickness through the dermis and into subcutaneous tissue.
    Shallow crater that may include exudates and necrotic tissue.
Stage 4: Deep penetration into fascia or bone.

Epidemiology
The incidence of pressure ulcers in skilled-care and nursing-home facilities approaches 23%.
Cause of lengthy hospital stays.
17%–56% in critically ill patients

Etiology
Moisture (incontinence).
Shear forces.
Pressure over a bony prominence.
Contributing factors include decreased mobility, decreased sensation, poor nutrition, and dementia.

Physiology and Pathophysiology
Injury occurs to the skin and underlying tissues. Ischemia and hypoxemia result as pressure is applied to the area. Waste products accumulate as ischemia continues. Toxins produced by the waste products further break down tissue.

Clinical Manifestation
Subjective
Pain over a bony prominence in Stage 1 or 2.
May be pain-free in Stage 3 or 4.
History should include:
    Chronic illness.

Hygiene status.
Nutritional status.
Immobility.
Constant skin moisture.
Incontinence.
Psychological factors.
Ability to perform activities of daily living.
Sources of support (family, friends, caregivers).

Objective

Skin examination reveals:
Erythema.
Exudate.
Ulcer crater.
Necrotic tissue.
Localized edema.

Differential Diagnosis

Venous stasis ulcer (edema, hyperpigmentation, usually found in lower extremity)

Diabetic ulcer (red, tender ulcerated tissue, usually found on forefoot and toes)

Ulceration from arterial insufficiency (pale atrophic skin, hair loss)

Skin cancer (atypical skin growth and/or mole)

Diagnostic Tests

Culture and sensitivity (to determine specific pathogen)
Albumin, CBC (to rule out malnutrition)
Sedimentation rate and x-ray examination (to rule out osteomyelitis)

Management/Treatment

Goals

Reduce pressure, moisture, shearing, friction.
Use debridement method least damaging to tissue.
Keep well humidified and protected with appropriate dressing.

Pharmacologic Management

Debriding methods:
Wet to dry dressings
Enzymatic ointments
Irrigate with saline
Whirlpool soaks
Dressings:
Semipermeable transparent film dressings: best for Stages 1–3 without heavy exudates.
Hydrocolloid: best for low- to moderate-exudate wounds.
Hydrogels: best for wounds with eschar or dry wounds.
Alginates: Stages 2–3 and bleeding wound.

Nonpharmacologic Management
Prevention: identify high-risk clients.

Nutritional support.

Reduce pressure and friction—make sure client moves/walks regularly.

Alternating air-pressure mattress pads.

Regular toileting and incontinence care.

Client Education
Prevention is key!

Discuss good hygiene—keeping skin clean and dry.

Proper positioning.

Nutrition.

Signs of secondary infection.

Follow-up
Clinic follow up weekly to monthly

Referral
Refer to plastic surgeon, infectious disease specialist, or dermatologist for pressure ulcers that fail to respond to treatment.

PSORIASIS

SIGNAL SYMPTOM ▶ scaling, silver skin

ICD-9 Codes	696.1	Psoriasis

Psoriasis is a common, heredity disorder of the skin with several clinical expressions. It is a papulosquamous eruption characterized by well-circumscribed erythematous macular and papular lesions with loosely adherent silvery white scale. Sites where it occurs are areas of repeated minor trauma: scalp, elbows, forearms, lumbosacral region, knees, hands, and feet.

Plaque-type psoriasis: Red, thick, scaly lesions with silvery scale.
  Precipitating factors: Stress, infection, trauma, medications, xerosis (dryness)
Guttate psoriasis: Teardrop-shaped, pink to salmon, scaly plaques; usually on trunk, with sparing of palms and soles.
  Precipitating factors: Streptococcal throat infection.
Pustular psoriasis, localized: Erythematous papules or plaques studded with pustules; usually on palms or soles.
  Precipitating factors: Stress, infection, medications.
Pustular psoriasis, generalized: Same as localized, but with more general involvement; associated with fever, malaise and diarrhea; may or may not have preexisting psoriasis.
Pustular psoriasis, generalized: Same as localized, but with more general involvement; associated with fever, malaise and diarrhea; may or may not have preexisting psoriasis.

Erythrodermic psoriasis: Severe, intense, generalized erythema and scaling covering entire body; often associated with systemic symptoms; may have had preexisting psoriasis.

Precipitating factors: Stress, infection, medications.

Epidemiology

Affects 2% of North Americans, with a mean age of onset of 20–30 years.

Lesions develop in 60% of clients before age 35.

Incidence in men equals that in women.

30% of clients have a family history.

Occurs worldwide, although the incidence is lower in warmer, sunnier climates.

Etiology

Chronic, relapsing hyperproliferative inflammatory disorder of the skin.

Cause unknown; may be due to a T-lymphocyte-mediated dermal immune response to an unidentified antigen.

Physiology and Pathophysiology

Psoriasis refers to a cluster of diseases of differing pathogeneses. The principal abnormality in psoriasis is an alteration of the cell kinetics of keratinocytes. The major change is a shortening of the cell cycle from 311 to 36 hours; this results in 28 times the normal production of epidermal cells.

Clinical Manifestations

Subjective

Duration of lesions: present for months or may be of sudden onset.

Skin symptoms: Seasonal pruritus.

Constitutional symptoms: Joint pain in arthritis. Ask about presence of nail pitting or arthritis, especially DIP joints of fingers and toes (psoriatic arthritis).

Ask about history of chronic dandruff, external ear scaling.

Recent streptococcal infection (pharyngitis).

Ask about HIV status/abrupt onset.

Previous treatment and results.

Medical history—focus on autoimmune disorders. Family history of psoriasis in first-degree relatives.

Assess impact on quality of life.

Objective

Type: papules and plaques, sharply marginated with marked silvery-white scale; removal of scale results in minute blood droplets (Ausspitz phenomenon); Pustules—presentation for erythroderma type.

"Salmon pink" color.

Round, oval, polycyclic, annular, linear.

Look for characteristic lesions, particularly on extensor surfaces.

CP 2–4 Clinical Pearl: Symmetry of distribution and silvery scale are hallmarks.

Use tongue blade to scrape over a lesion surface to elicit the pinpoint bleeding. Estimate body-surface area (BSA) affected (to determine local or generalized condition).

Differential Diagnosis

Plaque-type psoriasis: Atopic, irritant, seborrheic dermatitis, pityriasis rubra pilaris, cutaneous T-cell lymphoma

Guttate psoriasis: Pityriasis rosea, second-stage syphilis, drug eruption

Pustular psoriasis, localized, generalized, erythrodermic: Pustular drug eruption, dyshidrotic, atopic dermatitis, subcorneal pustular dermatosis, mycosis fungoides, pityriasis rubra pilaris

Diagnostic Tests

Usually none necessary.

Shave biopsy may be necessary for differential diagnosis.

Management/Treatment

Goals: Maximize treatment efficacy and client's quality of life, low side effects. Control of lesions is central. Most often treatment does not completely clear lesions. A positive response to therapy is noted as "normalization" of involved areas measured by reduced erythema and scaling as well as reduction of plaque elevation.

Pharmacologic Management

LOCALIZED

Corticosteroids: Topical steroids are drugs of choice; most commonly prescribed medicine for this condition. Classified as low-, medium-, high-, and super-high-potency. Low-potency agents used on the face, thinner skin areas, and on the groin and axillary areas. Associated with rapid flare-ups after discontinuation.

Most clients with psoriasis over <10% of their body-surface area can be treated with topical therapy alone, except for those with hand and foot psoriasis.

First-line—topical steroids; high-potency classification for initial therapy (new recommendation) e.g.: betamethasone dipropionate (Diprolene), 0.05% cream or triamcinolone acetonide (Aristocort), 0.5% cream or ointment.

Apply no more frequently than BID.

Instruct on steroid use; use only the amount that will easily rub into skin in 1–2 minutes. Apply gently. Always wash hands afterward to avoid inadvertently applying to other areas such as face and groin.

Use for 2 weeks only.

Calcipotriene: A vitamin D_3 analog available in cream, ointment, and solution.

Slow onset, not noticeable for 6–8 weeks; monotherapy is moderately effective in reducing the thickness, scaliness, and erythema. Maximum benefit is seen when used in combination with potent topical corticosteroids.

Coal tar: A black viscous fluid; thought to suppress epidermal DNA synthesis; most effective in combination with ultraviolet B light, and corticosteroids. Generally safe, but messy and smelly.

Anthralin or tazarotene: Antipsoriatic topical preparations derived from wood tar (second-line agent). Irritating to the skin and stains. 0.1 % to 1 % ointments (anthralin); 0.05–0.1 gel concentrations (tazarotene), creams, and solutions. Treatment graduation is done by increasing concentration and duration of contact, up to maximum of 30 minutes; can combine with UVB

Emollients.

LOCALIZED: FACE, PLEURAL FOLDS, AND GENITALIA

Low-potency agents such as hydrocortisone 1% cream or intermediate agent such as desonide (Tridesilon), 0.05% cream or lotion; BID; treat for no longer than 2 weeks.

Explain pulse therapy (once or twice a week) for maintenance.

Daily sunlight exposure helps four out of five people; avoid burning.

GENERALIZED PSORIASIS

Disease-modifying therapies (referral needed)
Phototherapy (e.g., UVB light phototherapy, natural sunlight)
Combination therapy (e.g., PUVA)
Systemic agents and possible hospitalization
  Retinoids (acitretin)
  Methotrexate
  Cyclosporine

REFRACTORY LESIONS

Intralesional injections of triamcinolone; inject directly into dermis of plaque, concentration, 3–10 mg/ml.

May need to be repeated injections Q4–6 weeks.

Complementary/Alternative Therapies

Flaxseed oil
Bayberry extract
Lecithin
Burdock
100% emulsion oil
Red clover
Terra maxa
Pumpkin extract
Dead sea salts

Client Education

Emphasize that the disorder is not contagious and that it can be controlled but not cured.

Provide client with opportunities to discuss feelings.

Counsel client regarding elements of a healthy lifestyle.

Discuss the role of stress and other exacerbating factors such as infection, trauma, xerosis, and use of medications such as angiotensin-converting–enzyme inhibitors, beta-adrenergic blockers, lithium, and antimalarials (Plaquenil).

Shaving affected areas may cause exacerbations.

Provide client with information about the National Psoriasis Foundation (NPF).

Follow-up

Follow up in 2–3 weeks; monitor for effectiveness of therapy and side effects every 2–3 months.

Referral

Refer to dermatologist to initiate treatment and/or if patient's disease does not respond to treatment.

SCABIES

SIGNAL SYMPTOMS ▶ itching, redness, burrowing

ICD-9 Code	133.0	Scabies

Scabies is caused by the mite *Sarcoptes scabiei* var. *hominis*. It is a contagious, parasitic disease.

Epidemiology

Estimated 300 million cases worldwide, with prevalence exceeding 50% in developing countries.

It is more common in communities where individuals are in close contact, such as schools or other institutions.

Etiology

Overcrowded conditions, immunocompromised states, and limited access to water are risk factors for scabies.

Young children and the elderly are more susceptible.

Physiology and Pathophysiology

The female mite burrows beneath the stratum corneum, depositing fecal pellets and eggs. These deposits cause intense pruritus. The larvae hatch and reach maturity in 14–17 days. Copulation of the adult mites repeats this cycle. Pruritus can remain several weeks after scabicide treatment is completed.

Clinical Manifestations

Subjective

Extreme pruritus, may be worse at night.

Rash.

Excoriation.

Affected sites (hands, feet, stomach, groin most common).

Previous treatments attempted.

History of overcrowded conditions.

Community outbreak.

Living conditions.

Immunocompromised state.

Objective

Burrows, appearing as a slightly raised, curved grayish line.

Tiny vesicles.

Excoriations.

Areas most commonly affected are interdigital areas, wrists, flexor surfaces, axillae, breasts, penis, skin folds, and buttocks.

Complete skin examination with concentration on the areas described above.

Examination for signs of secondary infection.

Differential Diagnosis

Neurodermatitis (inflammation of the skin, often associated with emotional disturbance)

Dermatitis herpetiformis (intensely pruritic red papular, vesicular, or pustular lesions in groups)

Atopic dermatitis (intensely pruritic red, swollen papules that become exudative and crusty)

Molluscum contagiosum (small, round, umbilicated elevated masses)

Flea bites (pruritic red, raised papules; history of exposure to pets/animals)

Lichen planus (small pruritic red papules that change to rough, scaly patches)

Diagnostic Tests

Usually none needed

Skin scraping of lesion (to examine for scabies mite egg—magnifying lens or microscope needed)

Management/Treatment

Pharmacologic Management

5% Permethrin (Elimite, Acticin) cream. Apply from chin to toes. Leave on 8–10 hours and follow with hot shower. One application usually suffices. Permethrin is safe for children >2 months old.

or

1% Lindane (Kwell) lotion. Apply from chin to toes. Leave on 8–10 hours and follow with hot shower. One application usually suffices. Lindane is not safe for young children (under 2 years old) or pregnant or lactating women because it is absorbed through the skin.

Treat secondary bacterial infections with oral antibiotics.

Antipruritics may be helpful.

Topical steroids may be helpful to reduce pruritic symptoms after scabicide treatment is complete.

Nonpharmacologic Management

Keep fingernails trimmed. Apply scabicide after handwashing.

Undergarments, linens, and towels must be laundered in hot water.

Household members and other close contacts must be treated concurrently.

Complementary/Alternative Therapies

Topical arnica flower may be helpful for itching.

Client Education

Educate clients regarding nonpharmacologic adjunctive treatment for scabies, while emphasizing the need for pharmacologic treatment as well.

Explain that pruritic symptoms can persist for weeks after scabicide treatment is complete; these symptoms do not mean the infestation is persisting.

Discuss notification and treatment of household members and other close contacts.

Follow-up

In clinic 2 weeks after treatment.

Follow client until infestation clears and symptoms resolve

Referral

To dermatologist in refractory cases, or in cases in which diagnosis is suspect or symptoms persist.

SKIN CANCER

SIGNAL SYMPTOMS ▶ atypical moles/growths on skin

ICD-9 Codes	172.9	Melanoma
		Squamous-cell carcinoma
	173.9	Basal-cell carcinoma
	173.9	Neoplasm, skin—malignant

Skin cancer is a malignancy of the skin. The three most skin cancers common are:

Basal-cell carcinoma—arising from basal-cell layer of the epidermis.

Squamous-cell carcinoma—arising from keratinizing cells of epidermis.

Melanoma—malignant transformation of epidermal melanocytes.

Epidemiology

Skin cancer accounts for one-third of all cancers in the United States.

Skin cancer develops at some point in one of six Americans.

Malignant melanoma accounts for 75% of all deaths associated with skin cancer and 1%–2% of all deaths from cancer.

Incidence of skin cancer is increasing in the United States: lifetime risk of having melanoma is 1 in 70.

Etiology

Risk factors include:

History of a changing mole.

Atypical nevi.

Cumulative sun exposure.

Intermittent intense sun exposure.

Family history (first-degree relative).

History of blistering sunburns.

Immunosuppression.

Stress may contribute to development and progression of skin cancer.

Physiology and Pathophysiology

Cancers develop as a complex interaction between exposure to carcinogens and gene mutations. This applies to the skin cancers as well as to other forms of cancer. Metastasis in basal-cell carcinoma is rare, whereas it is more common in squamous-cell carcinoma and especially malignant melanoma. Malignant melanoma is an aggressive cancer and should always be treated as such.

Clinical Manifestations

Subjective

Basal-cell carcinoma and squamous-cell carcinoma are generally asymptomatic.

Malignant melanoma: changing mole, bleeding, itching or burning, new pigmented lesion.

History

Risk factors

New lesions/change in moles

Objective

 CP 2–5 Clinical Pearl: Use good light, examine ALL areas of the skins, including under the arms, bottom of the feet and genital area. Use a magnification lens for close or detailed examination. Use a rule to measure the exact size of lesion. Palpate lesions to help in differential diagnosis. Draw lesion on chart for future reference.

Basal-cell carcinoma

Translucent, white papule ("pearly" in appearance)

Scaly patch with crust

Telangiectasia

Ulceration centrally

Face and upper back

Squamous-cell carcinoma
  Scaly erythematous macule or plaque
  Firm papule or plaque
  Telangiectasia
  Central ulceration
  Face, dorsal hand, and lower lip
Malignant melanoma
  Asymmetry
  Border irregularity
  Color variability
  Diameter greater than 6 mm (the size of a pencil eraser)

Differential Diagnosis

Actinic keratosis (single or multiple dry, rough, scaly lesions due to sun exposure; can lead to squamous-cell carcinoma)
Melanocytic nevus (small, round pigmented papules, macules, or nodules)
Blue nevus (solitary, benign dark-blue to black defined papule or nodule)
Lentigo simplex (benign brown macules, often seen in whites)
Solar lentigo (round macule varying from yellow to dark brown)
Seborrheic keratosis (benign skin tumor that range from flat to irregular shape)
Vascular lesions (lesions caused by vascular changes: include, but are not limited to hemangiomas, nevus flammeus, angiomas, and telangiectasias)

Diagnostic Tests

Biopsy (to rule out malignancy), includes punch biopsy, saucerization biopsy, elliptic excision

Management/Treatment

Excision (performed by dermatologist)

Client Education

Do a thorough skin examination monthly.
If any suspicious lesions are found, see health-care provider immediately.
Stress importance of sunscreen of at least SPF 15 (use regularly [every 2–3 hours] and liberally!)
Avoid exposure to midday sun and burning.
Protect children.
Wear protective clothing and broad-brimmed hats.
Avoid tanning beds.
Provide references and resources

Follow-up

Periodic for skin examination and per recommendation of dermatologist

Referral

Promptly refer all suspicious lesions to dermatologist.

SKIN INFECTIONS, BACTERIAL (Impetigo)

SIGNAL SYMPTOM ▶ oozing lesions on the skin

ICD-9 Code	684	Impetigo

Impetigo is a common contagious superficial skin infection caused by strepto-cocci, staphylococci, or both. It is characterized by thin-walled, fragile seropurulent vesicles.

Epidemiology

Most common in infants and children; peak incidence in late summer and early fall.

Etiology

May be a complication of insect bites, abrasions, or dermatitis. May be spread by direct contact or may be a complication of upper respiratory infection.

Physiology and Pathophysiology

Normally, intact skin is resistant to colonization or infection by pathogen, but skin injury interferes with this protective function. The disease is generally self-limited, but poststreptococcal glomerulonephritis has been reported to follow impetigo.

Clinical Manifestations

Subjective
Itching
Crusting
Blisters
Upper respiratory infection
History of skin breakdown
Immunocompromised state

Objective
Vesicles and pustules
Honey-colored crusts
Regional lymphadenopathy
Possible fever

Differential Diagnosis
Varicella (clear vesicles on erythematous base that crust and heal)
Herpes simplex (vesicles, usually found on mucous membranes)
Eczema (red, pruritic, scaly lesions)
Other vesicular or ulcerating skin lesions (can vary in size and site)

Diagnostic Tests
Generally not needed
Culture can be obtained (to determine specific pathogen)

Management/Treatment

Pharmacologic Management

TOPICAL ANTIBIOTIC THERAPY:

Indicated in immunocompromised clients with few, localized lesions. Mupirocin (Bactroban) ointment applied TID topically.

SYSTEMIC ANTIBIOTIC THERAPY:

Indicated in clients with widely disseminated or inaccessible lesions or those who are immunocompromised.

Cephalexin (Keflex), 250–500 mg QID PO; pediatric dose: 50 mg/kg/day Q6H **or** erythromycin (PCE) 1 g/day in divided doses; pediatric dose 40 mg/kg/day Q6H **or** dicloxacillin 250 mg QID PO; pediatric dose, 25 mg/kg/day Q6H.

Nonpharmacologic Management

Debridement of crust with wet soaks TID

Client Education

Impetigo is extremely contagious.

Keep fingernails short to prevent scratching and spread of infection.

Children should be removed from day care until 24 hours after antibiotic treatment is started.

Follow-up

Clinic follow up in 3–5 days if no improvement occurs.

Referral

Refer to dermatologist or infectious disease specialist if impetigo does not resolve.

SKIN INFECTIONS, FUNGAL (Candida)

SIGNAL SYMPTOM red, shiny, itchy lesions

ICD-9 Codes	117.9	Fungal infections
	112.9	Monilia NOS, Candidiasis NOS
	110.9	Ringworm NOS

Superficial fungal infections of the skin are those due to various fungi. Discussed here are dermatophyte infections, which include tinea capitis (scalp), tinea pedis (feet), tinea corporis (body), onychomycosis (nails), and infections due to candida (intertrigo—infections in body folds).

Epidemiology

Prevalent and often recurring.

Can occur at any age.

Tinea pedis is the most common.

Etiology

Immunocompromised states often lead to infections caused by *Candida*.

Moist, warm environments such as within body folds also facilitate excessive growth of candida. Pregnancy and oral-contraceptive use can also increase the risk of candidiasis.

Physiology and Pathophysiology

Some fungi are considered normal flora. However, a disruption in the host's homeostasis may result in infection. Infections that are typically superficial may exhibit deep involvement in immunosuppressed individuals. A candidal infection can be differentiated from a tinea infection by the presence of satellite lesions.

Clinical Manifestations

Subjective

Itching
Tenderness (occasionally)
Inflammation
Alopecia
Scaling
History
    Immunosuppressed state
    Oral contraceptives
    Recent exposure to kittens, puppies, or other children

Objective

Annular plaque with central clearing
Alopecia
Erythema
Broken hairs
Dry, thickened soles
Yellow, thickened nails
Satellite pustules (candida)
Cheesy exudates (candida, especially vaginal)
Physical examination
    Obesity/examination of skin folds and underneath breasts
    Inspection of lesions
    Location of lesions
    Characterization of discharge

Differential Diagnosis

Contact dermatitis (red, scaly plaques, usually localized to specific area of contact)
Psoriasis (silvery, scaly plaques, can be generalized all over the body)
Seborrheic dermatitis (dry, white to yellow greasy plaques on red base)

Diagnostic Tests

Potassium hydroxide (KOH) preparation (to rule out fungal infection)
Fungal culture (to determine specific pathogen)

Wood's light shone on affected site in darkened room (yellow or green fluorescence of hair shafts suggests fungal infection)

Management/Treatment
Pharmacologic Management

TINEA CAPITIS

Griseofulvin (ultramicrosize) (GriFulvin V), 500 mg QD PO for 4–6 weeks; pediatric dose: 10–20 mg/kg/day PO until hair regrows (6–8 weeks)
Terbinafine (Lamisil), 250 mg QD PO for 4–8 weeks (not approved by FDA)

TINEA CORPORIS

Limited area: Topical imidazole for 2–3 weeks. Continue for 1 week after clinical cure.
Extensive: Refer to dermatologist.

TINEA PEDIS

Topical imidazole for 4 weeks

ONYCHOMYCOSIS

Terbinafine (Lamisil), 250 mg QD PO for 12 weeks (toenail)
Terbinafine (Lamisil), 250 mg QD PO for 6 weeks (fingernail)
Itraconazole (Sporanox), 200mg QD PO for 12 weeks (toenail)
Itraconazole (Sporanox) 200mg BID PO for 1 week, then 3 weeks without treatment; repeat for 3 months.

Nonpharmacologic Management

Wear 100% cotton socks.
Protect feet in shared bathing areas (wear flip-flops).
Keep feet dry.
Treat chronic health conditions such as diabetes.

Client Education

Stress importance of treatment for entire course (fungi are stubborn).
Explain side effects of medications.
Avoid sharing socks or footwear with others.
Keep feet clean and dry, with attention to interdigital areas.
Wear cotton socks.
Protect feet in shared bathing areas.
Keep skin folds dry with powder such as corn starch.
Frequent candidiasis can be a sign of HIV infection.

Follow-up

1–2 weeks

Referral

Refer to dermatologist if no response to treatment.
Consider referral if lesion is present on the scalp, especially in children.
Refer in cases of widespread infection.

URTICARIA

ICD-9 Codes	708.9	Urticaria

Also known as hives, urticaria are pruritic, red, raised plaques or welts. They are frequently an allergic reaction. Urticaria can be acute (lasting hours to weeks) or chronic (lasting for more than 6 weeks).

Epidemiology

Approximately 20% of the population will have at least one episode.
Of patients who have chronic urticaria, 20% will have it for 10 years or more.

Etiology

In chronic urticaria, a cause can be found only about 20% of the time. It can be induced by physical factors:

Dermographism (writing on the skin).
Vibratory (vibration is the predominant motion).
Solar urticaria (exposure to sun).
Cold-induced urticaria (noted minutes after cold exposure).
Pressure urticaria (site of pressure application).
Cholinergic urticaria (after hot shower or exercise).
Acute urticaria is often an allergic reaction to a food, insect bite, inhalant, or injection. Often a cause cannot be found, especially in children.

Physiology and Pathophysiology

Urticaria usually involves the epidermis and the upper portions of the dermis. The release of mediators leads to vasodilation with extravasation of fluid and edema into the interstitial region. Histamine is the most important chemical mediator in urticaria.

Clinical Manifestations

Subjective

Itching (usually intense)
Edema (especially lips, around eyes, hands, and feet)
Ingestion of certain foods (peanuts and shellfish are common culprits)
Ask client about:
Diet history.
Wheezing, shortness of breath, difficulty breathing.
Previous episodes of urticaria.
Any identified pattern to urticaria (especially important in chronic urticaria).

Objective

Red, raised plaques with sharp borders.

Plaques can be migratory.

Cardiopulmonary examination (chest should be clear and free of wheezing). Assess for signs of angioedema.

Differential Diagnosis

Erythema multiforme (macular eruption with dark red papules, often on extremities)

Multiple insect bites (point of entry found on plaques; ask patient about recent travel or exposure to insects)

Contact dermatitis (red, scaly, dry, pruritic plaques)

Acute exanthem (may also have systemic symptoms such as fever/chills, fatigue, malaise)

Diagnostic Tests

Generally none needed, but consider CBC (which reveals increased eosinophils).

Management/Treatment

Pharmacologic Management

Hydroxyzine (Atarax), 25–50 mg PO QID
   Pediatric dose: <6 years, 50 mg PO daily in divided doses; >6 years, 50–100 mg PO daily in divided doses.

Diphenhydramine (Benadryl), 25–50 mg PO Q4–6H
   Pediatric dose: 2–6 years, 6.25 mg PO Q4H; 6–12 years, 12.5–25 mg PO Q4–6H.

Loratadine (Claritin), 10 mg PO QD
   Pediatric dose: <6 years, not recommended; >6 years, 10 mg PO QD.

Cetirizine (Zyrtec), 10 mg PO QD
   Pediatric dose: <2 years, not recommended; 2–5 years, 2.5mg PO QD; 5–10 years, 5–10 mg PO QD.

Nonpharmacologic Management

Cool or tepid soaks

Colloidal oatmeal (Aveeno) in bath water

Client Education

Stress careful attention to possible precipitating factors. It is often helpful to keep a journal.

Follow-up

Clinic follow-up in 48 hours if lesions persist

Referral

Immediate referral to emergency services:
   For evidence of anaphylaxis (hypotension, wheezing, tachycardia, coughing, severe anxiety, cyanosis).
   For evidence of edema of the larynx (hoarseness, inspiratory stridor).

Referral to dermatologist for chronic or recurrent urticaria lasting more than 6 weeks.

WARTS (Human Papillomavirus)

SIGNAL SYMPTOM fleshy growth on extremities

| ICD-9 Codes | 078.10 | Viral warts NOS and verruca vulgaris |
| | 078.11 | Condyloma acuminatum |

Human papillomavirus (HPV) is tropic to squamous epithelial cells, lies latent in the basal-cell layer, and replicates at the granular level. Replication is linked to keratinocyte differentiation.

In benign lesions viral DNA is not incorporated into the cell DNA. Oncogenic HPV does alter host-cell DNA.

Warts are classified into distinct classes as described in Table 2–4.

Epidemiology

Prevalence: 5 million health-care visits a year; 5%–10% of children have contracted common warts.

Anogenital HPV infects 24–40 million people in the United States. with 500,000–1 million new cases a year.

2% of all sexually active people have visible genital warts, and far more have subclinical infection; it is the most common sexually transmitted disease (STD).

Reports of up to 99% of cervical cancers are attributable to HPV infections.

81 million people, or 60% of the U.S. population aged 15–49, have had a prior infection, and, therefore, probably antibodies to HPV.

Etiology

A DNA virus. Member of the papovaviridae family. Over 100 types of HPV identified to date.

The virus is spread through direct contact. It is postulated that it enters through breaks in the skin. When new lesions appear in cutaneous trauma it is called the Koebner phenomenon.

Common (verrucae plantaris), flat (verrucae planae), anogenital (condylomata acuminata), cervical, laryngeal and other mucous membrane forms, and epidermodysplasia verruciformis.

Risk factors for HPV include: a large number of sexual partners, an increased rate of sexual intercourse, an increased rate of alcohol consumption, smoking, anal sex, and being black or of Hispanic ethnicity (risk factors for genital HPV).

Risk factors for common warts: Finger sucking, hangnail biting, and trauma.

Physiology and Pathophysiology

Incubation time ranges from 1 month to more than 3 years. Latent HPV also occurs. Two-thirds of cases in immunocompetent persons spontaneously regress within 2 years. HPV causes hyperproliferation of epithelial cells. Transmission

Table 2–4 Types of Warts

Common Warts	HPV types 1, 2, 4, and 26. Skin-colored hyperkeratotic papules found most often on the back of the hands, knees and periungal areas. Filiform variant usually found on the face; they have fine, finger-like projections.
Plantar Warts	HPV 1,2, and 4 are found on pressure areas they are skin-colored hyperkeratotic papules or plaques which are often studded and covered by black pinpoints that represent thrombosed capillaries. These warts often coalesce into plaques. This papule inverts in its growth. This is the one wart that is associated with pain and significant morbidity.
Flat Warts	HPV types 3 and 10 mainly affect children. Occur on the face and extremities in crops of 1–2 mm papules that are smooth, flat, and skin-colored. Koebner phenomenon is associated with this type.
Anogenital Warts	Range from small, skin-colored papules to large cauliflower-like growths. Bowenoid papulosis are small pigmented papules that are associated with HPV 6 and 16. Premalignant type is associated with cervical, melanoma, squamous cell cancer, leukoplakia, and oral carcinoma. Condylomea acuminata are attributed to HPV 6 & 11 and are a low malignant potential. Penile warts are smooth and flat. Perianal warts have cauliflower appearance. Warts in men are dry and keratinized; in women the vagina is moist without keratinization. It thrives at the transformation zone of the cervix. Symptoms include irritation, itching, burning, bleeding or pain. Laryngeal papilloma: Vertical transmission from mothers with anogenital warts to their infants. Can develop in adults via oral sex. HPV types 6 and 11 are the source. Present with hoarseness and stridor, can be life-threatening if large enough to obstruct airway. Also found on the oral and nasal mucous membranes and on conjunctivae
Cervical Warts	Inconspicuous white patches or flat plaques. Application of acetic acid and colposcopy aid in visualization. These types have been implicated as the cause of cervical dysplasia and neoplasia. HPV types associated with high risk of malignant transformation are 16, 18, 31, 33, 35, 45, 51, 52, & 56. Types 6, 11, 42, 43, and 44 are low risk.
Epidermodysplasia verruciformis	Rare autosomal receptive condition characterized by numerous flat verrucous papules and erythematous macules. They are refractory to treatment and are associated with 30% increased risk of developing squamous cell carcinoma. Types 5 and 8 are the offending types

depends on the number of viral particles, location of warts, preexisting skin injury, and T-cell-mediated immunity.

Clinical Manifestations

Subjective

Visible lesions on hands/fingers, feet/toes, and/or genital area.

Usually asymptomatic, but can be painful if present over pressure areas.

Obtain history, including social and sexual history.

Any recent group exposure.

Objective

COMMON WARTS

Round, elevated growths
Usually isolated
Usually found on hands, fingers

PLANTAR WARTS

Round, rough plaque with black dot in center
Often found on feet
Tender on palpation

FLAT WARTS

Flat, round pinkish papules

GENITAL WARTS

Fleshy, cauliflowerlike growths
Found on genital and/or anal area

Differential Diagnosis

Folliculitis
Lichen planus (flat, shiny, pink plaques, usually grouped together)
Milia (small, white papules, usually found in infants)
Molluscum (small, raised, umbilicated growths)
Granuloma annulare (red, raised circular plaques)
Corns, calluses (raised hyperkeratotic thickening of skin, usually over bony areas)
Herpes simplex virus (HSV) type 2 infection (vesicles usually found on mucous membranes)
Neoplasms (growths of varied size and shape)

Diagnostic Tests

Usually none needed
Biopsy (to rule out neoplasm)
Polymerase chain reaction (PCR) (to rule out specific viral infection)
For genital warts (see also, Chapter 14, "Infectious Diseases"):
Pap smear (screening tool for presence of HPV)
Acetowhitening (done during a colposcopy to determine HPV infection)
Serology (determines specific type of HPV infection)

Management/Treatment

Pharmacologic Management

EXTERNAL WARTS

Current treatment includes treatments applied by both patient and provider: ablative chemicals, immunomodulators, and surgical options. Warts on moist surfaces respond better to topical treatment than do warts on dry surfaces.

Note: Treated warts may appear to be resolved, but may just be in a latent phase; the epidermal tumor is resolved, but the virus is not eradicated.

Patient applications include compound W (salicylic acid). Topical 5-fluorouracil (5-FU), podofilox, 0.5% gel or 0.5% solution (antimitotic), applied BID for 3 days, followed by four days of no treatment (may repeat 4 times). Initial treatment to be performed by care provider. Imiquimod, 5% cream (immune enhancer-stimulates interferon), 3 times a week for up to 16 weeks QHS) is the most effective therapy.

Practitioner applications include podophyllin resin, trichloroacetic acid (TCA) or bichloroacetic acid (BCA) (caustic agent is quite effective) 80%–90%, liquid nitrogen (once a week, until resolved), curettage, electrosurgery, desiccation, laser surgery, tangential scissors/shave excision.

During pregnancy only option is surgical removal.

PLANTAR WARTS

Nonsurgical intervention preferred to limit scarring:

Liquid nitrogen or 10% formalin or 25% glutaraldehyde compresses for mosaic.

Salicylic acid suspended in karaya gum.

Curettage if prior therapy is ineffective.

ANOGENITAL AND CERVICAL WARTS (SEE ALSO, "EXTERNAL WARTS")

TCA, BCA, or podophyllum

Cryotherapy

Complementary/Alternative Therapies

Virxcan black salve

Birch park tea or rub

Client Education

Prevention (Anal intercourse is a common transmission activity).

Condom use (Cannot completely prevent transmission. This is due to possible transmission during foreplay or other nonintercourse sexual contact. It does reduce risk slightly).

Genital warts are highly contagious (90% of pediatric cases of anogenital warts are spread via nonsexual contact, such as changing diapers, bathing, etc.).

Regular Pap smears.

Length of treatment, cost, discomfort, risk of scarring, and likely failure of therapy.

Follow-up

No consensus on follow up period.

General rule: If applied therapy fails (three attempts by the provider and three by the patient), treatment method should be changed.

Regular follow-up for clients with persistent infections should be performed to help monitor and prevent HPV related to cancer

Referral

Refer to dermatologist:
Anogenital warts in a young child
Warts that are refractory to therapy
Warts in clients with diabetes or compromised circulation
Disfiguring warts or warts with hair or on the face
Refer to gynecologist:
Pap smear with dysplasia

REFERENCES

General

Buttaro, T.M. (1999). *Primary care: A collaborative practice.* St. Louis: Mosby Year-Book.

Corwin, E.J. (2000). *Handbook of pathophysiology.* Philadelphia: Lippincott Williams & Wilkins.

Dipiro, J.T. (1999). *Pharmacotherapy: A pathophysiologic approach.* Stamford, CT: Appleton & Lange.

Ferri, F. (2002). *Ferri's clinical advisor 2002: Instant diagnosis and treatment.* St. Louis: Mosby-YearBook.

Fitzpatrick, T.B., Johnson, R.A., Wolff, K., Polano, M.P., & Suurmond, D. (1997). *Color atlas and synopsis of clinical dermatology: Common and serious diseases.* New York: McGraw-Hill.

Porth, C.M. (1998). *Pathophysiology: Concepts of altered health states* (5th ed.) New York: Lippincott.

Uphold, C.R., & Graham, M.V. (1998). Clinical guidelines in family practice (3rd ed.). Gainesville, FL: Barmarrae Books.

Acne

Berson, D.S., Draelos, Z.D., & Webster, G.F. (1999). Saving face: A treatment update for acne. *Patient Care, 33,* 257–278.

Cooley S., Atkinson, P., Parks, D., & Hebert, A. (1998). Management of acne vulgaris. *Journal of Pediatric Health, 12,* 38–40.

Forster, J. (1997). Managing acne in adult women. *Patient Care, 31*(10), 30–43.

Johnson, B.A., & Nunley, J.R. (2000). Use of systemic agents in the treatment of acne vulgaris. *American Family Physician, 62,* 1823–1830.

Pogue, S. (1999). Acne in adolescents: Need for treatment is more than skin deep. *Advance for Nurse Practitioners, 7,* 53 55.

Russell, J.J. (2000). Topical therapy for acne. *American Family Physician, 61,* 358–366.

Acne Rosacea

Binder, R. (2001). The demographics of rosacea. *Rosacea Briefs, 2*(1), 1–8.

Chalmers, D.A. (1997). Rosacea: Recognition and management for the primary care provider. *Nurse Practitioner, 22*(10), 18–30.

Fried, R.G. (2000). The psychology of rosacea and its treatment. *Rosacea Briefs, 1*(5), 1–8.

Sturm, R.L. (2001). Topical treatments for rosacea. *Rosacea Briefs, 2*(2). 1–8.

Bites (Animal and Human)

Presutti, R.J. (2001). Prevention and treatment of dog bites. *American Family Physician, 63,* 1567–1572.

Burns

Morgan, E.D., Bledsoe, S.C. & Barker, J. (2000). Ambulatory management of burns. *American Family Physician, 62,* 2015–2026.

Cellulitis

Barg, N., Gantz, N. & Jarvis, W. (1998). Common and potentially fatal staph infections. *Patient Care, 32*(6), 25–49.

Corns and Calluses

Dale, S.J. (1997). Effective approaches to common foot complaints. *Patient Care, 31*(5), 158–180.

Singh, D., Bentley, G., & Trevino, S. (1996). Fortnightly review: Callosities, corns, and calluses. *British Medical Journal, 312,* 1403–1406.

Dermatitis (Atopic, Contact, Seborrheic)

Correale, C.E., & Walker, C. (1999). Atopic dermatitis: A review of diagnosis and treatment. *American Family Physician, 60,* 1191–1210.

Johnson, B.A., & Nunley, J.R. (2000). Treatment of seborrheic dermatitis. *American Family Physician, 61,* 2703–2710, 2713–2714.

Landow, K. (1997). Atopic dermatitis: Current concepts support old therapies and spur new ones. *Postgraduate Medicine, 101*(3), 101–117.

Nicol, N.H. (2000). Managing atopic dermatitis in children and adults. *Nurse Practitioner, 25*(4), 58–69.

Peters, S. (1997). Treating dermatitis in children: The role of topical corticosteroids. *Advance for Nurse Practitioners, 5*(2), 50–51.

Tramp, C., & Kaplan, D.L. (2000). Atopic dermatitis : How to recognize, how to treat. *Consultant, 40,* 2221–2233.

Herpes Simplex Infections/Herpes Zoster Infection

Cohen, J.I., Brunell, P.A., Straus, S.E., Krause, P.R. (1999). Recent advances in varicella-zoster virus infection. *Annals of Internal Medicine, 130,* 922–932.

Emmert, D.H. (2000). Treatment of common cutaneous herpes simplex virus infections. *American Family Physician, 61,* 1697–1704, 1705–1706, 1708.

Landow, K. (2000). Acute and chronic herpes zoster. *Postgraduate Medicine, 107*(7), 107–118.

Stankus, S.J., Dlugopolski, M., Packer, D. (2000). Management of herpes zoster (shingles) and postherpetic neuralgia, *American Family Physician, 61,* 2437–2444, 2447–2448.

Pressure Ulcers

O'Dell, M.L. (1998). Skin and wound infections: An overview. *American Family Physician, 57,* 2424–2432.

Psoriasis

Pardasani, A.G., Feldman, S.R., & Clark, A.R. (2000). Treatment of psoriasis: An algorithm-based approach for primary care physicians. *American Family Physician, 61,* 725–733, 736.

Scabies

Lim, D. (2000) Photo essay: Parasitic infections. *Consultant 40,* 2386.

Mukkavilli, G. (2000) Photo essay: Parasitic infections. *Consultant 40,* 2385.

Skin Cancer

Burke, C.C. (2000). In the sun: Tools for skin cancer prevention and early detection. *Advance for Nurse Practitioners, 8*(5), 33–47.

Edman, R.L., & Wolfe, J.T. (2000). Prevention and early detection of malignant melanoma. *American Family Physician, 62,* 2277–2284.

Goldstein, B.G. & Goldstein, A.O. (2001). Diagnosis and management of malignant melanoma. *American Family Physician, 63,* 1359–1368.

McEldowney, S. (1997). Malignant melanoma: Familial, genetic and psychosocial risk factors. *Clinician Reviews, 7*(7), 65–82.

Miller, S.J., Tsao, H., & Weinstock, M.A. (1999). Preventing mortality in cutaneous melanoma. *Patient Care, 33*(9), 34–60.

Skin Infections, Bacterial (Impetigo), Fungal (Candida)

Barg, N., Gantz, N., & Jarvis, W. (1998). Common and potentially fatal staph infections. *Patient Care, 32*(6), 25–49.

Bisno, A.L., Chapnick, E.K., & Panacek, E.A. (1999). Rapid responses to skin and soft tissue infections. *Patient Care, 33*(3), 114–127.

Haskal, Z.J., & Lutwick, L.I. (1998). Deep-tissue abscesses: Evolving approaches. *Patient Care, 32*(10), 18–38.

O'Dell;, M.L. (1998). Skin and wound infections: An overview. *American Family Physician, 57,* 2424–2432.

Skin Infections, Viral (Herpes Simplex, Herpes Zoster)

Bjorgen, S. (1998). Herpes zoster: How to recognize and manage this painful, self-limiting viral infection. *American Journal of Nursing, 98*(2), 46.

Centers for Disease Control and Prevention (1998). Guidelines for treatment of sexually transmitted diseases, *MMWR Morb Mortal Wkly Rep, 47*(RR-1), 1–116.

Emmert, D.H. (2000). Treatment of common cutaneous herpes simplex virus infections. *American Family Physician, 61,* 1697–1704.

Grin, C.M., & Rothe, M.J. (2000). Clinical theme and variations: Typical and atypical herpes zoster. *Consultant, 40*(12), 2351–2355.

Stankus, S.J., Dlugopolski, M., & Packer, D. (2000). Management of herpes zoster (shingles) and postherpetic neuralgia. *American Family Physician, 61,* 2437–2444.

Warts

Cohen, B.A. (1997). Are warts and children inseparable? *Patient Care, 4,* 163–184.

Ordoukhanian, E., & Lane, A.T. (1997). Warts and molluscum contagiosum: Beware of treatments worse than the disease. *Postgraduate Medicine, 101*(2), 223–232.

Rodgers, P., & Bassler, M (2001). Treating onychomycosis. *American Family Physician, 63,* 663–672.

Saunders, C. (2000). Monitoring HPV infection. *Patient Care, 34*(5), 142–171.

Woodward, C., & Fisher, M.A. (1999). Drug treatment of common STD's. Part II. Vaginal infections, pelvic inflammatory disease and genital warts. *American Family Physicians, 60,* 1716–1722.

RESOURCES

General

American Academy of Dermatology
   930 N. Meacham Rd.
   Schaumburg, IL 60173-4965
   Telephone: 847-330-0230
   Fax: 847-330-0050
   http://www.aad.org/

Acne
www.acne-site.com

Acne Rosacea
National Rosacea Society
Telephone: 888-NO-BLUSH
Rosacea Review
www.rosacea.org

Burns
Burn Survivor Resource Center
Telephone: 800-669-7700
www.burnsurvivor.com

Dermatitis (Atopic, Contact, Seborrheic)
National Eczema Association for Science and Education
1220 SW Morrison, St. 433
Portland, OR 97205
Telephone: 800-818-7546 or 503-228-4430
Fax: 503-224-3363
www.eczema-assn.org
E-mail: nease@teleport.com
National Eczema Society
www.eczema.org

Herpes Simplex Infection/Herpes Zoster Infections
Herpes Resource Center /HPV Support Program
American Social Health Association
P.O. Box 13827
Research Triangle Park, NC 27709
Telephone: 919-361-8488 or 800-227-8922
www.ashastd.org

National Herpes Hotline
Telephone: 919-361-8488

National STD Hotline
800-227-8922

VZV Research Foundation
36 E. 72nd St.
New York, NY 10021
Telephone: 212-472-3181

Pediculosis/Scabies
National Pediculosis Association, Inc.
www.headlice.org

Psoriasis
National Psoriasis Foundation/USA
http://www.psoriasis.org/
Psoriasis Research Association
107 Vista del Grande
San Carlos, CA 94070
Telephone: 415-593-1392

Skin Cancer

www.skin-cancer.com

www.aad.org

www.melanoma.com

The Skin Cancer Foundation
Box 561 DT
New York, NY 10156
Telephone: 800-SKIN-490

Urticaria

American Academy of Allergy, Asthma & Immunology
Telephone: 800-822-2762
www.aaaai.org

BLEPHARITIS

SIGNAL SYMPTOMS ▶ erythematous eyelid margins, crusting

ICD-9 Code	373.00	Blepharitis, unspecified

Blepharitis is ulcerative or nonulcerative inflammation of the eyelids characterized by redness, scaling, crusting, and swelling of the lid margin, often with acute flare-ups.

Epidemiology

More common in fair-skinned people.

Seen in childhood and often continuing throughout adulthood.

Occasionally seen in children with psoriasis, eczema, allergies, seborrhea, or lice infestation.

Etiology

Ulcerative blepharitis is caused by bacterial infection, usually by *Staphylococcus aureus* or *Staphylococcus epidermidis.*

Nonulcerative cause is often unknown; possibly psoriasis, seborrhea, acne rosacea, or allergic response.

Other causes include:

Eyelash infestation by lice

Contaminated makeup or contact lens solution

Poor hygiene

Tear deficiency

Physiology and Pathophysiology

Blepharitis is an inflammation of the lash follicles and meibomian glands of the eyelids.

Clinical Manifestations

Subjective

Redness, crusting, swelling, burning of eyelids.

Itching, tearing, mild mucous discharge, or conjunctival redness may also be present.

Objective

Erythematous eyelid margins with crusting within the lashes.

May have conjunctival injection or mucus discharge.

If caused by the ulcerative form: hard scales at the base of the lashes. When the crust is removed, ulceration of the hair follicles is noted and the lashes fall out.

If caused by acne rosacea the presence of telangiectatic blood vessels on the lid margins, cheeks, nose, and chin may be observed.

Differential Diagnosis

Conjunctivitis (conjunctival inflammation vs. eyelid inflammation)

Chalazion frequently associated with blepharitis, but more nodular in appearance.

Keratitis (inflammation of the cornea vs. eyelid inflammation).

Hordeolum (tender, erythematous, swollen furuncle at eyelid margin).

Sebaceous-cell carcinoma (rare, but suspect if intractable blepharitis).

Diagnostic Tests

None

Management/Treatment

Pharmacologic Management

Antibiotic ointment rubbed into lid margins: Sulfacetamide sodium (Sodium Sulamyd) ophthalmic ointment, 10% TID or QID for 7 days, **or** polymyxin B–bacitracin (Polysporin) ophthalmic ointment TID or QID for 7 days.

Oral antibiotics (if resistant or if client has ocular rosacea): Tetracycline 250 mg TID **or** erythromycin 250 mg TID

Nonpharmacologic Management

Eyelid soak or scrub:

Warm compresses for 15 minutes BID to loosen debris.

Scrub eyelids with wet washcloth or cotton-tipped applicator using a weak solution of baby shampoo and water (1:2) BID, or more frequently, depending on severity of symptoms.

Rinse eyelids.

If associated with seborrheic dermatitis:

Selenium sulfide shampoo to affected areas

If associated with lice infestation:

Apply thick petroleum jelly to eyelashes BID. The nits can then be removed in about 1 week.

Treat lice infestation of the head with an appropriate shampoo.

Client Education

Advise client that this is a chronic condition and that eyelid soaks or scrubs may need to be continued indefinitely.

Wear no contact lenses during treatment period.

Cleanse or sterilize contact lenses before use.

Use new eye makeup.

Practice good hygiene.

Follow-up

Usually none needed if condition is mild; if severe, reevaluate in 2 weeks.

If unresponsive to treatment, eyelid cultures should be obtained to determine antibiotic resistance.

Referral

None if mild; if severe or refractory to antibiotics refer to ophthalmologist.

CATARACTS

SIGNAL SYMPTOM ▶ progressive, painless loss of visual acuity

| ICD-9 Code | Cataract, unspecified |

Cataracts are an opacity of the lens of the eye, which results in visual impairment.

Epidemiology

An estimated 1.7 million people worldwide are blinded by cataracts each year.

The incidence of cataracts increases with age; 95% of individuals over age 65 have some degree of lens opacity.

Cataracts are the most common cause of age-related visual loss in the world.

Etiology

Senile cataract: Most common form of cataracts as a result of aging.

Traumatic cataract: Most often caused by blunt trauma to the eye or foreign-body injury to the lens. Can also be caused by overexposure to heat and radiation.

Cataracts may also be formed by infection, medications (corticosteroids, chlorpromazine) and as a complication of diseases such as diabetes, Down's syndrome, and other metabolic diseases. Cataracts are also linked to cigarette smoking.

Prolonged, unprotected exposure to ultraviolet (UV) B sunlight is also a cause of cataracts.

Congenital cataracts: Present at birth. Causes include genetic defects, toxic environmental agents, rubella infection during first trimester, and radiation exposure.

Half of children with congenital cataracts have other ocular problems such as nystagmus, strabismus, and microphthalmia (Fox, 1997).

Physiology and Pathophysiology

Cataracts may occur in one or both eyes. In age-related opacity of the lens, there is an alteration in the metabolism and transport of nutrients within the lens. In individuals with diabetes, excess glucose results in changes in the osmotic load and proteins within the lens. The presenile type of cataract, which forms during the fourth or fifth decade of life, often forms centrally at the back of the lens. It is often the result of systemic or topical steroid use or diabetes. Traumatic cataracts are the result of foreign bodies that penetrate the lens, causing the proteins within it to opacify. Congenital cataracts begin to form during the sixth to seventh week of fetal development.

Clinical Manifestations

Subjective

ADULTS

Gradual, progressive, painless loss of vision. The most common symptom is loss of visual acuity. Initially, vision is distorted, especially at night when driving, or in bright light (photophobia). Impairment of distance vision is noticed first.

Cloudy blurred vision.

Altered color vision with loss of contrast sensitivity; may gradually see a yellow cast.

CHILDREN

Congenital cataracts are difficult to assess because children may have difficulty verbalizing their visual difficulties. Ask about behavioral changes, changes in school performance, hand–eye coordination, and injuries to the eyes. Ask about a history of prenatal drug exposure or hypocalcemia.

Objective

Assess near and distance vision.

Do a full eye assessment, including: extraocular movements (EOMs) peripheral visual fields, pupillary reaction to light. PERLA (pupils equal, react to light and for accommodation) should be intact since it is the lens, not the pupil that is affected by cataracts. Visual acuity deficits may vary.

Funduscopic examination: Cataract formation is seen by a disruption of the red reflex; a black lens opacity is noted.

Congenital cataract: Abnormal eye movements in one or both eyes; strabismus; decreased visual acuity; red reflex not present; funduscopic shows white reflex (leukokoria); unable to visualize retinal details (Fox, 1997).

Differential Diagnosis

Macular degeneration (Abnormal funduscopic examination would include drusen, macular pigmentation irregularities, hemorrhage and scarring.)

Diabetic neuropathy (Proliferative retinal vessels would be visible on funduscopic examination.)

Retinal hemorrhage (Visible on funduscopic examination.)

Retinal scarring (Visible on funduscopic examination.)

Diagnostic Tests

None

Management/Treatment

Nonsurgical treatment is available for early cataracts, and changes in prescription lenses may be the initial treatment until the cataract progresses and visual impairment affects normal activities of daily living (ADL).

According to the American Academy of Ophthalmology, cataract surgery should be performed when corrected visual acuity is 20/50 or worse in the affected eye, when there is a work-related disability, or when it causes severe glare.

Client Education

Wear sunglasses and hat when exposed to sunlight; surgery is not indicated unless vision impairment interferes with ADL, education regarding pathophysiology of cataract formation.

If surgery is indicated, instruct client on postoperative use of eye shield and postoperative administration of eye drops (as prescribed by ophthalmologist).

Follow-up

As indicated

Referral

Refer to ophthalmologist for slit-lamp examination, evaluation, and treatment plan.

CHALAZION

SIGNAL SYMPTOMS ▶ initial mild erythema, followed by round painless mass

ICD-9 Code	379.90	Eye disorder, unspecified

Chalazion is a chronic inflammation of a meibomian gland that may follow an internal hordeolum.

Etiology

May be associated with blepharitis

May occur as a result of a chronic hordeolum

Physiology and Pathophysiology:

Chalazia are chronic granulomas, analogous to a sebaceous cyst that develops in the eyelids caused by distention of the meibomian glands (Taber's, 1997). Chalazia may become secondarily infected; usually with staphylococcus.

Clinical Manifestations

Subjective

Pain, tenderness, erythema and slight swelling of lid

History regarding visual acuity changes and previous history of chalazia, hordeolum, or blepharitis

Objective

Complete eye examination, including: visual acuity; inspection and palpation of lids for tenderness and redness; eversion of upper lid for pointing, sclera, and conjunctiva.

After a few days the inflammation resolves and a slow-growing, round, painless mass remains.

Chalazia point on the conjunctival side of the eyelid and typically do not affect the eyelid.

Perform funduscopic examination.

Assess for preauricular lymphadenopathy.

Differential Diagnosis

Blepharitis (inflammation of eyelids)

Hordeolum (inflammation of eyelash follicle)

Diagnostic Tests

None

Management/Treatment

Pharmacologic Management

Treat the condition if the chalazia are large or a secondary infection is suspected:

Erythromycin (Ilocytin), 5 mg/g ophthalmic ointment BID for 7 days **or** sulfacetamide sodium (Sodium Sulamyd) 10% (1–2 drops or 2 inches of ointment into each eye QID)

Nonpharmacologic Management

Warm compresses applied for 15 minutes QID for 2–3 days.

Scrub eyelash and eyelids with cotton-tipped applicator with 50% solution of no-tears shampoo 1–2 times/day.

Client Education

Good eye hygiene

Follow-up

As indicated; usually none for small chalazia that respond to treatment

Referral

Refer to ophthalmologist for clients not responsive to antibiotics after 4 weeks of treatment; incision and drainage may be indicated.

CONJUNCTIVITIS

SIGNAL SYMPTOMS ► conjunctivitis, unspecified: red conjunctiva, matted discharge; conjunctivitis, chronic allergic: seasonal, bilateral redness

| ICD-9 Codes | 372.30 | Conjunctivitis, unspecified |
| | 372.14 | Conjunctivitis, chronic allergic |

Conjunctivitis is inflammation of the conjunctiva, which can be infectious (bacterial or viral), environmental, chemical, or allergenic in nature. It is the most common eye disease and may be acute or chronic.

Epidemiology

Most common cause of red eye.

Most common acute disease of the eye seen in children.

Conjunctivitis in the newborn (formerly called ophthalmia neonatorum): Occurs during first month of life and in many states is a reportable infectious disease (Burns, 2000, p. 763).

Chlamydial conjunctivitis: Associated with poor hygiene; it is the leading cause of preventable blindness in the world. Seen in both adults and infants. Typically seen in 18- 30-year-old sexually active adults (Morrow & Abbott, 1998).

Viral conjunctivitis: Often occurs in community epidemics, with virus transmitted in schools, workplace, or swimming-pool water (Morrow & Abbott, 1998, paragraph 54).

Etiology

May be infectious (bacterial or viral), environmental, chemical, or allergic.

In children cases of conjunctivitis are approximately 50% bacterial and 50% adenoviral (Noble, 2001).

In adults cases of conjunctivitis are approximately 85% adenoviral and 15% bacterial.

Conjunctivitis caused by viruses and bacteria (including chlamydia) are transmissible by eye–hand contact (Morrow & Abbott, 1998, paragraph 14).

Chemical conjunctivitis can be caused by prolonged use of ophthalmic medication, contact lens solutions, cosmetics, over-the-counter (OTC) medications, and artificial tears.

Chlamydial conjunctivitis may be transmitted from the genitourinary tract during birth or may be seen in sexually active adults as a result of accidental contact with genital secretions.

Physiology and Pathophysiology

Infectious conjunctivitis, both bacterial and viral, initially presents in one eye and transmits to other eye within 3–5 days. Bacterial conjunctivitis is commonly caused by *Staphylococcus aureus, Streptococcus, Haemophilus influenzae, Neisseria gonorrhoeae, Chlamydia; Proteus;* and *Klebsiella pneumoniae.* Chlamydial conjunctivitis can occur in two forms: trachoma and inclusion conjunctivitis. Trachoma is a chronic conjunctivitis associated with serotypes A through C. This type of conjunctivitis is a health concern in developing countries. Trachoma is uncommon in North America; however, clients who have immigrated to North America from these countries may present with *Chlamydial trachomatis* infections; inclusion conjunctivitis is associated with serotypes

D through K. This is a common condition seen in both newborns and adults and is predominantly a sexually transmitted disease (Morrow & Abbott, 1998). Viral conjunctivitis is usually caused by adenovirus or herpes simplex virus.

Noninfectious conjunctivitis includes allergic and chemical conjunctivitis. Allergic conjunctivitis is associated with environmental antigens. It is often seasonal and presents bilaterally. It is an IgE-mediated hypersensitivity reaction that is initiated by small airborne allergens (Morrow & Abbott, 1998). Chemical or drug-induced conjunctivitis is due to various topical medications. Use of contact lenses and dry eyes can also cause inflammation of the conjunctiva.

Conjunctivitis in the newborn is most commonly caused by *Chlamydia* or chemical irritation from silver nitrate instillation. It may also be caused by herpes simplex virus (HSV), *Staphylococcus, Streptococcus, Haemophilus,* or *Neisseria gonorrhoeae* (Burns, 2000).

Clinical Manifestations

Subjective

GENERAL

Ask if inflammation is acute, chronic, or recurrent.

Ask about contact with other individuals with "pink eye."

Ask about itching.

If client is experiencing pain and photophobia, which are not typical of conjunctivitis, or blurred vision that fails to clear with blinking, consider more serious causes such as uveitis, keratitis, acute glaucoma, and refer to a specialist.

Objective

GENERAL

Evaluate eyelids for inflammation, tenderness and presence of discharge along the lash or lid line.

Evaluate drainage or crusting as mucopurulent, serous, or thin, watery secretions, and determine if unilateral or bilateral.

Evaluate for palpebral and bulbar conjunctival hyperemia.

Physical examination includes visual acuity, peripheral vision, pupillary constriction, and EOMs.

Evaluate cornea for clarity,

Assess for lymphadenopathy of the head and neck, especially the preauricular node, which often becomes enlarged with conjunctivitis. (See Table 3–1.)

Differential Diagnosis

Blepharitis (symptoms similar as conjunctivitis, except lid margins are inflamed with blepharitis)

Acute glaucoma (extreme ocular pain, visual loss, dilated pupil)

Corneal ulceration (pain, tearing, decreased vision, circumcorneal injection, and possibly purulent or watery discharge)

Table 3-1 Conjunctivitis: Clinical Manifestations and Treatment

Conjunctivitis	Clinical Manifestations: Subjective	Clinical Manifestations: Objective	Treatment
Bacterial Conjunctivitis	Acute, mucopurulent discharge from one or both eyes, tearing, itching. May have edematous eyelids and matting along lash line, especially in the morning. Usually no blurring of vision present. Often begins in one eye and spreads to other eye within 2–5 days.	Copious purulent discharge in one or both eyes. Increased inflammation of the palpebral conjunctiva versus bulbar conjunctiva. Lymphadeno-pathy is rare in acute bacterial conjunctivitis, except in gonococcal and chlamydial conjunctivitis	-No single broad-spectrum antibiotic covers all potential conjunctival pathogens. Consider the most likely pathogens when chosing one of the following broad spectrum antibiotic therapies: Erythromycin 0.5% (Ilotycin) children and adults: apply small amount of ointment qid OR polymyxin/trimethoprim (Polytrim) children >2 months and adults: 1 drop every 3–4 hours for 7–10 days (max. 6 doses/day) OR sulfac-etamide sodium ophthalmic oint-ment or solution (Sulamyd), 10%, 5 times daily for 7–10 days OR bacitracin oph-thalmic ointment -Neomycin should be avoided if possible. Aminoglycosides and fluoroquinolones should not be used in the first line treatment of routine conjunctivitis. -Wash lids and lashes gently with shampoo to remove crusting and discharge
Bacterial Conjunctivitis (Gonococcal)	*Adult:* Copious bilateral purulent yellow-green discharge that re-accumulates after being wiped away.	*Newborn:* Serosanguinous discharge at birth; purulent discharge 24–48 hours after birth.	*Adult and Newborn:* Ocular emergency due to possibility of rapid corneal ulceration and permanent loss of vision.

Table continued on following page.

Table 3-1   Conjunctivitis: Clinical Manifestations and Treatment (*Continued*)

Conjunctivitis	Clinical Manifestations: Subjective	Clinical Manifestations: Objective	Treatment
Viral Conjunctivitis (Adenovirus)	Other signs include: erythema and edema of conjunctiva and lids Burning, itching, conjunctival redness, copious tearing with little exudate. Recent URI, sometimes fever, malaise, pharyngitis.	Acute onset of watery discharge, small amount of exudate, with mild to moderate injection of the palpebral conjunctiva.	-Highly contagious for at least 7 days Avoid contact with other persons during this time; scrupulous handwashing -Topical antibiotics rarely needed because secondary bacterial infection is uncommon. -Supportive treatment: cold compresses, topical vasoconstrictors may alleviate symptoms.
Viral Conjunctivitis (Herpes Simplex Virus)	May present with vesicles on skin of face or eyelids.	May observe herpes labialis in conjunction with preauricular lymphadenopathy.	-Immediate ophthalmologic referral is required. -Topical and systemic antiviral agents are used for treatment.
Chlamydial Conjunctivitis (Adult)	Ask about sexual contact May be acute or chronic; unilateral or bilateral symptoms Thin mucus discharge and photophobia Often with foreign body sensation in the eye.	Chlamydial conjunctivitis in young adults and adults: acute redness, thin, mucoid discharge and eye irritation often with photophobia. Lymphadenopathy of pre-auricular nodes. Presents in sexually active individuals due to accidental contact with genital secretions.	-Treatment should be started based on basis of clinical signs and symptoms without waiting for laboratory confirmation. A genital work-up of the client and his or her sexual contacts is indicated before antibiotics are started. -Oral doxycycline, 300 mg initially followed by 100 mg bid, $\times$ 2 weeks, OR, Oral tetracycline or erythromycin, 250–500 mg qid for 2 weeks (do not use tetracycline in pregnancy or young children). Erythromycin should be used in pregnant and lactating women, 250 mg qid $\times$ 21 days.

Table continued on following page.

Table 3-1 Conjunctivitis: Clinical Manifestations and Treatment (*Continued*)

Conjunctivitis	Clinical Manifestations: Subjective	Clinical Manifestations: Objective	Treatment
Chlamydial Conjunctivitis (Newborn)	Watery discharge which turns purulent Occurs 5–12 days after vaginal delivery to women with chlamydial cervicitis	Consider as cause if seen within first 3 weeks of life; typically seen in infants 5–12 days after vaginal birth. Profuse exudate present and preauricular lymphadenopathy present.	-Ophthalmic referral is essential -Oral erythromycin 50 mg/kg/day divided qid × 14 days. -Local treatment is not necessary
Allergic Conjunctivitis	Bilateral intense itching (hallmark symptom), watery or mucoid discharge, swollen eyelids, rhinorrhea Often seasonal Ask about family history of atopic condition such as asthma, exzema, allergic rhinitis	Itchy, bilateral, watery eyes. May observe edema of lids and cobblestone appearance	-Topical vasoconstrictors -Mast cell stabilizers such as: cromolyn sodium (Crolom) 4 % ophthalmic solution, 1–2 drops OU 4–6 times daily at regular intervals in clients older than age 4 years OR lodoxamide (Alomide) 1% ophthalmic solution, over 2 years of age: 1–2 drops qid for up to 3 months -Topical antihistamines such as levocabastine (Livostin) for adults only. 1drop qid. OR -Topical antihistamine and mast cell stabilizer combination (Panatol) 0.1% solution in children > 3 years old and adults, 1–2 drops OU, BID at 6–8 hour intervals. -Topical NSAIDs such as tromethamine (Acular) 0.5% solution in adults only, 1 drop qid; may also use diclofenac sodium (Voltaren) -Systemic antihistamines and/or decongestants may also be successful such as loratadine (Claratin) 10 mg orally QD in children > 6 years old and adults.

Table continued on following page.

Table 3-1   Conjunctivitis: Clinical Manifestations and Treatment—*Continued*

Conjunctivitis	Clinical Manifestations: Subjective	Clinical Manifestations: Objective	Treatment
			-Topical corticosteroids (severe cases) but only prescribed under supervision of an ophthalmologist. -Allergen avoidance -Cold compresses -Refrigerated artificial tears -Avoid eye rubbing which causes trauma to mast cells located in the eye lids, causing them to release more histamine and increasing itching symptoms
Kerato-conjunctivitis Sicca (Dry Eyes)	Ask about collagen vascular disease and diuretic or antidepressant use which can cause dry red eyes.	Dry, red eyes, without discharge.	
Contact Lens Conjunctivitis	History of soft contact use	Erythema, mucoid discharge present with papillae present on the upper tarsal conjunctiva	

Corneal abrasion (bulbar injection usually associated with trauma)

Iritis (uveitis) (pain, decreased vision, photophobia, lacrimation; iris swollen, dull, and pupil contracted, with sluggish reaction)

Dacryocystitis (pain, redness, tearing, swelling of lacrimal sac, which may extend to lids and conjunctiva; may express purulent drainage from lacrimal sac)

Foreign bodies

Infants and children:

Kawasaki syndrome (acute illness accompanied by rash, no discharge from eyes) Measles (maculopapular rash, coryza, and Koplik spots)

Juvenile rheumatoid arthritis (fever, rash, arthralgia)

Diagnostic Tests

Culture (Recommended if there is a severe inflammation, if the condition is chronic or recurrent, if gonorrhea or chlamydia is suspected, or if client does not respond to treatment regimen. Discharge should be cultured on all infants under 1 month of age to determine the causative organism.)

Gram stain (If gonococcal infection is suspected cause, immediate Gram stain for gram-negative intracellular organisms and cultures for *Neisseria.*)

Management/Treatment

(See Table 3–1 for pharmacologic and nonpharmacologic management.)

Pharmacologic Management

In general, ointments are better tolerated by young children, while solutions are better tolerated by adults because of the blurring of vision that occurs with ointments.

Do not prescribe ophthalmic steroids unless under the direction of an ophthalmologist because of the risk of steroid-induced ocular complications.

Client Education

Advocate frequent handwashing, use of separate towels and washcloths, cleansing eye from inner to outer canthus, and using a new, clean washcloth to cleanse other eye to avoid spreading.

Clean eyelashes several times/day with weak solution of no-tears shampoo and water.

Warm soaks may help to relieve itching and burning.

Demonstrate correct instillation of ophthalmic ointments and solutions.

Bacterial conjunctivitis is contagious for 24–48 hours after the antibiotic treatment begins.

Symptoms of viral conjunctivitis usually resolve within 2–4 days, but client is contagious for at least 1 week (Goolsby, 2000, p 16).

Follow-up

None if client shows improvement within 24–72 hours and condition resolves within 2–3 weeks.

If the condition worsens, reevaluate, culture discharge, and seek consultation with ophthalmologist as needed.

Referral

Refer to ophthalmologist if:

Client has hyperacute, purulent infection.

Infection is suspected from herpes simplex, gonorrhea, or chlamydia.

Client has an abnormal eye examination.

Topical steroids are indicated (should be prescribed only by ophthalmologist).

Conjunctivitis fails to resolve within 2–3 weeks.

There is no improvement of symptoms within 24–48 hours of treatment.

Symptoms worsen.

EYE INJURIES

ICD-9 Codes	918.1	Corneal abrasion
	370.0	Corneal ulcer, unspecified
	940.9	Eye burn, unspecified
	379.90	Eye disorder, unspecified
	930.9	Eye foreign body, external, unspecified

Eye injuries can include corneal abrasion or injury, foreign bodies, fractures, abrasions, burns, contusions, and lacerations.

Epidemiology

40% of all eye injuries occur in the home.

Estimated that 90% of eye injuries are preventable.

One-third of all blindness in children is the result of trauma.

Eye injuries occur more often in boys.

High-risk sports include: wrestling, martial arts, baseball, basketball, and other sports with a rapidly moving ball or puck.

Etiology

Individuals may be at risk if occupational hazards exist and no eye protection is worn.

Individuals who wear contact lenses may be at risk for corneal injury.

Corneal abrasions often caused by scratches from fingernails, contact lenses, or foreign bodies.

Burns can be caused by thermal injuries (steam or intense heat) or by chemical products (cleaning products) or induced by bright light (bright snow, laser pointers, sunlamps) (MacDonald & Starr, 2000, p 777).

Orbital fractures can be caused from a blow or blunt trauma to the orbit with a ball or fist.

Retinal detachment seen with severe ocular trauma, child abuse; may also occur as an congenital abnormality.

Physiology and Pathophysiology:

Corneal ulcers are often caused by infection due to bacteria, viruses, fungi, or noninfectious causes such as inadequate eyelid closure, dry eyes, allergic eyes, and inflammatory disorders (Tierney, McPhee, & Papadakis, 2000). Corneal ulcers originate as a well-defined infiltration at the center or edge of the cornea, it then suppurates and forms an ulcer that can spread over the width of the cornea, or penetrate deep into the cornea (MacDonald & Starr, 2000, p 774).

Corneal injury is damage to the epithelial lining of the cornea; it can be caused by scratches, poorly fitting contact lenses or contact lenses worn too long, or foreign bodies. With foreign bodies, a superficial foreign body is typically lodged in the surface of the eye or superficially in the cornea.

Uveal-tract inflammation (iris, ciliary body, choroid) is often called uveitis. Inflammation can be anterior (iris, ciliary body, or both) or posterior, affecting the choroid. The retina, vitreous, and optic nerve can also be involved (MacDonald & Starr, 2000, p 774).

Clinical Manifestations

Subjective

Pain, photophobia, redness & ciliary flush & pupillary condraction (spasm) (Garoll, p 1078).

GENERAL

Obtain a history of the event preceding the symptoms, duration of symptoms, history of trauma, foreign body, and pain associated with symptoms. Investigate contact lenses.

Objective

GENERAL

Manifestations include redness with ciliary flush and papillary contraction from spasm. Flashlight examination shows a slightly cloudy anterior chamber. Slip-lamp examination discloses increased aqueous humor protein, causing a "flare" (Garoll, 2000, p 1078).

Perform a complete eye examination to include external eye (conjunctiva, cornea, lacrimal apparatus), visual acuity, EOMs, PERLA, and funduscopic examination. (See Table 3–2.)

Differential Diagnosis

Corneal abrasion (cornea not shiny, appearance irregular)

Foreign body (visible on examination)

Laceration (based on history and physical examination)

Burns (based on history and opacity of corneal tissue, visual impairment, photophobia, swollen corneas)

Iritis (circumcorneal redness, pupillary irregularity, photophobia, constricted pupil, throbbing pain; immediate referral indicated)

Diagnostic Tests

Fluorescein staining (for suspected corneal injury or foreign body if not visualized)

Slit-lamp examination (for suspected hyphema)

Management/Treatment

(See Table 3–2.)

Client Education

Eye safety and use of eye protection at home, work, around fireworks, etc.

Education of children regarding safe use of home chemicals with sprays or nozzles.

Safety regarding sports with sticks, rapidly moving balls or pucks, use of pellet guns and projectile toys.

Follow-up

For minor injuries (corneal abrasions, extraocular foreign bodies, mild thermal or UV burns), follow-up in 24 hours.

Table 3-2   Eye Injuries: Clinical Manifestations and Treatment

Injury	Clinical Manifestations	Treatment
Burns	Complaints of decreased visual acuity; no complaints of pain unless a UV burn when pain may be present about 6 hours after exposure; tearing 12 hours after exposure; photophobia Opacity of corneal tissue; decreased visual acuity; photophobia; swollen corneas; pale or necrotic appearance to surrounding skin; tearing within 12 hours of exposure	*Thermal Burns* Treat as a corneal abrasion Topical antibiotics (sulfacetamid 10% QID × 5 days, OR polymyxin-bacitracin) Rest and patch for 24 hours, then re-evaluate *Chemical Burns* Must be irrigated with saline or water for 20–30 minutes with the eyelids held apart, then immediate referral to ophthalmologist *UV Burns* Topical antibiotic (sulfacetamid 10% QID × 5 days OR polymyxin-bacitracin) Patch Re-evaluate in 24 hours. Typically heals in 1–2 days.
Corneal Injury or Ulceration	Severe pain, evidence and sensation of a foreign body, photophobia, tearing and decreased vision, conjunctival erythema, blepharospasm Eye is red with circumcorneal injection, decreased vision, pain, photophobia, and watery or purulent discharge. Positive fluorescein staining: irregular ridges visible and a yellow-green branching present.	*Severe* Refer to an ophthalmologist. *Mild* Topical antibiotic (sulfacetamid 10% QID × 5 days OR polymyxin-bacitracin) Rest and patching for 24–48 hours. Patch fit so that eye is held closed. The client should rest at home and follow-up in 24 hours. If patching an infant's eye, discuss with ophthalmologist regarding length of patching. According to Fox (1997), amblyopia can develop within 24 hours if continuously patched.
Foreign Body	Foreign body sensation and tearing. Irregular or peaked pupil; may see perforating wound to cornea.	*Intraocular foreign body* Do not attempt to remove; refer to an ophthalmologist *Extraocular foreign body* Evert eyelid, inspect for foreign body. Irrigate with sterile saline. Do not use a moistened cotton swab to remove the foreign body. This can cause damage to the cornea or scratching. After removal of extraocular foreign body, use ophthalmic antibiotic solution (e.g. sulfacetamid 10% QID × 5 days OR polymyxin-bacitracin) Patch for 5–7 days
Hyphema	History of traumatic injury; pain, photophobia, tearing, decreased visual acuity, somnolence (if associated with intracranial trauma)	Immediate referral to ophthalmologist Make client comfortable; place eye shield (not patch) over the eye avoiding pressure; elevate HOB 35 degrees; NPO until seen by ophthalmologist

Table continued on following page.

**Table 3-2   Eye Injuries: Clinical Manifestations and
Treatment (*Continued*)**

Injury	Clinical Manifestations	Treatment
	Blood in anterior chamber; diminished or absent red reflex in affected eye; decreased visual acuity; pupillary response to light abnormal	
Lacerations	Visible laceration present	Immediate referral to ophthalmologist.
Orbital Fractures	Pain; diplopia; difficulty chewing; ecchymosis of lids; nosebleed Decreased sensation along upper lip and ipsilateral cheek; ecchymosis of lids; epistaxis; decreased ocular movement; sunken or protruding appearance of globe; bony discontinuity; subcutaneous emphysema	Ophthalmologic emergency; immediate referral Ice injury for 24 hours then heat for 2–3 days. This allows swelling to decrease before surgery which is most often done within 2 weeks of injury
Orbital Hematoma/ Contusion	Decreased visual acuity, bruising of eyelids	Immediate referral to an ophthalmologist Cold compresses for first 48 hours, then warm compresses.
Retinal Detachment	Blurred vision that becomes progressively worse; showers of floaters. Blurred vision; darkened retinal vessels on ophthalmoscopic exam; may see gray elevation at site of detachment	Immediate referral to ophthalmologist NPO

Referral

Refer to ophthalmologist after initial assessment and evaluation.
Immediately refer to ophthalmologist as indicated in Table 3–2.

GLAUCOMA

SIGNAL SYMPTOMS▶ asymptomatic/mild to excruciating eye pain, halos around lights

ICD-9 Codes	365.9	Glaucoma, unspecified

Glaucoma is a group of intraocular diseases characterized by increased intraocular pressure, which cause damage to the optic nerve and can lead to blindness. Classified as acute-angle closure, chronic open-angle, infantile or congenital (before age 3), and juvenile (ages 3–30 years) glaucoma.

Epidemiology

Glaucoma is the third most prevalent cause of blindness in the United States. (The primary causes are cataracts and macular degeneration.)

1%–2% of individuals over age 40 years have glaucoma; 25% of these are not detected (Riordan-Eva & Vaughan, 1999).

Most common cause of age-related visual loss.

Cataracts are present in 50% of individuals between the ages 65 and 74 and in 70% of individuals over the age of 75 (Garoll, pg 1098).

90% of glaucoma cases are chronic open-angle type.

Increased incidence in elderly, those of African-American and Asian ancestry, and family history of glaucoma.

Infantile cataracts occur in 1 in 250 newborn infants Burs (pg 760).

Etiology

Open-angle: Insidious onset in older adults.

Closed-angle: Rapid onset in older adults, especially in hyperopic individuals; may also be caused by prolonged anterior uveitis or dislocation of the lens (Riordan-Eva & Vaughan, 1999). Associated with pupillary dilation; could potentially occur during times of stress, while sitting in a darkened room or movie theatre, or from systemic anticholinergic medications such as atropine, or inhaled ipratropium bromide (Riordan-Eva & Vaughan, 1999).

Infantile: Occurs in first 3 years of life, and is an anomaly of the drainage system of the aqueous humor. Also seen in association with developmental anomalies such as neurofibromatosis, facial nevus flammeus, Marfan or Hurler syndrome (Nelson, 1996).

Juvenile: Occurs as a result of the aqueous humor becoming obstructed after trauma, ocular infection, neoplasm, or long-term corticosteroid use (Burns, 2000, p 760). Occurs when aqueous humor drains too slowly to keep up with production in the anterior chamber.

Physiology and Pathophysiology

The essential feature of glaucoma is intraocular pressure (IOP) that is too high for the optic nerve. Increases in production of aqueous humor or obstruction to outflow will cause an elevation in IOP.

Acute closed-angle glaucoma is caused by a shallow anterior chamber and a narrowed angle through which the aqueous humor normally passes. The rate of the aqueous humor is impaired and the intraocular pressure increases.

Open-angle glaucoma (90% of cases) typically affects both eyes. The obstruction that causes increased IOP exists at the microscopic level in the trabecular meshwork, a connective-tissue filter at the angle between the iris and the cornea (Porth, 1995 pg 1034). The IOP is consistently elevated, and over a long period (months to years) cupping of the optic disk occurs, causing loss of peripheral vision. This type of glaucoma may also develop as a result of other eye trauma or uveitis.

Infantile glaucoma is an anterior-angle defect caused by an abnormal differentiation of embryonic tissue.

Juvenile glaucoma occurs between 3 and 30 years, when the drainage network for aqueous humor becomes obstructed after ocular infection, trauma, neoplasm, or long-term corticosteroid use.

Secondary causes of glaucoma include inflammation, neoplasm, corticosteroid therapy, and inflammation.

Clinical Manifestations

Subjective

GENERAL

Glaucoma may not cause any symptoms. Clients may note frequent need to change lenses, mild headaches, vague visual disturbances, and difficulty with night vision.

OPEN-ANGLE GLAUCOMA

Mild aching in eyes, loss of peripheral vision, headache, photophobia, blurring of vision, haloes around lights, decreased visual acuity that is increased at night and not improved with use of corrective lenses. Gradual loss of vision over years, causing tunnel vision.

ACUTE CLOSED-ANGLE GLAUCOMA

Excruciating unilateral eye pain and pressure, decreased visual acuity, blurred vision, diplopia, lacrimation, and haloes around lights. Because of increased IOP there may be associated nausea and vomiting. THIS IS AN OPHTHALMIC EMERGENCY.

INFANTILE GLAUCOMA

Excessive lacrimation and photophobia

Objective

OPEN-ANGLE GLAUCOMA

Central visual field testing, tonometry, and ophthalmoscopic assessment are the three key areas of assessment for glaucoma.

Assess visual acuity, peripheral vision, funduscopic examination looking for slight cupping of the disk, differences in cup to disc ratio between the eyes.

ACUTE CLOSED-ANGLE GLAUCOMA

Client is in extreme pain; blurred vision is present. Conjunctiva is red, cornea is cloudy, and the pupil is dilated midway and nonreactive to light (Riordan-Eva & Vaughan, 1999). Palpation of the globe of the eye reveals a hard globe.

 ES 3–1   Emergency Situation: Glaucoma. Acute closed-angle glaucoma is a medical emergency. REFER IMMEDIATELY. Severe, permanent vision loss occurs within 2–5 days after the onset of symptoms.

INFANTILE GLAUCOMA

Enlarged, hazy corneas, corneal edema, conjunctival injection, and visual impairment.

Differential Diagnosis

Conjunctivitis (conjunctiva erythematous, but no visual changes; cloudy cornea)

Acute uveitis (inflammation of uveal tract [iris, ciliary body, choroid]; IOP not increased; pupil small, with poor reactivity)

Corneal trauma or damage (normal IOP, normal pupil and reaction to light)

Macular degeneration (bilateral loss of central visual acuity)

Diagnostic Tests

Screening tonometry (shows increased IOP; normal pressures are 10–20 mm Hg)

Management/Treatment

Refer to ophthalmologist for management and treatment.

Client Education

Indications for eye examination (yearly for clients with diabetes or family history of glaucoma; every 2 years for family members of clients with infantile glaucoma; IOP measurement every 3–5 years for clients over age 40, especially black clients).

Need to wear medical identification jewelry (necklace or bracelet).

Follow-up

As indicated; usually followed by ophthalmologist.

Referral

Refer to ophthalmologist immediately if acute closed-angle glaucoma is suspected.

HORDEOLUM

SIGNAL SYMPTOMS ▶ erythematous, tender lump within eyelid

ICD-9 Codes	373.11	Hordeolum (stye)

Hordeolum is an infection of the sebaceous or sweat glands of the eyelids. It is commonly referred to as a stye.

Epidemiology

More common in children and adolescents

Etiology

Internal hordeolum caused by infection of meibomian gland.

External hordeolum occurs with infection of glands of Zeiss or Moll just anterior to the lash line.

Physiology and Pathophysiology

Typically a *Staphylococcus aureus* infection of the sweat, sebaceous, or meibomian glands.

Clinical Manifestations

Subjective

Sudden onset of erythematous, tender lump within eyelid.

Duration of less than a few weeks.

Ask about visual changes, previous episodes, duration of symptoms.

Objective

Assess of visual acuity

Eyelid assessment: Invert eyelid to assess for inflammation, masses, and pointing, which would be present with chalazia (a hordeolum that does not heal and forms granulation tissue). External eyelid: erythema, masses, tenderness, especially along lash line.

Examine conjunctiva and sclera for erythema and drainage.

Assess for lymphadenopathy, especially the preauricular area.

Differential Diagnosis

Conjunctivitis (conjunctival inflammation and discharge versus inflammation in eyelid or along lash line)

Chalazion (point on the conjunctival side of the eyelid; does not usually affect the eyelid margin and not usually erythematous or painful)

Diagnostic Tests

None

Management/Treatment

Pharmacologic Management

TOPICAL ANTIBIOTICS

Erythromycin (Ilotycin), 5mg/g ophthalmic ointment BID for 7 days **or** polymyxin B–trimethoprim drops (Polytrim) BID for 7 days

Nonpharmacologic Management

Warm compresses for 15 minutes, QID for 7 days

Client Education

Avoid rubbing eyes.

Use scrupulous periorbital hygiene.

Avoid eye makeup during this time, throw out old makeup.

Follow-up

Usually none indicated; should resolve and drain spontaneously after 7 days of compresses and topical antibiotics.

Referral

Refer to ophthalmologist if nonresolving lesion; incision and drainage may be required.

NASAL-LACRIMAL-DUCT OBSTRUCTION (Dacryostenosis, Dacryocystitis)

SIGNAL SYMPTOMS▶ persistent tearing of affected eye, mucopurulent discharge, crusting of lashes

| ICD-9 Codes | 379.90 | Eye disorder, unspecified |

Nasal-lacrimal-duct obstruction is an abnormal stricture or defect of the nasal lacrimal duct or sac.

Epidemiology

Occurs in up to 6% of infants, with most cases clearing during the first year (Hay, Hayward, Levin, & Sondheimer, 2000).

Etiology

Possibly due to the failure of the duct to canalize.

Symptoms appear 3–12 weeks after birth; characterized by tearing, crusting of lashes, mucopurulent discharge.

Physiology and Pathophysiology

Nasal-lacrimal-duct obstruction is the congenital failure of the duct to canalize; it may be unilateral or bilateral. If this condition is seen in older children, it may be caused by nasal polyps or dacrolithiasis. If inflammation is present, it is usually caused by *Staphylococcus aureus*.

Clinical Manifestations

Subjective

Persistent tearing, mucopurulent discharge, crusting of lashes.

When taking history, include unilateral or bilateral involvement, description of the discharge, vision changes, and when condition is the worst (i.e., after sleeping, with allergic symptoms).

Objective

External eye evaluation includes lids, lashes, conjunctiva, cornea, sclera for inflammation or discharge.

Palpate the lacrimal gland, apparatus, puncta; while wearing gloves, press against the nasolacrimal sac for evaluation of regurgitation.

Assess visual acuity

Differential Diagnosis

Blepharitis (inflammation would be along the lash line)

Conjunctivitis (inflammation and injection of the conjunctiva)

Dacryocystitis (inflammation of the nasolacrimal duct)

Periorbital cellulitis (inflammation of the tissues surrounding the involved eye)

Diagnostic Tests

Usually none; if associated with severe inflammation, obtain white blood count and culture discharge.

Management/Treatment

Pharmacologic Management

Topical ophthalmic ointment for concurrent conjunctivitis or purulent discharge, such as erythromycin ointment 0.5% (two inches in each eye)

QID for 7 days or until the inflammation clears (MacDonald & Starr, 2000).

Nonpharmacologic Management

Nasolacrimal-duct massage (to facilitate drainage of the duct): Exert firm pressure over the nasolacrimal sac and exert downward pressure toward the nose 10 times; repeat four times a day.

Saline drops into the nose before feeding and at bedtime (helps remove nasal congestion).

Warm compresses QID (if there is inflammation of nasolacrimal duct [dacrocystitis]).

Client Education

Teach parents to perform pharmacologic and nonpharmacologic management techniques (ointment application, nasolacrimal-duct massage, and application of saline drops and warm compresses).

Follow-up

Follow up in 2 weeks if client is placed on an antibiotic regimen.

Referral

Refer to ophthalmologist if persistent obstruction continues, especially after 6 months of age.

STRABISMUS

SIGNAL SYMPTOMS ▶ deviation of one eye from the other

ICD-9 Codes	368.10	Visual disturbance, unspecified

Strabismus is abnormal ocular alignment; the optic axes are not directed at the same object.

Epidemiology

Occurs in 2%–3% of children. In these, amblyopia or a secondary vision loss may develop in 40% (Larvich & Nelson, 1993).

Often a family pattern of strabismus.

Occurs equally in males and females.

Ethnicity is not a factor in development.

Leading cause of monocular vision loss in clients between the ages of 20 and 70 (Simons, 1996).

Etiology

Paralytic strabismus: Caused by paresis of extraocular muscle.

Nonparalytic strabismus: Most common, may be caused by various mechanisms, including muscle weakness, visual defects such as unilateral refractive errors, anatomical differences between the eyes.

Transient strabismus in children younger than 6 months of age is considered normal.

Physiology and Pathophysiology

Strabismus may be caused by cerebral hemisphere disease, head injury, febrile illness, thyroid disease, or neuromuscular disorders of the eye muscles.

Strabismus is the deviation of one eye from the other when the client looks at an object. Types of deviation may be upward, downward, inward, or outward. The classification of strabismus is based on the direction of deviation of the affected eye and whether it is constant or intermittent. Phoria is intermittent deviation; tropia is deviation of eyes away from the visual axis when the eyes are open and uncovered (Taber's, 1997).

Horizontal phorias or tropias are classified as "eso" if there is inward, or convergent, deviation of the eyes and "exo" if there is outward deviation, or deviation away from the nose.

Untreated strabismus can cause permanent visual damage or amblyopia (decreased vision in the affected eye). Disconjugate vision is caused because one eye deviates, causing diplopia. The brain then suppresses the visual stimuli from the affected eye and vision declines. Early detection and treatment is essential to prevent visual loss and maximize visual function.

Pseudostrabismus occurs when it appears that visual axes are not aligned because of factors such as an epicanthal fold, flattened nasal bridge, or decreased interpupillary distance.

Clinical Manifestations

Subjective
Expect normal alignment of the eyes by 3 months of age. If not, consider infantile (congenital) esotropia.

Child unable to follow or fixate on an object (eye squinting, head tilting, face turning, awkwardness).

Ask parents about family history of visual problems or strabismus, age symptoms were noticed, if child has reported diplopia, if child has reached developmental tasks at expected intervals.

Objective
Visual acuity testing appropriate for client's age.

Complete eye assessment includes: external structures, equality of palpebral fissures, presence of epicanthal folds, conjunctiva, eyelids, cornea, PERLA.

Assess EOMs: corneal light reflex, cover–uncover test, cardinal positions of gaze.

Funduscopic examination.

Differential Diagnosis

Pseudostrabismus (sclera between cornea and inner canthus is obstructed and inner canthus is obstructed by closely placed eyes, flat nasal bridge or prominent epicanthal folds).

If sudden onset, consider increased intracranial pressure, lead poisoning, encephalitis.

Diagnostic Tests

Performed by ophthalmologist

Management/Treatment

Refer to ophthalmologist.

Treatment may consist of corrective lenses, patching of the fixating eye, orthoptic exercises, and surgical repair.

Assess for strabismus at every visit, even after ophthalmology referral and treatment.

Client Education

Teach parents, and child (as appropriate for age) importance of wearing corrective lenses, orthoptic exercises, patching and other treatment regimens. Also advise parents on the need for siblings to be evaluated.

Follow-up

As indicated

Referral

Refer to ophthalmologist if client is under age 6 months and has fixed or constant strabismus; or if client is over age 6 months and strabismus is suspected.

VISION LOSS

ICD-9 Codes	367.9	Refractive errors, unspecified
	369.9	Visual loss, unspecified
	368.10	Visual disturbance, unspecified

Vision loss is a decrease in visual acuity in one or both eyes, which may be caused by refractive or nonrefractive errors.

Epidemiology

Approximately one in three elderly persons has some form of vision-reducing eye disease by age 65 (Quillen, 1999).

Etiology

Refractive errors are caused by conditions such as myopia (near-sightedness), hyperopia (farsightedness), presbyopia, and astigmatism. These conditions can usually be corrected with lenses.

Nonrefractive errors are caused by conditions such as glaucoma, cataract, retinal abnormalities, and other conditions that cannot be corrected by lenses alone (Uphold & Graham, 1998).

Physiology and Pathophysiology

The most common visual problem is alterations in refraction.

Myopia (nearsightedness): Light rays focus in front of the retina, causing the person to see near objects more clearly than distant objects.

Hyperopia (farsightedness): Light rays focus behind the retina, causing the person to see distant objects more clearly and to have difficulty with near vision.

Astigmatism: Caused by an unequal curvature of the cornea. The light rays do not focus on a single spot on the retina. This condition may occur with myopia, hyperopia, or presbyopia.

Presbyopia: A loss of accommodation in clients over the age of 40. The aging process causes the lens to become less elastic and unable to accommodate for near vision. Does not affect distance vision.

Clinical Manifestations

Subjective

MYOPIA

Blurred distance vision or difficulty seeing at a distance.

Children may report difficulty seeing the blackboard in the classroom. School-age children may have difficulty with performance or reading. Younger children may lag behind in fine-motor developmental. milestones if there is a visual problem.

HYPEROPIA

Difficulty with near vision; may be accompanied by blurred vision, headache.

PRESBYOPIA

Symptoms begin around age 40, and include the need to extend reading distance to accommodate for near vision; difficulty in focusing on close objects; increased light needed to visualize object.

GENERAL

Additional questions include eye watering, eye pain or discomfort, problems with glare (cataracts); flashing lights (retinal detachment); gradual vision loss (macular degeneration); nystagmus; wandering of eyes; rubbing eyes; eye pain; and family history of visual problems.

Objective

ADULTS

Assess the external eye, including the cornea, conjunctiva, and lacrimal apparatus.

Assess EOMs (corneal light reflex; six cardinal positions of gaze; and cover–uncover test).

Near-vision testing using Jaegar or Rosenbaum card, or varying sizes of print.

Distance-vision testing of each eye separately (OD, OS), then together (OU) using the Snellen alphabet or Snellen E chart.

Peripheral vision using the confrontation test.

Funduscopic examination.

CHILDREN

Assess the external eye, including the cornea, conjunctiva, and lacrimal apparatus.

Assess EOMs (corneal light reflex; six cardinal positions of gaze; and cover–uncover test).

Near-vision testing using Jaegar or Rosenbaum card, or varying sizes of print.

Distance-vision testing of each eye separately (OD, OS), then together (OU) using the Snellen alphabet or Snellen E chart for children over 6 years of age. For preschoolers (ages 3–6) use the Tumbling E or Allen (picture cards) test. Examine preschoolers at 10 feet from the chart, using an appropriate chart. The Allen picture cards may be reliable in screening cooperative toddlers as early as age 2. Testing for or children younger than 2 years of age is difficult and may best be done using a book with familiar pictures and asking the child to identify the pictures.

Peripheral vision using the confrontation testing children older than 3 years.

Funduscopic examination.

(See "Age-Related Considerations: Pediatric Eye Evaluation Screening Recommendations.")

Differential Diagnosis

Myopia (problem with distance vision)

Hyperopia (problems with near vision in children and young adults)

Presbyopia (problems with near vision and accommodation in 40–60-year-olds)

Cataracts (clouding of lens)

Glaucoma (changes in peripheral vision in open angle/eye pain with acute angle)

Retinal detachment (abrupt vision loss with changes in funduscopic examination)

Macular degeneration (gradual central vision loss)

Strabismus (deviation of eye axes with EOM testing)

Diagnostic Tests

None

Management/Treatment

Refer to ophthalmologist.

Client Education

Additional education based on etiology of vision loss

Follow-up

As indicated

Referral

Refer to ophthalmologist.

Age-Related Considerations: Pediatric Eye Evaluation Screening Recommendations

Age	Screening Recommendations	Criteria for Referral to Ophthalmologist
Newborn to 3 months*	Red reflex Inspection	Abnormal or asymmetrical Structural abnormality
6 months to 1 year	Fix and follow with each eye Alternate occlusion Corneal light reflex Red reflex Inspection	Failure to fix and follow in cooperative infant Failure to object equally to covering each eye Asymmetrical Abnormal or asymmetrical Structural abnormality
3 years (approximately)	Visual acuity Corneal light reflex/cover-uncover Red reflex Inspection	20/50 or worse or 2 lines of difference between eyes Asymmetrical/ocular refixation movements Abnormal or asymmetrical Structural abnormality
5 years (approximately)	Visual acuity Corneal light reflex/cover-uncover Red reflex Inspection	20/40 or worse or 2 lines of difference between eyes Asymmetrical/ocular refixation movements Abnormal or asymmetrical Structural abnormality
Older than 5 years	Visual acuity Corneal light reflex/cover-uncover Red reflex Inspection	20/30 or worse or 2 lines of difference between eyes Asymmetrical/ocular refixation movements Abnormal or asymmetrical Structural abnormality

*Normal visual acuity in infants:
-Birth to 2 weeks: May fixate on an object, poor following, may have intermittent strabismus
-One month: Can fixate on an object, normal alignment; can follow a brightly colored object to midline.
-Over 3 months: Horizontal and vertical following; normal alignment; can fixate and follow, reach for object.
Adapted from American Academy of Ophthalmology: Pediatric Eye Evaluations Preferred Practice Pattern, 1997, American Academy of Ophthalmology.

 ES 3–2   Emergency Situation: Vision Loss. IMMEDIATE referral is indicated if client has an abrupt episode of visual impairment.

REFERENCES

General

Behrman, R., & Kliegman, R. (1998). *Nelson essentials of pediatrics* (3rd ed.). Philadelphia: Saunders.

Burns, C., Brady, M., Dunn, A., Starr, N. (Eds.) (2000). *Pediatric primary care: A handbook for nurse practitioners* (2nd ed.). Philadelphia: Saunders.

Carter, S. (1998). Eyelid disorders: diagnosis and management. *American Family Physician.* Available at www.aafp.org/afp/9980600ap.carter.html.

Fauci, A., Braunwald, E., Wilson, J., Martin, J., Kasper, D., Hauser, S., & Longo, D. (1999) *Harrison's principles of internal medicine* (14th ed.). New York: McGraw Hill.

Fenstermacher, K., & Hudson, B. (1997). Practice guidelines for family nurse practitioners. Philadelphia: Saunders.

Fox, J. (1997). *Primary health care of children.* St. Louis: Mosby.

Gorroll, A., May, L., & Mulley, A. (1995). *Primary care medicine office evaluation and management of the adult patient* (3rd ed.). Philadelphia: Lippincott-Raven.

Hay, W., Hayward, A., Levin, M., & Sondheimer, J. (Eds.) (1999). Current pediatric diagnosis and treatment (14th ed.). (pp 360–383). Stamford, CT: Appleton & Lange.

Hill, N., & Sullivan, L. (1999). *Management guidelines for pediatric nurse practitioners.* Philadelphia: F.A. Davis.

Jarvis, C. (2000). *Physical examination and -health assessment* (3rd ed.). Philadelphia: Saunders.

McCance, K., & Huether, S. (1998). *Pathophysiology: The biologic basis for disease in adults and children* (3rd ed.). St. Louis: Mosby.

Nelson, L. (1996) Nelson Textbook of Pediatrics. (15th ed). Philadelphia: WB Saunders.

Rakel, R., (1996). *Saunders manual of medical practice.* Philadelphia: Saunders.

Taber's cyclopedic medical dictionary (18th ed.). (1997). Philadelpia: F.A. Davis.

Tierney, L., McPhee, S., Papadakis, M. (Eds.) (1999). Current medical diagnosis and treatment. (38th ed.). Stamford, CT: Appleton & Lange.

Uphold, C., & Graham, M. (1998). Clinical guidelines in family practice. (pp 305–306). Gainsville, FL: Barmarrae Books.

Conjunctivitis

Goolsby, M. (2000). The red eye: Differential diagnosis and management. *American Journal for Nurse Practitioners, 14*(6), 7–19.

Morrow, G., & Abbott, R. (1998). Conjunctivitis. *American Family Physician.* Available at www.aafp.org/afp/980215ap/morrow.html.

Nobel, J. (1996). Textbook of Primary Care Medicine(3rd ed). St. Louis: Mosby Yearbook.

Glaucoma

Lewis, P., Phillips, G., & Sassani, J. (1999). Topical Therapies for Glaucoma: What family physicians need to know. *American Family Physician.* Available at www.aafp.org/afp/990401ap/1871.html.

Porth, C.M. (1998). Pathophysiology: Concepts of Altered Health States. (5th ed.) Philadelphia: Lippincott.

Strabismus

Broderick, P. (1998). Pediatric vision screening for the family physician. *American Family Physician.* Available at www.aafp.org/aft/9809011ap/ broderic.html.

Larvich, J. & Nelson, L. (1993) Diagnosis and treatment of strabismus disorders. *Pediatric Clinics of North America, 40,* 737–752.

Mills, M. (1999). The eye in childhood. *American Family Physician.* Available at www.aafp.org/afp/990901ap/907.html.

Simons, K. (1996) Preschool vision screening: Rationale, methodology and outcome. *Survey of Ophthalmology, 41,* 3–30.

Vision Loss

Broderick, P. (1998) Pediatric vision screening for the family physician. *American Family Physician.* Available at www.aafp.org/aft/9809011ap/ broderic.html.

Mills, M. (1999). The eye in childhood. *American Family Physician.* Available at www.aafp.org/afp/990901ap/907.html.

Quillen, D., (1999), Common causes of vision loss in elderly patients. *American Family Physician.* Available at www.aafp.org/afp/990700ap/ 99.html.

Simons, K. (1996). Preschool vision screening: Rationale, methodology and outcome. *Survey of Ophthalmology, 41,* 3–30.

Vaughan, D.G.,Asburn, T., Riordoan-Eva, P. (1999). General Ophthamology (15th ed). Stamford, Appleton and Lange.

RESOURCES

American Academy of Ophthalmology:
  Telephone: (415) 561-8500
  www.eyenet.org

American Foundation for the Blind:
  Telephone: (800) 232-5463
  www.afb.org/

National Association for the Visually Handicapped:
  Telephone: (212) 889-3141
  www.navh.org/

National Eye Institute
  2020 Vision Pl.
  Bethesda, MD 20892-3655
  Telephone: (301) 496-5248
  www.nei.nih.gov/

Chapter 4

EAR, NOSE, AND THROAT DISORDERS

CERUMEN IMPACTIONS

SIGNAL SYMPTOMS ► hearing loss, possibly pain and itching

ICD-9 Codes	380.4	Impacted cerumen
	931	Foreign body in ear

Cerumen impaction is an excessive buildup of cerumen (or ear wax) in the external auditory canal.

Epidemiology

Common cause of hearing loss

Can occur in all ages

Etiology

Overproduction of cerumen.

Use of cotton-tipped applicators, which push ear wax further into the ear canal rather than removing it, can lead to impaction in the ear canal.

Physiology and Pathophysiology

The cerumen-secreting glands of the external auditory canal produce wax to protect the ear, and more specifically, the tympanic membrane (TM). In some individuals, these glands produce excessive amounts of wax, which can become hard and thus become impacted in the ear canal.

Clinical Manifestations

Subjective

"Stuffy" ears

Often can't hear well, or hearing is muffled

Objective

Unable to visualize tympanic membrane.

Obvious wax in the external auditory canal; may be orange to dark brown, soft or hard, thick or sticky.

Differential Diagnosis

Foreign body in ear canal (usually diagnosed visually and/or removed)

Otitis externa (infection of external ear canal; patient reports pain, discharge)
Otitis media (infection of inner ear; patient reports pain, usually no discharge)

Diagnostic Tests

Usually none; however, if hearing loss persists after initial removal of wax, an auditory examination is warranted.

Management/Treatment

Pharmacologic Management

First soften ear wax

Carbamide peroxide, 6.5% (Debrox) otic drops, 1–2 drops in each ear QD–BID for 1 week

Triethanolamine polypeptide oleate condensate 10% (Cerumenex) otic drops, 1–2 drops each ear QD–BID for 1 week

 CP 4–1   Clinical Pearl: Colace suspension, 1–2 drops each ear QHS for 1 week also works very well.

May irrigate ears with water after use with either.
These treatments may be used for primary prevention of impaction as well.

Nonpharmacologic Management

Irrigate ears with warm water.

30–50 gauge syringes
"Water picks"

Can also use "ear spoon."

Must have a steady hand, so as not to rupture TM.
Can be painful for the patient.

Client Education

When using eardrops, pull ear up and out, and hold head at a 45-degree angle.

May put cotton balls in outer external canal to keep drops in ear.

Do NOT use cotton-tipped applicators in the inner auditory canal!

Follow-up

Usually none, unless impactions continue. Some patients return for removal on a regular basis.

Referral

Refer to otolaryngologist (ENT [Ear/Nose/Throat]) for known tympanic membrane perforation, mastoidectomy, or persistent hearing loss after removal of wax.

DIZZINESS/VERTIGO

SIGNAL SYMPTOM▶ dizziness

| ICD-9 Code | 780.4 | Vertigo NOS or dizziness |

Dizziness/vertigo is the subjective sensation of dizziness, spinning falling, or rocking or the sensation that the patient is moving or spinning. Can also be objective, where a person senses that his/her surroundings are moving (true vertigo).

Epidemiology

Accounts for more than 7 million visits per year

Etiology

Can have a wide variety of causes:

Vestibular etiology (44%).

Benign positional vertigo (16%).

Acute labyrinthitis (9%).

Meniere's disease (5%).

Other (less common) causes include: acoustic neuroma, multiple scerosis, vertebrobasilar insufficiency, headache-associated vertigo, cardiovascular disease, cerebrovascular disease (stroke, transient ischemic attack [TIA]), psychiatric disease, metabolic disturbances

Physiology and Pathophysiology

Normal balance is a function of the vestibular system, with input from other systems, including visual and cerebellar. Information from the vestibular system to the brain that does not correspond with other bodily systems that help maintain balance results in dizziness/vertigo.

Clinical Manifestations

Subjective

A thorough history is imperative in determining the cause of the vertigo. Symptoms might include:

Sensation of dizziness, spinning, lightheadedness.

Tinnitus.

Ear fullness.

Difficulty hearing.

Pallor/sweating.

Nausea/vomiting.

Weakness/numbness.

Syncope.

Objective

A thorough physical examination should also be conducted, including:

Vital signs.

Ear examination.

Hearing/auditory examination.

Neck examination, including listening for bruits.

Neurologic examination, including cranial nerves and cerebellar function.

Differential Diagnosis

Any of the following diagnoses can present with dizziness:

Vestibular etiology.

Benign positional vertigo.
Labyrinthitis.
Meniere's disease.
Acoustic neuroma.
Multiple sclerosis.
Vertebrobasilar insufficiency.
Headache-associated vertigo.
Cardiovascular disease.
Cerebrovascular disease (stroke, TIA).
Psychiatric disease.
Metabolic disturbances.

Diagnostic Tests

Possible laboratory tests include:

Complete blood count (CBC) (to rule out anemia).
Sedimentation (SED) rate (to rule out possible infection/inflammation).
Thyroid panel (to rule out hypothyroid and hyperthyroid conditions).

Diagnostic tests might include:

Computed tomography (CT) scan or magnetic resonance imaging (MRI) (to rule out suspected lesion).

Management/Treatment

Note: Treatment depends largely on the etiology of the diagnosis.

Pharmacologic Management

Meclizine (Antivert), 25 mg Q6–8H as needed for vertigo.
Benzodiazepines are occasionally helpful, if anxiety is also present (e.g., diazepam [Valium], 2–10 mg BID–QID).

Nonpharmacologic Management

Prescribe positional/vestibular exercises (Cawthorne exercises).
Reassure patient.
Salt-restricted diet and thiazide diuretics may be helpful in Meniere's disease.

Client Education

Discuss nature/etiology of symptoms.
Reassure patients that treatment takes time.

Follow-up

Best to follow up patients, especially initially in a couple of weeks.

Referral

Refer to ENT if symptoms do not fully resolve.
Refer to neurologist if lesions or neurologic disease is present.

DYSPHAGIA

SIGNAL SYMPTOM▶ difficulty swallowing

ICD-9 Code	787.2	Dysphagia

Dysphagia is difficulty swallowing and the sensation of food being "trapped" in the esophagus; often divided into oropharyngeal and esophageal dysphagia.

Epidemiology

Affects 7%–10% of adults over 50 years of age.

May affect up to 25% of hospitalized patients, and up to 40% of nursing-home patients.

Etiology

Often indicative of another underlying cause.

ADULTS

Structural (tumors, strictures)

Gastroesophageal reflux disease (GERD)

Neuromuscular

CHILDREN

Malformations

Neuromuscular

GERD

Physiology and Pathophysiology

Swallowing involves four phases: oral preparatory, oral propulsive, pharyngeal, and esophageal. Depending on the location and swallowing phase, and the underlying etiology and/or disease process, the pathophysiology of dysphagia will vary.

Clinical Manifestations

Subjective

Difficulty swallowing

Sensation of choking

Pressure in mid-chest (under sternum)

Possible symptoms of GERD (heartburn, abdominal pain/burning, pressure under sternum)

Coughing or choking with swallowing

Food sticking in throat

Drooling

Unexplained weight loss

Objective

Masses inspected and/or palpated in neck

Possible abnormal voice/speech

Changes in oral cavity or pharynx (integrity, masses)

Position of soft palate

Possible change in gag reflex

Drooling

Differential Diagnosis

GERD (diagnosed via esophagogastroduodenoscopy [EGD] and pH testing) (reveals esophageal irritation; pH acidic)

Chest pain (history, examination, and possible positive electrocardiogram, to rule out cardiac origin)

Esophageal tumor (diagnosed with computed tomography CT scan)

Esophageal inflammatory changes (related to diet, stress, pregnancy)

Diagnostic Tests

X-ray examination of head/chest (to rule out obstruction, skeletal deformity)

Barium swallow (videofluorographic swallowing study [VFSS]) (to rule out esophageal stricture, hernia)

EGD (rule out GERD)

pH testing (rule out GERD)

CT scan of chest (rule out lesions, neoplasms)

Management/Treatment

It is important to ensure adequate hydration and nutrition, and to ensure adequate pulmonary function and rule out cardiac disease

Pharmacologic Management

FOR GERD-RELATED SYMPTOMS

H_2 blockers [cimetidine (Tagamet), famotidine (Pepcid), ranitidine (Zantac), nizatidine (Axid)]

Proton-pump inhibitors [omeprazole (Prilosec), lansoprazole (Prevacid), Rabeprazole (Aciphex), pantoprazole (Protonix)]

Antacids (Tums, Rolaids, Gaviscon)

FOR SPASMS

Nitrates

Calcium-channel blockers

Nonpharmacologic Management

Surgical intervention (esophageal dilatation/stent) may be necessary.

Swallow therapy:

  Compensatory techniques.

  Indirect therapy.

  Direct therapy.

Client Education

Encourage eating soft solid food, with uniform consistency.

Instruct to take small bites of food.

Explain that eating at 90-degree angle facilitates swallowing.

Referral

Refer to ENT or surgeon if symptoms are severe or continue to be problematic.

EPIGLOTTITIS

SIGNAL SYMPTOMS▶ sore throat, difficulty swallowing

ICD-9 Code	464.30	Epiglottitis

Epiglottitis is a life-threatening upper airway obstruction caused by a bacterial infection of the epiglottis, epiglottic folds, and surrounding tissues.

Epidemiology

May occur at any age, with peak incidence at 2–7 years of age.

Incidence is decreasing with the use of the *Haemophilus influenzae* type b (HIB) vaccine.

Emergence of group A beta-hemolytic streptococci (GABHS) as a causative agent has increased.

Etiology

Causative agent is *Haemophilus influenzae* type b.

Other causes:
  GABHS
  Staphylococcus aureus
  Streptococcus pneumoniae

Physiology and Pathophysiology

The looser connective tissue and multiple glands on the lingual surface of the epiglottis swell, causing the epiglottis to direct downward, which can obstruct the laryngeal introitus. The prodrome can last hours (as compared with days, as in croup) and airway obstruction can occur rapidly.

Clinical Manifestations

Subjective

Moderate to high fever
Sore, painful throat
Drooling
Marked difficulty swallowing
Tongue protrusion
Decreased appetite
Fright or anxiety

Objective
(*Note:* Do not attempt to visualize epiglottis, as respiratory arrest can occur immediately!)

High fever
Rapid pulse, rapid respirations
Classic "tripod" position (leaning forward)
Toxic, agitated, restless
Signs of dehydration: dry mucous membranes, poor tear production, decreased skin turgor

Muffled voice
Markedly erythematous pharynx
Drooling
Possible sternal retractions

Differential Diagnosis

Viral croup ("barky" cough, stridor)
Foreign-body aspiration (seen on x-ray examination)
Asthma (chest tightness and wheezing relieved with nebulized albuterol)
Bronchiolitis (hacking cough, fever, tachypnea, often seen in children)

Diagnostic Tests

Make sure airway is established and secured first!
CBC (may be elevated).
Cultures (to determine specific pathogen).
X-ray examination shows characteristic swollen epiglottis ("thumb sign").

Management/Treatment

 ES 4–1   Emergency Situation: Epiglottitis
Epiglottitis is a Medical Emergency

- Immediate referral to ENT or emergency department.
- Do not attempt to visualize epiglottis, as respiratory arrest can occur immediately!
- Do not move or lay a child down unless prepared to manage obstructed airway!
  - Bag, valve, or mask can buy time.
  - Needle cricothyrotomy, if needed.
  - Tracheostomy if unable to intubate.
  - Intubation (usually extubated 48–72 hours after antibiotics are started).

Pharmacologic Management

Cefotaxime (Claforan), 50–200 mg/kg/24 hours, divided Q6H.
Ceftriaxone (Rocephin), 75 mg/kg/24 hours.
Trimethoprim/sulfamethoxazole (TMP/SMX; Bactrim/Septra) is a second-line agent.
Continue antibiotics 7–10 days after extubation.

Client Education

Prevention: HIB vaccine
Emotional support to parents/family due to rapid onset

Referral

Medical emergency; refer immediately to ENT because of potential for respiratory arrest.

EPISTAXIS

SIGNAL SYMPTOMS▶ bleeding from nose possibly difficulty breathing

ICD-9 Codes	784.7	Epistaxis
	931	Foreign body in nose

Epistaxis is bleeding from the nostril or nasal cavity; divided into anterior and posterior bleeds.

Epidemiology

Majority are due to local irritation, and originate from Kiesselbach's plexus. Most adults report having at least one nosebleed in their lifetime.

Etiology

Trauma/irritation:
    Nose-picking (most common)
    Blunt trauma to nasal area
    Foreign body
    Dry nasal mucosa
Infection:
    Sinusitis (acute/chronic)
    Upper respiratory infection
Coagulation disorder (rare)
Vascular abnormalities
Septal deviation/perforation

Physiology and Pathophysiology

Kiesselbach's plexus, in the anterior region of the nasal cavity, is a, fragile, highly vascular area; it is susceptible to bleeding if irritated or injured.

Clinical Manifestations

Subjective

Usually rapid onset.
Bleeding from the nasal cavity (amount will vary).
Blood clots may also be present.
History of trauma and/or repeated episodes of epistaxis.

Objective

Wait for bleeding to stop before examining.
Palpate external nasal area for fractures, if history of trauma.
Attempt to locate site of bleeding via internal nasal examination.

Differential Diagnosis

Any of the following diagnoses can present with epistaxis:
Trauma
Infectious process (observe for fever, pain. and discharge)
Medications (review patient history)

Coagulation problem (review patient history and laboratory tests [elevated prothrombin time/partial thromboplastin time {PT/PTT}])
Neoplasm (diagnosed via CT scan)
Hypertension (review patient history, medications and current vitals)
Osler–Weber–Rendu syndrome (a hereditary hemorrhagic condition)

Diagnostic Tests

Complete blood count (CBC) (if infection is suspected, increased WBCs)
Coagulation studies, if copious bleeding and underlying pathology is suspected (increased PT/PTT)

Management/Treatment

Pharmacologic Management

Nasal sprays/topical decongestants may alleviate blood flow.
Primary prevention:
Petroleum-based ointment keeps nasal passages moist.
Application of estrogen cream can thicken nasal mucosa.

Nonpharmacologic Management

Application of direct pressure ("pinching") of anterior nose.
Most bleeds stop after 10 minutes.
Patient should be sitting in upright position, and leaning forward, to avoid swallowing blood.

Client Education

Avoid picking nose!
Avoid aspirin-containing medications.
Avoid vigorous nose blowing.
Humidified air can be helpful.

Referral

ENT if site of bleeding is inaccessible, or unable to stop bleeding completely

HEARING LOSS

SIGNAL SYMPTOM difficulty hearing

ICD-9 Codes	388.12	Noise-related sensorineural hearing loss
	389.18	Viral sensorineural hearing loss
	389.8	Hereditary sensoineural hearing loss
	389.9	Hearing loss NOS or deafness
	V72.1	Auditory testing
	744.04	Congenital conductive loss
	794.15	Abnormal auditory function study

Hearing loss is partial or complete loss of hearing that is either sensorineural or conductive in nature:

Sensorineural hearing loss (95%) involves abnormal structures of the inner ear, or damage to its neural components; it is often permanent.

Conductive hearing loss (5%) is the decreased ability of the external or middle ear to conduct sound waves to inner ear; the loss is mechanical.

Epidemiology

Ten percent of the U.S. population (~28 million Americans) have a hearing problem.

As many as 10 million persons have hearing loss caused by excessive noise levels.

Fifteen percent of school-age children have significant conductive hearing loss (Otitis media and its sequelae are the most common cause of conductive hearing loss in children.)

Profound hearing loss occurs in 1 in 1000 children.

Hereditary hearing loss occurs in 1 in 4000 live births.

An estimated 60% of people over 65 years of age have some degree of gradual and progressive bilateral sensorineural hearing loss. (Cerumen impaction is responsible for over 30% of hearing loss in adults over age 60.)

At least 30 million Americans are exposed to potentially harmful sound levels in their workplace.

Etiology

Genetic or hereditary factors.

Environmental/acquired diseases.

Malformations.

Causes of sensorineural hearing loss:

Congenital: Rubella, cytomegalovirus, syphilis, toxoplasmosis, exposure to ototoxic drugs, anoxia, birth trauma, erythroblastosis fetalis, albinism.

Acquired: Central nervous system embolism, thrombosis, vasculitis, viral infections (mumps, measles, influenza, chickenpox, mononucleosis), meningitis, prolonged exposure to loud noise, ototoxic drugs.

Causes of conductive hearing loss:

Impacted cerumen, foreign body, otitis externa, tympanic membrane perforation, chronic otitis media, congenital malformations of ossicles, trauma.

Physiology and Pathophysiology

Sensorineural: Continuous exposure to either ototoxic substances or excessive noise, causes "wear and tear" on the hair cells of the basilar membrane of the cochlea. As a result, cell damage, and even cell death, occurs, causing hearing loss.

Conductive: Due to either a blockage or mechanical trauma; sound waves cannot be conducted from the external ear to the inner ear.

Clinical Manifestations

Subjective

<u>HISTORY QUESTIONS</u>

Symptoms (may have to ask other family members too)

Speaks loudly or softly
Mispronounces words
Ringing in ears
Chronic infections
    Pulling on ears
    Frequent earaches, upper respiratory infections, sore throats
    Discharge from ears
Medical history
Noise exposure (home, work)

<u>SIGNS OF HEARING LOSS</u>

Shouting
Asking people to repeat themselves
Social withdrawal
Misunderstanding conversations
Ringing/buzzing in ears
Favoring one ear
TV/radio turned too loud for others
Inappropriate answers
For children, see "Age-Related Considerations: Signs of Hearing Loss in
    Children"

<u>SENSORINEURAL HEARING LOSS</u>

High-tone perception impaired.
May be able to hear people, but unable to decipher words.
May have difficulty hearing high-frequency sounds: telephones, doorbells,
    timers, ticking watches.
May report tinnitus.
Often speaks very loudly.

<u>CONDUCTIVE HEARING LOSS</u>

Diminished perception of sound, especially with low tones and vowels.
Often speaks very softly.

Objective

Inspect ear canal for infection, trauma, cerumen impaction, tympanic membrane perforation.

<u>HEARING TESTS</u>

Whisper tests

 Age-Related Considerations 4–1: Signs of Hearing Loss in Children

Says "What?" or "Huh?"
Sits close to the TV with high volume.
Infants/children do not turn head toward sounds.
Not startled by loud sounds.
Speech does not appear to be developing (∼12 months).

Tuning forks test:
    Weber (sound heard equally in both ears)
    Rinne (air conduction > bone conduction)

SENSORINEURAL HEARING LOSS

During Weber test, tuning fork is heard more loudly in unaffected ear.
During the Rinne test, air conduction will be better than bone conduction.

CONDUCTIVE HEARING LOSS

During Weber test, tuning fork is heard more loudly in problematic ear.
During Rinne test, bone conduction is better than air conduction.

Differential Diagnosis

Sensorineural Hearing Loss

Presbycusis
Noise-induced deafness
Meniere's disease
Acoustic neuroma
Diabetes
Multiple sclerosis

Conductive Hearing Loss

Impacted cerumen
Foreign body in the ear canal
Occlusive edema of auditory canal
Perforation of tympanic membrane
Chronic otitis media
Cholesteatoma

Diagnostic Tests

Audiography (audiometry testing) (to confirm hearing loss)
Tympanometry (confirms presence of fluid in inner ear)
CT scan (for tumors or cholesteatoma))
MRI (for tumors, multiple sclerosis)
Screening blood tests: chemistry panel (to rule out diabetes mellitus), CBC
    (to rule out infecton)

Management/Treatment

90%–95% of hearing impairment can be corrected, usually with the help of hearing aids at the discretion of an ENT. Hearing aids cannot totally restore hearing, but can dramatically improve quality of life
    5%–10% can be corrected either medically or surgically

Pharmacologic Management

Sensorineural hearing loss: Referral is warranted.
Conductive hearing loss: Treat either infection, trauma, or obstruction.

Client Education

Type of hearing loss
Prognosis

Treatment options

Education regarding hearing aids

Community/national resources

Follow-up

Audiometry is the primary method to monitor progress.

Referral

If any degree of hearing loss is found, patients should be referred to ENT for full audiologic evaluation immediately.

Referral to ENT might also be warranted if pathology is found concurrently.

LARYNGITIS

SIGNAL SYMPTOM ➤ loss of voice

ICD-9 Codes	464.0	Laryngitis
	478.75	Laryngospasm

Laryngitis is inflammation of the mucous membranes in the lining of the larynx that may be acute or chronic; often associated with an upper respiratory infection.

Epidemiology

Most often seen in people who regularly use their voice, such as professional speakers or singers.

Etiology

Result of a bacterial or viral agent that attacks the larynx, subglottic area, and epiglottis. (Viral causes: influenza A and B, rhinovirus, adenovirus, coronavirus; bacterial causes: GABHS, *Streptococcus pneumomiae*).

Often not an isolated disorder, but part of an upper respiratory infection.

Excessive use of voice.

Trauma from irritants (smoking).

Endotracheal intubation.

GERD.

Alcohol ingestion (chronic laryngitis).

Physiology and Pathophysiology

Hoarseness results from interference of normal apposition of vocal cords; voice quality indicatitive of pathophysiology:

"Raspy"—due to edema or inflammation.

"Breathy"—due to air escaping from nonapproximating vocal cords.

"Shaky"—due to decreased respiratory force.

Clinical Manifestations

Subjective

Hoarseness; may progress to aphonia.

Scratchy throat.

Pain on swallowing.

Constant need to clear throat.

Fever.

Malaise.

In severe cases, difficulty breathing and stridor may be present.

Objective

Voice quality.

Erythematous oropharynx.

Possible enlarged regional lymph nodes.

If patient has been hoarse for more than 2–3 weeks, laryngoscopy is warranted, which in most cases, provides an immediate diagnosis:

Reddened, enlarged, inflamed vocal cords.

Hemorrhaging may be present.

Polyps may also be present.

Consider biopsy in chronic laryngitis (smokers).

Differential Diagnosis

Croup (often seen in children; "barky" cough with stridor)

Diphtheria (gray membrane on oropharynx and positive culture)

Vocal nodules (seen on laryngoscopy)

Laryngeal carcinoma (laryngoscopy and positive biopsy)

Diagnostic Tests

Fiberoptic laryngoscopy (see above)

Management/Treatment

Pharmacologic Management

Usually self-limiting.

Antibiotics are not needed unless there is a bacterial infection.

Vasoconstricting sprays and analgesics are used by singers when use of their voice is absolutely necessary.

Steroids should not be used unless there is an underlying allergic component.

Analgesics for pain.

Antipyretics for fever.

Throat lozenges (avoid use in children because of the possibility of aspiration).

Nonpharmacologic Management

Rest voice.

When speaking is necessary, use moderate voice and avoid whispering.

Warm drinks.

Humidifier/steam inhalations.

Saline gargles.

Client Education

Encourage voice rest; provide nonverbal alternatives to communication.

Explain the need for no antibiotics.

Prescribe adequate rest and hydration.

Encourage avoidance of smoking and smoky environments.

Encourage decreased alcohol intake.

Follow-up

Generally not needed, unless voice does not return.

Referral

Refer to ENT if hoarseness persists for longer than 3 weeks; any patient with concurrent dyspnea; history of surgical vocal stripping

MASTOIDITIS

SIGNAL SYMPTOMS ▶ ear pain, fever

ICD-9 Codes	383.0	Acute or subacute mastoiditis
	383.9	Coalescent mastoiditis

Mastoiditis is an inflammatory process in the mastoic air cells, which can be acute (usually after otitis media) or chronic (often associated with cholesteatoma and/or chronic ear disease); may also involve an infectious process.

Epidemiology

Usually occurs concurrently with acute otitis media.

Etiology

Acute otitis media pathogens (*Streptococcus pneumoniae, Haemophilus influenzae, Moraxella catarrhalis*)

Cholesteatoma

Physiology and Pathophysiology

The air-cell system surrounding the mastoid bone is confluent with the middle ear. Bacteria in the middle ear, which causes an inner-ear infection (e.g., otitis media), moves into the air-cell system, causing inflammation and infection in and around the mastoid bone.

Clinical Manifestations

Subjective

Fever (usually over 103°F)

Ear pain

Possible swelling behind the ear

Objective

Red, bulging tympanic membrane

Postauricular mass and/or swelling

Postauricular tenderness

Possibly increased white-cell count

Clouding of mastoid air cells on plain films

Differential Diagnosis

Postauricular lymphadenopathy (nodes palpated behind ear)
Postauricular cellulitis (redness, warmth behind ear; possibly fever)
Severe otitis externa (ear drainage, pain)
Neoplasm, benign or malignant (persistent signs/symptoms despite treatment)

Diagnostic Tests

Plain films (to rule out infection, masses)
CT scan (to rule out tumors, masses)
CBC (to rule out infection)
Audiography (to rule out hearing loss)

Management/Treatment

Pharmacologic Management

Often warrants hospitalization
Broad-spectrum intravenous antibiotics (to cover GABHS, *Pseudomonas, Strep. pneumonia, Staph. aureus,* and *H. influenzae*)
Topical antibiotics (cortisporin, gentamicin) often used with pressure-equalization (PE) tubes

Nonpharmacologic Management

Placement of PE tubes
Mastoidectomy needed if patient does not respond to above measures

Client Education

Discuss disease process.
Discuss importance of keeping PE tubes patent.
Discuss water precautions: keep ear dry.
Discuss possibility of hearing loss.

Follow-up

Audiography to determine long-term hearing loss

Referral

Refer to ENT or neurologist for treatment and surgery.

OTITIS EXTERNA

SIGNAL SYMPTOMS▶ ear pain and discharge

ICD-9 Codes		
	380.10	Otitis externa, bacterial
	112.82	Otitis externa, fungal
	380.11	Swimmer's ear
	380.22	Allergic otitis externa
	388.60	Ear discharge, otorrhea

Otitis externa is an external auditory canal infection or inflammation, outside of the tympanic membrane, also referred to as "swimmer's ear." The infection is usually caused by bacteria, but can also have a fungal or eczematous etiology.

Epidemiology

Usually occurs in summer months (more exposure to water).
Affects 4 of 1000 people (usually teenagers and young adults).

Etiology

Bacterial:
> *Pseudomonas* (67%)
> *Staphylococcus aureus*
> *Streptococcus*
> Gram-negative rods

Fungal (rare):
> *Aspergillus* (90%)
> *Phycomycetes*
> *Rhizopus*
> *Actinomyces*
> *Penicillium*
> Yeast

Eczematous:
> History of eczema or seborrhea
> Purulent otitis media

Trauma to external canal

Chronic
> Usually *Pseudomonas* bacterial infection

Physiology and Pathophysiology

Cerumen, produced by the sebaceous glands, is usually bacteriostatic. However, continuous abrasion by heat, moisture, or water causes damage to the epithelium. Organisms can then invade the damaged, wet skin.

Clinical Manifestations

Subjective

Painful to move or touch ear
Pain with chewing
Colored, copious drainage from ear
Itching inside of ear
Plugged ear(s)
Hearing loss (rare)

Objective

TM usually not visualized because of ear drainage.
Erythema of auditory canal present.
Purulent drainage obvious in auditory canal:
> If yellow/white—*Staphylococcus aureus*.

If green/sticky—*Pseudomonas*.
Positive tragus sign—palpating and slightly pulling pinna of ear.
Possible presence of preauricular adenitis.

Differential Diagnosis

Eczema (history of allergic rhinitis and/or asthma; auditory canal itching, flaking)

Acute otitis media (documented inner ear infection; see "Otitis media" above)

Upper respiratory infection (cough, rhinitis, ear pain, congestion, fever)

Cerumen impaction (excessive cerumen)

Foreign body (foreign body in ear canal)

Diagnostic Tests

Usually none needed.

Management/Treatment

Pharmacologic Management

ACUTE

Polymyxin B plus neomycin (Cortisporin) otic drops, 3–4 drops QID for 7–10 days

CHRONIC

Eardrops: (polymixin B plus neomycin plus hydrocortisone QID) plus (selenium sulfide)

Nonpharmacologic Management

Protect ears from water, keep ear canals dry; use ear plugs.
Do not stick anything in ears.
Avoid manipulation of ear canal.

Complementary/Alternative Therapies

After swimming, apply acetic drops (1:1 solution of rubbing alcohol and vinegar) in each ear.

Client Education

Finish entire prescription of ear drops.

Follow-up

Usually none, unless infection persists and/or does not clear.

Referral

Recurrent or resistant infections may need ENT referral.

OTITIS MEDIA (Acute)

SIGNAL SYMPTOM ▶ ear pain

ICD-9 Codes	382.9	Otitis media NOS
	382.0	Otitis media, acute suppurative
	381.00	Otitis media, nonsuppurative otitis
	388.70	Earache, otalgia NOS

Acute otitis media (AOM) is an infection of the middle ear (bacterial, viral, or fungal etiology); it is often accompanied by a viral upper respiratory infection.

Epidemiology

Occurs most often in children 6–36 months, and 4–6 years (rare in adults)
Accounts for ~25 million office visits per year.
By 7 years of age, 93% of children have had at least one episode of AOM.

Etiology

Streptococcus pneumoniae (most common, 25%–50%)
Hemophilus influenzae (15%–30%)
Moraxella catarrhalis (3%–20%)
Staphylococcus aureus (1%)
Enterobacteriaceae (1%)
Rarely fungal (in immunocompromised persons)
Viral causes
Risk factors (see "Risk Factors: Acute Otitis Media")

Physiology and Pathophysiology

Eustachian-tube dysfunction:
Children have shorter, more horizontal eustachian tubes. (As fluid and secretions accumulate and remain in the eustachian tubes, pathogens enter and multiply.)
Smoking or exposure to second-hand smoke may also predispose a child to otitis media (because of the increased of risk upper respiratory infection and decreased mucocilliary function in the eustachian tubes).

Clinical Manifestations

Subjective
Rapid onset
Ear pain or fullness

 RF 4–1 Risk Factors: *Acute Otitis Media*

Risk Factors: Acute Otitis Media
Children in day care
More common in boys than in girls
Formula-fed infants
Smoking and children exposed to second-hand smoke
Children with Down's syndrome
Increased incidence in Native American/Alaskan and Canadian Inuits

Pulling at ears

Irritability

Not sleeping or eating well (especially in children)

Symptoms of upper respiratory infection (congestion, cough, sneezing, headache)

Fever, chills

Objective

Low- to high-grade fever

(*Note:* Redness alone is not indicative of AOM, especially in a crying child.)

Decreased mobility of TM (number 1 indicator)

Full, bulging TM

Decreased or absent bony landmarks

Distorted light reflex

Increased vascularity of TM

Differential Diagnosis

Otitis media with effusion (excessive serous fluid behind TM; good TM mobility)

Sinusitis (facial pain, purulent nasal drainage, possible fever)

Mastoiditis (jaw or ear pain, possible fever)

Temporomandibular joint (TMJ) dysfunction (TM normal; pain over TMJ on palpation and opening/closing of jaw)

Upper respiratory infection (cough, rhinitis, ear pain, congestion, fever)

Allergic rhinitis (itchy/watery eyes, clear rhinitis, sneezing)

Foreign body (foreign body in ear canal)

Head/ear trauma (review patient history)

Diagnostic Tests

Usually none needed. If hearing loss persists, auditory examination is warranted. Can refer for tympanometry to measure presence of middle ear fluid.

Management/Treatment

Pharmacologic Management

Analgesics/antipyretics for pain/fever (acetaminophen/ibuprofen)

Antibiotics (most symptoms resolve within 48 hours; if not, consider switching antibiotics (See Table 4–1.)

Nonpharmacologic Management

Warm compresses or light warm air (via blow dryer) may temporarily relieve pain.

Client Education

Cease smoking and decrease exposure to second-hand smoke.

Finish all antibiotics, even if feeling better.

Breast-feeding infants decreases the risk of AOM developing.

Follow-up

Recheck ears in 3–4 weeks.

Table 4–1   Antibiotics for Acute Otitis Media

Antibiotic	Adult Dose	Pediatric Dose
Amoxicillin (Amoxil/Trimox)	250–500 mg PO TID × 10 days	40–80 mg/kg divided in three daily doses
TMP/SMX (Bactrim/Septra)	1 double strength tablet PO BID × 10 days	Not a good choice in children, has proved to be resistant.
Amoxicillin plus Clavulanate (Augmentin)	500–875 mg PO BID × 10 days (with food)	45 mg/kg divided in two daily doses
Erythromycin (E.E.S./E-mycin)	PCE: 500 mg PO BID × 10 days EES: 400 mg PO BID × 10 days	
Erythromycin plus Sulfisoxazole (Pediazole)		50 mg/kg of erythromycin and 150 mg/kg of sulfisoxazole 1–2 g Q12H
Ceftriaxone (Rocephin)		50–75 mg/kg/day
Clarithromycin (Biaxin)	250–500 mg PO BID × 10 days	
Azithromycin (Zithromax)	500 mg PO Day 1; 250 mg PO Days 2–5	10 mg/kg once on day 1; 5 mg/kg once on days 2–5

Referral

Refer to ENT if recurrent OM, or if meningitis or mastoiditis is suspected.

OTITIS MEDIA (with Effusion)

SIGNAL SYMPTOMS ear pain, fullness

ICD-9 Codes	381.01	Serous otitis media
	381.81	Eustachian dysfunction
	388.70	Earache, otalgia NOS

Otitis media with effusion (OME) is an inflammation of the middle ear, with an accumulation of serous or mucoid fluid. It is also known as serous otitis media.

Epidemiology

Accounts for more than one-third of all early childhood visits to primary care providers.

Predominantly seen from October to May.

Etiology

Poor eustachian-tube function

"Silent" bacterial infection (in 20%–40% of cases)

Concurrent allergic causes

Barotrauma (airplane, scuba diving)

Risk factors:

Exposure to second-hand smoke

Exposure to environmental toxins

Presence of infection

Physiology and Pathophysiology

Poor eustachian-tube function and position allows for accumulation of fluid in the middle ear; fluid can be either serous or mucoid.

Clinical Manifestations

Subjective
Usually asymptomatic
Possible decreased hearing
Feeling of fullness in ears
"Popping" in ears when chewing, swallowing

Objective
TM may be dull, but not bulging.
TM mobility may be decreased.
Fluid (bubbles) present behind TM.
Decreased hearing often not measurable.

Differential Diagnosis

Otitis media (usually bacterial infection of inner ear) (See "Otitis media," above.)
Otitis externa (infection of external ear canal) (See "Otitis externa," above.)
TMJ pain/dysfunction (jaw pain, tenderness)

Diagnostic Tests

Usually none needed
Tympanometry (indicates presence of fluid in middle ear)
Audiometry (helps in determining extent of hearing loss)

Management/Treatment

Pharmacologic Management
Antibiotics often not warranted. (The debate continues, as antibiotics were the mainstay of treatment for many years; however, treatment is moving away from antibiotic use, unless OME has existed for >3 months.)
Decongestants may provide some relief.
Steroids have also been used, but their effectiveness has not been documented.

Nonpharmacologic Management
Surgical management consists of myringotomy and tube placement, to enable fluid to drain from eustachian tube.

Client Education
Cease smoking cessation and limit exposure to second-hand smoke.
Avoid, or limit exposure to, known allergens.
Breast-feeding decreases risk of OME developing.

Follow-up
Follow up in 1 month.

Referral

Refer to ENT if symptoms persist for longer than 3–6 months or if treatment fails

Refer to ENT or audiologist if there has been hearing loss.

PERITONSILLAR ABSCESS

SIGNAL SYMPTOMS sore throat, difficulty swallowing

ICD-9 Code	475	Peritonsillar abscess

Peritonsillar abscess is an abscess formed behind one of the tonsils, causing asymmetrical swelling of the tonsils and difficulty swallowing.

Epidemiology

Incidence rate, ~30 per 100,000 persons

45,000 cases annually

Recurrence rate, 0%–20%

Etiology

GABHS (most common)

Anaerobic bacteria

Staphylococci

Physiology and Pathophysiology

After bacterial invasion of the superior or inferior tonsil(s), localization of the infection results in the formation of an abscess.

Clinical Manifestations

Subjective

Unilateral throat pain

Possible same-side ear pain

Dysphagia, often severe

Dysphonia

Drooling

Fever/chills (often 102°F or higher)

Fatigue, malaise

Objective

Fever

One-sided marked erythema

Affected tonsil enlarged

Uvula displaced to one side; does not rise midline

Enlarged, tender cervical lymph nodes on affected side

Trismus (spasms of masticatory muscles)

Drooling

Differential Diagnosis

Infectious mononucleosis (CBC would reveal increased white-cell count with
  atypical lymphocytes, and a positive mono-spot test would be positive.)
Epiglottitis (confirmation via x-ray) (*Note:* Medical emergency) (See
  "Epiglottitis," above.)
Pharyngeal tumor (confirmed via CT scan and/or biopsy)
Cervical adenitis (palpable lymphadenopathy)
Mastoid infection (confirmed via x-ray examination)

Diagnostic Tests

Usually none needed. CBC, mono spot, rapid strep

Management/Treatment

 ES 4–2 Emergency Situation: Peritonsillar Abscess
Peritonsillar abscess is a medical emergency. Refer to ENT or ER
immediately for needle aspiration, antibiotic, and pain treatment. Hospitalization may
be necessary.

PHARYNGITIS/TONSILLITIS

SIGNAL SYMPTOM ▶ sore throat

ICD-9 Codes		
	462	Pharyngitis, bacterial or viral
	463	Tonsilitis, bacterial or viral
	472.1	Chronic pharyngitis
	474.0	Chronic tonsillitis
	34.0	Strep throat
	795.3	Positive throat culture

Pharyngitis/tonsillitis is an inflammation and/or infection of the pharynx or
tonsils or both.

Epidemiology

Sore throat is one of the four most common reasons that patients in the
  United States seek ambulatory care.
Approximately 11% of school-age children seek health care annually for
  sore throat.
Streptococcal pharyngitis is particularly prevalent in patients ages 6–12.
GABHS accounts for 30%–40% of cases of pharyngitis in children.

Etiology

Usually nonbacterial (presumed to be viral)
GABHS uncommon in children under 3 years of age
Less common causes:
  Mycoplasma pneumoniae
  Corynebacterium diphtheriae
  Neisseria meningitis/Neisseria gonorrhoeae
  Chlamydia trachomatis

Physiology and Pathophysiology

Invasion of pharyngeal mucosa usually begins by droplet transmission.

Incubation period varies from a few hours to several days, depending on organism.

Mucous membranes become inflamed and edematous; often tonsils are involved.

Clinical Manifestations

Subjective

Rapid onset

Sore throat, often with dysphagia

Fever exceeding 100–101°F

Usually no cough and rhinorrhea

Nausea and possibly vomiting (especially in children)

Decreased appetite

Headache

History of recent exposure

Objective

Elevated temperature

Marked erythema and swelling of throat and tonsils

Tonsillar exudate (Only 50% of patients with strep throat have exudate.) (See Table 4–2.)

Tender anterior cervical lymph nodes

Possible palatial petechiae

Possible scarlatiniform rash on the trunk, that spreads centrifugally (sand paper rash)

Differential Diagnosis

Upper respiratory infection (negative strep test/culture; presence of cough, congestion)

Influenza (negative strep test/culture; presence of high fever, body aches)

Infectious mononucleosis (positive mono-spot test; atypical lymphocytes and increased white-cell count on CBC)

Stomatitis (herpetic lesions in mouth) (positive HSV culture)

Diphtheria (gray, adherent membrane over tonsils; positive culture)

Table 4–2 Strep Score

Symptom Give one point for each symptom to estimate the probability of strep throat.	Score
Tonsillar exudate	
Anterior cervical lymphadenopathy	
Absence of cough	
Presence of fever	
Total A strep score of 3 indicates ~20% of sore throats have streptococci as the cause A strep score of 4 indicates ~40% of sore throats have streptococci as the cause	Total

Peritonsillar abscess (uvula does not rise midline; tonsils asymmetrical—refer to ENT)

Epiglottitis (child usually in tripod position, drooling, not talking, looks "toxic")

(*Note:* This is a medical emergency; do not attempt to visualize pharynx.)

Diagnostic Tests

Rapid strep-antigen testing:
 Sensitivity (~80%).
 Specificity.
 Requires proper technique.
Throat cultures:
 Sensitivity (~90%).
 Specificity.
 Can take 24–48 hours for confirmation.

Management/Treatment

Pharmacologic Management

Antibiotic therapy for GABHS:
 Benzathine penicillin (Bicillin): patients <25 kg, 600,000 units IM once; patients >25kg, 1.2 million units IM once
 Oral penicillin V, 250 mg PO TID for 10 days (adults)
 Amoxicillin (Amoxil/Trimox), 40 mg/kg/day PO TID for 10 days (children)
 Erythromycin (E.E.S., E-mycin, Ery-Tab/PCE), 500 mg PO BID for 10 days (adults), 30–50 mg/kg/day q 6–8hrs 10 days
 Erythromycin (Eryped), 50 mg/kg/day PO BID–QID for 10 days (children)
 Azithromycin (Zithromax), 250 mg, 2 PO on day 1, 1 PO on days 2–5 (adults)
 Cefpodoxime (Vantin), 200 mg PO BID for 5 days
Other pharmacology:
 Acetaminophen or ibuprofen for fever and sore throat pain
 Decongestants for congestion
 Prednisone (for severe mononucleosis)
Note: If GABHS is left untreated, complications can arise:
 Scarlet fever
 Peritonsillar abscess
 Glomerulonephritis
 Rheumatic fever

Nonpharmacologic Management

Increase fluid intake.
Rest.
Aspirate nasal secretions with bulb syringe.

Complementary/Alternative Therapies

Warm salt water gargles to alleviate sore throat pain.

Client Education

Finish all of antibiotic.

Throw out toothbrush 2 days after starting antibiotic therapy.

Wash hands often and well.

Do not share cups or utensils.

Limit exposure to others.

Referral

Refer to ENT for peritonsillar abscess, retropharyngeal abscess, or prolonged toxic course.

RHINITIS, ALLERGIC

SIGNAL SYMPTOMS ▶ rhinitis, sneezing, watery eyes

ICD-9 Codes	477.9	Allergic rhinitis
	472.0	Rhinorrhea, rhinitis

Allergic rhinitis is a chronic disease of the entire upper airway. It is characterized by rhinorrhea, sneezing, nasal congestion, pruritus of the eyes and nose, sore throat (or throat clearing), congestion of the ears, and coughing. The "classic triad" consists of nasal congstion, sneezing, and clear rhinorrhea.

Epidemiology

Affects 30–35 million Americans ($\sim$30% of the population)

Annual estimated cost of treatment (along with comorbid conditions) was $10 billion in 1995.

Annual cost of pharmacologic management of allergic rhinitis exceeds $2 billion.

Onset is usually before age 30, but can occur at any age.

Etiology

The most common allergens include:

Pollen

Weeds

Trees

Animal dander

Mold spores

Insects

Food

Dust mites

Risk factors (See "Risk Factors: Allergic Rhinitis.")

Physiology and Pathophysiology

The allergic response is caused by an immunoglobulin (IgE) response to allergens in the environment, especially over time. With continuous exposure, mast cells (in the upper respiratory system) become coated with IgE antibodies and release histamines, prostaglandins, and bradykinins, which are responsibe for symptoms.

RF 4–2 Risk Factors: *Allergic Rhinitis*

Risk Factors: Allergic Rhinitis
Family history (26% increase if one parent has allergic rhinitis; 52% increase if both parents have it)
Repeated exposure to allergens
Presence of other allergic morbities: asthma, atopic dermatitis, urticaria

Allergic rhinitis can be an immediate, as described above, or a delayed response, which involves infiltration of eosinophils, neutrophils, basophils, and mononuclear cells to the affected area. Symptoms can be either seasonal or perennial.

Clinical Manifestations

Subjective

Nasal congestion and stuffiness, with or without rhinorrhea
Sneezing
Sensation of fullness in ears
Itchy, watery eyes
Fatigue, malaise
Scratchy throat
Voice change
Postnasal drip
Constant cough (and even wheezing)
Change in taste and/or smell
Pressure over cheeks, forehead
A thorough history includes:
    Timing of symptoms
    Location of symptoms
    Comorbidities (rashes, asthma)
    Past and current use of medications (prescription and over-the-counter)
    Use of any alternative therapies
    Home environment
    Work environment
    Pets at home
    Recent travel
    Presence of allergic rhinitis in family members

Objective

Pale, gray, boggy nasal mucosa
Nasal polyps
"Allergic shiners" (dark circles under eyes)
"Dennie Morgan" lines (lines below inferior eyelid)
Clear rhinorrhea in nasal passages
Transverse nasal crease from rubbing nose
Dull facies

Differential Diagnosis

Seasonal allergic rhinitis (symptoms occur at specific times of year)

Perennial allergic rhinitis (symptoms present all year long)

Infectious rhinitis (bacterial [usually purulent], viral [usually clear]) (CBC may reveal increased white-cell count, nasal smear)

Nasal polyps (present on visual examination)

Obstructive sleep apnea (sleep studies; deep, low soft palate)

Upper respiratory infection (symptoms resolve in 7–10 days)

Diagnostic Tests

Skin testing can identify specific allergens, as well as degree of sensitivity (less expensive).

RAST (radioallergosorbent) testing determines serum levels of allergen-specific IgE titers (more specific).

Nasal smear may reveal increased eosinophils.

Table 4–3 Pharmacologic Management: Allergic Rhinitis

Tablets	
Antihistamines: First-generation (inexpensive and available over the counter, but cause significant drowsiness)	Diphenhydramine (Benadryl), 25-50 mg Q6H
	Hydroxyzine (Atarax, Vistaril), 25 mg TID–QID
	Chlorpheniramine (Chlortrimeton), 4 mg Q4–6H
	Brompheniramine (Dimetapp), 4 mg Q4–6H
Antihistamines: Second-generation (more expensive, need prescription; less drowsiness)	Loratadine (Claritin), 10 mg QD
	Fexofenadine (Allegra), 60–180 mg BID
	Cetirizine (Zyrtec), 10 mg QD
Nasal Sprays (Note: Nasal sprays are not generally recommended in children under age 6.)	
Corticosteroids	Fluticasone propionate (Flonase), 2 sprays in each nostril once daily
	Mometasone furoate (Nasonex), 2 sprays in each nostril once daily
	Triamcinolone acetonide (Nasacort AQ), 2 sprays in each nostril once daily
	Beclomethasone dipropionate (Beconase AQ, Vancenase), 1-2 sprays in each nostril twice daily
Antihistamines	Azelastine (Astelin), 2 sprays in each nostril twice daily (works well, but leaves bitter taste in mouth)
Anticholinergics	Ipratropium (Atrovent), 2 sprays in each nostril 2-3 times daily (helps controls excessive runny nose)
Mast-cell stabilizers	Cromolyn sodium (Nasalcrom), 1 spray in each nostril 3-4 times daily

Note: Terfenadine (Seldane) and Astemizole (Hismanal) have been removed from the U.S. market.

Management/Treatment

Pharmacologic Management
See Table 4–3.

Client Education
Environmental management:
> Wash curtains and bedsheets frequently in hot water.
> Remove carpets, if possible.
> Keeping heating ducts clean.
> Keep pet contact to a minimum, or avoid altogether.
> Use allergy control covers on mattresses and pillows.

Allergen avoidance:
> Avoid cigarette smoke.
> Avoid known allergens.

Pharmacologic Treatment and side effects
Compliance

Follow-up
Necessary until regimen that works is found.

Referral
Refer to ENT or allergist, depending on severity of symptoms, and/or treatment response.

SINUSITIS

SIGNAL SYMPTOMS purulent rhinitis, facial pain

ICD-9 Codes	461.9	Acute sinusitis
	473.9	Chronic sinusitis
	478.1	Sinus pain

Sinusitis is an inflammation of the mucous membranes lining the paranasal sinuses. It involves an accumulation of mucus and pus in the sinus cavities.

There are two different types of sinusitis

Acute: abrupt onset, with complete resolution after treatment ($>$10 days, but $<$30 days)

Chronic: episodes of prolonged inflammation and/or repeated (or inadequately treated) infections ($>$30 days)

Epidemiology
Accounts for more than 15 million office visits per year.
More than $2 billion is spent on sinus medications per year.

Etiology
Streptococcus pneumoniae
Haeomophilus influenza
Moraxella catarrhalis (25% of pediatric cases)
Streptococcus species (8% of adult cases)

Staphylococcus aureus (6% of adult cases)
Neisseria specis
Anaerobes (more common in chronic infections)
Gram-negative rods
Viruses
Fungal (immunocompromised/diabetic patients)
Risk factors:
  Upper respiratory infection
  Allergic rhinitis
  Anatomical abnormalities (deviated septum)
  Tonsillar/adenoid hypertrophy
  Cystic fibrosis
  Neoplasms/polyps
  Trauma
  Foreign bodies
  Mechanical ventilation
  Nasogastric tubes

Physiology and Pathophysiology

Lack of effective mucous transport and slowed sinus ventilation (often caused by sinus obstruction) allow for accumulation of organisms, leading to inflammation and infection.

Clinical Manifestations

Subjective

ACUTE

Yellow-green, thick nasal discharge
Congestion
Facial pain under or above the eyes
Increased facial pain when leaning forward
Fever
Sore teeth
Possible cough, often worse at night

CHRONIC

Thick, colored nasal discharge/congestion
Cough lasting longer than 30 days
Headache
Postnasal drip
Halitosis

Objective

Possible fever
Inflamed, boggy nasal mucosa
Mucopurulent rhinorrhea
Frontal and/or maxillary sinus tenderness with palpation
Poor transillumination of sinus cavities

Differential Diagnosis

Upper respiratory infection (cough, rhinitis, congestion, ear pain, fever)
Allergic rhinitis (see "Rhinitis, Allergic," above)
Foreign body/tumors (consider if signs/symptoms persist despite treatment)
Migraine/tension/cluster headache (Refer to Chapter 12, "Nervous System.")
TMJ pain (jaw or ear pain, "clicking")
Dental infection (tooth pain, possible drainage, fever)

Diagnostic Tests

CBC (possibly elevated white-cell count)
Nasal culture (to identify resultant organism)
X-ray examination (reveals air-fluid levels, thickened mucosa, and cloudiness)
Four views:
  Waters' position (often alone gives good diagnostic information)
  Lateral (side) view
  Submentovertex view (under the chin)
  Occipital–mental 30 degrees
CT scans—rule out chronic sinusitis or treatment failures
MRI—rule out tumors

Management/Treatment

Pharmacologic Management

Antibiotics (see Table 4–4)

Decongestants
  Pseudoephedrine, 60–120 mg PO Q12H
Expectorants/mucolytic agents
  Guaifenesin, 600–1200 mg PO Q12H
Topical sprays. *Maximum use:* 3 days to avoid rebound congestion (rhinitis medicamentosa)

Table 4–4 Antibiotics for Sinusitis

Antibiotic	Adult Dose	Pediatric Dose
Amoxicillin (Amoxil/Trimox)	500 mg PO TID × 10 days	40 mg/kg/day PO TID × 10 days
TMP-SMX (Bactrim/Septra)	DS tablet PO BID × 10 days	8/40 mg/kg/day PO BID × 10 days
Amoxicillin plus clavulanate (Augmentin)	500–875 mg PO BID × 10 days (with food)	45 mg/kg/day PO BID × 10 days (with food)
Cefuroxime (Ceftin)	250–500 mg PO BID × 10 days	30 mg/kg/day PO BID × 10 days
Cefprozil (Cefzil)	250–500 mg PO QD-BID × 10 days	7.5–15 mg/kg/day PO BID × 10 days
Ciprofloxacin (Cipro)	500 mg PO BID × 10 days	Not for use in children
Clarithromycin (Biaxin)	500 mg PO BID × 10 days	15 mg/kg/day PO BID × 10 days

Oxymetazoline (Afrin), 2–3 sprays in each nostril Q12H
Phenylephrine (Neo-Synephrine), 2–3 sprays in each nostril Q12H
Nasal corticosteroid sprays
Antihistamines—not recommended for treating sinusitis because they dry nasal secretions. Use only if there are components of severe concurrent allergic rhinitis.
Analgestics/Antipyretics
Tylenol
Ibuprofen

Nonpharmacologic Management
Saline/salt water nasal rinses
Warm/hot compresses to face/nasal area
Humidified air/steam inhalations

Client Education
Finish all of antibiotics, even if feeling better.
Drink plenty of warm/hot fluids, to increase movement of secretions.
Stop smoking.
Avoid known allergens.
Wash hands often and well.

Referral
Refer to ENT if there is treatment failure, periorbital edema, or cellulitis.

TINNITUS

SIGNAL SYMPTOM▶ ringing in ears

ICD-9 Code	388.30	Tinnitus NOS

Tinnitus is a ringing, buzzing, whistling, or hissing noise in one or both ears that is often benign, but it may also signal a more serious underlying disease.

Epidemiology
As many as 50 million Americans experience tinnitus.
Ninety percent of cases have an otologic cause.
Tends to worsen with age.

Etiology
Noise trauma
Toxins
Chronic otitis infections
Excessive cerumen
Perforation of the tympanic membrane
Fluid in the inner ear
Acoustic neuroma
Other medical causes: uncontrolled hypertension, hypercholesterolemia, or hypothyroidism

Physiology and Pathophysiology

Cause is often unknown (idiopathic).

Clinical Manifestations

Subjective

Some medications, such as aspirin, can cause tinnitus.

Ringing or buzzing in one or both ears.

Some hearing loss.

Patients usually present with concurrent frustration, depression, and/or insomnia.

Objective

Complete physical examination of head, ears, nose, mouth, throat, and neck usually shows normal results.

Audiometry testing may reveal some degree of hearing loss.

Differential Diagnosis

Otitis media (ear pain, fever) (Refer to "Otitis media," above.)

Labyrinthitis (dizziness) (Refer to "Dizziness/Vertigo," above.)

Noise exposure (Review patient history.)

Vascular disorders (Review patient history.)

Acoustic neuroma (Consider if sign/symptoms persist despite treatment.)

Transient ischemic attacks or cerebrovascular accident (if cranial-nerve dysfunction or weakness exists)

Diagnostic Tests

Hearing tests (to rule out hearing loss)

Screening laboratory tests (CBC, chemistry panel, thyroid panel, lipid profile to identify underlying acute/chronic conditions)

MRI (to determine structural abnormalities)

Management/Treatment

Pharmacologic Management

If infection exists, treat appropriately.

If obstruction exists, remove.

If hearing loss exists, referral to ENT or audiologist.

No medication exists to "treat" or "cure" tinnitus, but amitryptyline and alprazolam may provide some relief in patients with severe tinnitus.

Nonpharmacologic Management

Use other noises to decrease sensation of tinnitus.

A hearing aid may suppress tinnitus.

Tinnitus "masking" devices may be helpful.

Complementary/Alternative Therapies

Biofeedback, acupuncture, and hypnotherapy may provide some relief, but there is no documented improvement.

Client Education

Discuss causes of tinnitus.

Provide resources.

Reassure that there is no serious underlying condition.

Referral

Refer to ENT if tinnitus is severe.

Refer to ENT or audiologist if concurrent hearing loss exists.

Refer to ENT or neurologist if signs and symptoms persist despite treatment.

REFERENCES

Cerumen Impaction

Sadovsky, R. (2000). Temperature of saline solution for ear irrigation. *American Family Physician, 61,* 192.

Dizziness/Vertigo

Herting, R.L., & Frohberg, N.R. (2000). *University of Iowa Family Practice Handbook* (3rd ed.). St. Louis: Mosby.

Walling, A.D. (2000). How common are various causes of dizziness? *American Family Physician, 62.* 179.

Dysphagia

Ahuja, V., Yencha, M.W., & Lassen, L.F. (1999). Head and neck manifestations of gastroesophageal reflux Disease. *American Family Physician, 60,* 873–886.

Palmer, J.B., Drennan, J.C., & Baba, M. (2000). Evaluation and treatment of swallowing impairments. *American Family Physician, 61,* 2453–2468.

Spieker, M.R. (2000). Evaluating dysphagia. *American Family Physician, 61,* 3639–3653.

Epiglottitis

Wheeler, D.S., Kiefer, M.L., & Poss, W.B. (2000). Pediatric emergency preparedness in the office. *American Family Physician, 61,* 3333–3347.

Hearing Loss

Better Hearing Institute (1998). A physician's guide for identifying hearing loss. Better Hearing Institute. Alexandria, VA.

Kochkin, S. (1997). FAQ about people with hearing loss. Better Hearing Institute. Alexandria, VA.

Leung, A.K.C., & Kao, C.P. (1999). Evaluation and management of the child with speech delay. *American Family Physician, 61,* 2749–2762.

Miller, K.E., Zylstra, R.G., & Standridge, J.B. (2000). The geriatric patient: A systematic approach to maintaining health. *American Family Physician, 61,* 2823–2831.

Rabinowitz, P.M. (2000). Noise-induced hearing loss. *American Family Physician, 61,* 2479–2462.

Smeltzer, C. (1993). Primary care screening and evaluation of hearing loss. *Nurse Practitioner, 18*(8), 50–55.

Zazove, P. (1997). Understanding deaf and hard-of-hearing patients. *American Family Physician, 56,* 1953–1956.

Laryngitis

Rosen, C.A., Anderson, D., & Murry, T. (1998). Evaluating hoarseness: Keeping your patient's voice healthy. *American Family Physician. Vol. 59:* 1571–1582.

Otitis Externa

Daiichi Pharmaceutical (2000). Otitis externa. *Sound Advice, 1*(1), 1–12.

LaRosa, S. (1998). Primary care management of otitis externa. *Nurse Practitioner, 23*(6), 125–133.

Otitis Media (Acute)

Bluestone, C.D. (1998). Otitis media: To treat or not to treat? *Consultant, 38*(6), 1421–1433.

Combs, J.T. (1997). Objective diagnosis of otitis media: Examining a new tool. *Advance for Nurse Practitioners, 5*(12), 50–52.

Dowell, S.F., et al (1999). Acute otitis media: Management and surveillance in an era of pneumococcal resistance. *Nurse Practitioner, 24*(10; Suppl), 1–9.

Dowell, S.F., Schwarts, B., & Phillips, W.R. (1998). Appropriate use of antibiotics for URIs in Children: Part I. Otitis media and acute sinusitis. *American Family Physician, 60.*

Fitzgerald, M.A. (1999). Management of otitis media in an era of drug resistance: Implications for NP practice. *Nurse Practitioner, 24*(10; Suppl), 10–14.

Pichichero, M.E. (2000). Acute otitis media: Part I. Improving diagnostic accuracy. *American Family Physician, 61,* 2051–2056.

Pichichero, M.E. (2000). Acute otitis media: Part II. Treatment in an era of increasing antibiotic resistance. *American Family Physician, 61,* 2410–2416.

Tigges, B.B. (2000). Acute otitis media and pneumococcal resistance: Making judicious management decisions. *Nurse Practitioner, 25*(1), 69–79.

Tully, S.B. (1998). The right angle: Otitis media and infant feeding position. *Advance for Nurse Practitioners, 6*(4), 45–48.

Otitis Media (with Effusion)

American Family Physician (2000). Clinical policy: Otitis media with effusion in young children: Diagnosis and hearing evaluation.therapeutic interventions. *American Family Physician,60.*

American Family Physician (1998). Otitis media with effusion. *American Family Physician, 60.* [Patient Information]

Calandra, L.M. (1998). Otitis media with effusion. *Advance for Nurse Practitioners, 6*(2), 67–70.

Peritonsillar Abscess

Leung, A.K.C., & Cho, H. (1999). Diagnosis of stridor in children. *American Family Physician, 60,* 2289–2300.

Pharyngitis/Tonsillitis

Connaughton, D. (2000). Experts examine common respiratory problems, solutions. *American Family Physician, 62,* 1513–1517.

Dowell, S.F., Schwartz, B., & Phillips, W.R. (1998). Appropriate use of antibiotics for URIs in children: Part II. Cough, pharyngitis and the common cold. *American Family Physician.* [Patient Information]

Ruppert, S.D. (1996) Differential diagnosis of common causes of pediatric pharyngitis. *Nurse Practitioner, 21*(4), 38–47.

Rhinitis, Allergic

Clinical Courier (1999). Expanding opportunities for the nurse practitioner in the management of upper respiratory allergic disease. *Clinical Courier, 17*(14), 1–7.

Kaiser, H.B., Kaliner, M.A., & Slavin, R.G. (1999). Asthma, rhinitis, sinusitis, urticaria. *Patient Care, 33*(1), 115–146.

Kupeca, D. (1999). Managing allergic rhinitis. *Nurse Practitioner, 24*(5), 107–120.

Leccese, C. (1998). Giving the allergic salute an honorable discharge: Diagnosing and treating rhinitis in children. *Advance for Nurse Practitioners, 6*(5), 59–62.

Luskin, A.T., Scherger, J.E., Ledgerwood, G.L., Nuckolls, J.F., & Prenner, B.M. (2000). *Allergic rhinitis: Impact and diagnosis in the primary care setting.* Madison: University of Wisconsin- Medical School.

Luskin, A.T., Scherger, J.E., Ledgerwood, G.L., Nuckolls, J.F., & Prenner, B.M. (2000). Allergic rhinitis: Management and treatment in the primary care setting. Madison: University of Wisconsin Medical School.

Sadovsky, R. (2000). Overview of methods for treating allergic rhinitis. *American Family Physician, 61.*

Sinusitis

Calhoun, K.H. (1997). Chronic rhinosinusitis: Cost-effective work-up, guidelines for treatment. *Consultant,* 3112–3122.

Connaughton, D. (2000). Experts examine common respiratory problems, solutions. *American Family Physician.*

Dowell, S.F., Schwartz, B., & Phillips (1998). Appropriate use of antibiotics for URIs in children: Part I. Otitis media and acute sinusitis. *American Family Physician.*

Duchene, T.M. (2000). Managing sinusitis in children. *Nurse Practitioner, 25*(9), 42–55.

Fagnan, L.J. (1998). Acute sinusitis: A cost-effective approach to diagnosis and treatment. *American Family Physician, 58*(8), 1795–1802.

Kaiser, H.B., Kaliner, M.A., & Slavin, R.G. (1999). Asthma, rhinitis, sinusitis, urticaria. *Patient Care, 33*(1), 115–146.

Sinus and Allergy Health Partnership (2000). Antimicrobial treatment guidelines for acute bacterial rhinosinusitis. *Otolaryngology—Head and Neck Surgery, 123*(1), S1–S32.

RESOURCES

General

American Academy of Otolaryngology, Head and Neck Surgery
1 Prince St.
Alexandria, VA 22314-3357
Telephone: (703) 836-4444
www.entnet.org

American Academy of Pediatrics
www.aap.org

American Speech-Language-Hearing Association
1081 Rockville Pike
Rockville, MD 20852
Telephone: (800) 638-8255 or (301) 897-8682

Center for Voice Disorders of Wake Forest University
www.bgsm.edu/voice/

Virtual Hospital
www.vh.org

Dizziness/Vertigo

Vestibular Disorders Association (VEDA)
> P.O. Box 4467
> Portland, OR 97208-4467
> Telephone: (503) 229-7705 or (800) 837-8428
> E-mail: evda@teleport.com

A support group for persons affected by long-term dizziness:
> http://members.xoom.com/dizzymates/index.html

Information:
> www.cochlea.com

Dysphagia

Dysphagia Resource Center
> www.dysphagia.com

Dysphagia Diet
> www.dysphagia-diet.com/

Hearing Loss

Alexander Graham Bell Association for the Deaf
> 3417 Volta Pl., NW
> Washington, DC 20007
> Telephone: (202) 337-5220

Better Hearing Institute
> Box 1840
> Washington, DC 20013
> Telephone: (703) 642-1580 or (800) EAR-WELL

League for Hard of Hearing
> 71 West 23rd St.
> New York, NY 10010-4162
> Telephone: (917) 305-7700
> www.lhh.org/noise

National Association for the Deaf
> 814 Thayer Ave.
> Silver Spring, MD 20910
> Telephone: (301) 587-1788

Rhinitis, Sinusitis

American Academy of Allergy, Asthma and Immunology
> 611 East Wells St.
> Milwaukee, WI 53202
> Telephone: (800) 822-ASTHMA or (414) 272-6071
> www.aaaai.org

American College of Allergy, Asthma and Immunology
> 85 West Algonquin Rd., Ste. 550
> Arlington Heights, IL 60005
> Telephone: (800) 842-7777 or (847) 427-1200
> www.allergy.mcg.edu

American College of Asthma, Allergy & Immunology
> www.acaai.org

American Rhinologic Society
    c/o Frederick J. Stucker, M.D.
    Dept. of Otolaryngology
    LSU School of Medicine in Shreveport
    1501 Kings Hwy.
    P.O. Box 33932
    Shreveport, LA 71130
    Telephone: (888) 520-9585 or (318) 675-6262

Asthma and Allergy Foundation of America
    1125 15th St., N.W.
    Washington, DC 20005
    Telephone: (800) 7-ASTHMA or (202) 466-7643
    www.aafa.org

National Institutes of Health; National Institute of Allergy and Infectious Diseases
    Bethesda, MD 20892
    www.nih.gov

Tinnitus

American Tinnitus Association
    www.ata.org

Chapter 5

RESPIRATORY DISORDERS

ASTHMA

SIGNAL SYMPTOMS chest tightness, wheezing

ICD-9 Codes	493.0	Extrinsic asthma
	493.1	Intrinsic asthma
	493.2	Chronic obstructive asthma
	493.9	Asthma, unspecified

Asthma is a chronic inflammatory disorder of the airways that involves many cells and cellular elements, in particular, mast cells, eosinophils, T lymphocytes, macrophages, neutrophils, and epithelial cells.

Epidemiology

Approximately 5.8%–7.2% of the population has asthma.

The prevalence is higher in children under 18 years of age.

The prevalence and mortality and hospitalization rates are higher in blacks than in whites.

The prevalence and mortality and hospitalization rates are higher in women than in men.

The cost related to asthma in the United States was $11.3 billion in 1998.

Etiology

Asthma is a complex disorder that involves biochemical, autonomic, immunologic, infectious, endocrine, and psychologic factors.

Physiology and Pathophysiology

Asthma is a chronic inflammatory disorder of the airways characterized by denudation of the airway epithelium, collagen deposition beneath the basement membrane, edema, mast-cell activation, and inflammatory cell infiltration by neutrophils, eosinophils and lymphocytes. Airway inflammation results in airway hyperresponsiveness and airflow limitation, including acute bronchoconstriction, airway edema, mucous plug formation, and airway wall remodeling. In some clients, subbasement membrane fibrosis may lead to persistent abnormalities in respiratory functioning. A variety of mediators secreted by mast cells, eosinophils, epithelial cells, macrophages, and activated T cells contribute to the inflammatory process.

Childhood-onset asthma is frequently associated with atopy, the genetic predisposition for the development of an immunoglobulin E (IgE)–mediated response to common allergens such as house-dust mites, animal proteins, or fungi. IgE antibodies sensitize mast cells and possibly other airway cells, which become activated with subsequent encounters with specific antigens.

Adult-onset asthma may be related to IgE antibodies, but is more likely associated with coexisting sinusitis, nasal polyps, and/or sensitivity to aspirin or other related nonsteroidal antiinflammatory agents. Occupational exposure to a variety of workplace materials also may result in airway inflammation and signs of asthma. Although the inflammatory response is similar in nonallergic, or intrinsic, asthma the underlying mechanisms are not clearly understood.

Bronchoconstriction occurs within minutes and subsides rapidly in extrinsic asthma. However, in some individuals, a late-phase response may develop 4 to 8 hours after the initial episode. Eosinophils predominate, causing increased bronchial inflammation, so that bronchodilator medications are less effective in the treatment of the late reaction.

Exercise-induced bronchospasm is caused by loss of heat, water, or both from the lungs during exercise because of hyperventilation. It occurs within minutes of exercise, peaks 5–10 minutes after stopping, and typically resolves within 20–30 minutes.

Clinical Manifestations

Symptoms are worsened by exercise, viral infection, changes in the weather, strong emotional response, menses, and/or exposure to animals with fur or feathers, dust mites, mold, smoke, pollen, or airborne chemicals or dusts.

Symptoms can be perennial, seasonal, continual, or episodic.

Diurnal variations are found, with symptoms increasing at night or early in the morning.

Subjective

Cough
Wheezing
Shortness of breath
Chest tightness
Sputum
In exercise-induced bronchospasm: cough, shortness of breath, chest pain or tightness, wheezing, or endurance problems associated with exercise.

Objective

Wheezing (may be absent between exacerbations or with mild intermittent asthma)
Absent or diminished respiratory sounds in severe exacerbations
Hyperexpansion of the thorax
Hunched shoulders
Chest deformity

Increased respiratory rate

Use of accessory muscles

Nasal flaring

Prolonged expiration

Mental status changes

Possibly signs of allergies/atopic disease that increase likelihood of asthma: increased nasal section, mucosal swelling, nasal polyps, or atopic dermatitis/eczema

Spirometry (See Table 5–1 for categorization of asthma based on symptoms and lung function.)

Table 5–1   Classification of Asthma Severity*

Classification	Symptoms	Nighttime Symptoms	Lung Function

Step 4
Severe
   persistent
	Continual symptoms
	Limited physical
	   activity
	Frequent
	   exacerbations
		Frequent	FEV_1 or PEF ≤60% of
			   predicted
			PEF variability
			   >30%

Step 3
Moderate
   persistent
	Daily symptoms
	Daily use of inhaled
	   short-acting β_2-
	   agonist
	Exacerbations affect
	   activity
	Exacerbations ≥2
	   times a week; may
	   last days
		>1 time a week	FEV_1 or PEF >60%
			   to <80% predicted
			PEF variability >30%

Step 2
Mild
   persistent
	Symptoms >2 times
	   a week but <1
	   time a day
	Exacerbations may
	   affect activity
		>2 times a month	FEV_1 or PEF ≥80%
			   predicted
			PEF variability 20–30%

Step 1
Mild
   intermittent
	Symptoms ≤2 times
	   a week
	Asymptomatic and
	   normal PEF between
	   exacerbations
	Exacerbations brief
	   (from a few hours
	   to a few days);
	   intensity may vary
		≤2 times a month	FEV_1 or PEF ≥80%
			   predicted
			PEF variability <20%

FEV_1 = forced expiratory volume in 1 second; PEF = peak expiratory flow.

*The presence of one of the features of severity if sufficient to place a patient in that category. An individual should be assigned to the most severe grade in which any feature occurs. The characteristics noted in this table are general and may overlap because asthma is highly variable. Furthermore, an individual's classification may change over time.

†Patients at any level of severity can have mild, moderate or severe exacerbations. Some patients with intermittent asthma experience severe and life-threatening exacerbations separated by long periods of normal lung function and no symptoms.

Source: National Heart, Lung, and Blood Institute (1997). *Guidelines for the diagnosis and management of asthma* (NIH Publication No. 97-4051). Washington, DC: US Department of Health and Human Services.

Differential Diagnosis

All Age Groups

Allergic rhinitis (characterized by recurrent clear, watery nasal discharge, sneezing, pruritus, and pale and boggy nasal mucosa)

Sinusitis (distinguished by purulent nasal discharge, sore throat, fever, facial pain, cough, and erythematous turbinates)

Vocal-cord dysfunction (characterized by chronic cough, weak, breathy voice, and inspiratory or expiratory stridor on exertion)

Gastroesophageal reflex (heartburn and sour taste in mouth along with cough)

Pneumonia (noisy cough, dyspnea, pleuritic chest pain, sputum production, chills, fever, tachypnea, inspiratory crackles, vocal fremitus, bronchophony, and egophony)

Infants and Children

Foreign body in trachea or bronchus (characterized by abrupt onset of coughing, gagging, and choking with unilateral wheezing, decreased air movement, and rhonchi)

Vascular rings or laryngeal webs (characterized by vascular anomalies that may cause stridor and dyspnea in infants; usually soft inspiratory stridor with expiratory wheeze, often accompanied by brassy cough and difficulty swallowing)

Laryngotracheomalacia, tracheal stenosis or bronchostenosis (characterized by onset in the first 4 weeks of life and inspiratory stridor)

Viral bronchiolitis or obliterative bronchiolitis (viral bronchiolitis is usually preceded by 1–2 days of fever, rhinorrhea and cough, followed by wheezing, tachypnea, tachycardia, nasal flaring, retractions, accessory muscle use, and shallow, rapid respirations; wheezes predominant with long expiratory phase)

Cystic fibrosis (distinguished by failure to thrive, chronic productive cough, bulky stools, positive family history, nasal polyps, clubbing of fingers, increased anteroposterior chest diameter, scattered and/or localized course rhonchi)

Bronchopulmonary dysplasia (typically in infants who were premature, had respiratory distress syndrome during neonatal period, or received high concentrations of inspired oxygen; characterized by intermittent bronchospasms, mucous plugging, and pulmonary hypertension)

Heart disease (persistent, nonproductive cough along with failure to thrive; may see cyanosis, tachypnea, hepatomegaly, and murmur)

Adults

Chronic bronchitis (characterized by 3-month history of rasping, hacking, productive cough, possible rhonchi that clear with cough, possible barrel chest, prolonged expiration and possible wheezing)

Congestive heart failure (characterized by cough, frothy sputum, fatigue, weight gain, peripheral edema, paroxysmal nocturnal dyspnea, orthopnea, and palpitations; jugular venous distention, anxiety, tachypnea, crackles, displaced point of maximal impulse [PMI], S3, and S4)

Pulmonary embolism (acute onset cough, dyspnea, mild to severe chest pain, hemoptysis, and diminished breath sounds, crackles, wheezes and pleural friction rub; possible history of deep venous thrombosis [DVT], recent surgery, or oral-contraceptive use)

Mechanical obstruction of the airways such as benign and malignant tumors (characterized by hemoptysis, weight loss, and shortness of breath)

Cough resulting from drugs such as angiotensin-converting–enzyme (ACE) inhibitors (occurs hours to months after starting ACE inhibitor, usually nonproductive, associated with irritating, tickling, or scratching sensation in throat; examination results normal)

Diagnostic Tests

Pulmonary function testing (PFT) (See Table 5–2.) Spirometry measurements before and after inhalation of short-acting bronchodilator recommended. Additional PFTs may be indicated if there are questions about coexisting chronic obstructive pulmonary disease, restrictive deficit, or possible central airway obstruction. Airflow obstruction is indicated by decreased forced expiratory volume in 1 second (FEV_1) or a ratio of FEV_1 to forced vital capacity (FVC) of <70%. Reversibility after administration of a bronchodilator of ≥12% and 200 ml FEV_1 is indicative of asthma.)

Chest x-ray examination (to rule out other diagnoses).

Allergy skin testing (clients with persistent asthma who require daily therapy should be evaluated to rule out possible allergies)

Table 5–2 Pulmonary Function Tests (Spirometry)

Measures	Description
FVC	Maximum amount of gas that can be displaced from the lung during a forced expiration
FEV_1	Maximum amount of air that can be expired from the lung in 1 second
FEV_1/FVC	Percentage of maximum inspiration that is expired in 1 second, usually 80% of FVC
FEV_3	Maximum amount of air that can be expired from the lung in 3 second
FEV_3/FVC	Percentage of maximum inspiration that is expired in 3 second, usually 95% of FVC
$FEF_{25\%-75\%}$	Sometimes reported as maximum mid-expiratory flow rate (MMFR)
Results	
Values over 80%	Normal
Reduced FEV_1 and FEV_1/FVC ratio (< 65%).	Indicative of an obstructive air flow defect
Reduced FVC with normal FEV_1/FVC	Indicative of a restrictive air flow defect

$FEF_{25\%-75\%}$ = forced expiratory flow rate during the middle 50% of expiration; FEV_1 = forced expiratory volume in 1 second; FEV_3 = forced expiratory volume in 3 seconds; FVC = forced vital capacity.

Management/Treatment

Goals

Prevent chronic and troublesome symptoms.

Maintain (near) "normal" pulmonary function.

Maintain normal activity levels (including exercise and other physical activity).

Prevent recurrent exacerbations of asthma and minimize the need for emergency department visits or hospitalizations.

Provide optimal pharmacotherapy, with minimal or no adverse effects.

Meet clients' and families' expectations of and satisfaction with asthma care.

Pharmacologic Management

Inflammation is hypothesized to be an early and persistent aspect of asthma. Therefore, early intervention with antiinflammatory agents may modify the course of the disease.

LONG-TERM-CONTROL MEDICATIONS

These medications are taken daily to achieve and maintain control of persistent asthma. See Table 5–3 for overview of medications, Table 5–4 for usual dosages, and Table 5–5 for comparative doses of corticosteroids.

Corticosteroids

Cromolyn sodium and nedocromil

Long-acting β_2-agonists

Methylxanthines

Leukotriene modifiers. Since publication of the National Heart, Lung, and Blood Institute's guidelines, another leukotriene modifier, montelukast, has been approved. However, the role of leukotriene inhibitors in asthma remains to be established.

QUICK-RELIEF MEDICATIONS

These medications are used to provide prompt relief of bronchoconstriction and the accompanying symptoms of cough, chest tightness, and wheezing. See Table 5–6 for overview of medications, and Table 5–7 for usual dosages.

Short-acting β_2-agonists

Anticholinergics

Systemic corticosteroids

STEPWISE APPROACH

A stepwise approach to pharmacologic therapy is recommended. For adults and children older than 5, see Table 5–8. For children 5 or younger, see Table 5–9.

TREAT ASSOCIATED CONDITIONS

Allergic rhinitis

Gastroesophageal reflux disease

EXERCISE-INDUCED BRONCHOSPASM

Short-acting β_2-agonists used as close as possible to exercise, e.g., albuterol, 2 puffs prior to exercise.

Cromolyn or nedocromil is also effective.

Table 5–3   Long-Term Control Medications for Asthma

Name/ Product	Indications/ Mechanisms	Potential Adverse Effects	Therapeutic Issues
Corticosteroids (Glucocorticoids)			
Inhaled: Beclomethasone dipropionate Budesonide Flunisolide Fluticasone propionate Triamcinolone acetonide	Indications Long-term prevention of symptoms; suppression, control, and reversal of inflammation Reduce need for oral corticosteroids Mechanisms: Antiinflammatory. Block late reaction to allergen and reduce airway hyperrespon-siveness. Inhibit cytokine production, adhesion protein activation, and inflammatory-cell migration and activation Reverse β_2-receptor down-regulation. Inhibit micro-vascular leakage.	Cough, dysphonia, oral candidiasis In high doses, systemic effects may occur, although studies are not conclusive, and clinical significance of these effects has not been established (e.g., adrenal suppression, osteoporosis, growth and suppression, and skin thinning and easy bruising).	Spacer/holder chamber devices and mouth wash-ing after inhalation decrease local side effects and systemic absorption Preparations are not absolutely inter-changeable on a microgram or per-puff basis. New delivery devices may provide greater delivery to airways, which may affect dose. The risks of uncon-trolled asthma should be weighed against the limited risks of inhaled corticosteroids. The potential but small risk of adverse events is well balanced by efficacy. Dexamethasone is not included because it is not highly absorbed and cause side effects from long-term suppression.
Systemic: Methylpred-nisolone Prednisolone Prednisone	Indications For short-term (3–10 days) "burst"; to gain prompt control of inadequately controlled persistent asthma. For long-term prevention of symptoms in severe persistent asthma: suppression, control, and	Short-term use: Reversible, abnormalities in glucose metabolism, increased appetite, fluid retention, weight gain, mood alteration, hypertension, peptic ulcer, and rarely, aseptic necrosis of femur. Long-term use: Adrenal axis suppression, growth suppression,	Use at lowest effective dose. For long-term use, alternate-day am dosing procedures produces least toxicity. If daily doses are required, one study shows improved efficacy with no increase in adrenal suppression when administered at 3 P.M. rather than in the morning.

Table continued on following page.

Table 5–3   Long-Term Control Medications for Asthma (*Continued*)

Name/ Product	Indications/ Mechanisms	Potential Adverse Effects	Therapeutic Issues
	reversal of inflammation. *Mechanisms:* Same as inhaled	dermal thinning, hypertension, diabetes, Cushing's syndrome, cataracts, muscle weakness, and—in rare instances— impaired immune function. Consideration should be given to coexisting conditions that could be worsened by systemic corticosteroids, such as herpes-virus infections, varicella, tuberculosis, hypertension, peptic ulcer and *Strongyloides.*	
Cromolyn Sodium and Nedocromil	*Indications* Long-term prevention of symptoms; may modify inflammation. Preventive treatment prior to exposure to exercise or known allergen. *Mechanisms:* Antiinflammatory. Block early and late reaction to allergen. Interfere with chlor-channel function. Stabilize mast-cell membranes and inhibit activation and release of mediators from eosinophils and epithelial cells. Inhibit acute response to exercise, cold, dry air, and sulfur dioxide	15 to 20% of patients report unpleasant taste from nedocromil.	Therapeutic response to cromolyn and nedocromil often occurs within 2 wk, but a 4- to 6-wk trial may be needed to determine maxi-mum benefit. Dose of cromolyn MDI (1 mg/puff) may be inadequate to affect airway hyperresponsive-ness. Nebulizer delivery (20 mg/ampule) may be preferred for some patients. Safety is the primary advantage of these agents.

Table continued on following page.

Table 5–3   Long-Term Control Medications for Asthma (*Continued*)

Name/ Product	Indications/ Mechanisms	Potential Adverse Effects	Therapeutic Issues
Long-Acting β$_2$-Agonists			
Inhaled: Salmeterol	*Indications* Long-term prevention of symptoms, especially nocturnal symptoms, added to anti-inflammatory therapy. Prevention of exercise-induced bronchospasms. *Not to be used to treat acute symptoms of exacerbations.* *Mechanisms* Bronchodilation: smooth-muscle relaxation following adenylate cyclase activation and increase in cyclic AMP, producing antagonism of bronchoconstriction. In vitro, inhibit mast-cell mediator release, decrease vascular permeability, and increase mucociliary clearance. Compared to short-acting inhaled β$_2$-agonists, salmeterol (but not formoterol) has slower onset of action (15 to 30 min) but longer duration (> 12 hr).	Tachycardia, skeletal muscle tremor, hypokalemia, prolongation of QT$_c$ interval in overdose. A diminished bronchoprotective effect may occur within 1 week of long-term therapy. Clinical significance has not been established.	Not to be used to treat acute symptoms or exacerbations. Clinical significance of potentially developing tolerance is uncertain because studies show symptom control and bronchodilation are maintained. Should not be used in place of antiinflammatory therapy. May provide more effective symptom control when added to standard doses of inhaled corticosteroids.

Table continued on following page.

Table 5–3 Long-Term Control Medications for Asthma (Continued)

Name/Product	Indications/Mechanisms	Potential Adverse Effects	Therapeutic Issues
Oral: Albuterol, sustained-release			Inhaled long-acting β_2-agonists are preferred because they are longer-acting and have fewer side effects than oral sustained-release agents.

Methylxanthines
    Theophylline, sustained-release tablets and capsules
	Indications:
	    Long-term control and prevention of symptoms, especially nocturnal symptoms.
	Mechanisms:
	    Bronchodilation. Smooth-muscle relaxation from phospho-diesterase inhibition and possibly adenosine antagonism. May affect eosinophilic infiltration into bronchial mucosa as well as decrease T-lymphocyte numbers in epithelium. Increase diaphragm contractility and mucociliary clearance.
		Dose-related acute toxicities include tachycardia, nausea, and vomiting, tachyarrhythmias (SVT), central nervous system stimulation, headache, seizures, hematemesis, hyperglycemia, and hypokalemia. Adverse effects at usual therapeutic doses include insomnia, gastric upset, aggravation of ulcer or reflux, increase in hyperactivity in some children, difficulty in urinating in elderly males with prostatism.	Maintain steady-state serum concentrations between 5 and 15 μg/ml. Routine serum concentration monitoring is essential because of significant toxicities, narrow therapeutic range, and individual differences in metabolic clearance.
			Absorption and metabolism may be affected by numerous factors, which can produce significant changes in steady-state serum theophylline concentrations.
			Not generally recommended for exacerbations. There is minimal evidence for added benefit to optimal doses of inhaled β_2 agonists. Serum concentration monitoring is mandatory.

Leukotriene Modifiers			
Zafirlukast tablets	Indications Long-term control and prevention of symptoms of mild persistent asthma for	No specific adverse effects to date. As with any new drug, there is the possibility of rare hypersensitivity or	Administration with meals decreases bioavailability; take at least 1 hr before or 2 hr after meals.

Table continued on following page.

Table 5–3 Long-Term Control Medications for Asthma (Continued)

Name/ Product	Indications/ Mechanisms	Potential Adverse Effects	Therapeutic Issues
	patients ≥ 12 yr of age. *Mechanisms:* Leukotriene (LT) receptor antagonist: selective competitive inhibitor of LTD_4 and LTE_4 receptors.	idiosyncratic reactions that cannot usually be detected in initial premarketing trials. One reported case of reversible hepatitis and hyperbilirubinemia; high concentrations may develop with liver impairment.	Inhibits the metabolism of warfarin and increases prothrombin time; it is a competitive inhibitor of CYP2C9 hepatic microsomal isoenzymes. (It has not affected elimination of terfenadine, theophylline, or ethinyl estradiol, drugs metabolized by CYP3A4 isoenzymes.)
Zileuton tablets	*Indications:* Long-term control and prevention of symptoms of mild persistent asthma for patients ≥ 12 yr of age. *Mechanisms:* 5-Lipoxygenase inhibitor.	Elevation of liver enzymes has been reported. Limited case reports of reversible hepatitis and hyperbilirubinemia.	Zileuton is a microsomal CYP3A4 enzyme inhibitor that can inhibit the metabolism of terfenadine, warfarin, and theophylline. Doses of those drugs should be monitored accordingly. Monitor hepatic enzymes (alanine aminotranferase).

Source: National Heart, Lung, and Blood Institute (1997). *Guidelines for the diagnosis and management of asthma* (NIH Publication No. 97-4051). Washington, DC: US Department of Health and Human Services.

ANNUAL INFLUENZA VACCINATION

Nonpharmacologic Management

ENVIRONMENTAL/ALLERGEN CONTROL MEASURES

Clients who have asthma should not smoke or be exposed to environmental tobacco.

Avoid exertion or exercise outside when levels of air pollution are highest.

Avoid fumes from unvented gas, oil or kerosene stoves, wood-burning appliances, or fireplaces.

Clients who have symptoms associated with eating processed potatoes, shrimp, or dried fruit or drinking wine or beer should avoid these foods.

Nonselective oral or ophthalmologic β-blockers should be avoided

Vacuum once or twice each week to decrease dust. Clients should avoid being in rooms while they are vacuumed. If clients must vacuum, recommend that they wear a dust mask or use a central cleaner with the collecting bag outside of the house or a cleaner fitted with a HEPA filter.

Table 5-4   Usual Dosages for Long-Term-Control Medications

Medication	Dosage Form	Adult Dose	Child Dose	Comments
Systemic Corticosteroids				
Methylprednisolone	Tablets of 2, 4, 8, 16, and 32 mg	7.5–6.0 mg daily in a single dose or QOD as needed for control. Short-course "burst": 40–60 mg/day as single or 2 divided doses for 3–10 days.	0.25–2 mg/kg/day in single dose or QOD as needed for control. Short course "burst": 1–2 mg/kg/day, maximum 60 mg/day, for 3–10 days.	For long-term treatment of severe persistent asthma, administer single dose in morning either daily or on alternate days (alternate-day therapy may produce less adrenal suppression). If daily doses are required, one study suggests improved efficacy and no increase in adrenal suppression when administered at 3:00 P.M. (Beam et al. 1992). Short courses or "bursts" are effective for establishing control when initiating therapy or during a period of gradual deterioration. The burst should be continued until patient achieves 80% PEF personal best or symptoms resolve. This usually requires 3–10 days but may require longer. There is no evidence that tapering the dose after improvement prevents relapse.

Table continued on following page.

Table 5-4 Usual Dosages for Long-Term-Control Medications (*Continued*)

Medication	Dosage Form	Adult Dose	Child Dose	Comments
Prednisolone	5 mg tablets, 5 mg/5 ml, 15 mg/5 ml	See above.	See above.	
Prednisone	Tablets of 1, 2.5, 5, 10, 20, 25 mg; 5 mg/ml, 5 mg/5 ml	See above.	See above.	
Cromolyn and Nedocromil				
Cromolyn	MDI, 1 mg/puff. Nebulizer solution, 20/ mg/ampule.	2–4 puffs TID-QID 1 ampule TID-QID	1–2 puffs TID-QID 1 ampule TID-QID	One dose prior to exercise or allergen exposure provides effective prophylaxis for 1–2 hr
Nedocromil	MDI, 1.75 mg/ puff	2–4 puffs TID-QID	1–2 puffs BID-QID	See Cromolyn above.
Long-Acting β_2-Agonists				
Salmeterol	*Inhaled* MDI, 21 μg/ puff, 60 or 120 puffs. DPI, 50 μg/blister	2 puffs Q12H 1 blister Q12H	1–2 puffs Q12H 1 blister Q12H	May use one dose nightly for symptoms. Should not be used for symptom relief or for exacerbations.
Sustained-release albuterol	*Tablet:* 4 mg tablet	4 mg Q12H	0.3–0.6 mg/ kg/day, not to exceed 8 mg/day	
Methylxanthines				
Theophylline	Liquids, sustained-release tablets, and capsules	Starting dose, 10 mg/kg/ day up to 300 mg maximum; usual maximum, 800 mg/ day	Starting dose 10 mg/kg/ day; usual maximum: <1 year of age: 0.2 (age in weeks) + 5 = mg/kg/ day. ≥1 year of age: 16 mg/kg/ day.	Adjust dosage to achieve serum concentration of 5–15 μg/ml at steady state (at least 48 hr on same dosage). Because of wide interpatient variability in theophylline metabolic clearance, routine monitoring of serum theophylline level is important.

Table continued on following page.

Table 5-4   Usual Dosages for Long-Term-Control Medications (*Continued*)

Medication	Dosage Form	Adult Dose	Child Dose	Comments
Leukotriene Modifiers				
Zafirlukast	20-mg tablet	40 mg daily (1 tablet BID)	10 mg BID for children 7–11 yr old	For zafirlukast, administration with meals decreases bioavailability; take at least 1 hr before or 2 hr after meals.
Zileuton	300-mg tablet, 600-mg tablet	2400 mg daily (two 300-mg tablets or one 600-mg tablet, QID)	Must be greater than or equal to 12 yr old	For zileuton, monitor hepatic enzymes. (alanine aminotrans-ferase).

Source: National Heart, Lung, and Blood Institute (1997). *Guidelines for the diagnosis and management of asthma* (NIH Publication No. 97-4051). Washington, DC: US Department of Health and Human Services.

Table 5–5   Estimated Comparative Daily Dosages for Inhaled Corticosteroids

Drugs	Low Dose	Medium Dose	High Dose
Adults			
Beclomethasone, dipropionate, 42 μg/puff; 84 μg/puff	168–504 μg (4–12 puffs— 42 μg) (2–6 puffs— 84 μg)	504–840 μg (12–20 puffs— 42 μg) (6–10 puffs— 84 μg)	>840 μg (>20 puffs— 42 μg) (>10 puffs— 84 μg)
Budesonide DPI: 200 μg/ dose	200–400 μg (1–2 inhalations)	400–600 μg (2–3 inhalations)	>600 μg (>3 inhalations)
Flunisolide, 250 μg/puff	500–1000 μg (2–4 puffs)	1000–2000 μg (4–8 puffs)	>2000 μg (>8 puffs)
Fluticasone, MDI: 44, 110, 220 μg/puff DPI: 50, 100, 250 μg/ dose	88–264 μg (2–6 puffs—44 μg) OR (2 puffs—110 μg) (2–6 inhalations— 50 μg)	264–660 μg (2–6 puffs—110 μg) (3–6 inhalations— 100 μg)	>660 μg (>6 puffs—110 μg) OR (>3 puffs—220 μg) (>6 inhalations— 110 μg) OR (>2 inhalations— 250 μg)
Triamcinolone acetonide 100 μg/puff	400–1000 μg (4–10 puffs)	1000–2000 μg (10–20 puffs)	>2000 μg (>20 puffs)

Table continued on following page.

Table 5–5 Estimated Comparative Daily Dosages for Inhaled Corticosteroids (*Continued*)

Drugs	Low Dose	Medium Dose	High Dose
Children			
Beclomethasone dipropionate, 42 mcg/puff; 84 mcg/puff	84–336 μg (2–8 puffs–42 μg) (1–4 puffs–84 μg)	336–672 μg (8–16 puffs–42 μg) (4–8 puffs–84 μg)	>672 μg (>16 puffs–42 μg) (>8 puffs–84 μg)
Budesonide DPI: 200 μg/ dose	100–200 μg	200–400 μg (1–2 inhalations– 200 μg)	>400 μg (>2 inhalations– 200 μg)
Flunisolide, 250 mcg/puff	500–750 μg (2–3 puffs)	1000–1250 μg (4–5 puffs)	>1250 μg (>5 puffs)
Fluticasone MDI: 44, 110, 220 μg/puff DPI: 50, 100, 250 μg/ dose	88–176 μg (2–4 puffs–44 μg) (2–4 inhalations– 50 μg)	176–440 μg (4–10 puffs–44 μg) OR (2–4 puffs–110 μg) (2–4 inhalations– 100 μg)	>440 μg (>4 puffs–110 μg) OR (>2 puffs– 220 μg) (>4 inhalations– 100 μg) OR (>2 inhalations– 250 μg)
Triamcinolone acetonide 100 μg/puff	400–800 μg (4–8 puffs)	800–1200 μg (8–12 puffs)	>1200 μg (>12 puffs)

Note: The most important determinant of appropriate dosing is the clinician's judgment of the patient's response to therapy. The clinician must monitor the patient's response on several clinical parameters and adjust the dose accordingly. The stepwise approach to therapy emphasizes that once control of asthma is achieved, the dose of medication should be carefully titrated to the minimum dose required to maintain control, thus reducing the potential for adverse effect.

The reference point for the range in the dosages for children is data on the safety of inhaled corticosteroids in children, which, in general, suggest that the dose ranges are equivalent to beclomethasone dipropionate, 200–400 μg/day (low dose), 400–800 μg/day (medium dose), and >800 μg/day (high dose).

Some dosages may be outside package labeling.

Metered-dose inhaler (MDI) dosages are expressed as the actuator dose (the amount of drug leaving the actuator and delivered to the patient), which is the labeling required in the United States. This is different from the dosage expressed as the valve dose (the amount of drug leaving the valve, all of which is not available to the patient), which is used in many European countries and in some of the scientific literature. Dry powder inhaler (DPI) doses are expressed as the amount of drug in the inhaler after activation.

Source: National Heart, Lung, and Blood Institute (1997). *Guidelines for the diagnosis and management of asthma* (NIH Publication No. 97-4051). Washington, DC: US Department of Health and Human Services.

For animal allergens, remove animals and products made of feathers from home. If unable to remove animal, keep pet out of client's bedroom, keep bedroom door closed, place dense filtering materials over forced air outlets to trap airborne dander, remove upholstered furniture and carpets from the home, and wash the pet weekly.

For house-mite allergen:

Encase mattress in allergen-impermeable cover.

Encase the pillow in an allergen-impermeable cover or wash it weekly.

Wash sheets, blankets, and stuffed toys weekly in water $\geq 130°F$.

Table 5–6 Quick-Relief Medications

Name/Product	Indications/ Mechanisms	Potential Advserse Effects	Therapeutic Issues
Short-Acting Inhaled β₂-agonists			
Albuterol, bitolterol, pirbuterol, terbutaline	*Indications* Relief of acute symptoms; quick-relief medication. Preventive treatment prior to exercise for exercise-induced bronchospasm. *Mechanisms:* Bronchodilation. Smooth-muscle relaxation following adenylate cyclase activation and increase in cyclic AMP producing functional antagonism of broncho-constriction.	Tachycardia, skeletal muscle tremor, hypokalemia, increased lactic acid, headache, hyperglycemia. Inhaled route, in general, causes few systemic adverse effects. Patients with preexisting cardiovascular disease, especially the elderly, may have adverse cardio-vascular reactions with inhaled therapy.	Drug of choice for acute broncho-spasm. Inhaled route has faster onset, fewer adverse effects, and is more effective than systemic routes. The less β_2-selective agents (isoproterenol, metaproterenol, isoetharine, and epinephrine) are not recommended because of their potential for excessive cardiac stimulation, especially in high doses. Albuterol liquid is not recommended. For patients with mild intermittent asthma, regularly scheduled daily use neither harms nor benefits asthma control. Regularly scheduled daily use is not generally recommended. Increasing use or lack of expected effect indicates inadequate control. >1 canister a month (e.g., albuterol has 200 puffs per canister) may indicate overreliance on this drug. $\geq$ 2 canisters in 1 month poses additional adverse risk.

Table continued on following page.

Table 5–6 Quick-Relief Medications (*Continued*)

Name/Product	Indications/ Mechanisms	Potential Advserse Effects	Therapeutic Issues
			For patients who use β_2-agonists frequently, antiinflammatory medication should be initiated or intensified.
Anticholinergics			
Ipratropium bromide	*Indications* Relief of acute bronchospasm. *Mechanism* Bronchodilation. Competitive inhibition of muscarinic cholinergic receptors. Reduces intrinsic vagal tone to the airways. May block reflex broncho-constriction secondary to irritants or to reflux esophagitis. May decrease mucous gland secretion.	Drying of mouth and respiratory secretions, increased wheezing in some individuals, blurred vision if sprayed in eyes.	Reverses only cholinergically mediated bronchospasm; does not modify reaction to antigen. Does not block exercise-induced bronchospasm. May provide additive effects to β_2-agonists but has slower onset of action. Is an alternative for patients with intolerance for β_2-agonists. Treatment of choice for bronchospasm due to β-blocker medication.
Corticosteroids			
Systemic:			
Methylprednisolone, prednisolone, prednisone	*Indications:* For moderate-to-severe exacerbations, to prevent progression of exacerbation, reverse inflammation, speed recovery, and reduce rate of relapse. *Mechanism:* Antiinflammatory.	Short-term use: Reversible, abnormalities in glucose metabolism, increased appetite, fluid retention, weight gain, mood alteration, hyper-tension, peptic ulcer, and rarely, aseptic necrosis of femur. Long-term use: Adrenal axis suppression, growth suppression, dermal thinning, hypertension,	Short-term therapy should continue until patient achieves 80% PEF personal best or symptoms resolve. This usually requires 3-10 days but may require longer. There is no evidence that tapering the dose after improvement prevents relapse.

Table continued on following page.

Table 5–6   Quick-Relief Medications (*Continued*)

Name/Product	Indications/ Mechanisms	Potential Advserse Effects	Therapeutic Issues
		diabetes, Cushing's syndrome, cataracts, muscle weakness, and, in rare instances, impaired immune function. Consideration should be given to coexisting conditions that could be worsened by systemic corticosteroids, such as herpesvirus infections, varicella, tuberculosis, hypertension, peptic ulcer and *Strongyloides*.	

Source: National Heart, Lung, and Blood Institute (1997). *Guidelines for the diagnosis and management of asthma* (NIH Publication No. 97-4051). Washington, DC: US Department of Health and Human Services.

Reduce indoor humidity to less than 50% and do not use humidifiers.
Remove carpets and avoid upholstered furniture.
For cockroach allergen:
Do not leave food or garbage exposed.
Use poison baits, boric acid and traps rather than chemical agents to trap the cockroaches.
Control dampness and fungal growth in home.
Outdoor allergens (tree, grass, weed pollens, seasonal molds):
Keep windows closed and use air conditioning, especially during midday and afternoon.
Conduct outdoor activities shortly after sunrise.
In exercise-induced bronchospasm, a lengthy warm-up period before exercise may preclude use of medication.

Complementary/Alternative Therapies
The effectiveness of many of these therapies has not been documented, so the nurse practitioner should consider safety and possible interactions with other treatments before recommending any of these.

Nutrition: Avoid foods that cause allergies. There is some evidence to support supplementation with ascorbic acid. Essential fatty acids, zinc, and magnesium supplementation has been proposed, but few data support this intervention at this point.

Table 5–7 Usual Dosages for Quick-Relief Medications

Medication	Dosage Form	Adult Dose	Child Dose	Comments
Short-Acting Inhaled β_2-Agonists				
Albuterol Albuterol HFA Bitolterol Pirbuterol Terbutaline	*MDI:* 90 μg/puff, 200 puffs 90 μg/puff, 200 puffs 370 μg/puff, 300 puffs 200 μg/puff, 400 puffs 200 μg/puff, 300 puffs	2 puffs 5 minutes prior to exercise; 2 puffs TID-QID PRN	1–2 puffs 5 minutes prior to exercise; 2 puffs TID-QID PRN	An increasing use or lack of expected effect indicates diminished control of asthma. Not generally recommended for long-term treatment. Regular use on a daily basis indicates the need for additional long-term-control therapy. Differences in potency exist, so that all products are essentially equipotent on a per-puff basis. May double usual dose for mild exacerbations. Nonselective agents (i.e., epinephrine, isoproterenol, metaproterenol) are not recommended because of their potential for excessive cardiac stimulation, especially in high doses.
Albuterol Rotahaler	*DPI:* 200 μg/capsule	1–2 capsules Q4–6H as needed and prior to exercise.	1 capsule Q4–6H as needed and prior to exercise.	
Albuterol	*Nebulizer solution* 0.5 mg/ml (0.5%)	1.25–5 mg (0.25–1 ml) in 2–3 ml of saline Q4–8H	0.05 mg/kg (minimum, 1.25 mg, maximum, 2.5 mg) in 2–3 ml of saline Q4–6H	May mix with cromolyn or ipratropium nebulizer solutions. May double dose for mild exacerbations.

Table continued on following page.

Table 5–7   Usual Dosages for Quick-Relief Medications (*Continued*)

Medication	Dosage Form	Adult Dose	Child Dose	Comments
Bitolterol	2 mg/ml (0.2%)	0.5–3.5 mg (0.25–1 ml) in 2–3 ml of saline Q4–8H	Not established.	May not mix with other nebulizer solutions.
Anticholinergics				
Ipratropium	*MDI:* 18 µg/puff, 200 puffs	2–3 puffs Q6H	1–2 puffs Q6H	Evidence is lacking for anti-cholinergics producing added benefit to β_2-agonists in long-term asthma therapy.
	Nebulizer solution 0.25 mg/ml (0.025%)	0.25 mg Q6H	0.25–0.5 mg Q6H	Evidence is lacking for anti-cholinergics producing added benefit to β_2-agonists in long-term asthma therapy.
Systemic Corticosteroids				
Methylpred-nisolone	Tablets of 2, 4, 8, 16, and 32 mg	Short course "burst": 40–60 mg/day as single or 2 divided doses for 3–10 days	Short course "burst": 1–2 mg/kg/day, maximum 60 mg/day, for 3–10 days	Short courses or "bursts" are effective for establishing control when initiating therapy or during a period of gradual deterioration. The burst should be continued until patient achieves 80% PEF personal best or symptoms resolve. This usually requires 3–10 days but may require longer. There is no evidence that tapering the dose after improvement prevents relapse.
Prednisolone	5 mg tablets, 5 mg/5 ml, 15 mg/5 ml	As above.	As above.	As above.

Table continued on following page.

Table 5–7 Usual Dosages for Quick-Relief Medications (*Continued*)

Medication	Dosage Form	Adult Dose	Child Dose	Comments
Prednisone	Tablets of 1, 2.5, 5, 10, 20, 25 mg; 5 mg/ml, 5 mg/5 ml	As above.	As above.	As above.

Source: National Heart, Lung, and Blood Institute (1997). *Guidelines for the diagnosis and management of asthma* (NIH Publication No. 97-4051). Washington, DC: US Department of Health and Human Services.

Botanicals: Many European, American, Chinese, Japanese, and Indian herbs have been used (e.g., Ma huang (ephedra), Gingko biloba, ginseng, and licorice). Some of these have been found to have a positive impact on pulmonary functioning in asthma. Need to be knowledgeable about these herbs and to consult with reputable herbalist.

Massage: One small study found that massage improved pulmonary function in children with asthma.

Biofeedback: May have some role in asthma treatment, although some relaxation therapies may have adverse effects in some patients with asthma (e.g., relaxation-induced bronchoconstriction).

Hypnosis: May have a role in asthma treatment.

Client Education

BASIC PRINCIPLES OF SUCCESSFUL ASTHMA EDUCATION

Education begins at diagnosis and is a regular part of asthma care.

Includes all members of the team, including the client and family, nurses, physicians, pharmacists, and respiratory therapists.

Tailor the approach to the unique needs of the client and family.

Jointly develop treatment goals.

Use written materials.

COMPONENTS OF ASTHMA EDUCATION

Basic facts about asthma

Role of medications for long-term control and quick-relief

SKILLS

Use of inhaler/spacer/holding chamber.

Symptom monitoring.

How to monitor peak flows:

Use if the client has moderate-to-severe persistent asthma.

Use to establish personal best (2–3 weeks of recording PEF 2–4 times per day).

Use in acute exacerbations to determine severity and to guide treatment decisions.

Table 5-8   Stepwise Treatment Approach for Managing Asthma in Adults and Children Older than 5 years of Age

Step	Long-Term Control	Quick Relief	Education
Step 4: Severe persistent	*Daily Medications:* Antiinflammatory: inhaled corticosteroid (high dose) AND Long-acting bronchodilator: either long-acting inhaled β_2-agonist, sustained-release theophylline, or long-acting β_2-agonist tablets AND Corticosteroid tablets or syrup long-term (make repeat attempts to reduce systemic steroids and maintain control with high-dose inhaled steroids).	Short-acting bronchodilator: inhaled β_2-agonists as needed for symptoms. Intensity of treatment will depend on severity of exacerbation; see component 3— Managing Exacerbations. Use of short-acting inhaled β_2-agonists on a daily basis, or increasing use, indicates the need for additional long-term-control therapy.	Steps 2 and 3 actions plus: Refer to individual education/ counseling.
Step 3: Moderate Persistent	*Daily Medication:* Either Antiinflammatory: inhaled corticosteroid (medium dose) OR Inhaled corticosteroid (low-medium dose) and add a long-acting bronchodilator, especially for nighttime symptoms; either long-acting inhaled β_2-agonist, sustained-release theophylline or long-acting β_2-agonist tablets. If needed: Antiinflammatory: inhaled corticosteroids (medium-high dose) AND Long-acting bronchodilator, especially for nighttime symptoms; either long-acting inhaled	Short-acting bronchodilator: inhaled β_2-agonists as needed for symptoms. Intensity of treatment will depend on severity of exacerbation; see component 3— Managing Exacerbations. Use of short-acting inhaled β_2-agonists on a daily basis, or increasing use, indicates the need for additional long term-control therapy.	Step 1 actions plus: Teach self-monitoring. Refer to group education if available. Review and update self-care plan.

Table continued on following page.

Table 5-8 Stepwise Approach for Managing Asthma in Adults and Children Older than 5 years of Age: Treatment (*Continued*)

Step	Long-Term Control	Quick Relief	Education
	β_2-agonist, sustained-release theophylline, or long-acting β_2-agonist tablets.		
Step 2: Mild Persistent	*One daily medication:* Antiinflammatory: either inhaled corticosteroid (low dose) or cromolyn or nedocromil (children usually begin with a trial of cromolyn or nedocromil). Sustained-release theophylline to serum concentration of 5–15 μg/ml is an alternative, but not preferred, therapy. Zafirlukast or zileuton may also be considered for patients ≥ 12 yr of age, although their position in therapy is not fully established.	Short-acting bronchodilator: inhaled β_2-agonists as needed for symptoms. Intensity of treatment will depend on severity of exacerbation; see component 3—Managing Exacerbations. Use of short-acting inhaled β_2-agonists on a daily basis, or increasing use, indicates the need for additional long-term-control therapy.	Step 1 actions plus: Teach self-monitoring. Refer to group education if available. Review and update self-care plan.
Step 1 Mild Intermittent	No daily medication needed.	Short-acting bronchodilator: inhaled β_2-agonists as needed for symptoms. Intensity of treatment will depend on severity of exacerbation; see component 3—Managing Exacerbations. Use of short-acting inhaled β_2-agonists more than 2 times a week may indicate the need to initiate long-term-control therapy.	Teach basic facts about asthma. Teach inhaler/spacer/holding chamber technique. Discuss roles of medications. Develop self-care plan. Develop action plan for when and how to take rescue actions, especially for patients with a history of severe exacerbations. Discuss appropriate environmental control measures to avoid exposure to known allergens and irritants (See component 4.)

Table continued on following page.

Table 5-8 Stepwise Approach for Managing Asthma in Adults and Children Older than 5 years of Age: Treatment (*Continued*)

Step down: Review treatment every 1 to 6 months; a gradual stepwise reduction in treatment may be possible.

Step up: If control is not maintained, consider step up. First, review patient medication technique, adherence, and environmental control (avoidance of allergens or other factors that contribute to asthma severity).

Note: The stepwise approach presents general guidelines to assist in clinical decision making; it is not intended to be a specific prescription. Asthma is highly variable; clinicians should tailor specific medication plans to the needs and circumstances of individual patients.

Gain control as quickly as possible; then decrease treatment to the least medication necessary to maintain control. Gaining control may be accomplished by either starting treatment at the step most appropriate to the initial severity of the condition or starting at a higher level of therapy (e.g., a course of systemic corticosteroids or higher dose of inhaled corticosteroids).

A rescue course of systemic corticosteroids may be needed at any time and at any step.

Some patients with intermittent asthma experience severe and life-threatening exacerbations separated by long periods of normal lung function and no symptoms. This may be especially common with exacerbations provoked by respiratory infections. A short course of systemic corticosteroids is recommended.

At each step, patients should control their environment to avoid or control factors that make their asthma worse (e.g., allergens, irritants); this requires specific diagnosis and education. Referral to an asthma specialist for consultation or comanagement is recommended if there are difficulties achieving or maintaining control of asthma or if the patient requires step 4 care. Referral may be considered if the patient requires step 3 care.

Source: National Heart, Lung, and Blood Institute (1997). *Guidelines for the diagnosis and management of asthma* (NIH Publication No. 97-4051). Washington, DC: US Department of Health and Human Services.

If using daily PEF monitoring, should measure in morning, before taking bronchodilator.

Minimize or eliminate environmental triggers (see "Nonpharmalogic Management" above).

Adult clients with severe persistence asthma, nasal polyps, or a history of sensitivity to aspirin or nonsteroidal antiinflammatory drugs should be counseled to avoid these drugs.

WHEN AND HOW TO TAKE RESCUE ACTIONS

How to recognize symptom patterns that indicate poor asthma control.

Measures to take to improve respiratory functioning.

Follow-up

Regular follow-up visits are essential and should be scheduled every 1–6 months, although the timing of follow-up visits depends on the severity of the initial exacerbation (anywhere from 1 day to several weeks).

Referral

Referral and/or consultation with an allergist or pulmonologist is indicated for the following:

Life-threatening exacerbation of asthma

Not meeting goals of asthma therapy after 3–6 months of treatment

Table 5–9 Stepwise Approach for Treating Infants and Young Children (5 years of Age and Younger) with Acute or Chronic Asthma Symptoms

Step	Long-Term Control	Quick Relief
Step 4: Severe persistent	Daily antiinflammatory medicine. High-dose inhaled corticosteroid with spacer/holding chamber and face mask. If needed, add systemic cortico-steroids 2 mg/kg/day and reduce to lowest daily or alternate-day dose that stabilizes symptoms.	Bronchodilator as needed for symptoms (see step 1) up to 3 times a day
Step 3: Moderate persistent	Daily antiinflammatory medication. Either: Medium-dose inhaled corticosteroid with spacer/ holding chamber and face mask OR Once control is established: Medium-dose inhaled corticosteroid and nedocromil OR Medium-dose inhaled corticosteroid and long-acting bronchodilator (theophylline).	Bronchodilator as needed for symptoms (see step 1) up to 3 times a day
Step 2: Mild persistent	Daily antiinflammatory medication. Either: Cromolyn (nebulizer is preferred; or MDI or nedocromil (MDI only) Infants and young children usually begin with a trial of cromolyn or nedocromil OR Low-dose inhaled corticosteroid with spacer/holding chamber and face mask.	Bronchodilator as needed for symptoms (see step 1)
Step 1: Mild intermittent	No daily medication needed.	Bronchodilator as needed for symptoms more than 2 times a week. Intensity of treatment will depend on severity of exacerbation (see component 3—Managing Exacerbations). Either: Inhaled short-acting β_2-agonist by nebulizer or face mask and spacer/holding chamber OR Oral β_2-agonist for symptoms with viral respiratory infection. Bronchodilator Q4–6H up to 24 hr (longer with physician consult) but, in general, repeat no more than once every 6 wk Consider systemic corticosteroid if: Current exacerbation is severe OR Patient has history of previous severe exacerbations

Table continued on following page.

Table 5–9 Stepwise Approach for Managing Infants and Young Children (5 years of Age and Younger) with Acute or Chronic Asthma Symptoms (*Continued*)

Step down: Review treatment every 1 to 6 months. If control is sustained for at least 3 months, a gradual stepwise reduction in treatment may be possible

Step up: If control is not maintained, consider step up. But first: review patient medication technique, adherence, and environmental control (avoidance of allergens or other precipitant factors).

Note: The stepwise approach presents general guidelines to assist in clinical decision making. Asthma is highly variable; clinicians should tailor specific medication plans to the needs and circumstances of individual patients.

Gain control as quickly as possible; then decrease treatment to the least medication necessary to maintain control. Gaining control may be accomplished by either starting treatment at the step most appropriate to the initial severity of the condition or starting at a higher level of therapy (e.g., a course of systemic corticosteroids or higher dose of inhaled corticosteroids).

A rescue course of systemic corticosteroids (prednisolone) may be needed at any time and step.

In general, use of short-acting β_2-agonist on a daily basis indicates the need for additional long-term-control therapy.

It is important to remember that there are very few studies on asthma therapy for infants.

Consultation with an asthma specialist is recommended for patients with moderate or severe persistent asthma in this age group. Consultation should be considered for all patients with mild persistent asthma.

Source: National Heart, Lung, and Blood Institute (1997). *Guidelines for the diagnosis and management of asthma* (NIH Publication No. 97-4051). Washington, DC: US Department of Health and Human Services.

Atypical signs and symptoms

Other conditions complicating asthma and/or its diagnosis (e.g., sinusitis, nasal polyps, aspergillosis, severe rhinitis, vocal-cord dysfunction, gastroesophageal reflux, or chronic obstructive pulmonary disease)

Additional diagnostic testing indicated (e.g., allergy skin testing, rhinoscopy, complete pulmonary function testing, provocative challenge, or bronchoscopy)

Immunotherapy needed

Severe persistent asthma, requiring step 4 care

Continuous oral corticosteroid therapy, high-dose inhaled corticosteroids, or more than two bursts of oral corticosteroids required in 1 year

Under age 3 and requires step 3 or 4 care (Referral should be considered if client is under age 3 and step 2 care of long-term daily therapy is being considered.)

Occupational or environmental inhalant or ingested substance thought to be provoking or contributing to the asthma

BRONCHIOLITIS

SIGNAL SYMPTOMS ▶ cough, rhinorrhea, dyspnea

| ICD-9 Code | 466.1 | Bronchiolitis |

Bronchiolitis is an inflammatory obstruction of the bronchioles caused by infection or in response to toxic fumes.

Epidemiology

Most common in infants and children (usually in infants 2–6 months, although it can occur in children up to 2 years of age).

Approximately 50% of infants will become infected with respiratory syncytial virus (RSV) in first year of life.

Reinfection is common, but subsequent infections are usually less severe.

Outbreaks of RSV usually occur annually during the late fall, winter, or early spring months.

RSV is spread through close contact with respiratory secretions or contaminated surfaces or objects.

Risk factors for severe RSV bronchiolitis include prematurity, low socioeconomic status, congenital heart disease, chronic lung disease, immunodeficiency and immunosuppressive therapy, age younger than 2 months, inborn errors of metabolism, and neuromuscular disease or impairment.

Etiology

Infectious, although can also be caused by exposure to noxious agents.

Usually viral, with RSV as the most common pathogen.

Other pathogens include parainfluenzaviruses and influenzaviruses, adenovirus, *Mycoplasma, Chlamydia, Ureaplasma,* and *Pneumocystis.*

Bronchiolitis obliterans does occur in adults and is related to toxic fumes or as a late response to mycoplasmal or viral lung infection.

Idiopathic bronchiolitis obliterans with organizing pneumonia (BOOP) is an idiopathic disorder that affects men and women, usually between the ages of 50 and 70.

Physiology and Pathophysiology

The bronchoalveolar epithelium is targeted by the microorganisms, leading to cell necrosis; bronchial infiltration of lymphocytes, plasma cells, and macrophages; and submucosal edema. Partial or complete airway obstruction results from mucous plugging and edema. Atelectasis and/or hyperinflation may be found.

Clinical Manifestations

Manifestations can range from very mild to life threatening disease.

Subjective

RSV bronchiolitis.

Usually begins with rhinorrhea and cough for 2–3 days.

Cough.

Can progress to severe illness with decreased oral intake, profuse rhinorrhea, lethargy, wheezing, and respiratory distress.

Fever is more common with concurrent otitis media.

Bronchiolitis obliterans.

Cough.

Dypsnea.

Objective

RSV bronchiolitis
Intercostal and subcostal retractions
Nasal flaring
Increased anteroposterior diameter of the chest
High-pitched and polyphonic wheezing
Fine crackles on inspiration.
Palpable spleen and liver because of chest hyperinflation
Bronchiolitis obliterans
Crackles on auscultation

Differential Diagnosis

Asthma (can be hard to differentiate; positive family history of atopy, dramatic improvement in symptoms with bronchodilators, episodic symptoms related to allergen exposure, and usually no crackles)
Bronchitis (dry hacking nonproductive paroxysmal cough; breath sounds usually normal, although wheezing and rhonchi can be heard)
Pneumonia (abrupt onset of fever and respiratory distress; localized dull percussion, crackles, and egophony or bronchophony present)
Croup/bacterial tracheitis (inspiratory stridor and barking cough)
Tracheomalacia and other anatomic abnormalities (continuous symptoms)
Gastroesophageal reflux (usually chronic symptoms)
Aspiration of foreign body (usually abrupt onset of unilateral wheezing)
Cystic fibrosis (usually associated with failure to thrive, chronic cough, bulky bowel movements, and malabsorption)

Diagnostic Tests

Chest x-ray examination (can be done if needed to aid in diagnosis)
Viral culture (the gold standard for diagnosis of RSV, but expensive)
RSV nasopharyngeal swab using rapid antigen test (to rule out RSV)
White-cell count (may be elevated)
Arterial blood gas sampling and/or pulse oximetry (can be used to assess the severity of the disease)

Management/Treatment

Most infants and children can be treated at home, although some will require hospitalization.

Pharmacologic Management

Bronchodilators (Use of bronchodilators is controversial without adequate efficacy data, but bronchodilators are usually recommended based on the individual client.)
β_2-agonists
Epinephrine
Corticosteroids (often used empirically but few data support their use)
Antibiotics (risk of secondary infection low, but dual infection should be considered if client presents with atypical clinical signs such as high fever or pleural effusions)

Ribavirin (Virazole) (should be considered in severely ill patients with PaO_2 of <90%, clients on mechanical ventilation, or in clients with underlying congenital heart disease or chronic lung disease)

Nonpharmacologic Management
Hydration and fluids
Adequate nutrition
Oxygen
Rest

Complementary/Alternative Therapies
Vitamin A therapy 12,500 to 25,000 IU has been recommended.

Client Education
Signs and symptoms of worsening illness, respiratory distress, and dehydration
Typical course of bronchiolitis
Strategies to decrease transmission
Use of bulb syringe
Ways to prevent repeat infections

Follow-up
Close follow-up needed after the initial diagnosis
Telephone calls and return visits within 24 hours recommended
Also may be warranted to follow-up within 10–14 days to evaluate resolution
Prevention: RSV immunoglobulin has been approved for prevention of RSV in high-risk populations (e.g., premature infants with chronic pulmonary disease)

Referral
The following criteria are for referral and/or hospital admission for infants/children with RSV:

Oxygen saturation <93% on room air
Any significant underlying illness such as bronchopulmonary dysplasia or immunosuppression
Any history of previous need for intubation with wheezing
Age <3 months
Retractions or tachypnea
Toxic appearance, dehydration, or tachycardia out of proportion to fever
Recent history of apnea or cyanosis
Social situation that makes follow-up or adequate home care unlikely
Consultation/referral recommended if bronchiolitis obliterans suspected

BRONCHITIS, ACUTE

SIGNAL SYMPTOM productive cough

| ICD-9 Code | 466.0 | Acute bronchitis |

Acute bronchitis is a generalized inflammation of the tracheobronchial tree, usually as a result of infection.

Epidemiology

Responsible for over 3 million physicians visits per year
Incidence rate of approximately 3.2 cases per 100 persons
Affects all age groups
Generally more common during winter months

Etiology

Usually infectious, with viral agents accounting for the majority of cases, but with the specific agent often unknown.
Organisms considered likely causes include influenza A and B, adenovirus, parainfluenzavirus, coronavirus, respiratory syncytial virus, coxsackievirus A21, *Bordetella pertussis, Mycoplasma pneumoniae,* and *Chlamydia pneumoniae.*
Noninfectious irritants (smoke, dust or common environmental pollutants) may also play a role.

Physiology and Pathophysiology

Acute bronchitis results in transitory inflammatory changes to the mucous membranes of the tracheobronchial tree. Bronchial edema and mucus formation lead to productive cough and signs of bronchial obstruction, such as wheezing or shortness of breath. Destruction of the bronchial epithelium is generally mild; however, it can be extensive with *M. pneumoniae* and influenzaviruses. Irritants such as smoking can worsen the severity of the infection.

Clinical Manifestations

Subjective

Hallmark symptom is cough
Clear or purulent sputum
Afebrile
Occasional wheezing
Substernal chest pain with increased cough and shortness of breath

Objective

Often normal
May find wheezing, rhonchi, and/or prolonged expiratory phase

Differential Diagnosis

Asthma (acute onset may be similar; suspect asthma in recurrent bronchitis and/or family history of atopy)
Chronic bronchitis (chronic cough with sputum production for a minimum of 3 months; usually associated with smoking)
Sinusitis (postnasal drip, headache, tooth pain, and tenderness over the sinuses)
Common cold (clear nasal discharge and cough, but no evidence of bronchial wheezing)

Pneumonia (can be difficult to differentiate; pneumonia often presents with abrupt onset of fever, chills, pleuritic chest pain, and rusty/bloody sputum; usually find crackles and respiratory rate greater than 20)

Croup (barking cough following viral upper respiratory infection [URI])

Pertussis (paroxysms of cough associated with characteristic inspiratory whoop)

Congestive heart failure (basilar crackles, orthopnea, signs of cardiomegaly, S3 gallop, and tachycardia)

Reflux esophagitis (heartburn and intermittent symptoms when lying down)

Bronchogenic tumor (constitutional symptoms such as weight loss with cough chronic and sometimes hemoptysis)

Other aspiration syndromes (usually a precipitating event such as smoke inhalation or vomiting; decreased level of consciousness)

Diagnostic Tests

Usually none indicated for acute bronchitis

Chest x-ray examination (if diagnosis unclear, to rule out pneumonia)

Pulmonary-function tests (not indicated in otherwise healthy adult, unless asthma is suspected)

Nasopharyngeal cultures (to rule out *Bordetella pertussis* or influenza)

Management/Treatment

Therapy is aimed at relieving the symptoms.

Pharmacologic Management

Antibiotics: Although frequently prescribed, they do not have a role in the treatment of acute bronchitis except in a few select cases. A recent meta-analysis of antibiotic treatment of acute bronchitis found no significant improvement in outcomes for those treated with antibiotics. Antibiotics are appropriate if *B. pertussis* is suspected and there is concern about possible transmission to nonimmune children and infants. Drug of choice is erythromycin (500 mg every 6 hours for 10–14 days for adults; 30–50 mg/kg per day in 3–4 divided doses for infants/children).

Bronchodilators: Albuterol 2 puffs QID is recommended (oral albuterol has been used in acute bronchitis and is cheaper, but is associated with more tremor, especially when used at 4 mg per dose. Leiner (1997) recommends albuterol, 2 mg PO TID to QID).

Antitussives/expectorants: Guaifenesin is often used, although its effectiveness is questionable. Dextromethorphan or codeine can help control cough and induce sleep.

Nonpharmacologic Management

Increase fluids, humidify air.

Rest.

Avoid smoking and/or exposure to smoke.

Client Education

Stop smoking, if client a smoker.

Most bronchitis is viral, so antibiotics are not necessary.

Alert clinician to symptoms of worsening illness.

Avoid antihistamines.

Teach how to use inhaler, if prescribed.

Follow-up

No follow-up needed unless client's symptoms have not resolved.

If cough continues beyond 3 weeks, consider further workup.

Referral

Consider referral/consultation for clients who are in acute respiratory distress, elderly clients, and clients with underlying chronic lung disease.

CHRONIC OBSTRUCTIVE PULMONARY DISEASE

SIGNAL SYMPTOMS ► dyspnea, shortness of breath, cough

ICD-9 Codes	491	Chronic bronchitis
	492	Emphysema
	493.2	Chronic obstructive disease with asthma

Chronic obstructive pulmonary disease (COPD) is characterized by chronic progressive alterations in expiratory flow and is caused by chronic bronchitis and emphysema. Clients with unremitting asthma also are classified as having COPD. Chronic bronchitis is defined by the presence of a productive cough for at least 3 months per year for 2 consecutive years. Abnormal airspace enlargement and destruction of the alveolar walls characterize emphysema.

Epidemiology

Approximately 14 million people in the United States have COPD; this incidence has increased by 42% since 1982.

It is the 4th leading cause of death in the United States.

Usually affects both men and women in fifth or sixth decade of life.

Most important risk factor for COPD is cigarette smoking.

Other risk factors include occupational exposure to tobacco, and α_1-antitrypsin deficiency.

Air pollution, childhood exposure to smoke, alcohol, and hyperreactive airways may also increase risk.

Etiology

Results from chronic irritation from cigarette smoking.

Primary emphysema, which accounts for only about 1%–2% of cases of COPD, results from an inherited deficiency of the enzyme α_1-antitrypsin.

Physiology and Pathophysiology

Inflammation and enlargement of mucus-secreting glands and goblet cells of the central airways characterize chronic bronchitis. Mucus is thicker and more tenacious. Ciliary function is also impaired and this, in combination with increased mucus production, increases susceptibility to pulmonary infection. Inflammation continues and increases with chronic infection and injury. Over time, not only are the larger airways involved, but eventually all airways are involved. The thick mucus and hypertrophied bronchial smooth muscle obstruct the airways, leading to closure, collapse, and airway trapping.

In emphysema, obstruction results from changes in the lung tissues, not from increased mucus production, as in chronic bronchitis. It starts with destruction of the alveolar walls, which increases air in the acinus. Elastic recoil is lost, making it more difficult to expire air passively. Hyperinflation of alveoli causes large air spaces called bullae and/or blebs, which are air spaces next to the pleura.

Clinical Manifestations

Subjective

Progressive exertional dyspnea.

Productive cough of mucoid sputum.

Intermittent acute chest illnesses characterized by cough, purulent sputum, wheezing, increased dyspnea, and occasional fever.

Later the exacerbations become more frequent, and cyanosis, morning headache, weight loss, and hemoptysis may develop.

Objective

Wheezes with forced expiration initially but progressing to diminished breath sounds and coarse crackles in the bases

Enlarged anteroposterior diameter

Prolonged expiratory phase, accessory muscle use

Pursed lip breathing

Forced contractions of the abdominal muscles

Leaning forward posture to relieve dyspnea

Diagnosis/Initial Impression

Pulmonary embolism (acute onset of pleuritic chest pain, dyspnea, hemoptysis, tachycardia, tachypnea, diminished breath sounds, crackles and wheezes; often associated with history of DVT, recent surgery, trauma or oral-contraceptive use)

Congestive heart failure (chronic progressive dyspnea, cough, frothy sputum, fatigue, weight gain, ankle edema, paroxysmal nocturnal dyspnea or orthopnea, jugular venous distention, tachypnea, use of accessory muscles, crackles, wheezes, displaced PMI, S3, S4, and liver enlargement)

Acute bronchitis (loose hacking cough typically preceded by URI; cough can become productive; low-grade fever, coarse to fine crackles or lung examination normal; symptoms present less than 3 months)

Asthma (cough, dyspnea, wheezing, tachypnea, use of accessory muscles, decreased vocal fremitus, diminished breath sounds, and inspiratory and expiratory wheezes; often associated with history of atopy)

Atelectasis (dyspnea, tachypnea, tachycardia, diminished chest-wall movement, absent or diminished breath sounds, cyanosis and intercostal retractions; fever and other signs of infection may develop)

Lung cancer (Chest pain, shortness of breath, hemoptysis, and cough in smoker; physical examination may be normal, although can find localized diminished breath sounds or dullness.)

Diagnostic Tests

Pulmonary-function tests are critical. The other tests should be done as indicated by individual case.

Spirometry: Early identification of COPD can be beneficial. The National Lung Health Education Program recommends that all smokers ≥ 45 and any client with cough, dyspnea, or wheeze should have spirometric measurements done to determine a base-line measurement and serially, if smoking cessation is not achieved and/or symptoms persist.)

FEV_1 >50%: Stage I Moderate

FEV_1 35%–49%: Stage II Severe

FEV_1 <34%: Stage III Very Severe

Chest x-ray examination (to rule out pneumonia)

α_1-Protease inhibitor deficiency testing (for clients 45 years of age or younger) (to rule out α_1-protease inhibitor deficiency)

Arterial blood gases/pulse oximetry (to rule out acidosis/alkalosis)

Electrocardiography (to rule out cardiac disease or advanced COPD)

Complete blood count (CBC) (to rule out infection)

Comprehensive metabolic panel (to rule out electrolyte imbalance)

Management/Treatment

Pharmacologic Management

Medications are for symptom control; they do not alter the course of COPD. See Table 5–10 for a stepwise approach to pharmacologic management of COPD.

β_2-agonists: A variety of inhaled agents are available: albuterol, bitolterol, isoetharine, metaproterenol, pirbuterol, salmeterol, and terbutaline. Albuterol, metaproterenol, and terbutaline are available orally. Cause less bronchodilation than in asthma. Older clients may be less tolerant of side effects of these medications and may be unable to use MDIs. A spacer may help facilitate inhalation of the drug.

Anticholinergic therapy: Once persistent symptoms are experienced, ipratropium MDI is recommended. It is available as an inhaler and as a solution for nebulization.

Theophylline therapy: This is a third-line agent for COPD.

Corticosteroids: In contrast to efficacy in asthma, steroids have not been found to have a significant role in the routine treatment of COPD. Can be useful in treating symptoms in some patients.

Mucokinetic agents: Use is not strongly supported. Potassium iodide has been used as an expectorant but has associated risks. Guaifenesin has been used, but there is little support for this. N-acetylcysteine (Mucomyst) can be inhaled via nebulization.

α_1-Antitrypsin replacement: If appropriate.

TABLE 5–10 **Step-wise to Approach Pharmacologic Management of COPD**

Step	Pharmacologic Management
1: Mild variable symptoms	Select β_2-agonist MDI aerosol, 1–2 puffs Q2–6H PRN (not to exceed 8 to 12 puffs/24 hr) OR Long-acting β_2-agonist, 2 puffs Q12H
2: Mild to moderate continuing symptoms	Ipratropium MDI aerosol, 2–6 puffs Q6–8H (not to be used more frequently) PLUS Selective β-agonist MDI aerosol, 1–4 puffs QID PRN (for rapid relief, when needed, or as regular supplement
3: Mild to moderate increase in symptoms (response to step 2 is unsatisfactory)	ADD Sustained-released theophylline sustained-released, 200–400 mg BID or 400–800 mg HS for nocturnal bronchospasm AND/OR Consider albuterol sustained-release, 4–8 mg BID or at night only AND/OR Consider mucokinetic agent
4: Suboptimal Control of Symptoms	Consider oral steroids (e.g., prednisone) up to 40 mg/day for 10 to 14 days. If no improvement occurs, wean down to low daily or alternate-day dosing, e.g., 7.5 mg. If no improvement occurs, stop abruptly. If steroid appears to help, consider possible use of aerosol MDI, particularly if patient has evidence of bronchial hyperreactivity.
5: Severe exacerbation	Increase β_2-agonist dosage, e.g., MDI with spacer, 6–8 puffs Q½–2H OR Inhalant solution, unit dose Q½–2H OR Epinephrine or terbutaline, 0.1–0.5 ml SQ AND/OR Increase ipratropium to 6–8 puffs Q3–4H OR Ipratropium inhalant solution 0.5 mg Q4–8H AND Theophylline IV to bring serum level to 10–12 μg/ml (rarely, 12–18 μg/ml) AND Methylprednisolone IV given 50–100 mg IV STAT, then Q6–8H; taper as soon as possible ADD Antibiotic, if indicated

Adapted from: Celli, B.R. (1998). Clinical aspects of chronic obstructive pulmonary disease. In G.L. Baum, J.D. Crapo, B.R. Celli, & J.B. Karlinsky (Eds.), *Textbook of pulmonary diseases* (6th ed.) (Vol. 2, pp. 843–863). Philadelphia: Lippincott-Williams & Wilkins.

Antimicrobial therapy: Recommendations for antibiotic use in acute exacerbations of chronic bronchitis are evolving. In a recent study, the outcomes of acute exacerbations were more related to client factors than to the antibiotic given. High risk clients (age ≥65, >4 exacerbations per year, comorbid disease, or FEV_1 ≤50%) with moderately severe exacerbations (characterized by at least two of the following: increased sputum, increased sputum volume, and purulent sputum) have been shown to benefit from antimicrobial therapy.

Should be given when there is evidence of infection (e.g., fever, leukocytosis, or a change on chest x-ray examination).

Most common pathogens include *Haemophilus influenzae, Moraxella catarrhalis,* and *Streptococcus pneumoniae. Pseudomonas aeruginosa* is a common nosocomial pathogen and is more common in clients with severe underlying disease. Viruses account for approximately one third of exacerbations; atypical causes account for less than 10%.

Selection of antibiotic should include client characteristics (e.g., underlying comorbidities), likely pathogens, local resistance patterns, individual antibiotic properties, and cost (older, less expensive drugs may be cost effective).

Tetracyclines (including doxycycline), trimethoprim/sulfamethoxazole, amoxicillin, and macrolides are appropriate first-line agents, depending on local resistance patterns and risk profile of client. Fluoroquinolones should be considered first-line agents for clients with an acute exacerbation complicated by comorbid illness or severe obstruction (FEV_1 <50%), who are older (>65 years), or who have recurrent exacerbations.

Immunizations: Pneumococcal and influenza vaccines should be strongly recommended.

Nonpharmacologic Management

Pulmonary rehabilitation

Upper-extremity exercise

Psychological support

Elimination of environmental irritants, if possible

Oxygen therapy:

Indications include:

PaO_2 ≤55 mm Hg or SaO_2 ≤88% breathing ambient air

OR

PaO_2 ≤56 to 59 mm Hg or SaO_2 ≤89% with either electrocardiographic evidence of cor pulmonale or erythrocytosis (hematocrit >56%)

OR

PaO_2 ≥60 mm Hg or SaO_2 ≥90% with compelling medical justification

Surgery: bullectomy, lung-volume-reduction surgery or lung transplantation

Complementary/Alternative Therapies

Aromatherapy

Guided imagery

Client Education

Smoking cessation: Essential first step in treatment. In the Lung Health Study (Kanner, 1996), middle-aged adults with mild obstruction had slight improvement and then only minimal decline in FEV_1 if they stopped smoking. See Table 5–11 for a general overview of smoking cessation techniques.

Medication regimen.

How to use oxygen and/or inhalers.

Signs and symptoms of worsening disease or acute exacerbations.

Nutrition: Frequent small meals, dietary supplements. High-lipid and low-carbohydrate diets have been recommended, although their effectiveness has not been proven.

Exercise.

Energy conservation.

Pursed lip breathing.

Postural drainage and cough techniques to remove thick mucus.

Travel cautions: Airplane travel may be problematic because can lead to hypoxia. Clients need supplemental oxygen to maintain PaO_2 at $\leq$55 mm Hg.

Sexual intercourse: Position to decrease exertion and pressure on chest, plan intercourse for periods when client is rested, use bronchodilators prior to intercourse, use oxygen as needed, and use waterbed to help propel client without excessive energy expenditure.

Advance directives.

Follow-up

Regular follow-up required. Every 3–6 months when stable and more frequently if disease is worsening or acute exacerbations are present.

Referral

Hospitalize patient if any of the following are present:

Table 5–11   Smoking Cessation Techniques: The 4 A's*

Ask	Ask about tobacco use at every encounter: Make smoking status a vital sign and have it recorded in each client's chart.
Advise	Advise all smokers to quit: Use strong, clear, and personalized language using the 4 R's (relevance, risks, rewards, and repetition) to help the client understand why it is important to quit.
Assist	Assist patients in quitting: • Develop a quitting plan. • Set quitting date. • Review preparations for quitting (e.g., let family, friends and co-workers know, and remove objects associated with smoking from environment (cigarettes, ashtrays, matches, etc.). • Recommend nicotine-replacement therapy: patch or gum. • Offer key advice (skills training and problem solving). • Provide educational materials. • Arrange for follow-up to prevent relapse.
Arrange	Arrange for follow-up: • Arrange for frequent follow-up visits or phone contacts to assess cessation, provide positive reinforcement and prevent relapse. • At each contact, ask patients if they've quit, provide positive reinforcement, and if smoking has resumed remind them that relapses are common. • Have the client use the 4D's (delay, distract, drink water, deep breathing) to prevent relapse.

*The Agency for Health Care Policy and Research Smoking Cessation Guidelines recommend using the 4 A's to help clients achieve smoking cessation.

Acute exacerbations (increased dyspnea, cough, and sputum production), with client exhibiting one or more of the following: unresponsive to outpatient management; unable to walk between rooms; unable to eat or sleep because of dyspnea; cannot manage at home, and home care resources not immediately available, presence of high-risk comorbid condition; prolonged, progressive symptoms; or worsening hypoxemia, new or worsening hypercarbia, or new or worsening cor pulmonale.

Acute respiratory failure.

New or worsening cor pulmonale unresponsive to outpatient management.

Plans for invasive procedures requiring analgesics or sedatives.

Comorbid condition that is worsening pulmonary functioning.

Refer to pulmonologist if concomitant cardiac, renal, or other organ impairment, e.g., cor pulmonale; signs of worsening respiratory function; failure to respond to standard treatment; severe dyspnea; bullous disease; suspected pulmonary neoplasia; sleep apnea; perioperative management.

Refer to endocrinologist if clients with suspected α_1-antitrypsin deficiency.

Other possible referrals: oxygen company; home health care; pulmonary rehabilitation (Individually, tailored, multidisciplinary programs that include client evaluation and education, psychological support, and exercise training); nutritionist

COMMON COLD

SIGNAL SYMPTOMS cough, rhinorrhea, sore throat, myalgias

ICD-9 Codes	465.9	Acute URI
	472.0	Rhinorrhea
	786.2	Cough

The common cold is an acute infection of the upper respiratory tract (characterized by rhinorrhea, sore throat, cough, myalgias and low-grade fever) that lasts several days.

Epidemiology

Occurs with greater frequency than any other infectious disease.

Approximately 75 million visits to medical offices in the United States are attributable to symptoms of the common cold.

Approximately 250 million restricted activity days, and 150 million lost work days in the United States are due to URIs.

Etiology

Rhinovirus accounts for 30–40% of cases

Other causes

Coronavirus

Parainfluenzavirus

Influenzavirus
Respiratory syncytial virus
Adenovirus
Enterovirus

Physiology and Pathophysiology

Mechanism of infection is poorly understood. Infection begins in the posterior nasopharynx. Chemical mediators of the immune system, such as interleukins and PMNs (polymorphonuclear neutrophils) lead to common symptoms such as rhinorrhea, cough, sore throat, and sneezing. Modes of transmission include hand-to-hand contact, aerosolization of virus-laden respiratory secretions, and direct mucous membrane contact with virus from contaminated hands and/or other skin surfaces.

Clinical Manifestations

Subjective

Prodromal symptoms
  Chills
  Low-grade fever
  Myalgias/arthalgias
Presenting symptoms
  Scratchy throat
  Dry cough
  Rhinorrhea
  Sneezing
  Nasal stuffiness
  Headache
  Hoarseness
  Watery eyes
  Decreased appetite (especially in children)

Objective

Erythematous, edematous nasal mucosa
Clear, thin nasal drainage (may become purulent)
Mildly erythematous pharynx
Mild conjunctivitis
Fever, usually low-grade

Diagnostic Tests

Usually none
CBC (to rule out bacterial infection)
Nasal culture (to determine specific pathogen, especially in infants with persisting symptoms)

Differential Diagnosis

Allergic rhinitis (itchy watery eyes, sneezing, runny nose)
Foreign body (unilateral nasal drainage that may be malodorous, purulent, or bloody)

Management/Treatment

Pharmacologic/Symptomatic Management

Antipyretics/analgesics (acetaminophen, ibuprofen) for fever and aches

Decongestants: Pseudoephedrine (Sudafed) 60 mg PO Q4–6H (infants and children: oral drops, 7.5/0.8 ml, use age appropriate dosing)

Nasal sprays: Afrin (over the counter) nasal spray, limit use to 3 days to prevent rebound rhinorrhea

Expectorants: Guaifenesin (Duratuss G) 2400 mg/day maximum in adults

Cough suppressants: Cough syrups with codeine (Histussin HC), 1–2 tsp PO Q4–6H

Antihistamines: Not recommended due to drying properties

Nonpharmacologic Management

Increased fluid intake

Aspiration of nasal secretions, especially in infants and children

Client Education

Explain that antibiotics have no role in viral URIs.

Avoid aerosol exposure.

Wash hands.

Keep hands away from mucous membranes.

Complementary/Alternative Therapies

Ecchinacea, 1.5–7.5 ml of tincture, or 2–5 g of dried root

Zinc, 15 mg/day for men, 12 mg/day for women

Vitamin C, 200–400 mg/day

Follow-up

Usually not necessary, unless symptoms persist or worsen

Referral

Usually none needed.

If underlying allergies exist, consider allergist or ENT (otolaryngologist).

CROUP

SIGNAL SYMPTOMS ▶ barky cough, rhinorrhea

ICD-9 Code	464.4	Croup

Croup is an acute laryngotracheobronchitis or an infection of the larynx, trachea, and bronchi.

Epidemiology

Usually seen in children 3 months to 5 years of age.

Typically seen in late fall and winter months.

Responsible for approximately 41,000 hospitalizations each year

Etiology

Infectious, usually viral.

Parainfluenzaviruses cause approximately 75% of cases.

Remaining cases caused by adenoviruses, respiratory syncytial virus, influenza A and B viruses, and measles virus.

Physiology and Pathophysiology

Croup is a laryngeal obstruction caused by inflammatory edema and fibrinous exudates in the subglottic area. This narrows the airway and causes inspiratory stridor. The inflammation often extends down the trachea and bronchi, resulting in thick viscid secretions and ventilation-perfusion mismatch. The subglottic edema and lower airway involvement can lead to respiratory distress and hypoxemia.

Clinical Manifestations

Usually benign and self-limiting

Subjective

Often follows an upper respiratory infection.

Rhinorrhea.

Coryza.

Hoarseness.

Low-grade fever.

Characterized by a barking cough advancing to stridor and slight dyspnea.

Symptoms worsen at night and lessen or subside with exposure to moist or cold air.

Objective

Will depend on the severity of the illness

Wheezing

Low-grade fever

Nasal flaring

Inspiratory stridor

Suprasternal and intercostal retractions

Increased respiratory rate

Differential Diagnosis

Epiglottitis (sudden onset with low-pitched stridor, difficulty swallowing, fever, drooling and anxiety; child appears more toxic and typical age range is 2 to 7 years of age; usually caused by *Haemophilus influenzae*)

Bacterial tracheitis (characterized by brassy cough, inspiratory stridor, high fever, and profuse, thick purulent secretions)

Congenital subglottic stenosis (prolonged or recurrent episodes of croup)

Bronchiolitis (usually child is less than 2 years of age and has rapid shallow breathing, wheezing, cough, and inspiratory retractions of lower ribs and sternum)

Aspiration of foreign body (sudden onset of unilateral wheezing)

Diphtheria (gray exudative pharyngeal membrane and acute dysphagia)

Laryngitis (hoarseness accompanied by symptoms of URI)

Retropharyngeal or peritonsillar abscess (severe sore throat, drooling, and unilateral tonsillar swelling)

Diagnostic Tests

Pulse oximetry (to assess oxygen saturation)

Chest x-ray and posteroanterior neck x-ray examinations (to rule out epiglottitis)

White-cell count (to rule out infection)

Management/Treatment

Pharmacologic Management

Epinephrine: For children with moderate to severe respiratory distress, epinephrine (0.5 ml of 1:1000 concentration) or racemic epinephrine (0.5 ml) should be considered.

Cortiosteroids: For infants and children in whom increased work of breathing is demonstrated, glucocorticoids are recommended. Nebulized budesonide (2 mg) or dexamethasone (0.15–0.6 mg/kg PO or IM) can be used.

Nonpharmacologic Management

Cool, moist air

Humidified oxygen if needed

Client Education

Signs/symptoms of worsening illness and when to seek emergency care

Hydration

Acetaminophen or ibuprofen for fever and discomfort

Use of cool, moist air

Follow-up

Telephone follow-up within 24 hours. Follow-up visit necessary if no improvement after 48 hours.

Referral

Hospitalization should be considered for children with severe symptoms, signs of dehydration, respiratory distress.

Refer to pulmonologist for suspected epiglottitis.

CYSTIC FIBROSIS

SIGNAL SYMPTOMS cough; greasy/foul smelling stools

ICD-9 Code	277.0	Cystic fibrosis

Cystic fibrosis is a chronic progressive exocrine gland disorder characterized by excessive concentrations of sodium chloride in sweat, chronic respiratory disease, and exocrine pancreatic insufficiency.

Epidemiology

Most common genetic disorder affecting Caucasians

Affects approximately 1 in 2500 to 3500 newborns

In the United States, 96% affected are white and 3.3% black

Almost 54% are male

Median survival approximately 30 years

Etiology

Genetic disorder (autosomal recessive)

Physiology and Pathophysiology

Clinically, cystic fibrosis is a triad of chronic respiratory disease, pancreatic exocrine insufficiency, and excessive sodium chloride in the sweat. The chronic respiratory disease is related to the accumulation of viscid mucus in the bronchi, impaired mucociliary function, and chronic lung infections. Impaired chloride ion transport and excessive active sodium resorption occur in the respiratory epithelial cells, resulting in thick mucus and impaired clearance of pulmonary secretions. Total obstruction of the airway and atelectasis can occur. Chronic infection and inflammation lead to lung destruction. *Staphylococcus aureus* and *Pseudomonas* infections are common.

Pancreatic function is abnormal in over 80% of people with cystic fibrosis because of alterations in chloride permeability. Obstruction of the small ducts, decreased fluid secretion, and subsequent release of pancreatic enzymes cause autodigestion of the exocrine pancreas and maldigestion. Infertility is common related to occlusion of the vas deferens, epididymis, and seminal vessels in males, and distended cervical glands and copious cervical secretions in females.

Clinical Manifestations

Subjective

Cough is the earliest and most prominent sign, often beginning as an infrequent and nonproductive cough, then progressing to a productive cough of thick sputum.

Chronic rhinitis.

Bulky, greasy, foul smelling stools.

Steatorrhea.

Failure to thrive.

Objective

Lungs can be clear on auscultation, with intermittent wheezing and/or crackles with acute exacerbations, until the disease is advanced.

In advanced disease, enlarged anteroposterior chest diameter, clubbing, cyanosis, hemoptysis, atelectasis, and pneumothorax may appear.

Pansinusitis occurs in many patients.

Concentrations of 60 mmol/L on two separate occasions on quantitative pilocarpine ion electrophoresis sweat test.

Differential Diagnosis

Usually diagnosed in first year of life, although atypical cases can be diagnosed later in childhood.

Asthma (recurrent, tight, typically nonproductive cough; can be accompanied by wheezing; not typically associated with gastrointestinal [GI] symptoms)

Bronchiolitis (episodic cough associated with URI that may be accompanied by wheezing; repeated episodes of bronchiolitis may indicate cystic fibrosis; not typically associated with GI symptoms)

Gastroenteritis (episodic watery diarrhea associated with nausea and vomiting; not accompanied by respiratory symptoms)

Celiac sprue/protein hypersensitivity (failure to thrive, abdominal distention, irritability, and muscle wasting; not accompanied by respiratory symptoms)

Gastroesophageal reflux (cough associated with reflux, worsening after feeding and possibly accompanied by vomiting, failure to gain weight, and irritability)

Food allergies (chronic intermittent diarrhea associated with specific foods; may have other systemic symptoms such as urticaria or angioedema; not typically associated with recurrent respiratory infections)

Diagnostic Tests

Quantitative pilocarpine ion electrophoresis sweat test: Positive test requires a sweat chloride concentration of 60 mmol/L on two separate occasions with one or more phenotype features consistent with cystic fibrosis or documented cystic fibrosis in a sibling.

Mutation analysis: DNA testing can be a substitute for sweat testing in circumstances in which suspicion of cystic fibrosis is high, but sweat test is repeatedly negative.

Management/Treatment

Best managed by a multidisciplinary team at an accredited cystic fibrosis center.

Pharmacologic Management

A variety of agents can be used:

Bronchodilators: Controversial although helpful in some clients

Antibiotics: Long-term medications (colistin M) and acute medications for lung infections

Mucus liquefying agents: Dornase alfa

Steroids

Vitamins

Pancreatic enzyme replacement

Nonpharmacologic Management

Chest percussion
Forced expiratory maneuvers
Vigorous exercise
High salt intake
Psychosocial support

Complementary/Alternative Therapies

Massage therapy
Biofeedback

Client Education

Early signs of worsening respiratory status, especially signs and symptoms of infection

Diet

Regular exercise

Breathing exercises

Instructions about medications

Follow-up

Regular follow-up (every 6–8 weeks) required in conjunction with cystic fibrosis specialty care.

Referral

Refer to cystic fibrosis treatment center necessary for initial treatment plan and ongoing follow-up.

Consider referral to nutritionist, mental health services, support groups, etc.

LUNG CANCER

SIGNAL SYMPTOMS cough, hemoptysis

ICD-9 Code	162.0	Lung cancer

Lung cancer, specifically bronchogenic carcinoma, originates in the tracheobronchial tree or the lung parenchyma.

Epidemiology

Second most common cancer.

Leading cause of death from cancer in both men and women, accounting for 28% of all cancer deaths.

From 1990 to 1996 the incidence of lung cancer in women has increased 0.1%, while that in men has decreased 2.6%.

Cigarette smoking is most important risk factor, responsible for approximately 90% of all lung cancers.

Exposure to other carcinogens, such as asbestos and radon, also plays a role.

Etiology

Neoplastic with the majority of cases related to tobacco exposure

Physiology and Pathophysiology

There are four major subtypes of lung cancer (accounting for about 95% of all primary bronchogenic carcinomas): squamous-cell carcinoma, adenocarcinoma, large-cell carcinoma, and small-cell (or oat-cell) carcinoma. Differentiating small-cell lung cancer (SCLC) from non-small-cell lung cancer (NSCLC, which includes squamous-cell carcinoma, adenocarcinoma, and large-cell carcinoma) is important in treatment decisions.

Squamous-cell carcinomas account for 30% to 40% of all lung cancers and are related almost exclusively to smoking. They arise from the bronchial epithelial cells with histologic hallmarks of keratin "onion pearls" and intercellular bridges. Adenocarcinomas occur more commonly in the periphery of the lung rather than in the central airways; they are more common in women than men. Tobacco use and exposure to ionizing radiation are risk factors. Because of their location, adenocarcinomas are less likely to be associated with pulmonary symptoms. Large-cell carcinomas, which account for approximately 10% of all lung cancers, occur as solitary bulky masses in the lung periphery. Finally, SCLC accounts for approximately 20% of all cancers and is strongly associated with smoking. SCLCs tend to be centrally located, arising in the peribronchial tissues.

Clinical Manifestations

Subjective

Usually nonspecific, with symptoms similar to other disorders, such as
chronic bronchitis
Persistent cough
Hemoptysis
Dull, intermittent chest pain
Weight loss
Dysphagia
Hoarseness
Frequent bouts of lower respiratory tract infections
Fatigue and malaise

Objective

Variable, depending on the type of cancer, location, and extent of spread.
Can be completely normal.
Localized wheezing.
Diminished sounds or dullness to percussion can be related to pleural
effusions and/or compressive atelectasis.
Supraclavicular or cervical adenopathy.
Jugular venous distention.
Papilledema.
Signs of cardiac tamponade (narrow pulse pressure, enlarged heart).
Other laboratory tests in consultation with oncologist or pulmonologist.
Lung cancer should be suspected in anybody who presents with a lung mass
on chest x-ray examination (even without any symptoms), or when
pneumonia fails to resolve after 6 to 8 weeks of appropriate therapy,
especially if the client is a smoker. Lung cancer should be suspected in
smokers who present with a chronic cough or a change in cough,
especially if hemoptysis is also present and even if chest x-ray yields
normal results.

Differential Diagnosis

COPD (chronic progressive shortness of breath, persistent cough, fatigue,
and history of smoking; increased thoracic diameter, use of accessory
muscles, pursed-lip breathing, and diminished breath sounds)

Pneumonia (productive cough of yellow, green, or rust-colored sputum, shortness of breath and fever; local inspiratory crackles, vocal fremitus, dull percussion, and bronchophony and egophony)

Interstitial pulmonary fibrosis (insidious onset of shortness of breath that occurs with exercise; rapid shallow respirations, nonproductive cough, and clubbing can occur in advanced stages)

Tuberculosis (history of exposure or high-risk group, fatigue, weight loss, cough, hemoptysis, and night sweats)

Pulmonary edema (pink, frothy sputum, diaphoresis, rapid shallow breathing, jugular venous distention, hepatomegaly, and ankle edema)

Diagnostic Tests

The following tests, with the exception of chest x-ray examination, would typically be done in consultation with an oncologist or pulmonologist:

Chest x-ray examination (initial diagnostic tool)

Sputum cytology (to identify organism)

Computed tomography (CT) scan of chest and abdomen (to rule out neoplasm)

Bone scan (to rule out metastasis)

Bronchoscopy (to localize neoplasm)

Management/Treatment

Nurse practitioners (NPs) are responsible for prevention, early identification, and prompt referral of clients with suspected lung cancer. The NP may be involved in symptom management of the client and smoking cessation (prevention) counseling. (See Table 5–11.)

Pharmacologic Management
Chemotherapy

Nonpharmacologic Management
Surgical resection
Radiation

Complementary/Alternative Therapies
Aromatherapy
Art and music therapy
Biofeedback
Massage therapy
Meditation
Prayer, spiritual practices
Tai chi
Yoga
Nutrition

Client Education
Emotional support
End-of-life planning: Advance directives

Follow-up

In collaboration with oncologist

Referral

Prompt referral to an oncologist or pulmonologist is required for clients with suspected lung cancer.

PNEUMONIA

SIGNAL SYMPTOMS ▶ purulent cough, fever, dyspnea

ICD-9 Codes	480.9	Viral pneumonia
	481	Pneumococcal pneumonia (*Streptococcus pneumoniae* pneumonia)
	482.0	Pneumonia due to *Klebsiella pneumoniae*
	482.2	Pneumonia due to *Haemophilus influenzae*
	482.9	Bacterial pneumonia, unspecified

Pneumonia is an acute infection of the pulmonary parenchyma associated with at least some symptoms of acute infection (fever, rigors, sweats, new cough, chest discomfort, or dyspnea) and the presence of acute infiltrate on chest x-ray examination or auscultatory findings consistent with pneumonia (e.g., localized crackles). The term *community-acquired pneumonia* (CAP) is used to describe pneumonias caused by organisms found in the community as opposed to the hospital or nursing home.

Epidemiology

There are 2 to 4 million cases of CAP each year.

Pneumonia prompts approximately 10 million office visits and 500,000 hospitalizations each year.

Sixth leading cause of death, with persons aged 65 and older accounting for 89% of deaths.

Advanced age, presence of leukocytosis, bacteremia, extent of radiographic changes, high alcohol use, active malignancies, immunosuppression, neurologic disease, congestive heart failure and diabetes mellitus increase risk of death from pneumonia.

Pneumonias caused by *Streptococcus pneumoniae, Haemophilus influenzae,* and influenzavirus typically occur during the winter months.

Pneumonias caused by *Chlamydia pneumoniae* occur year-round.

Legionnaires' disease is more common in the summer months.

Pattern of mycoplasma infection is not clearly documented.

Etiology

Infectious.

Agent cannot be determined in 40%–60% of cases.

Most common pathogen is *S. pneumoniae*

Other pathogens include *H. influenzae, Mycoplasma pneumoniae, C. pneumoniae, Staphylococcus aureus, Streptococcus pyogenes,*

Neisseria meningitidis, Moraxella catarrhalis, Klebsiella pneumoniae, Legionella species, influenzavirus, respiratory syncytial virus, adenovirus, and parainfluenzavirus. See ARC 5–1 for age-specific causes of pneumonia in children.

Physiology and Pathophysiology

Most pneumonia is caused by aspiration of bacteria from the tracheobronchial tree or bacteria inhaled into the lung. Typically, aspirated or inhaled bacteria do not cause pneumonia because of the body's extensive defense mechanisms (cough reflex, mucociliary clearance, and phagocytosis). In individuals with compromised defense mechanisms (due to alcohol or drug use, tumors, etc.), the invading pathogen releases damaging toxins, stimulating inflammatory and immune responses. The terminal bronchioles and acini are filled with infectious debris and exudate from inflammation and edema. This leads to ventilation-perfusion abnormalities. Necrosis of lung parenchyma may occur if *Staphylococcus* or gram-negative bacteria cause the pneumonia.

Clinical Manifestations

Subjective

Classic symptoms include abrupt onset of cough, sputum, dyspnea, fever and pleuritic chest pain.

Elderly clients often do not present with classic symptoms. They may present with changes in mental status, falls, worsening underlying disease, metabolic derangement, incontinence, or failure to thrive.

In general infants and young children may not present with classic symptoms. Symptoms may be nonspecific, such as lethargy, poor feeding, vomiting, abdominal pain, cough, fever, and respiratory distress. In infants, pneumonia can usually be ruled out by the absence of tachypnea.

Age-Related Considerations: Causes of Pneumonia

Age	Causes
1–3 months (Pneumonitis syndrome, usually febrile)	*Chlamydia trachomatis*, respiratory syncytial virus (RSV), other respiratory viruses, *Bordetella pertussis*
1–24 months (Mild to moderate pneumonia)	RSV, other respiratory viruses, *Streptococcus pneumoniae*, *Haemophilus influenzae* type b(Hib), nontypable *H. influenzae* (NTHI), *C. trachomatis*, *Mycoplasma pneumoniae*
2–5 years	Respiratory viruses, *S. pneumoniae*, Hib, NTHI, *M. pneumoniae*, *Chlamydia pneumoniae*
6–18 years	*M. pneumoniae*, *S. pneumoniae*, *C. pneumoniae*, NTHI, influenza A or B, adenovirus, other respiratory viruses
All ages (Severe pneumonia)	*S. pneumoniae*, *Staphylococcus aureus*, Group A streptococci, Hib, *M. pneumoniae*, adenovirus

Adapted from: Jadavji, T., Law, B., Lebel, M. C., Kennedy, W. A., Gold, R., & Wang, E. E. L. (1997). A practical guide for the diagnosis and treatment of pediatric pneumonia. *Canadian Medical Association Journal, 156,* S703–S711.

Chest indrawing, signs of respiratory distress such as nasal flaring and abnormal breath sounds (crackles or decreased breath sounds) aid in ruling in pneumonia.

Differentiating the specific etiologic agent in CAP can be difficult because of lack of sound data. See Table 5–12 for typical clinical manifestations of common pneumonias.

Objective

Fever

Localized dullness

Crackles

Wheezes

Table 5–12   Clinical Manifestations of Common Pneumonias

Type of Pneumonia	Clinical Manifestations
Streptococcus pneumoniae (pneumococcal pneumonia)	Prior URI, fever (100° to 106°F), cough, rust-colored or green sputum, pleuritic chest pain relieved with rest, shaking chills, myalgia, tachycardia, and localized dullness/flatness, crackles, egophony, bronchophony, friction rub.
Streptococcus pyogenes pneumonia	Abrupt onset of shaking chills, fever, cough, sputum, and chest pain. May see hemoptysis. Crackles and dullness may be found, although signs of consolidation are not always found on examination.
Staphylococcus pyogenes pneumonia	Rarely causes pneumonia in healthy adults, and clinical manifestations vary depending on the setting. Almost all patients have fever. May also see chest pain, shaking, chills, productive cough of purulent sputum, tachycardia, and tachypnea.
Haemophilus influenzae pneumonia	In infants and/or patients with alcoholism or underlying immunodeficiency may present similarly to classic bacterial pneumonia. Adults with chronic lung disease usually have gradual onset, with low-grade fever, cough, increasing sputum production, worsening dypsnea, and occasionally myalgia.
Moraxella catarrhalis pneumonia	Typically occurs in adults with chronic lung disease. Usually mild symptoms with weakness and dyspnea and minor change in cough,
Legionellosis	Clinical manifestations vary from self-limited, influenzalike illness to fulminant pneumonia with malaise, muscle aches, headache, confusion, high fever, chills, cough, and thin to purulent sputum. Findings on examination also vary from a few crackles to evidence of significant consolidation.
Mycoplasma pneumonia	More common in adolescents and young adults (<30 years). Can have either an insidious or an acute onset. Persistent, hacking, nonproductive cough and fever greater than 101°F common. May also see myalgia, coryza, sore throat, shaking chills. Early in disease findings on examination may be negative but can progress to crackles and/or wheezes.
Chlamydia pneumonia	Similar to *M. pneumoniae*. Generally mild, but can last for 3–6 weeks.
Viral pneumonia	Usually symptoms more mild. Dypsnea and cough accompanied by scant sputum.

Egophony
Bronchophony

Differential Diagnosis

Viral upper respiratory tract infection (cough, nasal congestion, sore throat, fever, chills, myalgia, enlarged anterior cervical nodes, and erythematous nasal and/or pharyngeal mucosa; lung examination normal)

Pulmonary embolism (acute onset of pleuritic chest pain, dyspnea, hemoptysis, tachycardia, tachypnea, diminished breath sounds, crackles and wheezes; often in person with history of deep-vein thrombosis (DVT), recent surgery, trauma or oral-contraceptive use)

Congestive heart failure (chronic progressive dyspnea, cough, frothy sputum, fatigue, weight gain, ankle edema, paroxysmal nocturnal dyspnea or orthopnea, jugular venous distention, tachypnea, use of accessory muscles, crackles, wheezes, displaced PMI, S3, S4 and liver enlargement)

Bronchitis (loose hacking cough that is typically preceded by URI; cough can become productive; low-grade fever; coarse to fine crackles or lung examination normal)

Asthma (cough, dyspnea, wheezing, tachypnea, use of accessory muscles, decreased vocal fremitus, diminished breath sounds, and inspiratory and expiratory wheezes; often in person with history of atopy)

Pleurisy (mild, localized chest pain that is worse with deep breathing and often following a URI, shallow respirations, local tenderness, and pleural friction rub)

Atelectasis (dyspnea, tachypnea, tachycardia, diminished chest wall movement, absent or diminished breath sounds, cyanosis and intercostal retractions; fever and other signs of infection may develop)

Lung cancer (chest pain, shortness of breath, hemoptysis, and cough in smoker; physical examination may be normal or localized, with diminished breath sounds or dullness)

Diagnostic Tests

The Infectious Diseases Society of America now recommends at minimum for clients with CAP to be treated on an outpatient basis, that a chest x-ray examination be done to confirm the pneumonia, and that a Gram stain/culture be attempted to identify the etiologic agent. Other diagnostic tests may be done as needed for specific cases:

Chest x-ray examinations are strongly recommended to substantiate the diagnosis of pneumonia, to rule out other possible diagnoses and to assess prognosis.

Gram stain/culture (to identify causative organism).

CBC (to rule out infection).

Glucose, liver enzymes, electrolytes, blood urea nitrogen (BUN), creatinine (to rule out hypoglycemia or hyperglycemia, liver dysfunction, electrolyte imbalance and kidney dysfunction, respectively).

Pulse oximetry or arterial blood gases (to rule out acidosis/alkalosis).

Human immunodeficiency virus (HIV) testing (to rule out HIV/AIDS).

Purified protein derivative (to rule out tuberculosis [TB] and/or exposure to TB).

Diagnostic thoracentesis for clients with a pleural effusion.

For hospitalized clients, the following should be considered: CBC with differential, glucose, liver enzymes, electrolytes, BUN, creatinine, arterial blood gases, two sets of blood cultures, HIV testing, sputum for Gram stain and culture, test for *Mycobacterium tuberculosis* with acid-fast stain and culture (for those with cough >1 month, other common symptoms, or suggestive radiologic features), and test for Legionnaires' disease (seriously ill, immunocompromised, unresponsive to therapy, common symptoms, or during outbreak).

Management/Treatment

Approximately 75% of clients with CAP can be treated appropriately at home.

Pharmacologic Management

See Table 5–13 for recommended antimicrobial regimes if the etiologic agent is known.

See Table 5–14 for empirical treatment of community-acquired pneumonia. Note that since 1998, when these guidelines were published by the Infectious Diseases Society of America, the Drug-Resistant *Streptococcus pneumoniae* Therapeutic Working Group has recommended reserving fluoroquinolones for adults in whom first-line agents have failed, who are allergic to alternative agents, or who have a documented infection with a highly-resistant pneumococci (minimal inhibitory concentration of penicillin, ≥4). They recommend a macrolide antibiotic (e.g., erythromycin, clarithromycin, or azithromycin), doxycycline (tetracycline), or an oral β-lactam antibiotic with good antipneumococcal activity (e.g., cefuroxime, amoxicillin or amoxicillin–clavulanate). For children younger than 5 years they recommend β-lactam antibiotics because doxycycline or fluoroquinolones should be avoided. Erythromycin (40 mg/kg daily divided into four doses) is also recommended for infants and children.

The duration of antimicrobial therapy is not clearly defined. Most recommendations are for 7 to 14 days.

Symptomatic treatment: Antipyretics and analgesics.

For patients with CAP hospitalized in a general ward: a β-lactam antibiotic (ceftriaxone, cefotaxime) with or without a macrolide antibiotic (azithromycin, clarithromycin, or erythromycin), or a fluoroquinolone alone.

Prevention

Pneumococcal vaccine recommended for the following groups:

Persons aged ≥65 years.

Immunocompetent persons aged ≥2 years who are at increased risk for illness and death associated with pneumococcal disease because of chronic illness.

Persons aged ≥2 years with functional or anatomic asplenia.

Table 5–13 Treatment of Pneumonia According to Pathogen

Pathogen	Preferred Antimicrobial	Alternative Antimicrobial
Streptococcus pneumoniae Penicillin-susceptible (MIC, <0.1 μg/ml)	Penicillin G or penicillin V, amoxicillin	Cephalosporins,* macrolides,[†] clindamycin, fluoroquinolones,[‡] doxycycline
Intermediate penicillin resistant (MIC, 0.1–1 μg/ml)	Parenteral penicillin G, ceftriaxone or cefotaxime, amoxicillin, fluoroquinolones,[‡] other agents based on in vitro susceptibility test results	Clindamycin, doxycycline, oral cephalosporins*
Highly penicillin resistant[§] (MIC, ≥2 μg/ml)	Agents based on in vitro susceptibility results, fluoroquinolones,[‡] vancomycin	
Empirical selection	Fluoroquinolones,[‡] selection based on susceptibility test results in community[¶]	Clindamycin, doxycycline, vancomycin
	Penicillin**	Cephalosporins,* macrolides,[†] amoxicillin, clindamycin
Haemophilus influenzae	Second- or third-generation cephalosporins, doxycycline, β-lactam/β-lactamase inhibitor, fluoroquinolones[‡]	Azithromycin, TMP/SMX
Moraxella catarrhalis	Second- or third-generation cephalosporins, TMP/SMX, amoxicillin-clavulanate	Macrolides,[†] fluoroquinolones,[‡] β-lactam/β-lactamase inhibitor
Anaerobes	Clindamycin, penicillin plus metronidazole, β-lactam-β-lactamase inhibitor	Penicillin G or penicillin V, ampicillin/amoxicillin with or without metronidazole
Staphylococcus aureus[§] Methicillin-susceptible	Nafcillin/oxacillin with or without rifampin or gentamicin[§]	Cefazolin or cefuroxime, vancomycin, clindamycin, TMP/SMX, fluoroquinolones[‡]
Methicillin-resistant	Vancomycin with or without rifampin or gentamicin	Requires in vitro testing; TMP/SMX
Enterobacteriaceae (coliforms: Escherichia coli, Klebsiella, Proteus, Enterobacter)[§]	Third-generation cephalosporin with or without aminoglycoside, carbapenems[††]	Aztreonam, β-lactam/β-lactamase inhibitor, fluoroquinolones[‡]
Pseudomonas aeruginosa[§]	Aminoglycoside plus antipseudomonal β-lactam: ticarcillin, piperacillin, mezlocillin, ceftazidime, cefepime, aztreonam, or carbapenems[††]	Aminoglycoside plus ciprofloxacin plus antipseudomonal β-lactam
Legionella species	Macrolides[†] with or without rifampin, fluoroquinolones[‡]	Doxycycline with or without rifampin
Mycoplasma pneumoniae	Doxycycline, macrolides,[†] fluoroquinolones[‡]	

Table continued on following page.

Table 5–13   Treatment of Pneumonia According to Pathogen (*Continued*)

Pathogen	Preferred Antimicrobial	Alternative Antimicrobial
Chlamydia pneumoniae	Doxycycline, macrolides,[†] fluoroquinolones[‡]	
Chlamydia psittaci	Doxycycline	Erythromycin, chloramphenicol
Nocardia species	Sulfonamide with or without minocycline or amikacin, TMP/SMX	Imipenem with or without amikacin, doxycycline, or minocycline
Coxiella burnetti[‡‡]	Tetracycline	Chloramphenicol
Influenza A	Amantadine or rimantadine	
Hantavirus	None[§§]	

*Intravenous: cefazolin, cefuroxime, cefotaxime, ceftriaxone; oral: cefpodoxime, cefprozil, cefuroxime.
[†]Erythromycin, clarithromycin, azithromycin.
[‡]Levofloxacin, sparfloxacin, grepafloxacin, trovafloxacin, or another fluoroquinolone with enhanced activity against *S. pneumoniae*; ciprofloxacin is appropriate for *Legionella* species, fluoroquinolone-susceptible *Staph. aureus,* and most gram-negative bacilli.
[§]In vitro susceptibility tests are required for optimal treatment; for *Enterobacter* species, the preferred antibiotics are fluoroquinolones and carbapenems.
[¶]High rates of high-level penicillin resistance, susceptibility strains unknown, and/or patient is seriously ill.
[**]Low rates of penicillin resistance in community and patient is at low risk for infection with resistant *Strep. pneumoniae.*
[††]Imipenem and meropenem.
[‡‡]Agent of Q fever.
[§§]Provide supportive care.
Note: TMP/SMX = trimethoprim/sulfamethoxazole
Adapted from: Bartlett, J.G., Breiman, R.F., Mandell, L.A., & File, T.M. (1998). Community-acquired pneumonia in adults: Guidelines for management. *Clinical Infectious Diseases, 26,* 811–838.

Persons aged ≥2 years living in environments in which the risk for disease is high.
Immunocompromised persons ≥2 years who are high risk for infection
Influenza vaccine.

Nonpharmacologic Management
Oxygen
Hydration
Rest

Client Education
Hydration and rest
Need to complete antibiotic treatment
Signs and symptoms of worsening illness
Smoking cessation
Pneumonia and influenza vaccines as appropriate

Follow-up
Follow-up within 24 to 72 hours in person or by phone depending on the severity of the pneumonia.

Table 5–14 Empirical Antibiotic Selection for Patients with Community-Acquired Pneumonia

Outpatients
  Generally preferred: Macrolides,* fluoroquinolones,† or doxycycline
  Modifying factors:
    Suspected penicillin-resistant *Streptococcus pneumoniae:* fluroquinolones†
    Suspected aspiration: amoxicillin/clavulanate
    Young adult (>17–40 years): doxycycline
Hospitalized Patients
  General medical ward
    Generally preferred: β-lactam‡ with or without a macrolide* or a fluoroquinoline† (alone)
    Alternatives: cefuroxime with or without a macrolide or azithromycin* (alone)
  Hospitalized in the intensive care unit for serious pneumonia
    Generally preferred: erythromycin, azithromycin, or a fluoroquinoline† *plus* cefotaxime, ceftriaxone, or a β-lactam/β-lactamase inhibitor§
  Modifying factors
    Structural disease of the lung: antipseudomonal penicillin, a carbapenem, or cefepime plus a macrolide* or a fluoroquinoline† plus an aminoglycoside
    Penicillin allergy: a fluoroquinoline† with or without clindamycin
    Suspected aspiration: a fluoroquinolone plus either clindamycin or metronidazole or a β-lactam/β-lactamase inhibitor§ (alone)

---

*Erythromycin, clarithromycin, azithromycin.
†Levofloxacin, sparfloxacin, grepafloxacin, trovafloxacin, or another fluoroquinolone with enhanced activity against *Strep. pneumoniae;* ciprofloxacin is appropriate for *Legionella* species, fluoroquinolone-susceptible *Staph. aureus,* and most gram-negative bacilli.
‡Cefotaxime, ceftriaxone, or a β-lactam/β-lactamase inhibitor
§Ampicillin/sulbactam, or ticarcillin/clavulanate, or piperacillin/tazobactam (for structural disease of the lung, ticarcillin or piperacillin).
Adapted from: Bartlett, J.G., Breiman, R.F., Mandell, L.A., & File, T.M. (1998). Community-acquired pneumonia in adults: Guidelines for management. *Clinical Infectious Diseases, 26,* 811–838. .

For clients older than 40 years and clients who are smokers, repeat chest x-ray examination in 4 to 8 weeks to rule out bronchogenic carcinoma.

Referral

Consult with physician for clients in severe respiratory distress, with significant comorbidity or with little improvement in condition after 72 hours of microbial therapy.

Hospitalization is required for some clients with CAP.

PULMONARY EMBOLISM

SIGNAL SYMPTOMS▶ cough, shortness of breath, tachycardia

ICD-9 Code	415.1	Pulmonary embolism

Pulmonary embolism (PE) is an acute obstruction of the pulmonary vessels by an embolism.

Epidemiology

Overall incidence is 139 per 100,000 or approximately 347,000 cases per year (some sources estimate up to 500,000 cases per year).

About 2% die in the first day.

10% have recurrent embolism.

PE is responsible for about 50,000 deaths each year.

A strong association exists between deep vein thrombosis and PE. PEs are detected in approximately 50% of clients with documented DVT, while asymptomatic venous thrombosis is found in about 70% of clients with confirmed PE.

Risk factors: See RF 5–1.

Etiology

Thromboembolic event.

About 80% of cases of PE have a definable cause.

Physiology and Pathophysiology

Pulmonary emboli arise from deep venous thromboses in the ileofemoral or pelvic veins or right side of the heart, tumors invading venous circulation, or other sources, such as amniotic fluid, air, fat, bone marrow, or foreign intravenous material. A partial or whole thrombus dislodged into the venous circulation can be transported to the right side of the heart and then into the pulmonary circulation, resulting in hemodynamic and pulmonary complications. A significant rise in pulmonary vascular resistance results from mechanical obstruction of the pulmonary vessels. In severe cases this can lead to pulmonary hypertension and right ventricular failure. The release of vasoactive amines, such as serotonin and thromboxane A_2, and the stimulation of baroreceptors also leads to vasoconstriction. The major respiratory complications of PE result from reflex bronchoconstriction in the embolized area (which accounts for the wheezing heard in some clients), increased alveolar dead space, and loss of alveolar surfactant. Actual pulmonary infarction is uncommon.

 RF 5–1 Risk Factors: *Pulmonary Embolism*

- History of previous thrombotic event(s)
- Age older than 40 years
- Recent surgery (especially orthopedic)
- Internal malignancy
- Prolonged bedrest or immobilization
- Fracture of pelvis, hip or long bones
- Serious burns
- Congestive heart failure
- Bacterial, fungal or viral septicemia
- Estrogen treatment (especially high dose oral contraceptives)
- Pregnant or post-partum
- Obese
- Hypercoagulability status (e.g., protein C deficiency, antithrombin III deficiency).

Clinical Manifestations

Can be fairly nonspecific.

Subjective

Acute pleuritic chest pain
Shortness of breath (preceding chest pain)
Cough
Apprehension
Diaphoresis
Hemoptysis

Objective

Tachycardia
Tachypnea
Increased jugular venous pressure
Abnormally split second heart sound with accentuation of the pulmonary component
In severe cases, signs of acute right ventricular failure, hypotension, and cyanosis

Differential Diagnosis

Angina/myocardial infarction (substernal chest pressure caused by exertion or emotion; in the case of angina, relieved by rest or nitroglycerin; in myocardial infarction, prolonged crushing substernal pain radiating to arm, neck or jaw and accompanied by diaphoresis and hypotension)

Pneumonia (productive cough or yellow, green, or rust-colored sputum associated with dyspnea, pleuritic chest pain, fever, localized dullness, fremitus, inspiratory crackles, and bronchophony and egophony)

Pneumothorax (acute pleuritic chest pain and dyspnea are primary symptoms; may have unilateral diminished breath sounds and decreased chest movement; tension pneumothorax characterized by rapidly developing shock and tracheal shift)

Aortic dissection (acute onset of severe tearing pain with restlessness, asymmetry of pulses, and murmur of aortic insufficiency)

Dysrhythmias (palpitations, dizziness, tachycardia, and irregular pulse)

Pericarditis (sharp, pleuritic chest pain worsened by twisting, coughing, deep breathing, swallowing or supine position; associated with fever, tachycardia, and pericardial friction rub)

Pleuritis (mild, localized pleuritic chest pain worsened by deep breathing, with history of previous URI, shallow respirations, and pleural friction rub)

Costochondritis (pain and tenderness along sternal border that increases with deep breathing; history of URI or physical activity common)

Panic attack (paroxysms of substernal heaviness, lightheadedness, palpitations, nervousness and weakness; may report feeling of panic and impending catastrophe)

Diagnostic Tests

Ventilation-perfusion scan: Initial imaging test. For those with normal results, likelihood of PE very low. For those with high probability, likelihood of PE very high. However, "indeterminate" or intermediate results are more difficult to interpret.

Pulmonary angiography: Gold standard. Used for clients with indeterminate results.

Compression ultrasonography: Also can be used for clients with indeterminate results.

Electrocardiography: Usually nonspecific ST–T-wave changes.

Chest x-ray examination: Usually normal.

Arterial blood gases: Usually reveal respiratory alkalosis.

Management/Treatment

Pulmonary embolism is a clinical emergency that requires hospitalization. The nurse practitioner's responsibilities include early identification and referral, prevention and/or risk reduction, and management of therapeutic anticoagulation therapy after the acute PE.

Pharmacologic Management

Heparin: For 5–7 days.

Low-molecular-weight heparin: Can be used in cases of PE that are hemodynamically stable.

Warfarin: Started on day 1 or day 2 and usually given for 3–6 months, with a target international normalized ratio of 2–3. May be given longer if underlying risk factors for thromboembolism cannot be eliminated or if recurrent thromboembolism occurs.

Prevention: High-risk clients may need prophylaxis.

Nonpharmacologic Management

Oxygen.

Inferior vena cava filter can be used in clients for whom anticoagulation is contraindicated.

Thrombectomy.

Complementary/Alternative Therapies

Vitamin E

Client Education

For those at risk, avoid prolonged standing or sitting with legs dependent.

There is a risk of a repeat thrombotic event.

Anticoagulation therapy needed.

Ongoing monitoring needed, especially with oral anticoagulants.

Some foods and medications can alter anticoagulation therapy.

Wear medical identification bracelet or necklace.

Use soft-bristle toothbrush.

Watch for signs and symptoms of increased bleeding, such as blood in stool or urine, headache, backache, bruising or excessive bleeding.

Follow-up

Will depend on the underlying pathology and treatment. If on oral anticoagulation therapy, weekly to monthly prothrombin/international normalized ratio monitoring.

Referral

Emergency referral for treatment and hospitalization.

SARCOIDOSIS

SIGNAL SYMPTOMS ► cough, wheezing, eye/skin changes

ICD-9 Code	135.0	Sarcoidosis

Sarcoidosis is a multisystem granulomatous disorder characterized by an exaggerated cellular immune response.

Epidemiology

Usually affects adults between 20 and 40 years of age.

Occurs in approximately 1 per 10,000 people each year; approximately 22,500 cases per year.

African Americans are 3–4 times more likely to have sarcoidosis than Caucasians.

Women are at slightly greater risk than men.

Disease will resolve in two thirds of clients; 15–20% of clients will suffer permanent lung damage and 5% will die of the disease.

Etiology

Unknown.

Evidence suggests that sarcoidosis results from exposure of genetically susceptible hosts to specific environmental agents—for example, infectious agents, tree pollen, and inorganic compounds such as aluminum or talc.

Physiology and Pathophysiology

A hyperimmune response to an unknown agent(s) at the affected areas has been found. Lesions can be found in any organ in the body, although the lungs and the intrathoracic lymph nodes are affected in about 90% of clients. In the lungs, macrophage–T-lymphocyte alveolitis precedes noncaseating, nonnecrotic epithelioid granuloma formation; these lesions tend to be peribronchial, interstitial, and subpleural in location. An interstitial pneumonitis may precede granuloma formation.

Clinical Manifestations

Subjective

Insidious

Cough

Exertional dyspnea

Systemic symptoms such as fever, fatigue, weight loss, and weakness
Up to 50% of people are asymptomatic at the time of diagnosis

Objective

Occasional wheezing
Can also present with ocular (acute uveitis, cataracts, lacrimal gland
swelling and inflammation, and retinal periphlebitis) and skin lesions
(erythema nodosum, maculopapular lesions, nodules, and ulcers).

Differential Diagnosis

Tuberculosis (productive cough, chest pain, hemoptysis, fatigue, weight loss,
night sweats in person with history of exposure or residing in high-risk area)
Fungal lower respiratory infections (often asymptomatic, but may report
flu-like symptoms of fever, chills, cough and scanty sputum)
Pneumonia (sudden onset of fever, productive cough, dyspnea, and
pleuritic chest pain)
Asthma (cough associated with intermittent or persistent wheezing)
Interstitial lung disease (cyanosis on exertion and clubbing of the fingers)
COPD (cough and progressive dyspnea in smoker; hyperresonant chest,
distant breath sounds, prolonged expiratory phase and enlarged anteroposterior diameter of the chest; onset usually later in 5th or 6th decade)
Congestive heart failure (chronic progress dyspnea, cough, fatigue
accompanied with ankle edema, orthopnea, jugular venous distention,
enlarged heart, and hepatomegaly)
Lung cancer (unilateral wheezing and/or dullness in smoker, weight loss)

Diagnostic Tests

Done in consultation with pulmonologist
Posteroanterior chest x-ray examination: Required in all clients. See
staging of disease based on radiographic findings in Table 5–15.
Lung biopsy (to rule out neoplasm)
Computerized tomography (CT) scan of chest (to rule out neoplasm)
Pulmonary-function tests (to assess pulmonary function)
White-cell-count (to rule out infection)
Serum chemistries: calcium, liver enzymes, creatinine, blood urea nitrogen
(BUN)
Urinalysis (to rule out urinary disorders)
Electrocardiography (to rule out cardiac disorders)
Routine ophthalmic examination (to rule out ocular dysfunction)

Table 5–15 Staging of Sarcoidosis

Stage	Radiographic Findings
Stage 0	No radiographic changes
Stage 1	Bilateral hilar lymphadenopathy without parenchymal infiltrates
Stage 2	Bilateral hilar lymphadenopathy with parenchymal infiltrates
Stage 3	Parenchymal infiltrates without hilar lymphadenopathy
Stage 4	Pulmonary fibrosis

Purified protein derivative (to rule out tuberculosis or exposure to tuberculosis)

Also can consider obtaining serum γ-globulin, serum angiotensin-converting enzyme

Management/Treatment

Pharmacologic Management

For those with stage 1 or asymptomatic disease: No treatment recommended.

NSAIDS: Can be used for fever and/or joint pain.

Oral corticosteroids: Usually reserved for those with stage 2, symptomatic disease. Typical starting dose is 20–40 mg per day of prednisone on alternate days. Treatment is required for a minimum of 12 months.

Nonpharmacologic Management

Many clients require only observation and monitoring.

Client Education

Nature of the disease

Medication regimen

Signs and symptoms of worsening disease

Follow-up

In connection with pulmonologist

Referral

Refer to pulmonologist or other appropriate specialist.

SLEEP APNEA

SIGNAL SYMPTOMS snoring, disrupted sleep, nocturnal gasping

ICD-9 Code	780.51	Sleep apnea

Sleep apnea is a breathing disorder characterized by repetitive collapse of the upper airway during sleep, with consequent apnea, or cessation of breathing.

Epidemiology

Prevalence of obstructive sleep apnea approximately 2% in women and 4% in men.

Common among people with obesity, acromegaly, asthma, arterial hypertension and heart disease, adult-onset diabetes, or craniofacial abnormalities.

Etiology

Structural abnormalities

Physiology and Pathophysiology

Two types of sleep apnea have been described. Central sleep apnea, which is associated with central nervous system disorders such as encephalitis and brain-stem infarction, is rare; it is characterized by a lack of respiratory drive and no airflow. Obstructive sleep apnea is more common; it is characterized by closure of the upper airway, usually at the oropharynx, leading to the cessation of airflow despite continued ventilatory effort. Mixed sleep apnea can occur with a combination of central and obstructive sleep apneas.

Clinical Manifestations

Subjective

Loud snoring
Sleep disrupted by gasping or choking episodes, insomnia, excessive daytime sleepiness
Morning headaches
Fatigue
Irritability
Memory and judgment problems
Automobile or work-related accidents
Personality changes

Objective

Often normal
High blood pressure, obesity, large neck girth (in men 17 inches or greater and in women 16 inches or greater), and nasopharyngeal narrowing
Pulmonary hypertension and cor pulmonale (both rare).

Differential Diagnosis

Narcolepsy (characterized by excessive daytime sleepiness, irresistible sleep attacks, and cataplectic episodes of brief, barely perceptible weakness of a muscle group, e.g., jaw dropping or losing one's grip)
Restless leg syndrome (prickling, tingling, creeping and crawling sensations of the legs escalating to irresistible urge to move the legs; symptoms occur at rest and are worse toward evening)
Medication use (sedatives, stimulants, or alcohol)
Hypothyroidism (fatigue is prominent symptom but often associated with weight gain, skin changes, constipation, cold intolerance, and decreased deep tendon reflexes)
Addison's disease (weakness, weight loss, and anorexia associated with hyperpigmentation especially of the palmar creases and buccal mucosa)
Depression (depressed or saddened mood and/or decreased pleasure associated with sleep disturbances or weight loss or gain)
Congestive heart failure (fatigue and nocturnal dyspnea associated with peripheral edema, S3, S4, displaced PMI, and crackles)

Diagnostic Tests

Epworth Sleepiness Scale: Greater scores on the scale indicate greater daytime sleepiness.
Polysomnography: Expensive and requires nighttime stay at sleep laboratory. Can consider home sleep studies, although these are less accurate.

Complete blood count (to rule out infection).

Electrocardiogram (to rule out cardiac disorders).

Thyroid function (to rule out hypothyroid and hyperthyroid conditions).

Oximetry (to assess oxygen saturation).

Management/Treatment

Pharmacologic Management

Currently there is no safe and effective medication for sleep apnea.

Nonpharmacologic Management

Nasal continuous positive airway pressure (CPAP) or biphasic positive airway pressure (BPAP)

Oral/dental devices

Surgical procedures to correct structural abnormalities

Client Education

Explain nature of sleep apnea.

Teach proper use of CPAP or BPAP.

Instruct about weight loss, if appropriate.

Avoid alcohol and sedatives in the evening.

Avoid sleeping in the supine position.

Stop smoking if smoker.

Sleep hygiene: Consistent bedtime, reserving bed for sleep, minimizing distractions.

Follow-up

Regular follow-up needed to evaluate response to treatment and compliance.

Referral

Refer to sleep specialist for sleep studies.

Refer to dentist or orthodontist if considering oral/dental devices.

Refer to otolaryngologist for possible surgery.

REFERENCES

General

Adams, P.F., Hendershot, G.E., & Marano, M.A. (1999). Current estimates from the National Health Interview Survey, 1996. *Vital and Health Statistics, 10*(200).

American Thoracic Society: Guidenlines for the management of adults with community-acquired pneumonia. American Journal of Respiratory and Critcal Care Medicine 2001; 162: 1730–1754.

Brashers, V.L., & Davey, S.S. (1998). Alterations of pulmonary function. In K.L. McCance & S.E. Huether (Eds.), *Pathophysiology. The biologic basis for disease in adults and children* (pp. 1158–1200). St. Louis: Mosby.

Chesnutt, M.S., Prendergast, T.J., & Stauffer, J.L. (1999). Lung. In LM. Tierney, S.J. McPhee, & Papdakis, M.A. (Eds.), *Current medical diagnosis and treatment* (38th ed., pp. 255–338). Stamford, CT: Appleton & Lange.

Dains, J.E., Baumann, L.C., & Scheibel, P. (1998). *Advanced health assessment and clinical diagnosis in primary care.* St. Louis: Mosby.

DerMarderosian, A. (Ed.) (1999). *A guide to popular natural products*. St. Louis, MO: Facts and Comparisons.

Fugh-Berman, A. (1997). *Alternative medicine: What works*. Baltimore: Williams & Wilkins.

Larsen, G.L., Accurso, F.J., Deterdeing, R.R., Halbower, A.C., & White, C.W. (1999). Respiratory tract & mediastinum. In W.W. Hay, A.R. Hayward, M.J. Levin, & J.M. Sondheimer (Eds.), *Current pediatric diagnosis and treatment* (14th ed., pp. 418–464). Stamford, CT: Appleton & Lang.

Levine, B.S., & Meredith, P. (2000). *Pulmonary health*. In P.V. Meredith & N.M. Horan (Eds.), *Adult primary care* (pp. 350–379) Philadephia: Saunders.

Pagana, K.D., & Pagana, T.J. (1998). *Manual of diagnostic and laboratory tests*. St. Louis: Mosby.

Porth, C.M. (1998). *Pathophysiology: Concepts of altered health status* (5th ed.). Philadelphia: Lippincott.

Schappert, S.M., & Nelson, C. (1999). National ambulatory medical care survey: 1995–1996 summary. *Vital and Health Statistics, 13*(142).

Smith, D.S. (1999). *Field guide to bedside diagnosis*. Philadelphia: Lippincott.

Tauer, K.M., & Hollis, L.E. (1999). Lower respiratory disorders. In E.Q. Youngkin, K.J. Swain, J.F. Kissinger, & D.S. Israel (Eds.), *Pharmacotherapeutics: A primary care clinical guide* (pp. 393–471). Stamford, CT: Appleton & Lange.

Asthma

Bielory, L., & Lupoli, K. (1999). Herbal interventions in asthma and allergy. *Journal of Asthma, 31*(1), 1–65.

Davis, P.A., Chang, C., Hackman, R.M., Stern, J.S., & Gershwin, M.E. (1998). Acupuncture in the treatment of asthma: A critical review. *Allergologia et Immunopathologia (Madrid) 26,* 263–271.

Drugs for asthma (1999). *Medical Letter, 41*(1044), 5–10.

Ducharme, F.M., & Hicks, G.C. (2000). Anti-leukotriene agents compared to inhaled corticosteroids in the management of recurrent and/or chronic asthma. *Cochrane Database System Review, 3,* CD002314.

Field, T., Henteleff, T., Hernandez-Reif, M., Martinez, E., Mavunda, K., Kuhn, C., & Schanberg, S. (1998). Children with asthma have improved pulmonary functions after asthma therapy. *Journal of Pediatrics, 132,* 852–858.

Forecasted state-specific estimates of self-reported asthma prevalence—United States 1998. (1998). *Morbidity and Mortality Weekly Report, 47,* 1022–1025.

Hackman, R.M., Stern, J.S., & Gershwin, M.E. (1999). Complementary/alternative therapies in general medicine: Asthma and allergies. In J.W. Spencer & J.J. Jacobs (Eds.), *Complementary/alternative medicine: An evidenced-based approach* (pp. 65–89). St. Louis: Mosby.

Kamholz, S.L. (1999). Understanding pulmonary function tests. *The Clinical Advisor, 2*(9), 30–47.

Lehrer, P.M. (1998). Emotionally triggered asthma: A review of research literature and some hypotheses for self-regulation therapies. *Applied Psychophysiology and Biofeedback, 23*(1), 13–41.

Mannino, D.M., Noma, D.M., Pertowski, C.A., Ashizawa, A., Nixon, L.L., Johnson, C.A., Ball, L.B., Jack, E., & Sang, D.S. (1998). Surveillance for asthma—United States, 1960–1995. *Morbidity and Mortality Weekly Report, 47*(SS-1), 1–27.

Miller, J.E. (2000). The effects of race/ethnicity and income on early childhood asthma prevalence and health care use. *American Journal of Public Health, 90,* 428–430.

National Heart, Lung, and Blood Institute (1997). *Guidelines for the diagnosis and management of asthma* (NIH Publication No. 97-4051). Washington, DC: U.S. Department of Health and Human Services.

National Heart, Lung, and Blood Institute (1999). *Data Fact Sheet: Asthma statistics.* Washington, DC: U.S. Department of Health and Human Services.

Newacheck, P.W., & Halfon, N. (2000). Prevalence, impact and trends in childhood disability due to asthma. *Archives of Pediatric and Adolescent Medicine, 154,* 287–293.

Spooner, C.H., Saunders, L.D., & Rowe, B.H. (2000). Nedocromil sodium for preventing exercise-induced bronchoconstriction. *Cochrane Database System Review, 2,* CD001183.

Taylor, D.R., Sears, M.R., & Cockcroft, D.W. (1999). The beta-agonist controversy. *Medical Clinics of North America, 80,* 719–748.

Ziment, I. (2000). Recent advances in alternative therapies. *Current Opinion in Pulmonary Medicine, 6,* 71–78.

Bronchiolitis

Baker, K.A., & Ryan, M.E. (1999). RSV infection in infants and young children. What's new in diagnosis, treatment, and prevention? *Postgraduate Medicine, 106*(7), 97–111.

Blinkhorn, R.J. (1998). Upper respiratory tract infections. In G.L. Baum, J.D. Crapo, B.R. Celli, & J.B. Karlinsky (Eds.), *Textbook of pulmonary diseases* (6th ed., vol. 1, pp. 493–502). Philadelphia: Lippincott-Raven.

Carlsen, K.C.L., & Carlsen, K.H. (2000). Inhaled nebulized adrenaline improves lung function in infants with acute bronchiolitis. *Respiratory Medicine, 94,* 709–714.

Jeng, M., & Lemen, R.J. (1997). Respiratory syncytial virus bronchiolitis. *American Family Physician, 55,* 1139–1146.

Klassen, T.P. (1997). Recent advances in the treatment of bronchiolitis and laryngitis. *Pediatric Clinics of North America, 44,* 249–261.

Levy, B.T., & Graber, M.A. (1997). Respiratory syncytial virus infection in infants and young children. *Journal of Family Practice, 45,* 473–481.

Bronchitis, Acute

Anmin, C. (1998). Traditional Chinese medicine in treatment of bronchitis and bronchial asthma. *Journal of Traditional Chinese Medicine, 18*(1), 71–76.

Becker, K.L., & Appling, S. (1998). Acute bronchitis. *Lippincott's Primary Care Practice, 2,* 643–646.

Bent, S., Saint, S., Vittinghoff, E., & Grady, D. (1999). Antibiotics in acute bronchitis: A meta-analysis. *American Journal of Medicine, 107,* 62–67.

Finkelstein, J.A., Metlay, J.P., Davis, R.L., Rifas-Shiman, S.L., Dowell, S.F., & Platt, R. (2000). Antimicrobial use in defined populations of infants and young children. *Archives of Pediatric and Adolescent Medicine, 154,* 395–400.

Gonzales, R., Wilson, A., Crane, L.A., & Barrett, P.H. (2000). What's in a name? Public knowledge and experiences with antibiotic use for acute bronchitis. *American Journal of Medicine, 108,* 83–85.

Harvey, S. (1999). Acute bronchitis. In T.M. Buttaro, J. Trybulski, P.P. Bailey, & J. Sandberg-Cook (Eds.), *Primary care. A collaborative practice* (pp. 282–283). St. Louis: Mosby.

Hueston, W.J., & Mainous, A.G. (1998). Acute bronchitis. *American Family Physician, 57,* 1270–1276.

Leiner, S. (1997). Acute bronchitis in adults: Commonly diagnosed but poorly defined. *Nurse Practitioner, 22*(1), 104–117.

Mainous, A.G., Zoorob. R.J., & Hueston, W.J. (1996). Current management of acute bronchitis in ambulatory care: The use of antibiotics and bronchodilators. *Archives of Family Medicine, 5,* 79–83.

Chronic Obstructive Pulmonary Disease

American Thoracic Society (1995). Standards for the diagnosis and care of patients with chronic obstructive pulmonary disease. *American Journal of Respiratory and Critical Care Medicine, 153,* S77–S120.

Ball, P. (1995). Epidemiology and treatment of chronic bronchitis and its exacerbation. *Chest, 108,* 43S–52S.

Calverley, P.M.A. (2000). COPD. Early detection and intervention. *Chest, 117,* 365S–371S.

Celli, B.R. (1996). Current thoughts regarding treatment of chronic obstructive pulmonary disease. *Medical Clinics of North America, 80,* 589–609.

Celli, B.R. (1998). Clinical aspects of chronic obstructive pulmonary disease. In G.L. Baum, J.D. Crapo, B.R. Celli, & J.B. Karlinsky (Eds.), *Textbook of pulmonary diseases,* (6th ed.) (Vol. 2, pp. 843–863). Philadelphia: Lippincott-Raven.

Celli, B.R. (1998). Standards for the optimal management of COPD: A summary. *Chest, 113,* 283S–287S.

Demetis, S. (1999). Chronic obstructive pulmonary disease. In J.K. Singleton, S.A. Sandowski, C. Green-Hernandez, T.V. Horvath, R.V. DiGregorio, & S.P. Holzemer (Eds.), *Primary care* (pp. 792–799). Philadelphia: Lippincott.

Dewan, N.A., Rafique, S., Kanwar, B., Satpathy, H., Ryschon, K., Tillotson, G.S., & Niderman, M.S. (2000). Acute exacerbation of COPD. Factors associated with poor treatment outcome. *Chest, 117,* 662–671.

Ferguson, G.T., Enright, P.L., Buist, A.S., & Higgins, M.W. (2000). Office spirometry for lung health assessment in adults. *Chest, 117,* 1146–1161.

Grossman, R.F. (2000). Cost-effective therapy for acute exacerbations of chronic bronchitis. *Seminars in Respiratory Infections, 15,* 71–81.

Heath, J.H., & Mongia, R. (1998). Chronic bronchitis: Primary care management. *American Family Physician, 57,* 2365–2372.

Hilleman, D.E., Dewan, N., Malesker, M., & Friedman, M. (2000). Pharmacoeconomic evaluation of COPD. *Chest, 118,* 1278–1285.

Kanner, R.E. (1996). Early intervention in chronic obstructive pulmonary disease: A review of the Lung Health Study results. *Medical Clinics of North America, 80,* 523–544.

Niederman, M.S. (2000). Antibiotic therapy for exacerbations of chronic bronchitis. *Seminars in Respiratory Infections, 15,* 59–70.

Niewoehner, D.E. (1998). Anatomic and pathophysiological correlations in COPD. In G.L. Baum, J.D. Crapo, B.R. Celli, & J.B. Karlinsky (Eds.), *Textbook of pulmonary diseases* (6th ed., vol. 2, pp. 823–842). Philadelphia: Lippincott-Raven.

O'Donohue, W.J. (1996). Home oxygen therapy. *Medical Clinics of North America, 80,* 611–622.

Petty, T.L. (1997). A new national strategy for COPD. *Journal of Respiratory Disease, 18,* 365–369.

Petty, T.L. (1998). Supportive therapy in COPD. *Chest, 113,* 256S–262S.

Sethi, S. (1999). Infectious exacerbations of chronic bronchitis: Diagnosis and management. *Journal of Antimicrobial Chemotherapy, 43*(Suppl A), 97–105.

Silverman, E.K., & Speizer, F.E. (1996). Risk factors for the development of chronic obstructive pulmonary disease. *Medical Clinics of North America, 80,* 501–522.

Witta, K.M. (1997, July).COPD in the elderly. Controlling symptoms and improving quality of life. Advances for Nurse Practitioners, pp. 18–23, 27.

Common Cold

Coakley-Maller, C. & Shea, M. (1997, September). Respiratory infections in children: Preparing for the fall and winter. Advances for Nurse Practitioners, pp. 20–23, 27.

Dowell, S.F., Schwartz, B. & Phillips, W.R. (1998). Appropriate use of antibiotics for URIs in children: Part II. Cough, pharyngitis and the common cold. *American Family Physician, 58,* 1335–1342, 1345.

Weiss, M., DeAbate, C.A., Blondeau, J.M., Guthrie, R.M., Iannini, P.B. & Tillotson, G.S. (2000). Respiratory tract infections: Is "first-line" therapy now second best? *Consultant, 40*(13), S1–S36.

Croup

Blinkhorn, R.J. (1998). Upper respiratory tract infections. In G.L. Baum, J.D. Carpo, B.R. Celli, & J.B. Karlinsky (Eds.), *Textbook of pulmonary diseases* (6th ed., vol. 1, pp. 493–502). Philadelphia: Lippincott-Raven.

Marx, A., Torok, T.J., Homan, R.C., Clarke, M.J., & Anderson, L.J. (1997). Pediatric hospitalizations for croup (laryngotracheobronchitis): Biennial increases associated with human parainfluenza virus 1 epidemics. *Journal of Infectious Diseases, 176,* 1423–1427.

Cystic Fibrosis

Cystic fibrosis: Guidelines for accurate diagnosis (1998, September). *Consultant,* pp. 2201–2210.

Delk, K.K., Gevirtz, R., Hicks, D.A., Carden, F., & Rucker, R. (1993). The effects of biofeedback assisted breathing retraining on lung functions in patients with cystic fibrosis. *Chest, 105,* 23–28.

Hernandez-Reif, M., Field, T., Krasnegor, J., Martinez, E., Schwartzman, M., & Mavunda, K. (1999). Children with cystic fibrosis benefit from massage therapy. *Journal of Pediatric Psychology, 24*(2) 175–181.

Wood, R.E., Schafer, I.A., & Karlinsky, J.B. (1998). Genetic diseases of the lung. In G.L. Baum, J.D. Carpo, B.R. Celli, & J.B. Karlinsky (Eds.), *Textbook of pulmonary diseases* (6th ed., vol. 2, pp. 1451–1468). Philadelphia: Lippincott-Raven.

Lung Cancer

Demetis, S. (1999). Carcinoma of the lung. In J.K. Singleton, S.A. Sandowski, Green-Hernandez, C., Horvath, T.K., DiGregorio, R.V., & Holzemer, S.P. (Eds.), *Primary Care* (pp. 785–791). Philadephia: Lippincott-Raven.

Lung cancer in women: Lessons for the next century. (1999). *Women's Health in Primary Care, 2,* 810–815.

Strauss, G.M. (1998). Bronchiogenic carcinoma. In G.L. Baum, J.D. Carpo, B.R. Celli, & J.B. Karlinsky (Eds.), *Textbook of pulmonary diseases* (6th ed., vol. 2, pp. 1329–1381). Philadelphia: Lippincott-Raven.

Pneumonia

American Lung Association (2000). Trends in morbidity and morality: Pneumonia, influenza and acute respiratory conditions. New York: Author. (Available at http://www.lungusa.org).

American Thoracic Association (1993). Guidelines for the initial management of adults with community-acquired pneumonia: Diagnosis, assessment of severity; and initial antimicrobial therapy. *American Review of Respiratory Disease, 148,* 1418–1426.

Bartlett, J.G., Breiman, R.F., Mandell, L.A., & File, T.M. (1998). Community-acquired pneumonia in adults: Guidelines for management. *Clinical Infectious Diseases, 26,* 811–838.

Centers for Disease Control and Prevention (1997). Prevention of pneumococcal disease. Recommendations of the Advisory Committee on Immunization Practices (ACIP). *Morbidity and Mortality Weekly Report, 46*(RR-8).

Gleason, P.P., Wishwa, N.K., Stone, R.A., Lave, J.R., Obrosky, D.S., Schulz, R., Singer, D.E., Coley, C.M., Marrie, T.J., & Fine, M.J. (1997). Medical outcomes and antimicrobial costs with the use of the American Thoracic Society Guidelines for outpatients with community-acquired pneumonia. *JAMA, 278,* 32–39.

Heffelfinger, J.D., Dowell, S.F., Jorgensen, J.H., Flugman, K.P., Mabry, L.R., Musher, D.M., Plouffe, J.F., Rakowsky, A., Schuchat, A., Whitney, C.G., & the Drug-Resistant Streptococcus pneumoniae Therapeutic Working Group (2000). Management of community-acquired pneumonia in the era of pneumococcal resistance. *Archives of Internal Medicine, 160,* 1399–1408.

Jadavji, T., Law, B., Lebel, M.C., Kennedy, W.A., Gold, R., & Wang, E.E.L. (1997). A practical guide for the diagnosis and treatment of pediatric pneumonia. *Canadian Medical Association Journal, 156,* S703–S711.

Margolis, P., & Gadomski, A. (1998). Does this infant have pneumonia? *JAMA, 279,* 308–313.

Pneumonia and influenza death rates—United States, 1979–1984. (1995). *Morbidity and Mortality Weekly Report, 44,* 535–537.

Pulmonary Embolism

American Thoracic Society (1999). The diagnostic approach to acute venous thromboembolism. *American Journal of Respiratory and Critical Care Medicine, 160,* 1043–1066.

Baker, W.F. (1998). Diagnosis of deep venous thrombosis and pulmonary embolism. *Medical Clinics of North America, 82,* 459–476.

Bick, R.L., & Kaplan, H. (1998). Syndromes of thrombosis and hypercoagulability. *Medical Clinics of North America, 82,* 409–458.

Calikyan, R. (1999). Pulmonary thromboembolic disease. In J.K. Singleton, S.A. Sandowski, C. Green-Hernandez, C., Horvath, T. K., DiGregorio, R.V., & Holzemer, S.P. (Eds.), *Primary care* (pp. 825–833). Philadelphia: Lippincott-Raven.

Davidson, B. L. (1999). Controversies in pulmonary embolism and deep venous thrombosis. *American Family Physician, 60,* 1969–1980.

Haas, S.K. (1998). Treatment of deep venous thrombosis and pulmonary embolism: Current recommendations. *Medical Clinics of North America, 82,* 495–510.

Hirsh, J., & Hoak, J. (1996). Management of deep vein thrombosis and pulmonary embolism. *Circulation, 93,* 2212–2245.

Sarcoidosis

American Thoracic Society (1999). Statement on sarcoidosis. *American Journal of Respiratory and Critical Care Medicine, 160,* 736–755.

Belfer, M.H., & Stevens, R.W. (1998). Sarcoidosis: A primary care review. *American Family Physician, 58,* 2041–2050.

Blackmon, G.M., & Raghu, G. (1995). Pulmonary sarcoidosis: A mimic of respiratory infection. *Seminars in Respiratory Infection, 10*(3), 176–186.

Rybicki, B.A., Maliarik, M.J., Major, M., Popovich, J., & Iannuzzi, M. C. (1998). Epidemiology, demographics, and genetics of sarcoidosis. *Seminars in Respiratory Infection, 13*(3), 166–173.

Tanoue, LT., & Elias, J. A. (1998). Systemic sarcoidosis. In G.L. Baum, J.D. Carpo, B.R.

Celli, & J.B. Karlinsky (Eds.), *Textbook of pulmonary diseases* (6th ed., vol. 1, pp. 407–430. Philadelphia: Lippincott-Raven.

Sleep Apnea

American Thoracic Association/American Sleep Disorders Association (1998). Statement on health outcomes research in sleep apnea. *American Journal of Respiratory and Critical Care Medicine, 157,* 335–341.

Dato, C. (1999). Sleeping disorders. In J.K. Singleton, S.A. Sandowski, C. Green-Hernandez, T.V. Horvath, R.V. DiGregorio, & S.P. Holzemer (Eds.), *Primary care* (pp. 686–691). Philadelphia: Lippincott.

Man, G.C.W. (1996). Obstructive sleep apnea. *Medical Clinics of North America, 80,* 803–820.

National Heart, Lung, and Blood Institute (1995). *Sleep apnea: Is your patient at risk?* (NIH Publication No. 95-3803). Bethesda, MD: Author.

Partinen, M. (1995). Epidemiology of obstructive sleep apnea syndrome. *Current Opinions in Pulmonary Medicine, 1,* 482–487.

Strohl, K.P. (1998). Sleep apnea syndrome and sleep-disordered breathing. In G.L. Baum, J.D. Carpo, B.R. Celli, & J.B. Karlinsky (Eds.), *Textbook of pulmonary diseases* (6th ed., vol. 2, pp. 867–882). Philadelphia: Lippincott-Raven.

Victor, L.D., (1999). Obstructive sleep apnea. *American Family Physician, 60,* 2279–2286.

Weinstein, R.A. (2000). Community-aquired pneumonia in adults. 38th annual meeting of the Infectious Diseases Society of America conference summary. Presented in August 2001. Chicago, IL.

RESOURCES

All Net Pediatric Critical Care Textbook
http://pedsccm.wustl.edu/All-Net/english/pulmpage/bronchio/intro.html

Alpha$_1$ National Association
8120 Penn Ave. S.
Ste. 549
Minneapolis MN 55431-1326
Telephone: (952) 703-9979 or 800-521-3025
http://www.alpha1.org

American Academy of Family Practice
11400 Tomahawk Creek Pky.
Leawood, KS 66211-2672
Telephone: (913) 906-6000
http://www.aafp.org/

American Cancer Society
Telephone: 1-800-ACS-2345
http://www.cancer.org/

American College of Allergy, Asthma & Immunology
85 W. Algonquin Rd.
Suite 550
Arlington Heights, IL 60005
http://allergy.mcg.edu/home.html

American College of Chest Physicians
3300 Dundee Rd.
Northbrook, IL 60062-2348
Telephone: (847) 498-1400
http://www.chestnet.org

American Heart Association National Center
    7272 Greenville Ave.
    Dallas, TX 75231
    Telephone: 1-800-AHA-USA1
    http://www.americanheart.org

American Lung Association
    1740 Broadway
    New York, NY 10019
    Telephone: (212) 315-8700
    http://www.lungusa.org/

American Sleep Apnea Association
    1424 K St. NW
    Washington, DC 20005
    Telephone: (202) 293-3650
    http://www.sleepapnea.org

American Thoracic Society
    1740 Broadway
    New York, NY 10019
    Telephone: (212) 315-8700
    http://www.thoracic.org

Children's Virtual Hospital
    http://www.vh.org/Providers/Textbooks/ElectricAirway/Text/MICCroupSymptoms.html

Cystic Fibrosis Foundation
    6931 Arlington Rd.
    Bethesda, Maryland 20814
    Telephone: (301) 951-4422
    http://www.cff.org

Infectious Diseases Society of America
    99 Canal Center Plaza
    Suite 210
    Alexandria, VA 22314
    Telephone: (703) 299-0200
    http://www.idsociety.org

JAMA Asthma Information Center
    http://www.ama-assn.org/special/asthma/asthma.htm

National Cancer Institute
    Bldg., 31, Rm. 10A03
    31 Center Dr.
    MSC 2580
    Bethesda, MD 20892-2580
    Telephone: (301) 435-3848
    http://www.nci.nih.gov/

National Center on Sleep Disorders
    2 Rockledge Centre
    Suite 7024
    6701 Rockledge Dr., MSC 7920
    Bethesda, MD 20892-7920
    Telephone: (301) 435-0199

http://www.nhlbi.nih.gov/about/ncsdr/index.htm

National Heart, Lung, and Blood Institute, National Institutes of Health
NHLBI Information Center
P.O. Box 30105
Bethesda, MD 20824-015
Telephone: (301) 592-8573
http://www.nhlbi.nih.gov/index.htm

National Jewish Medical and Research Center
1400 Jackson St.
Denver, CO 80206
Telephone: 1-800-222-LUNG
http://www.njc.org/

National Lung Health Education Program
HealthONE Center
1850 High St.
Denver, CO 80218
Telephone: (303) 839-6755
http://www.nlhep.org

National Sarcoidosis Foundation
St. Michael's Medical Center
268 Dr. Martin Luther King Blvd.
Newark, NJ 07102
Telephone: 1-800-223-6429

National Sarcoidosis Resource Center
Telephone: (908) 699-0733
http://www.nsrc-global.net/

National Sleep Foundation
1522 K St., NW
Suite 500
Washington, DC 20005
http://www.sleepfoundation.org

Oncolink, University of Pennsylvania
http://www.oncolink.upenn.edu

Sarcoidosis Center
http://www.sarcoidcenter.com/

Sarcoidosis Online Resources
http://www.blueflamingo.net/sarcoid/

UC Davis Center for Complementary & Alternative Medicine Research in Asthma
Department of Nutrition
3150 Meyer Hall
University of California, Davis
1 Shields Ave.
Davis, CA 95616-8669
Telephone: (530) 752-6575
http://www-camra.ucdavis.edu/

Chapter 6

CARDIOVASCULAR SYSTEM

ANEMIA

SIGNAL SYMPTOMS ▶ fatigue, weakness, dyspnea

ICD-9 Codes	280.0	Anemia of chronic disease
	285.9	Atypical (primary)
	281.1	Pernicious anemia
	281.1	Vitamin B_{12} deficiency
	281.2	Folate deficiency
	280.9	Iron-deficiency anemia
	280.0	Blood loss anemia
	272.4	Hemolytic anemia
	282.60	Sickle-cell anemia
	282.4	Thalassemia
	285.9	Anemia NOS
	285.9	Low HCT

Anemia is a group of diseases characterized by a significant reduction in red-blood-cell (RBC) mass or hemoglobin (Hgb), which corresponds to a decrease in the oxygen-carrying capacity of the blood. The World Health Organization (WHO) defines anemia as a peripheral hemoglobin level less than 13 g and a hematocrit less than 42% for men, and a hemoglobin level less than 12 g and a hematocrit less than 36% for women.

A decline in circulating RBCs can be a result of inadequate production or increased RBC destruction or loss. Inadequate production may be caused by ineffective erythropoiesis related to an erythrocyte maturation defect or a hypoproliferative state.

Anemia is classified according to morphology, pathophysiology, or etiology:

Morphology: Describes whether cell sizes are normochromic, hypochromic, or hyperchromic.

Normocytic, normochromic: RBC size is normal, with normal hemoglobin content, but circulating numbers are decreased. Examples include blood loss, hemolysis, chronic disease (infection, inflammation, renal failure, aplastic anemia, hypothyroidism), bone marrow failure, and myeloplastic anemias.

Microcytic, hypochromic: RBCs are smaller than normal, with a decrease in the amount of hemoglobin. Examples include iron-deficient, genetic abnormalities such as sickle-cell anemia, thalassemia, and other hemoglobinopathies.

Macrocytic: RBCs are larger than normal. Examples include megaloblastic anemias (vitamin B_{12} deficiency, folic acid deficiency) hemolytic, hemorrhagic.

The cells are classified as macrocytic when they are oversized, normocytic when they are normal sized, and microcytic when they are smaller than normal.

Anemias are classified on the basis of three mechanisms: deficiency (iron, vitamin B_{12}, folic acid, pyridoxine); central—caused by impaired bone marrow function (anemia of chronic disease, anemia of the elderly, malignant bone disorders); and peripheral (bleeding [hemorrhage] hemolysis [hemolytic anemias]).

Epidemiology

2% of the U.S. population is anemic.

Iron-deficiency anemia is single most common cause; it represents 50–75% of all cases.

Anemia is more common in young women (as a result of menstrual bleeding and pregnancy); 10%–20% of menstruating women and 20%–60% of pregnant women suffer from iron-deficiency anemia (IDA).

Folate deficiency is common in pregnancy and alcoholic liver disease; it is the most commonly observed problem in the elderly.

African-Americans have a higher incidence of anemia.

Iron deficiency is the most common nutritional deficiency in the world; the second most common anemia is that resulting from chronic disease.

Pernicious anemia is the most common form of anemia of vitamin B_{12} deficiencies.

Thalassemia minor—mild anemia in people of Mediterranean or Far Eastern extraction.

Sickle-cell disease and trait—most common hemoglobinopathy, found primarily in people of African extraction and in a wide area including the Mediterranean region.

Etiology

Excessive blood loss (recent hemorrhage)

Trauma

Peptic ulcer disease

Gastritis

Hemorrhoids (chronic hemorrhage)

Vaginal bleeding

Peptic ulcer

Intestinal parasites

Drugs (aspirin, nonsteroidal antiinflammatory drugs)

Excessive cell destruction

Extracorpuscular/intracorpuscular (inadequate production of mature RBCs)

Deficiency of nutrients (vitamin B_{12}, folic acid, iron, protein)

Deficiency of erythroblasts

Conditions with bone marrow infiltration
Endocrine abnormalities
Chronic renal disease
Chronic inflammatory disease
Hepatic disease

Physiology and Pathophysiology

Abnormality of Hemoglobin Synthesis

A defect in hemoglobin synthesis results in an abnormal hemoglobin molecule.

Under normal conditions, the body produces 6.25 g of hemoglobin/day. The survival time for the normal RBC is 120 days.

The delivery of iron to the bone marrow is accomplished by a specific plasma transport protein (globulin), called transferrin.

The average adult body contains approximately 4 g of iron about two thirds of which exists as myoglobin; the remainder is a combination of ferritin and hemosiderin.

Iron is absorbed more effectively from the duodenum and upper portion of the jejunum.

Intestinal absorption is sensitive to the number of RBCs, not to total iron stores in the body. Under normal conditions the loss of iron is around 1 mg in men and postmenopausal women—the same as the amount absorbed from the intestine. In menopausal women, the requirement is between 1.5 and 3 mg. Pregnant women and children have increased iron needs. A menstruating woman needs to absorb iron at a rate of 2 mg/day to compensate for blood loss. Pregnancy results in a need for 2.5 to 3 mg/day to meet demands of the fetus.

The normal Western diet contains 12–15 mg of iron mainly in the ferric (Fe^{3+}) unabsorbed form. The average American diet contains 12 mg of iron in 2000 calories (Goroll, 2000, p 532).

Bone Marrow Failure

Usually identified as an anemia that occurs gradually over weeks to months.

Underproduction anemias can be a result of bone marrow failure or a failure to produce erythropoietin.

Conditions with infiltration of the bone marrow include lymphoma and leukemia.

Hemolysis of RBCs

Hemolytic anemias are classified into an intrinsic defect of red cells, usually congenital and those involving an extrinsic defect, usually acquired. They can also be categorized at the level of cell destruction. Two locations are primarily responsible—the circulation (intravascular) and the spleen (extravascular). In the absence of the spleen, the liver becomes the predominant hemolytic organ. The usual response of the bone marrow to hemolysis is an increase in erythropoiesis up to eightfold, seen in the laboratory results as an elevated reticulocyte count. Hemolysis should be suspected whenever the reticulocyte count is elevated with no evidence of blood loss. Unconjugated bilirubin is usually increased in hemolytic states because of the release of the hemoglobin breakdown pigments from the macrophages. Other laboratory abnormalities may include decreased serum haptoglobin, hemoglobinemia, hemoglobinuria, hemosiderinuria, and increased lactate dehydrogenase.

Clinical Manifestations

See Table 6–1 for the clinical manifestations and management of the various types of anemias.

> Diagnostic tests: Men: Hgb, <13 g, Hct, $<42\%$; women: Hgb, <12 g, Hct, $<36\%$)
>
> Differential Diagnosis (Any of the following can present with signs and symptoms of anemia)
> Microcytic Anemias (mean corpuscular volume [MCV], <80)
> Iron-deficiency anemia
> Thalessemia
> Sideroblastic anemia
> Anemia of chronic disease (e.g., HIV, malignancy)
> Lead poisoning
> Macrocytic anemia (MCV, >100)
> Pernicious anemia
> Folic acid (folate) deficiency
> Anemia of liver disease
> Myeloblastic syndromes
> Normocytic anemia
> Anemia of chronic disease (e.g., renal failure, hypothyroidism, HIV)
> Aplastic anemia
> Hemolytic/hemorrhagic:
>> Pure red-cell aplasia
>> Infiltration marrow diseases
>> Exclude reversible causes
>> Sickle-cell anemia
>> Other hemoglobinopathies
>> Acute pain syndrome (bone, joints)

Diagnostic Tests

It is best to start with a complete blood count (CBC), RBC indices, and a reticulocyte count. If you are unable to make your diagnosis from these tests, proceed to the other diagnostic tests listed.

> CBC.
> RBC Indices.
>> MCV (mean corpuscular volume) measured in femtoliters, is the volume of space occupied by one red cell; it is the basis for the classification of anemia.
>> MCHC (mean corpuscular hemoglobin concentration) measured in grams per deciliter; measures the average concentration of hemoglobin in the RBCs; calculated with the MCH.

Table 6–1   Clinical Manifestations and Management of Anemia

Type of Anemia	Clinical Manifestations	Diagnostic Tests	Treatment
Microcytic Anemia (MCV, <80 μg)			
Iron-deficiency anemia	Fatigue, listlessness, faintness, weakness, pallor, headaches, dyspnea on exertion, angina, tachycardia, pica, anorexia, bone pain, sensitivity to cold, pallor, dry skin, brittle nails and hair, increased pulse/ respirations, wide pulse pressure, heart murmurs, myocardial hypertrophy	MCHC: Low Reticulocyte count: Low RDW: Increased TIBC: Increased Ferritin: Low Iron: Low	Ferrous sulfate, 300–325 mg for 6 months (levels should return to normal within 2 months). If nausea occurs, give smaller amounts of iron with each administration. Food affects iron absorption—give 1 or 2 hours before meals. *Note:* In women in whom iron deficiency is suspected, CBC should be done during menstrul cycle.
Thalassemia	Weakness, faintness, fatigue, pallor or bronze appear-ance, head-ache, dyspnea on exertion, angina, anorexia, tachycardia, widening pulse pressure, systolic murmur, tachypnea, may have bone deformity of face (chipmunk deformity)	Reticulocyte count: Normal or increased Iron: Normal or increased TIBC: Normal Ferritin: Normal or increased RDW: Normal Hgb electrophoresis: Decreased α- or β-hemoglobin chains	Refer to hematologist Iron supplementation contraindicate Stress good nutrition
Macrocytic Anemia (MCV, >100 μg)			
Pernicious anemia	Weakness, sore tongue or glossitis, palpitations, dizziness, peripheral paresthesias, swelling of legs, anorexia, diarrhea, mucositis, premature aging, tachycardia, hepatomegaly, splenomegaly, increased or decreased DTRs,	Reticulocyte count: Normal or low MCHC: Normal Serum vitamin B_{12}: <100 pg/ml Folate: Normal or low Bilirubin: Increased Urobilinogen: Increased on Schilling test	Vitamin B_{12} (cyanoco-balamin) IM daily for 1 wk; decrease frequency and give a total of 2000 μg during first 6 wk of therapy; mainte-nance dose, 100 μg IM monthly

Table continued on following page.

**Table 6–1 Clinical Manifestations and Management:
Anemia (*Continued*)**

Type of Anemia	Clinical Manifestations	Diagnostic Tests	Treatment
	diminished position sense, ataxia, poor coordination, positive Romberg and Babinski signs, mental status changes		
Folic acid deficiency	Easily fatigues, dizziness, listlessness, dyspnea on exertion, pallor, faintness, weakness, headaches, tachycardia, angina, anorexia, pica, pale, lethargic, Increased pulse/respirations, dry skin, brittle nails and hair, functional murmurs, may have hepatic enlargement	Reticulocyte count: Normal Or decreased MCHC: Normal Folate: <3 ng/ml Serum vitamin B_{12}: Normal Shilling test: Normal	Folate 1 mg PO or IM daily
Normocytic Anemia			
Anemia of chronic disease	Fatigue, weakness, dyspnea on exertion, light-headedness, anorexia, increased pulse/respirations, pale skin, skin may be jaundiced, sclera may be icteric, tongue may be coated	MCV: Normal or slightly low Serum iron: Low TIBC: Normal or low Serum ferritin: Normal or increased	Treat underlying disease Adequate nutritional intake, rest Some respond to erythropoietin 25–250 U/kg given subcutaneous three times per week or 150–600 U/kg twice per week
Other			
Sickle-cell anemia	Fever and pallor, arthralgia, scleral icterus, abdominal pain, weakness, anorexia, skin ulcers, jaundice, cardiomegaly, systolic murmur hepatomegaly, degenerative arthritis Adults experience delays in growth and sexual maturation,	Reticulocyte count: Increased Platelets: Increased Hemoglobin electrophoresis RBC cellular morphology: Shows evidence of sickling	Therapeutic Supportive Long-term folic acid supplementation with folic acid 1 mg/day Acute episodes (painful) Analgesia High-volume IV fluids Oxygen Antibiotic Blood transfusion Long-term Management

Table continued on following page.

Table 6–1   Clinical Manifestations and Management: Anemia (*Continued*)

Type of Anemia	Clinical Manifestations	Diagnostic Tests	Treatment
	height and weight below average; for women, reduced level of fertility, menstrual abnormalities		Pneumococcal vaccine Pentoxifylline (Trental) Bone marrow transplantation Prophylactic heparin

DTR = deep tendon reflex; MCHC = mean corpuscular hemoglobin concentration; MCV = mean corpuscular volume; RDW = red-cell size distribution width; TIBC = total iron-binding capacity.

MCH (mean corpuscular hemoglobin); measures the average weight of hemoglobin per RBC; measurement significant for clients with severe anemia.

RDW (red-cell size distribution width) detects red cell heterogeneity (variation in size).

Reticulocyte count.

Platelet count.

Review RBC cellular morphology.

Further testing may include:

Schilling test (to diagnose vitamin B_{12} deficiency anemia)

Iron concentration (serum iron level): men, 75–175; women, 65–165; newborns 100–250

Ferritin (determine iron stores): <15 mg/L indicates IDA

Total iron-binding capacity (TIBC): 240–450 mg/dl is normal

Folate and vitamin B_{12}

Transferrin saturation <16% indicates IDA nml 10–50 ♂ 15–50 ♀

Bone marrow aspiration

Electrophoresis (to differentiate thalassemia)

Management/Treatment

Pharmacologic Management
See Table 6–1.

Client Education
Teach clients to identify signs and symptoms of anemia.

Provide medical instruction (when, where, how, with what).

Inform about the possible side effects of medication (such as constipation with iron administration).

Teach about diet therapy.

Develop management strategies.

Identify safe activity level; restore activity slowly.

Accidental iron overdoses are often fatal for young children. Keep all medications out of reach of children.

Follow-up

Follow-up depends on type of anemia:

For less acute anemias (e.g., iron deficiency), initial follow-up may be 4–8 weeks, and then 3–6 months after treatment stabilization.

For more acute anemias (e.g., sickle-cell anemia), follow-up will be much sooner, as patients are often hospitalized.

Referral

Refer to a hematologist if unable to reach adequate blood levels with treatment plans or for more complicated, less common anemias.

ANGINA PECTORIS

SIGNAL SYMPTOM▶ chest pain

ICD-9 Code	413.9	Angina Pectoris

Angina is a symptomatic manifestation of myocardial ischemia—a paroxysmal thoracic pain with a feeling of suffocation and impending death due to anoxia of myocardium. Ischemia is defined as a lack of oxygen and decreased or no blood flow in the myocardium. Anoxia results when oxygen demand exceeds available supply. Vasoconstriction responses to decreased oxygen increases vascular resistance and reduces myocardial perfusion (Goroll, 2000, p 194).

In a chronic stable setting angina occurs when demand exceeds vascular supply.

Epidemiology

Gender prevalence depends on age: Overall it is more prevalent in men than in women (4·1); under age 40, the ratio is 8:1, and over age 70 it is 1:1.

For chronic stable angina the annual risk of death is 2% to 12%.

Etiology

Atherosclerosis is the most common cause.

Cholesterol deposition and reactive endothelial injury leads to acute thrombosis.

Pain occurs when demand exceeds supply.

Vasospastic disease.

Restriction of coronary blood flow.

Related to loss of endothelial vasoregulatory activity.

Coronary endothelium stops producing vasoactive peptides and prostaglandin, leaving vascular smooth muscle unopposed and susceptible to spasm.

Documented in patients both with and without disease.

Coronary stenosis: Hemodynamically significant stenosis or calcific obstruction of coronary ostia results in inadequate perfusion.

Coronary microvascular dysfunction: Vasoconstrictive responses to autonomic and biochemical stimuli can increase total resistance and reduce myocardial perfusion (also known as microvascular angina or syndrome X).

Silent myocardial ischemia: Documented ischemia in the absence of symptoms; mechanism unknown.

Metabolic contributors: Hyperthyroidism, fever, severe anemia, respiratory insufficiency

Circadian susceptibility: Chest pain occurs more typically in early morning, with surge of catecholamines.

Physiology and Pathophysiology

The pathophysiology of angina pectoris is dynamic. It is based on determinants of oxygen demand (heart rate, contractility, and intramyocardial wall tension) and regulation of coronary blood flow (extrinsic anatomic factors, such as resistance and perfusion pressure, and intrinsic factors, such as metabolic and myogenic responses, neural reflexes, and humoral substance).

Clinical Manifestations

Subjective

RISK FACTORS (REVIEW WITH PATIENT)

Increased cholesterol
Increased low-density lipoprotein (LDL) cholesterol
Decreased high-density lipoprotein (HDL) cholesterol
Hypertension
Smoking
Male gender
Postmenopausal woman
Advanced age
Family history of premature heart disease
Diabetes

QUALITY OF DISCOMFORT

Tightness, squeezing, heaviness, burning, indigestion, or an aching sensation.
Only rarely described as pain (client will correct you).
Lasts for a few minutes (<10).

LOCATION AND RADIATION

Levine sign—Fist to chest.
Angina is usually diffuse rather than localized.
Most intense in the retrosternal or anterior chest (left), jaw, and abdomen.
Anginal pattern in each patient is different, but in the same patient, the pattern will be similar with each episode.

PRECIPITATING FACTORS

Exertion
Emotional stress
Eating

ASSOCIATED SYMPTOMS

Dyspnea

Diaphoresis

Nausea

Fatigue

Palpitations

Resolve quickly along with chest pain; typically lasts 15–20 minutes; if more than 30 minutes—unstable angina

FREQUENCY

Level of exertion needed to precipitate angina remains fairly constant.

Patient recognizes this and avoids activities that stimulate pain.

Unstable development occurs when frequency or duration (or both) increases, and it also occurs at rest or with minimal activity.

RELIEVING FACTORS

Rest

Nitroglycerin

Objective

GENERAL VASCULAR EXAMINATION

Equality of blood pressure

Palpation and auscultation of carotid arteries

CARDIAC EXAMINATION

May have no remarkable physical findings.

S_4 common with coronary artery disease (CAD), but not indicative.

Abdominal examination to rule out abdominal aortic aneurysm.

Observe for evidence of congestive heart disease.

Differential Diagnosis

Gastroesophageal reflux disease (GERD; pain is usually epigastric, and burning in quality; worse after eating)

Anxiety (pain difficult to localize; timing can be very random, and often coincides with symptoms of anxiety)

Depression (similar to anxiety)

Costochondral pain (pain usually substernal, can often be reproduced on palpation)

Pneumothorax (patient presents with sudden difficulty breathing)

Congestive heart failure (patient unable to lie flat; wakes in the middle of night breathing fast; possible peripheral swelling)

Pneumonia (chest congestion, productive cough, fever/chills)

Pericarditis (fever, precordial pain, dry cough dyspnea and palpitations)

Asthma (chest tightness, difficulty breathing, audible wheezing)

Myocardial infarction (squeezing chest pain made worse with exertion and relieved by rest, diaphoresis)

Diagnostic Tests

Lipids

Increased cholesterol

Increased LDL (cholesterol:HDL ratio >4.5%)

Fasting blood sugar (to rule out hypoglycemia or hyperglycemia)

Hemoglobin/hematocrit (may exacerbate symptoms if anemic)

Chemistry profile (to rule out electrolyte imbalances)

Thyroid studies (to rule out hypothyroid or hyperthyroid disorders, which can exacerbate myocardial ischemia)

Isoenzymes/troponin I (to rule out myocardial infarction for angina more than 20 minutes)

Electrocardiogram (ECG) during episode demonstrates elevation or depression of ST-segment or T-wave peak or inversion during episode; reversal after attack; normal in 25% of clients)

Further testing (beyond primary care setting) may include:

Coronary angiography (definitive test for diagnosis of coronary artery disease)

Thallium 201

Exercise ECG (stress test) (ischemic changes or angina during test; clinically diagnostic)

Nuclear medicine studies (to evaluate presence, extent, and location of disease)

Echocardiography/stress echocardiography (during attack can determine abnormalities at ventricular wall—suggestive of disease; with exercise can detect ventricular-wall abnormalities)

Radionuclide ventriculography (can help evaluate infarction and ischemic segments of the heart)

Ambulatory ECG

Management/Treatment

Pharmacologic Management

ACUTE ATTACK

Administer sublingual or buccal nitroglycerin.

If pain unrelieved after three doses at 5-minute intervals, evaluate in emergency room.

MEDICATIONS

Lipids: Lower LDL cholesterol to <100 mg/dl; if after 3 months of dietary modification LDL is >160 or 130 mg/dl, pharmacologic therapy is recommended.

Nicotinic acid: Start slow and then increase; usual dose 1000–3000 mg/day. Usual rate of titration is 100 mg TID for 1 week, 200 mg TID for 1 week, 300 mg TID for 1 week, 500 mg TID for 1 week, then 1000 mg TID.

Bile-acid-binding resins: Start with 1 package/day; increase to achieve results.

Statins: Start with low dose; titrate to achieve goals.

Aspirin therapy: For all clients, 81–325 mg/day with food.

β-Blockers: Prevent angina by reducing myocardial oxygen requirements; use with caution in clients with ejection fraction <35%, lung disease, or bradycardia.

Metoprolol, 50–200 mg daily in two divided doses.

Atenolol, 25–200 mg daily.

Calcium-channel blockers: Prevent angina by reducing myocardial oxygen demand and effecting vasodilation; use with caution in clients with congestive heart failure.

Nifedipine (Procardia XL) (long-acting form), 30–60 mg once daily.

Verapamil (Isoptin, Calan, Verelan), 180–480 mg daily.

Diltiazem (Cardizem, Tiazac, Dilacor XR), 120–360 mg daily.

Long-acting nitrates: Prevent angina by effecting vasodilation.

Isosorbide dinitrate (Isordil, Sorbitrate), 10–40 mg TID.

Mononitrate form (Imdur, ISMO, Monoket), 30–60 mg up to 160 mg daily.

Nitroglycerin patch (NitroDur, Transderm), 0.2–0.6 mg/min (worn only 12 hours/day to avoid tolerance).

Sustained-release nitroglycerin (NitroBid), 2.5–18 mg BID–QID.

Treat underlying cause.

Nonpharmacologic Management

RISK MODIFICATION

Decrease activities that provoke angina.

Exercise.

Stop smoking.

Complementary/Alternative Therapies

Tai chi

Meditation

Relaxation therapy

Yoga

Client Education

Teach client how to take his or her own pulse.

Complete medication education.

Develop exercise plan.

Have client keep diary of symptoms and precipitating events.

Encourage family members to take cardiopulmonary resuscitation (CPR) training; teach family members when and how to activate 911 and EMS system.

Follow-up

Depends on frequency and severity of symptoms. If patient has angina that is stable, follow-up should be 3–6 months.

Referral

Refer to cardiologist if angina is new in onset or its characteristics are changing, or if client's disease fails to respond to pharmacologic therapy.

Hospitalize if client with stable angina develops pain while at rest (likelihood of impending myocardial infarction).

ATRIAL FIBRILLATION

SIGNAL SYMPTOMS ▶ fatigue, irregular heartbeat

ICD-9 Codes	427.31	Atrial fibrillation
	427.9	Rhythm disorder—arrhythmia, NOS

Atrial fibrillation is an irregular, rapid, and randomized contraction of the atria working independently of the ventricles. It is a type of supraventricular tachycardia that is characterized by fibrillatory atrial activity, an erratic ventricular response, and loss of the atrial kick (contraction); it may indicate underlying heart disease.

See Table 6–2 for types of atrial fibrillation.

Table 6–2   Types of Atrial Fibrillation

Type	Description
Lone atrial fibrillation	Appears without clinical evidence of heart disease, usually in persons <60. Is harmless in young people and is usually caused by stress, alcohol, stimulants, or smoking. No chamber enlargement. In elderly, problem is different, underlying heart disease, even if not apparent.
Tachycardia-bradycardia syndrome (sick sinus syndrome)	Important and subtle cause of atrial fibrillation. Cause is unknown—could be related to degenerating conduction system. Atrial tachycardia alternates with bradycardia and sinus arrest. Symptoms: Palpitations, lightheadedness, and syncope. Identification is very important because of the presence of bradycardia. Paroxysmal atrial fibrillation due to "sick sinus" is associated with increased risk of thromboembolism.
Apathetic hyperthyroidism of the elderly	Can appear without evidence of heart disease. Signs: Apathy, impressive weight loss, severe depression. Signs and symptoms of thyrotoxicosis are usually absent. Hard to control with standard therapy. Need to correct hyperthyroid state.
Wolff-Parkinson-White (WPW) syndrome	Characterized by rapid ventricular response >200 beats/min. May be partially congenital. Rapid atrioventricular conduction over an accessory pathway (Kent bundle branch). Conduction bypasses the atrioventricular node and causes preexcitation. May have normal base-line ECG. Irregular narrow QRS complex. Widening of the QRS toward flutter. Mimics ventricular fibrillation in 11%–39% of clients with WPW. Digitalis therapy may worsen and cause the client to go into ventricular tachycardia and/or ventricular fibrillation.
Alcohol cardiomyopathy	In early stages of alcohol cardiomyopathy a client may experience paroxysms of atrial fibrillation triggered by binge drinking. Difficult to distinguish from lone fibrillation because of its presentation Treatment—abstinence from alcohol.

Epidemiology

Atrial fibrillation.

Incidence is greater in men than in women.

Frequency increases with age.

Most common sustained arrhythmia; most common rhythm disturbance seen in clinical practice.

Most common cause of ischemic stroke in elderly.

Incidence.

Overall incidence of atrial fibrillation is about 2%; this approximately doubles in elderly men (Dipiro, 1999).

Seen in 2% of clients over 60 and 10% over 70 years of age.

Although common, morbidity is significant even in the absence of valvular disease.

Affects more than 2 million Americans (Noble, 2001).

Etiology

Occurs in clients with valvular and nonvalvular heart disease and in those with cardiac and noncardiac causes.

Can be acute or chronic and has numerous potential causes.

Acute atrial fibrillation lasts for only 24–48 hours, after which the heart spontaneously converts back to sinus rhythm.

Chronic atrial fibrillation: Most frequently associated with coronary artery disease, congestive heart failure, rheumatic heart disease, cardiomyopathy, pericarditis, ischemic heart disease, nonrheumatic mitral-valve disease, hypertensive cardiovascular disease, chronic lung disease, atrial septal defect, and other cardiac abnormalities.

Most common cause of atrial fibrillation is hypertension with evidence of left ventricular hypertrophy.

Physiology and Pathophysiology

Presents as persistent or paroxysmal form.

Usually related to hypertension, coronary artery disease, rheumatic heart disease, heart failure, hyperthyroidism, congestive heart failure, or hypoxia.

Common arrhythmia after heart surgery, emotional stress, exercise, or acute alcohol intoxication.

Clinical Manifestations

Subjective

Clients may be asymptomatic or may experience palpitations, difficulty breathing, fatigue, chest pain, and even dizziness and/or syncope.

During history-taking include family history of Wolff–Parkinson–White syndrome or heart disease; assess for alcohol, stress, stimulants, fever, infections, heart murmur, chest pain, preexisting heart disease, hypertension, dyspnea, cough, calf pain, edema, risk of embolization, medication history (alcohol, digitalis), other (weight loss, depression, level of consciousness, lightheadedness).

Objective
Irregular pulse
Possible hypotension
Tachycardia
Dyspnea
Auscultation of irregular heartbeat

Differential Diagnosis

Many of these have similar symptoms. They are diagnosed by ECG and/or other diagnostic tests:

Multifocal atrial tachycardia (atrial arrhythmias from many different locations)

Paroxysmal atrial tachycardia (rapid atrial arrhythmias occurring suddenly and periodically)

Atrial flutter (regular, rapid atrial activity noted on ECG)

Sinus arrhythmia

Premature ventricular beats (irregular ventricular contraction)

Ingestion of stimulants or drugs (elicited via patient history)

Hypoglycemia (fatigue, sweating, weakness, palpitations; diagnosed via measurement of serum blood glucose)

Hyperthyroidism (nervousness, weight loss, heat intolerance, sweating; diagnosed via thyroid-stimulating hormone [TSH] and free thyroxine [T_4] blood tests)

Mitral-valve prolapse (chest pain, shortness of breath, palpitations; diagnosed via cardiac ultrasound)

Wolff–Parkinson–White syndrome (an abnormal cardiac rhythm, often presenting as supraventricular tachycardia; diagnosed via ECG)

Coronary artery disease (diagnosed via angiogram and lipid testing)

Diagnostic Tests

The ECG is essential to correctly diagnose atrial fibrillation. The atrial rate is typically very fast (more than 300 beats per minute) and is usually irregular and disorganized. The corresponding ventricular rate (QRS complex) is often also irregular, and is based on the ability of the atrioventricular node to conduct impulses to the ventricles.

CBC (to rule out anemia or hematologic causes).

Chemistry panel (may show causes, such as hypomagnesemia, hypokalemia, or renal or liver disease).

TSH levels (to rule out secondary causes).

ECG (shows irregular rhythm, absent P waves, narrow QRS complexes unless bundle branch is present; distinguishing features are absence of P waves and irregular ventricular response; may see group beating; may see regular ventricular response rate indicating a drug-induced junctional tachycardia).

Holter monitor (24-hour; endless-loop recorder) (to diagnosis intermittent or infrequent arrhythmia).

Chest x-ray examination.

Echocardiography (to determine extent of structural heart disease).

Management/Treatment

See Figure 6–1

Pharmacologic Management

Rate and rhythm control.

Digitalis, calcium-channel blockers, β-blockers.

Calcium-channel blockers and β-blockers can be more useful at times due to the ability to slow the ventricular rate more quickly and effectively.

Caution with cardiac output and blood pressure.

Antithrombotic therapy (primary prevention of stroke; long-term therapy indicated)

Warfarin in nonvalvular atrial fibrillation reduces the risk of stroke for clients by 68%; not indicated in lone atrial fibrillation.

Treatment of underlying precipitants.

Nonpharmacologic Management

Radiofrequency ablation/modification with uncontrolled chronic atrial fibrillation

Cardioversion

Permanent pacemaker may be necessary

Atrial fibrillation confirmed

↓

Discuss with collaborating physician
Anticoagulate if client has sustained atrial fibrillation
    or structural heart disease
If heart rate is controlled, observe
If heart rate is not controlled, consider beta blockers,
    digoxin, calcium channel blockers

↓

If pharmacologic treatment is successful, observe
If pharmacologic treatment is unsuccessful, anti-
    coagulate for 3–4 week after effective INR
    (2.0–3.0), then perform electrical cardioversion to
    convert atrial fibrillation to sinus rhythm
Anticoagulate 4 weeks after cardioversion; maintain
    INR between 2.0 and 3.0

Figure 6–1 Treatment of Atrial Fibrillation in Office Setting

Client Education

Health promotion: stop smoking, take medications correctly, exercise, diet, limit use of alcohol or other stimulants, decrease stress.

Educate about when to call health-care provider.

Follow-up

Once patient is stabilized on treatment (usually with a cardiologist), follow-up can be 3–6 months. However, if patient is treated with antithrombotics (such as coumadin), follow-up for blood work (prothrombin time) may be weekly to monthly.

Referral

Refer to cardiologist if client is experiencing syncope or near-syncope, has a structural heart defect, complex dysrhythmias, arrhythmia that may cause cardiovascular embarrassment, is not responsive to pharmacologic agents, or is a child.

CHEST PAIN

SIGNAL SYMPTOMS heaviness or tightness in the chest

ICD-9 Codes	786.50	Chest pain, NOS
	786.52	Chest-wall pain

Cardiac chest pain is described as severe, oppressive, nagging, constrictive retrosternal discomfort. It often radiates to the left shoulder and down the left arm. It is often associated with anxiety, restlessness, diaphoresis, nausea, or dyspnea.

In general, chest pain is any type of pain or discomfort in the anterior thoracic area. This can include cardiac, pulmonary, musculoskeletal, gastrointestinal, psychiatric, and even drug abuse/overdose causes. Thus, a thorough history and physical examination are essential to a correct diagnosis.

Epidemiology

Adults

50% of patients presenting with chest pain with classic symptoms have disease.

Myocardial infarction (MI) is the cause of symptoms in 23% of patients who present with burning pain or indigestion.

MI was identified in 13% of patient describing chest ache, and in 5% with sharp, stabbing pain; in those with nonspecific chest discomfort, such as numbness or tugging, the incidence of MI was 23%.

Goroll (2000, p 110) found that between 18% and 31% of patients with angina-like symptoms and normal coronary arteries have esophageal disease. And at least 30% of patient admitted to the coronary-care unit do not have confirmed MIs.

Children

Fox (1997) found that the most common cause (20%–75%) is costochondritis.

The most common arrhythmia causing chest pain in children is supra-ventricular tachycardia (SVT).

In 21%–39% of children with chest pain it is idiopathic; in 30% it is musculoskeletal.

Anxiety and emotional distress account for 9%–20% of chest pain in adolescents.

Etiology

Depends on the underlying cause (cardiac, pulmonary, gastrointestinal, musculoskeletal, psychiatric, etc.). See "Angina Pectoris."

Physiology and Pathophysiology

Chest structures with sensory nerve fibers include the skin, fascia, skeletal muscle, periosteal lining of the ribs, parietal pleura, rib cartilage, and the inferior portion of the pericardium.

Clinical Manifestations

Subjective

History of previous similar episodes
History of presenting symptoms
    Pain brought on by excitation and relieved by rest
    Responds to nitroglycerin
    Brought on by eating
    Pain increased with respiration, cough, deep breathing, or position change
    Sudden onset of maximally severe pain
Classic symptoms of cardiac chest pain
    Squeezing, heaviness, or pressure (although may be burning or sharp)
    Radiating pattern—jaw, neck, shoulder, arm, back, or upper abdomen
    Nausea and vomiting may occur, with or without dyspnea
    Episodes last 2–20 minutes; prompt relief with nitroglycerin within 5 minutes; ischemic pain lasts longer, suggesting coronary insufficiency or MI

Objective

General appearance.
Vital signs (blood pressure in both arms).
Skin.
Eye examination—fundi.
Carotid pulses.
Jugular venous distention (JVD).
Chest-wall examination with pleuritic chest pain.
Auscultation of heart and lungs.
Abdominal examination.
Examination of legs for edema and phlebitis.
Peripheral pulses.
Palpate spine for tenderness.
Neurological—Check for new focal defects/deficits.

Differential Diagnosis

Cardiac

Cardiac chest pain is usually squeezing in quality, exacerbated by activity and relieved with rest; patient often cannot pinpoint pain. Causes include angina pectoris, myocardial infarction, arrhythmia, mitral-valve prolapse, aortic aneurysm, aortic dissection (sudden onset, severe chest pain, tearing/ripping quality, diminished peripheral pulses), pericarditis (sharp pain aggravated by respiration, activity, position; ECG shows ST-segment and T-wave changes).

Pulmonary

Causes include pneumonia (chest congestion, productive cough, fever/chills, aches), pleurisy (chest pain, fever, dry cough, anxiousness), pulmonary embolism (shortness of breath, tachycardia), pulmonary hypertension (chest pain, dyspnea, ventricular lift, increased JVD), and asthma (chest tightness, difficulty breathing, wheezing).

Gastrointestinal

Causes include GERD (substernal, burning pain, often worse after eating), esophagitis (substernal, burning pain), peptic ulcer (gnawing, burning epigastric pain, often 1–3 hours after eating), duodenal ulcer (right upper quadrant pain; patient often has positive test for *Helicobacter pylori*), gallbladder disease (stabbing right upper quadrant pain, often after eating; enlarged gallbladder/gallstones present on ultrasound), pancreatitis (sudden abdominal pain, nausea, vomiting).

Musculoskeletal

Causes include muscle strain (patient often able to pinpoint pain; reproducible on palpation), costochondritis (often substernal; patient able to pinpoint pain), bruised/fractured rib (tenderness at location; occasional difficulty breathing; diagnosed via x-ray examination), bursitis (in shoulder) (limited range of motion of shoulder, inflamed bursa).

Psychiatric

Chest pain is usually generalized and coincides with signs and symptoms of anxiety and depression). Causes include anxiety, panic attacks, and depression.

Drug Abuse

Elicited via patient history. Causes include cocaine use or abuse.

Other

Neoplasm or growth diagnosed via x-ray examination or computed tomographic scan; may have systemic symptoms such as fever/chills, fatigue, aches that do not improve.

Diagnostic Tests

Based on the working differential diagnosis

Management/Treatment

Pharmacologic Management

Depends highly on diagnosis. See other chapters for management of differential diagnoses. For pharmacologic management of cardiac chest pain, see "Angina Pectoris."

Nonpharmacologic Management
Decrease, or ideally discontinue, smoking
Low-fat diet
Regular aerobic exercise

Complementary/Alternative Therapies
Relaxation therapy
Meditation
Yoga
Tai chi

Client Education
Health promotion: Stop smoking, take medications correctly, exercise, diet, limit use of alcohol or other stimulants, decrease stress.
Educate about when to call health-care provider.
Diagnosis disease-process information.
Medication information (side effects, proper dosage).

Follow-up
Follow-up depends on diagnosis. See "Angina Pectoris."

Referral
Refer to cardiologist.

CORONARY ARTERY DISEASE

SIGNAL SYMPTOM chest pain (most common)

ICD-9 Codes	414.0	Coronary artery disease
	414.9	Ischemic heart disease
	414.0	Coronary atherosclerosis

Cardiovascular disease refers to a variety of diseases and conditions affecting the heart and blood vessels principally, high blood pressure, heart disease, and stroke.

Epidemiology
More than 960,000 Americans die of cardiovascular disease each year, accounting for more than 40% of all deaths.
Ischemic heart disease (coronary heart disease) death rates are estimated at 135.2 per 100,000 people.
Risk factors:
Positive family history (2–5 times greater risk than in general population).
Age.
Male gender (male:female ratio, 4:1; over age 70 ratio is 1:1).
Blood-lipid abnormalities (total serum cholesterol >260 mg/dl doubles risk).
Hypertension (doubles risk).
Physical inactivity/sedentary lifestyle.

Cigarette smoking (doubles risk; may triple risk in females).
Diabetes mellitus (doubles risk).
Elevation of homocystine levels.
Obesity.
Stress/personality type.

Etiology

Fatty streak.
Macrophages migrate into subendothelial space and take up lipids.
Plaque progresses, with smooth-muscle cells migrating into plaque.
Fibrous cap forms, with calcification; lumen narrows.
Rupture of plaque results in partial or complete occlusion of blood vessel.

Physiology and Pathophysiology

CAD occurs as a result of fatty streaks that deposit on coronary artery endothelium and may progress to form atherosclerotic plaques, depending on the absence or presence of specific risk factors. If progression occurs, plaques develop, proliferate, and eventually disrupt the integrity and function of the endothelium.

Clinical Manifestations

Subjective

Characteristic chest discomfort
    Sensation of tenderness, squeezing, burning pressure.
    80%–90% of clients experience discomfort behind or slightly to left of midsternum.
    Radiates most often to left shoulder and upper arm down inner aspect of arm.
    May be felt in lower jaw, back of neck, upper left side of back.
    Typically lasts 15–20 minutes.
Anxiety
Diaphoresis
Dyspnea
Nausea

Objective

Systolic and diastolic pressures may be elevated during attack.
May hear transient systolic murmur with mitral insufficiency.
Transient S_3 or S_4.
Evidence of cardiovascular risk factors.
Pulse and respirations may be elevated.
Levine's sign (highly suggestive of angina).
May not have any remarkable physical findings.

Differential Diagnosis

GERD (burning, epigastric pain, usually worse after eating)
Anxiety (generalized chest pain, often coinciding with anxiety symptoms)
Depression (similar to above)

Costochondral pain (patient usually able to localize pain; reproducible on palpation)

Pneumothorax (shortness of breath, difficulty breathing, same-sided chest pain)

Congestive heart failure (shortness of breath, nocturnal dyspnea, peripheral edema)

Pneumonia (chest congestion, productive cough, fever/chills, aches)

Pericarditis (fever, precordial chest pain and tenderness, dry cough, dyspnea, palpitations)

Asthma (chest tightness, difficulty breathing, wheezing)

Aortic dissection (sudden chest pain, weakness)

Myocardial infarction (squeezing chest pain, exacerbated with activity and relieved with rest, diaphoresis)

Diagnostic Tests

Initial testing includes:

CBC (to rule out anemia)

Chemistry panel (to rule out electrolyte imbalance)

Serum lipids (LDL >160 mg/dl indicates risk) (to rule out elevated cholesterol and/or triglycerides)

ECG (to rule out any cardiac electrical abnormalities; normal in 25% of clients; characteristic findings of myocardial infarction are ST-segment depression or T-wave inversion during attack; reverses after attack; may see evidence of old infarction)

Chest x-ray examination (to rule out infection, neoplasms, or fractures)

Further diagnostic testing includes:

Echocardiogram (to rule out valvular changes and determine cardiac functioning)

Exercise electrocardiogram (stress test) (to rule out coronary artery disease)

Thallium scan (abnormal base-line ECG indicates hypoperfusion)

Radionuclide ventriculography

Coronary angiography (indicated in clients with high probability of disease to aid in treatment)

Management/Treatment

Pharmacologic Management

Control elevated blood pressure (see "Hypertension")

Maintain normal range lipids (see "Lipid Disorders")

Manage angina (see "Angina Pectoris")

Nonpharmacologic Management

Decrease, or ideally discontinue, smoking.

Eat low-fat, low-salt diet.

Lose weight, if necessary.

Perform regular aerobic exercise.

Limit alcohol use.

Reduce stress.

Complementary/Alternative Therapies
Stress reduction
Meditation
Relaxation therapies
Yoga
Tai chi

Client Education
Educate about disease process.
Inform about risk factors, and teach about how to reduce risks.
Stress the importance of lifestyle modifications.
Health promotion: stop smoking, take medications correctly, exercise, diet,
limit use of alcohol or other stimulants, decrease stress.
Teach when to call health-care provider.
Teach client how to take his or her own pulse.
Develop exercise plan.
Have client keep diary of symptoms and precipitating events.
Encourage family members to take CPR training; teach family members
when and how to activate 911 and EMS system.

Follow-up
Initially, follow-up may need to be weekly to monthly; however, once stabilized,
follow-up can be 6–12 months.

Referral
Refer to cardiologist if angina is new in onset or its characteristics are changing, if
client's disease fails to respond to pharmacologic therapy, or if LDL goal is not
achieved after diet and/or medication.

HEART FAILURE

SIGNAL SYMPTOMS chest pain, dyspnea, paroxysmal nocturnal
dyspnea (PND), swelling

ICD-9 Codes	428.9	Congestive heart failure (CHF), NOS
	429.0	CHF, right
	428.1	CHF, left

New York Heart Association Classification Summarization
Class I—Cardiac disease, but without physical limitation.
Class II—Cardiac disease resulting in slight limitation of physical activity
(i.e., fatigue, palpitation, dyspnea, anginal pain).
Class III—Cardiac disease resulting in marked limitation of physical
activity (less than ordinary activity—results in fatigue, palpitation,
dyspnea, or anginal pain).
Class IV—Cardiac disease resulting in inability to carry on any physical
activity without discomfort. Symptoms of heart failure or the anginal

syndrome may be present even at rest. With any physical activity discomfort increases (AHA, 1994.).

Epidemiology

An estimated 4.8 million Americans are affected, with an estimated 400,000 new cases each year.

Most common diagnosis in hospital patients aged 65 and older.

Incidence of congestive heart failure is equal in men and women.

Incidence two times more common in patients with hypertension and in patients with coronary heart disease.

Fatality is high (one in five people die within 1 year); sudden death most common cause, occurring at a rate of six to nine times that of the general population.

Etiology

Systolic dysfunction (decreased contractility)

Dilated cardiomyopathies

Ventricular hypertrophy

Pressure overload (e.g., systemic or pulmonary hypertension, aortic or pulmonic valve)

Volume overload (e.g., valvular regurgitation, shunts, high-output states)

Reduction in muscle mass (e.g., MI)

Diastolic dysfunction (restriction in ventricular filling)

Increased ventricular stiffness

Ventricular hypertrophy (e.g., hypertrophic cardiomyopathy, other examples above)

Infiltrative myocardial diseases (e.g., amyloidosis, sarcoidosis, endomyocardial fibrosis)

Myocardial ischemia and infarction

Mitral- or tricuspid-valve stenosis

Pericardial disease (e.g., pericarditis, pericardial tamponade)

Physiology and Pathophysiology

Myocardial failure begins with various types of overload to which the heart cannot adequately adapt. Congestive mechanisms (e.g.. leg edema, paroxysmal nocturnal dyspnea, crackles, and jugular venous distention) represent elevations in right or left ventricular filling pressures.

Systolic dysfunction results in the backup of blood into pulmonary and systemic venous systems; the hallmark is a reduced ejection fraction.

Diastolic dysfunction is manifested by increased resistance to diastolic ventricular filling.

Mechanisms include impairment of diastolic myocardial relaxation, valvular dysfunction, loss of myocardial distensibility, ventricular remodeling, and intracellular calcium overload.

Heart failure triggers a number of neurohumoral factors as compensatory mechanisms.

Clinical Manifestations

Subjective

Objective

Right ventricular dysfunction: Abdominal pain, anorexia, nausea, bloating, constipation, ascites, peripheral edema, jugular venous distention, hepatojugular reflux, hepatomegaly

Left ventricular dysfunction: Dyspnea on exertion, paroxysmal nocturnal dyspnea, orthopnea, tachypnea, cough, hemoptysis, bibasilar crackles, pulmonary edema, S_3 gallop, pleural effusion, Cheyne–Stokes respirations

Nonspecific findings: Exercise intolerance, fatigue, weakness, nocturia, central nervous system symptoms, tachycardia, pallor, cyanosis of digits, cardiomegaly

Differential Diagnosis

Any of the following can present with similar signs and symptoms; differentiation is usually determined through diagnostic testing:

Right heart failure (increased JVD, peripheral swelling)

Left heart failure (cough, dyspnea, PND)

Pulmonary edema (difficulty breathing; fluid in bases of lungs on chest x-ray examination)

Enlarged liver (palpable liver edge; possible elevated hepatic enzymes)

Peripheral edema (tightness, swelling of extremities)

Nephrotic syndrome (proteinuria, electrolyte imbalances, fatigue, weakness)

Diagnostic Tests

Chemistry panel (including renal function, to rule out any electrolyte imbalances and/or kidney dysfunction)

Chest x-ray examination (to determine pulmonary edema or infection)

ECG (to determine chamber enlargement or electrical abnormalities)

Cardiac ultrasound (more specific for chamber enlargement)

Management/Treatment

Initial Therapy

Low-sodium diet: 85 mEq/day, 2000–3000 mg/24 hr

Measures to improve myocardial function

Reduce systemic blood pressure

Correct anemia if present

Digoxin—inotropic effect

Decrease pulmonary vascular resistance and central vasodilation

Nitrates

Angiotensin-converting–enzyme (ACE) inhibitors

Increase renal excretion of sodium and water

Oral diuretics

Hydrochlorothiazide, 25–50 mg every morning.

Furosemide, 20–40 mg every morning.

Bumetanide 0.5–2 mg PO daily.

Spironolactone, 25–100 mg PO daily.

Metolazone, 1.25–5 mg PO daily.

Higher doses may be given; however, provider should be consulted. If client's disease is refractory with above doses, consultation and/or referral is warranted.

IV diuretics require supervision by physician (Hoole, 1999).

Inotropic—Increase contractility.

Digoxin, 0.25 mg QD.

ACE inhibitors: Lisinopril (Zestril) 5 mg QD, etc.

Other agents that may be started by provider:

Carvedilol (Coreg) 3.125 mg daily, increasing to 25 mg PO BID.

β-Blockade—although controversial, may be protective for neuro-humoral effects.

Pharmacologic Management

Treat underlying cause as indicated

Client Education

Disease and disease process, including signs and symptoms to watch for and complications

Complete medication information

How and when to contact health care provider and activate EMS (911) system

Risk factors

Diet

Exercise

Weight loss, if needed

Follow-up

Usually 2–3 weeks after treatment is initiated.

Once patient and treatment are stabilized, follow-up may be monthly to every 3–6 months, depending on severity and patient response.

Referral

May need to refer to cardiologist, especially if not responding to treatment or if patient has worsening of symptoms.

HEART MURMURS

SIGNAL SYMPTOM ▶ irregular heartbeat

ICD-9 Codes	785.2	Murmur (undifferentiated)
	424.1	Aortic insufficiency
	396.1	Aortic stenosis
	785.2	Midsystolic
	396.2	Mitral stenosis
	424.0	Mitral insufficiency
	424.3	Pulmonic
	785.2	Tricuspid

Heart murmurs are produced when vibrations occur with the movement of blood with the heart and/or adjacent large blood vessels. Murmurs are heard on auscultation and are characterized by a soft blowing or swooshing sound.

Epidemiology

Fairly common in young children, pregnant women, and adults.

50%–70% of healthy children have murmurs.

Can be found in all age groups.

Classified as systolic or diastolic; systolic are often benign; diastolic are always indicative of valvular or structural abnormality.

Etiology

Innocent murmurs or physiologic murmurs occur due to rapid turbulent flow of blood into left ventricle during atrial systole and through the aorta during ventricular systole.

Vibrations are produced by movement of blood within heart and/or adjacent large blood vessels,

Valves do not close tightly (incompetent heart valve).

Aortic aneurysm or narrowed orifice present, as in mitral or aortic stenosis.

Physiology and Pathophysiology

Systolic murmurs are ejection, regurgitant, and nonorganic ejection.

Ejection

Heard as a crescendo–decrescendo.

Pitch is medium to low.

Heard at base of heart, after first heart sound and ending before second heart sound.

Radiate to neck and down to apex.

Heard with bell of stethoscope.

Calcific aortic stenosis may have a higher pitch and maximum sound at apex.

Changes in intensity with heart rate and cardiac cycle.

Soft with increased heart rate.

Loud with decreased heart rate.

The louder and longer the sound the greater the obstruction.

Classified as innocent, physiologic, aortic, or pulmonic.

Regurgitant

High-pitched.

Localized to apex or left sternal border.

Pansystolic or late systolic.

Sometimes preceded by a click.

Handgrip markedly augments intensity (mitral regurgitation and ventral septal defect).

Nonorganic ejection

Fever

Anxiety

Pregnancy

Hyperthyroidism
Exercise
Hypertension, aging
Aortic regurgitation, bradycardia, atrial septal defect

Significant Murmurs

DIASTOLIC

All diastolic murmurs are considered pathologic and require immediate referral to a cardiologist. These include the murmurs of mitral stenosis and aortic regurgitation.

SYSTOLIC

Ventricular septal defect
Atrial septal defect
Patent ductus arteriosus
Pulmonary stenosis
Aortic stenosis
Coarctation of the aorta
Mitral-valve prolapse

Clinical Manifestations

Subjective

Obtain a thorough history
Often asymptomatic, or may have associated signs and symptoms (see Table 6–11 for specific clinical manifestations associated with selected cardiac-valve disorders)

Objective

Perform thorough cardiac examination (see Tables 6–3 and 6–4).

Differential Diagnosis

Determine if murmur is innocent or physiologic.

Innocent Murmurs

Still's murmur (midsystolic; heard with ejection of blood from the ventricle; heard best between the apex and third intercostal space; characteristic musical quality; commonly heard in toddlers, older children, and adolescents)

Physiologic pulmonary ejection murmur (harsh; midsystolic mid- to low-frequency; heard best over the pulmonary region; probably due to turbulence of flow out of the right ventricular outflow tract)

Supraclavicular arterial bruit (result of turbulence referred to carotid from the subclavian artery; heard over the carotid artery in early systole over the right carotid artery; distinguished from a carotid bruit by extending the client's arms backward as though to touch the elbows together, which causes it to disappear; common in adolescence)

Cervical venous hum (continuous murmur or hum; best heard at the base of the neck on the right side; hum will characteristically diminish with the client in a supine position; disappears when you place gentle pressure on the jugular vein; common in children 3–8 years of age)

Table 6–3 Heart Murmurs

Murmur	Type	Location	Pitch	Radiation	Quality
Mitral stenosis	Diastolic	Apex	Low	Little to none	Rumbling
Mitral regurgitation	Pansystolic	Apex	Medium/high	Left axilla	Blowing
Mitral-valve prolapse	Late-systolic	Second left intercostal space	Medium	Left sternal border to apex	Harsh
Aortic stenosis	Midsystolic	Second left intercostal space	Medium	Neck at sternal border	Harsh
Aortic regurgitation (aortic insufficiency)	Diastolic	Second to fourth left intercostal space	High	Apex	Blowing
Triscupid stenosis	Diastolic	Left of the lower sternum	High	Little to none	Rumbling
Triscupid regurgitation	Pansystolic	Lower left sternal border	Medium	Right sternum	Blowing

Physiologic Murmurs (see Table 6–4)

Aortic murmurs
Pulmonic murmurs
Mitral regurgitation murmurs
Tricuspid regurgitation murmurs
Ventricular septal defect

Diagnostic Tests

CBC (to rule out anemia)
Chemistry and thyroid studies (to rule out electrolyte imbalances)
Chest x-ray examination (to rule out infection and/or neoplasm)
Cardiac ultrasound (to determine chamber size and valve function)
ECG (to determine electrical and/or rhythm abnormalities)
Echocardiogram (to further determine chamber and valve function)
Cardiac catheterization (to rule out coronary artery disease)

Management/Treatment

Innocent (hemodynamically insignificant) murmurs: No treatment necessary
Physiologic murmurs: Treat underlying cause

Client Education

Provide support for client and family.
Assess client's knowledge and understanding.
Explain possible causes for murmur.
Offer referrals and resources, such as American Heart Association and Healthy Heart Program.

Table 6–4 Listening for a Murmur

First listen for S_1 and S_2.
Listen for change in intensity or loudness of murmur.
Note any splits.
Listen for S_3 and S_4.
Change client position.
Listen for bruits (carotids, femoral, renal arteries).
Last longer than other heart sounds.
Describe murmur characteristics:

  Murmurs last longer than other heart sounds. Eight factors should be considered when assessing heart murmurs:

  Timing—Is it systolic between S_1 and S_2 or diastolic between S_3 and S_4?
  Duration—Is it early, mid, or late systolic or diastolic, or does it last the entire cycle? The prefix pan- or holo- before systolic or diastolic describes a murmur that lasts throughout the cycle.
  Quality—Define quality as "soft," "harsh," "blowing," "musical," etc.
  Intensity—Intensity is measured on a graded scale of I to VI:
    Grade I: Barely audible
    Grade II: Audible but quiet
    Grade III: Moderately loud, without thrill
    Grade IV: Loud, with or without thrill
    Grade V: Very loud, with thrill; audible with stethoscope partially off chest
    Grade VI: Louder still, with thrill: audible with stethoscope completely off chest
  Pitch—Heard better with the bell if it is low-pitched; heard better with the diaphragm if it is high-pitched.
  Location—Valve area where murmur is heard best.
  Radiation of sound—Aortic murmurs are heard best at the second intercostal space just to the right of the sternum. They usually radiate upward and into the carotid. Mitral murmurs are generally heard best over the fourth to fifth intercostal space to the left of the sternum and usually radiate toward the axilla.
  Changes—Position changes usually intensify some volume-dependent murmurs.

Counseling may be indicated for feeding infants, antibiotic prophylaxis, exercise and activities of daily living.

Follow-up

Depends on type and severity of murmur. Most murmurs can be followed up on an annual basis,

Referral

Refer to cardiologist if uncertain of significance of any murmur; immediate referral if murmur is pathologic.

HYPERTENSION

SIGNAL SYMPTOM ► elevated blood pressure

ICD-9 Codes		
	403.90	Unspecified
	401.1	Hypertension, benign
	402.90	Hypertensive heart disease, with congestive heart failure (CHF)
	402.92	Hypertensive heart disease, without CHF

Hypertension is a common, often asymptomatic disorder characterized by elevated blood pressure. It is described as persistent elevation of systolic blood pressure to more than 140 mm Hg or diastolic blood pressure to more than 90 mm Hg, based on the average of two or more blood pressure recordings on two or more visits after an initial screening visit. Blood pressure recording of more than 186/110 mm Hg or accompanied with end-organ damage requires immediate treatment (Joint National Committee on Prevention, Detection, Evaluation, and Treatment of High Blood Pressure, 1997). (See Table 6–5)

Types of hypertension include:

Primary hypertension: Has no identifiable cause (most common in adults); also called essential or idiopathic.

Secondary hypertension: Related to an ongoing organic process.

Labile hypertension: Blood pressure that intermittently rises above the normal levels for each given age group and sex. Established hypertension has been shown to develop more commonly in such clients.

White-coat hypertension: Blood pressure elevations that occur in the healthcare provider's office, elevation is seen in the systolic blood pressure.

Pseudorefractory hypertension: Elevation in the diastolic blood pressure from using a cuff that is too small; may be confused with refractory, but no end-organ damage.

Resistant hypertension: Persistence of diastolic blood pressure above 95 mm Hg despite the concomitant use of three antihypertensive drugs.

Pregnancy-induced hypertension: Hypertension that occurs during pregnancy.

Epidemiology

50 million Americans aged 6 and older have high blood pressure (Joint National Committee on Prevention, Detection, Evaluation, and Treatment of High Blood Pressure (1997).

Table 6–5 Blood Pressure Levels

Category	Systolic (mm Hg)	And/or	Diastolic (mm Hg)	Follow-up Recommended
Optimal*	<120	and	<80	Recheck in 2 yr
Normal	<130	and	<85	Recheck in 2 yr
High normal	130–139	or	85–89	Recheck in 1 yr
Hypertension stage 1 (mild)	140–159	or	90–99	Confirm within 2 mo
Hypertension stage 2 (moderate)	160–179	or	100–109	Evaluate within 1 mo
Hypertension stage 3 (severe)	180 or higher	or	110 or higher	Evaluate immediately or within 1 wk depending on clinical situation

*Unusually low readings should be evaluated for clinical significance.
From the Sixth Report of the Joint National Committee on Detection, Evaluation, and Treatment of High Blood Pressure, NIH Publication, 1997.

35% of clients do not know they have high blood pressure; 52% are not on therapy; 27% are on inadequate therapy; 21% are on adequate therapy.

High blood pressure is easily detected and usually controllable.

Blacks, Puerto Ricans, Cubans, and Mexican-Americans are more likely to suffer from high blood pressure than are non-Hispanic whites.

People with lower education and income levels tend to have higher levels of blood pressure.

1995 data: Prevalence of high blood pressure: 26% white men, 44% black men, 17% white women, 37% black women. In the elderly (over age 65) hypertension is not more prevalent in one gender; 63% in whites, 76% in blacks (Joint National Committee on Prevention, Detection, Evaluation, and Treatment of High Blood Pressure (1997).

High blood pressure increases the risks of coronary disease, heart failure, renal failure, and stroke.

Health-care costs attributable to heart disease in the United States are more than $259 billion in direct and indirect costs per year. The high prevalence of hypertension in society makes this a public health concern.

Etiology

The cause of 90%–95% of the cases of high blood pressure is not known. Hypertension is a heterogeneous disorder.

In adults:

Primary, essential, idiopathic refers to an increase in peripheral vascular resistance or cardiac output of unknown origin (95%).

It seems to run in families (genetic)

Traits include high sodium–lithium countertransport, increased aldosterone and other adrenal steroids, and high angiotensinogen levels.

Secondary hypertension (specific cause) from some underlying pathophysiologic mechanism accounts for less then 5% of cases of hypertension; causes include pheochromocytoma, Cushing's syndrome, primary aldosteronism, and coarctation of the aorta.

Exogenous substances include estrogens, glucocorticoids, licorice, sympathomimetic amines, nonsteroidal antiinflammatory agents, long-term alcohol use, and tyramine-containing foods in combination with monoamine oxidase inhibitors.

In children:

Primary, essential idiopathic refers to an increase in peripheral vascular resistance or cardiac output of unknown origin.

Secondary is related to ongoing organic process. The three most common are parenchymal disease, renal artery disease, and coarctation of the aorta. Other causes include endocrine disorders (hyperthyroidism, adrenal dysfunction, hyperparathyroidism), neurogenic disorders, drugs, and miscellaneous such as hypovolemia and hypernatremia and Stevens–Johnson syndrome. (Fox, 1997).

See RD: ARC 6–1 Age-Related Considerations: Hypertension in Children.

Physiology and Pathophysiology

The physiology of blood pressure is a complex process, affected by numerous mechanisms. Thus, hypertension, or high blood pressure, can be due to a change in any of these various mechanisms.

Vasculature: Peripheral vascular resistance

Neural components:

Central nervous system

Autonomic nervous system (sympathetic and parasympathetic systems, baroreceptors)

Peripheral autoregulatory components (renal, tissue)

Humoral mechanisms (renin–angiotensin–aldosterone system, natriuretic hormone, hyperinsulinemia)

Clinical Manifestations

Subjective

Often no symptoms; known as the "silent killer."

Symptoms of underlying cause may present in secondary hypertension (e.g., pallor, tremor, flushing, profuse perspiration, palpitations).

Age-Related Considerations: Hypertension in Children

Hypertension in children is defined as an average systolic or diastolic blood pressure equal to or greater than the 95th percentile for age and sex with measurements obtained on at least three separate occasions.

Children can have high blood pressure, even very young babies. The American Heart Association (1998) recommends that all children have yearly blood pressure measurements. Early detection of high blood pressure will improve the health care of children.

Primary hypertension includes factors such as heredity, stress, obesity, high salt intake, or increased sensitivity to salt, and poor diet (Loggie and Sardegna, 1997).

Secondary hypertension results from renal and cardiac anomalies (most common), others being ventral nervous system disorders or illnesses, renal trauma, drug-induced causes, and miscellaneous causes such as anxiety, pain, fractures, burns, leukemia, Stevens–Johnson syndrome, hypercalcemia, inappropriate cuff size, and heavy-metal poisoning.

Threshold for Significant and Severe Hypertension in Children
(American Heart Association [1998] Recommendations)

Age (in years)	Significant Hypertension (mm Hg)	Severe Hypertension (mm Hg)
<2	112/74 or higher	118/82 or higher
3–5	116/76 or higher	124/84 or higher
6–9	122/78 or higher	130/86 or higher
10–12	126/82 or higher	134/90 or higher
13–15	136/86 or higher	144/92 or higher
16–18	142/92 or higher	150/98 or higher

Headache (suboccipital), pulsating, occurring early in morning, improving throughout the day.

Oliguria, nocturia, or hematuria may be present.

Epistaxis (severe hypertension).

Hypertensive encephalopathy (severe hypertension) with associated symptoms.

Objective

Elevated systolic and/or diastolic blood pressure.

Hematuria and/or proteinuria may occur with renal disorders.

Ventricular hypertrophy (chronic hypertension).

Differential Diagnosis

Primary hypertension (95% of clients with new hypertension)

Secondary hypertension (5% of clients with new hypertension; 2.4% renal failure, 1% renal vascular disease, 1% primary aldosteronism, 0.8% drugs, 0.2% pheochromocytoma, 0.1% Cushing's syndrome)

Systolic hypertension: Arteriosclerotic vascular disease, hyperthyroidism, anxiety

Diastolic hypertension: Renal disease, coarctation of aorta, pheochromocytoma, Cushing's syndrome (Joint National Committee on Prevention, Detection, Evaluation, and Treatment of High Blood Pressure (1997).

 CP 6–1 Clinical Pearl: Suspect secondary hypertension in the following cases: drug therapy ineffective in compliant client, high blood pressure in client aged 25 or younger, occurrence of associated symptoms (perspiration, hirsutism, edema, abnormal heart sounds, stria, palpitations, dizziness).

Diagnostic Tests

Laboratory tests may be performed to assess cardiovascular risk factors as well as to evaluate end-organ function or secondary causes of hypertension. Tests may include urinalysis, chemistry panel, blood glucose, TSH level, plasma lipids (to rule out kidney disorders, electrolyte imbalances, hypoglycemia or hyperglycemia, hypothyroidism or hyperthyroidism, and/or elevated lipids, respectively).

ECG (to rule out electrical or rhythm abnormalities).

Other tests are ordered based on differential diagnosis and index of suspicion and may include nuclear renal isotope scan—flow and clearance (to rule out renal artery stenosis), and chest x-ray examination (may show aortic coarctation and ventricular hypertrophy in chronic states).

Management/Treatment

Goal is to firmly establish the diagnosis, ruling out secondary causes, and determining the severity of pressure elevation, the degree of end-organ damage, and the presence of associated risk factors.

CP 6–2   Clinical Pearl: Things to Remember

Try lifestyle modification for 3 months before initiating drug therapy in mild hypertension.

Start medications at low doses and increase gradually, adjusting at 3–4 week intervals.

When blood pressure is controlled, try reducing number or dosage of drugs.

Individualize therapy: Consider factors such as quality of life, cost, compliance, etc.

Consider concomitant disorders.

Pharmacologic Management

SINGLE-DRUG THERAPY

Diuretics
    β-Blockers
    Calcium-channel blockers
    ACE inhibitors

COMBINATION DRUG THERAPY

ACE inhibitor/diuretic combination
Angiotensin II antagonist/diuretic combinations
β-Blocker/diuretic combinations
Calcium antagonist/β-blocker combinations
Calcium antagonist/ACE inhibitor combinations
Dual calcium antagonist therapy
(See Table 6–6.)

Nonpharmacologic Management

Lifestyle modifications
    Smoking cessation
    Weight reduction/low-salt diet
    Reduction of alcohol consumption
    Regular exercise
    Stress reduction

Complementary/Alternative Therapies

Tai chi
Meditation
Relaxation therapy
Yoga
Biofeedback

Client Education

Disease process known as "silent killer."
Blood pressure is controllable.
Modify lifestyle.
Elicit client's personal beliefs; determine level of understanding; develop a mutually agreeable plan; involve family and/or significant other.

Address modifiable risk factors: Smoking cessation, alcohol reduction, diet modifications, weight reduction.

Review cardiovascular effects of hypertension.

Teach blood-pressure-taking techniques.

Supply complete medication education.

Provide written materials and resource information.

Follow-up

Recheck and confirm blood pressure of 140–150/90–99 within 2 months.

Recheck low normal in 2 years; high normal in 1 year.

Assess for end-organ damage.

Table 6–6   Antihypertensive Drug Therapy

Drug Class	Drugs
β-Blockers	Atenolol, 25–200 mg daily Labetalol, 200–1200 mg daily in two divided doses Metoprolol, 50–200 mg in 1 or 2 divided doses
	Contraindications: CHF, type 1 diabetes, asthma Cautions: Clients with conduction disorders, hypertriglyceridemia
Calcium-channel Blockers	Diltiazem, 90–360 mg daily in two divided doses Verapamil, 180–480 mg daily in two divided doses
	Contraindications: Conduction-system disorders, sick sinus syndrome, second- and third-degree atrioventricular block, CHF
ACE inhibitors	Captopril, 50–300 mg in two to three divided doses Lisinopril, 5–40 mg daily
	Contraindications: Bilateral renal artery stenosis
α₂-Agonists	Second-line agents
Angiotensin II receptor antagonists	Used for clients who have side effects with ACE inhibitors
Individualizing Therapy	(Listed in order of preference)
Age less than 70; healthy	β-blocker Diuretic, ACE inhibitor Calcium-channel blocker Children: β-blockers
Age 70 and over; healthy	Diuretic, calcium-channel blocker β-blocker, ACE inhibitor Elderly: For drug therapy, dose should be half the usual first-line drug dose (thiazide, ACE inhibitors, calcium-channel blocker, β-blocker). Start low and go slow. Drugs likely to cause postural hypotension should be avoided (α-blockers) or daytime sedation (methyldopa, clonidine) are less desirable (Goroll et al., 2000).
Benign prostatic hypertrophy	α-Blockers
Blacks	Diuretic Calcium-channel blocker ACE inhibitor Diuretics, calcium-channel blocker. "Two rules of thumb are that blacks may respond better to diuretics than to beta-blocking agents, and that blacks with cardiac involvement may benefit from calcium antagonists as initial therapy" (Fine-tuning antihypertension therapy, 1997).

Table continued on following page.

Table 6–6   Antihypertensive Drug Therapy (*Continued*)

Drug Class	Drugs
Cerebral ischemia	β-blocker ACE inhibitor, calcium-channel blocker Diuretic (central agent)
Chronic lung disease	Diuretic, ACE inhibitor, calcium-channel blocker. (for asthma/chronic obstructive pulmonary disease: Calcium channel blocker)
Diabetes	ACE inhibitor Calcium-channel blocker *Note:* If client is taking insulin and a β-blocker is indicated, select atenolol or metroprolol (less likely to mask catecholamine-induced hypoglycemic symptoms). If a diuretic is indicated, avoid use of thiazide diuretics (may worsen hyperlipidemia and glucose intolerance).
Gout	If diuretic is indicated, allopurinol is an excellent choice.
Heart failure	Diuretic ACE inhibitor
Ischemic heart disease	β-Blocker Calcium-channel blocker Diuretic, ACE inhibitor
Left ventricular hypertrophy	β-Blocker, ACE inhibitor, calcium-channel blocker Calcium-channel blocker Diuretic (central agent)
Lipid disorder (HDL, <35%)	β-Blocker, ACE inhibitor, calcium-channel blocker α-blocker Hyperlipidemia: α_1-blockers
Migraine headache	β-Blocker
Myocardial infarction (history of)	β-Blocker
Osteoporosis	β-Blocker, diuretic ACE inhibitor, calcium-channel blocker
Pregnancy	β-Blocker (methyldopa, labetalol)
Renal failure	Diuretic (fursoemide, metolazone, others) β-Blocker, vasodilator, calcium-channel blocker

Referral

Consult physician or refer to cardiologist when initiating therapy or when client does not respond to first-line pharmacotherapy.

LIPID DISORDERS

SIGNAL SYMPTOM ▶ elevated lipids, usually asymptomatic

ICD-9 Codes	272.5	Hyperlipidemia
	272.1	Carbohydrate-induced
	272.4	Combined
	272.1	Endogenous
	272.3	Exogenous
	272.3	Fat-induced
	272.2	Mixed

Hyperlipidemia is defined as an elevation of one or more of the following: cholesterol, cholesterol esters, phospholipids, or triglycerides. (Dipiro, 1999.)

Epidemiology

It is estimated that approximately 52 million Americans are candidates for dietary intervention to lower their cholesterol levels.

About 12.7 million Americans may be candidates for lipid-lowering pharmacotherapy—4 million with coronary artery disease and 8.7 with no established coronary artery disease, which represents 3.1 million over 65 years of age (Dipiro, 1999.)

Risk factors for hyperlipidemia (a major risk factor for coronary heart disease):
Age, gender
Genetic factors
Diet, exercise, weight, smoking
Medications
Concurrent illnesses/diseases

Etiology

Plasma lipids: cholesterol, triglyceride, phospholipids, and free fatty acids are derived from dietary sources and lipid synthesis.

Cholesterol and triglyceride are the two lipids important to atherogenesis.

Physiology and Pathophysiology

There are four major classifications of lipoprotein, as described below:

Chylomicrons

Lowest density—Will float to the top of plasma when left overnight in refrigerator.

Derived from diet.

Carry triglycerides throughout the body.

Removed by the action of lipoprotein lipase.

Deficiency of this enzyme elevates triglyceride levels which increases the risk of pancreatitis (Goroll et al., 2000).

Very-Low-Density Lipoproteins (VLDL)

Function is to carry triglycerides made in liver and intestines to capillary beds in fat and muscle where they are hydrolyzed.

Once triglyceride is removed, VLDL metabolizes further to LDL.

Serves as acceptors of cholesterol transferred from HDL—may account for inverse relationship between HDL and VLDL

LDL

Major carrier of cholesterol in humans.

Implicated in atherogenesis.

Increased in persons consuming larger amounts of saturated fat and/or cholesterol, with familial hypercholesterolemia, structural defects, or polygenic form of increased LDL.

After threshold exceeded, LDL can become trapped in arterial intima causing injury, stimulating atherogenesis.

HDL

Thought to function as acceptor of free cholesterol in peripheral tissue, where the cholesterol is esterified and stored in the core of the HDL.

Apolipoprotein A-I major apoprotein of HDL and level correlates inversely with risk of coronary heart disease.

Women, until menopause, with higher HDL level. Exercise increases level. Smoking, obesity, and hypertriglyceridemia lower levels.

HDL cholesterol concentration is the single most powerful predictor of coronary heart disease risk.

Clinical Manifestations

Subjective

May be asymptomatic and have normal presentation, or presentation of coronary artery disease, including chest pain and even myocardial infarction or stroke

Family history (positive)

Objective

Usually none, but can include xanthoma/xanthelasma—flat, elevated yellowish plaques or nodules, usually occurring on the eyelids and even on the Achilles tendons.

Differential Diagnosis

Congenital hypercholesterolemia (familial hypercholesterolemia, elicited via patient history)

Syndrome X (a cluster combination of hypercholesterolemia, hypertriglyceridemia, impaired glucose tolerance/diabetes and hypertension)

Diagnostic Tests

Fasting lipid profile (total cholesterol, LDL, HDL, and triglycerides) (to determine lipid levels)

After confirmation of hyperlipidemia, further treatment is based on coronary heart disease risk factor and total cholesterol level (Dipiro, 1999),

Further testing may include:

Chemistry panel (to include fasting glucose, to rule in/our concurrent diabetes mellitus)

ECG (to rule out cardiac electrical or rhythm abnormalities)

Liver-function tests (to rule out hepatic dysfunction; especially important for base-line information if initiating statin therapy)

Thyroid function studies (to rule out hypothyroid or hyperthyroid disorders)

Management/Treatment

Goal is to reduce coronary heart disease risk.

Reduction of LDL, total cholesterol, and increase HDL.

Should be based on repeat measurements of serum lipid levels

Management and Treatment

Lipid evaluation.

Define category of lipid abnormality.

Cholesterol level >175–200 mg/dl—nutritional counseling, exercise; rule out secondary causes of hyperlipidemia.

Cholesterol >200 mg/dl—above interventions, including family nutritional counseling and family screening.

Cholesterol >230 mg/dl—all previously described management and referral to lipid specialist.

Hyperlipidemia >6 months, consider bile acid sequestrant as follows: cholestyramine, 4–16 g active resin per day, or colestipol resin, 5–10 mg/day.

Hyperlipidemia screening is indicated with presence of any risk factors. Screen all children after 2 years of age for base-line cholesterol level; if cholesterol is <175 mg/dl, repeat in 3 to 5 years. Children treated with cholesterol-lowering medication should be monitored for retardation of growth and development.

Treatment in Elderly

Dietary measures are first line with maintaining adequate nutritional minimal requirements.

Goal is to have LDL cholesterol <130 mg/dl.

Medication added as needed, but as in this population, with caution (Goroll et al., 2000).

Hyperlipidemia in Children

5%–25% of children and teens have cholesterol in excess of 200 mg/dl.

Higher incidence of hyperlipidemia with family history of coronary artery disease and hyperlipidemia.

Can be due to genetic disorders.

About 80% of children with coronary artery disease have symptoms before age 20 (Fox, 1997).

(See Table 6–7.)

Pharmacologic Management

Used when target levels of LDL or increases in HDL are not effective by lifestyle modifications alone.

Involves assessing risk:benefit ratio.

Degree of coronary heart disease determined.

Niacin:

Effective and inexpensive.

Affects fatty acid mobilization.

Lowers LDL and VLDL (very-low-density lipoprotein), raises HDL.

May be used in combination with colestipol or as monotherapy.

3-Hydroxy-3-methylglutaryl–coenzyme A reductase inhibitors (statins):

One of the drugs most often prescribed when a person has a coronary heart disease and needs hypolipidemic medication.

Table 6–7   Treatment Decisions Based on LDL Cholesterol*

Dietary Therapy	Initiation Level (mg/dl)	LDL Goal (mg/dl)
Without CHD and <2 risk factors	160 and higher	<160
Without CHD and ≥2 or more risk factors	130 and higher	<130
With CHD	>100	100 or less
Drug Treatment	**Consideration Level (mg/dl)**	**LDL Goal (mg/dl)**
Without CHD and <2 risk factors	190 and higher†	<160
Without CHD and ≥2 risk factors	160 and higher	<130
With CHD	130 and higher‡	100 or less

*Desirable/normal: Total cholesterol <200 mg/dl; LDL <130 mg/dl; HDL >35 mg/dl; triglycerides <200 mg/dl.
†In men <35 years old and premenopausal women with LDL cholesterol levels of 190–219 mg/dl, drug therapy should be delayed except in high-risk clients, such as those with diabetes.
‡In clients with CHD and LDL cholesterol levels of 100–129 mg/dl, the clinician should exercise clinical judgement in deciding whether to initiate drug treatment.
CHD = coronary heart disease.
From National Cholesterol Education Program (NCEP) Guidelines (1998).

Increases hepatic removal of LDL and slows production of cholesterol.
Bile-acid sequestrants:
    Have been first-line therapy for years.
    Cost may be concern for client.
    Bind bile acid in gut and interrupt normal enterohepatic circulation.
Fibrates:
    Decreased VLDL synthesis
    Most potent of triglyceride-lowering medications
    Variable effect of LDL
    Gemfibrozil generally well tolerated
In children:
    Medication not recommended for children <10 years of age; may use bile sequestrant only after diet treatment for 6 to 12 months.
    (See Table 6–8.)

Nonpharmacologic Management

DIETARY MODIFICATIONS

Reduction in daily total fat, saturated fat, and cholesterol
Dietary guidelines: Adults
    American Heart Association (1994) recommends following a step by step plan:
    Step 1 is recommended for the American population >2 years of age and maintains total fat at <30%.

Step 2 is for those at highest risk for coronary heart disease or who are not responding adequately to step 1. Requires slightly more effort to follow.

Dietary guidelines: Children

The following pattern of nutrient intake is recommended:

Saturated fatty acids—less than 10% of total calories

Total fat—an average of no more than 30% of total calories

Dietary cholesterol—less than 300 mg per day

LIFESTYLE MODIFICATIONS

Increase exercise.

Lose weight.

Stop smoking.

Reduce stress.

Consume alcohol only in moderation.

Complementary/Alternative Therapies

Omega-3 fish oil supplements are popular, but they interfere with blood clotting at high doses.

Antioxidant vitamins (E and C and β-carotene) may increase LDL resistance to oxidative process, reducing risk of arterial injury, but do not lower cholesterol levels (Goroll et al., 2000).

Garlic: Average daily dose—4 g fresh garlic or equivalent preparations (Mandelbaum-Schmid, 1998); 1 clove can produce modest reduction (5%–10%) as can psyllium (10 g/d) (Goroll et al., 2000).

Soy lecithin: 3.5 g (3-sn-phosphatidyl)choline.

Table 6–8   Drugs Commonly Used in the Treatment of Hyperlipidemia*

Drug	Usual Daily Dose	Maximum Daily Dose
Atorvastatin (Lipitor)	10–80 mg QD	80 mg per day
Atorvastatin (Lipitor)	10–80 mg a day	80 mg/day
Cholestyramine (Questran, Questran Light)	8 g TID	32 g
Cholestyramine (Cholybar)	8 g TID	32 g
Clofibrate (Atromid-S)	1 g BID	2 g
Colestipol (Colestid)	10 g BID	30 g
Dextrothyroxine (Choloxin)	6 mg QD	8 mg
Gemfibrozil (Lopid)	600 mg BID	1.5 g
Fluvastatin (Lescol)	20–40 mg	80 mg
Lovastatin (Mevacor)	20–40 mg	80 mg
Neomycin sulfate	1 g BID	2 g
Niacin	2 g TID	9 g
Pravastatin (Pravachol)	20–40 mg	40 mg
Simvastatin (Zocor)	10–20 mg	40 mg

*When prescribing an antibiotic, stop lipid-lowering medications during the time the antibiotic is being taken in order to avoid drug-drug interaction and the chance of liver toxicity.

Soy phospholipid: 1.5–2.7 g phospholipids from soybean with 73%–79% 3-sn-phosphatidylcholine in a single dose (Mandelbaum-Schmid, 1998).

Client Education

Education is the mainstay of this diagnosis.

Encourage client to change/modify diet and exercise.

Encourage client to keep food diary and activity log.

Provide educational materials.

Teach client about medications, side effects, signs and symptoms to report, and compliance.

Follow-up

Normal cholesterol level: Screen every 3–5 years.

Cholesterol 175–200 mg/dl: Screen every 6–12 months until level is normal.

Cholesterol >200 mg/dl: Screen every 6–12 months during treatment until acceptable level is achieved.

Referral

Refer to cardiologist or lipid specialist if cholesterol level is greater than 230 mg/dl, there is a significant family history of premature heart disease or sudden death, or if hyperlipidemia persists with appropriate treatment.

MYOCARDIAL INFARCTION

SIGNAL SYMPTOM ▶ chest pain

ICD-9 Codes	410.9	Acute myocardial infarction
	412	Old myocardial infarction

Acute myocardial infarction (AMI) most commonly occurs in an area of an atherosclerotic coronary artery when plaque disruption leads to platelet aggregation, thrombus formation, and spasm, causing an immediate reduction in blood to the myocardium and resulting in ischemia. When ischemia is prolonged, cell death may ensue.

Epidemiology

One of the most common serious health problems in Western society

In the United States approximately 1.5 million persons are diagnosed annually

500,000 deaths occur annually/

Accounts for one fourth of all deaths in the United States annually.

Etiology

Caused by occlusion of coronary artery

Plaque rupture with thrombus formation

Usually occurs at an area with atherosclerotic arterial disease

Physiology and Pathophysiology

Coronary occlusion is usually the result of instability of underlying atherosclerotic plaque and its interaction with mediators of vascular tone, prostaglandins, platelets, and the clotting cascade. Disruption of the plaque by fracture, fissure, or hemorrhage can result in vascular occlusion. Acute thrombotic occlusion occurs in 80%–90% of cases. Platelet aggregation further leads to vasoconstriction by thromboxane A_2 and overwhelming endogenous vasodilators, such as prostacyclin and endothelial-derived nitric oxide. Activation of intrinsic and extrinsic coagulation results in thrombin activation, fibrin deposition, and entrapment of erythrocytes into an expanding thrombus. Luminal obstruction depends on atheromatous plaque, intraluminal thrombi, aggregated platelets, and a variable degree of spasm.

Other causes include nonatherosclerotic causes, coronary spasm, coronary artery embolus, coronary artery abnormalities, and hypercoagulable states.

Clinical Manifestations

Subjective

Typical presentation:
- Severe substernal chest pain
- Intolerable crushing or constricting pain
- Located beneath the sternum, with radiation to the inner aspect of the left arm
- Pain in the jaw, neck, epigastrium, arm only, or back
- Indigestion
- Diaphoresis
- Weakness
- Feeling of impending doom
- Vagal symptoms (nausea, abdominal cramping)

Objective

New or worsening angina preceding the infarction by hours to weeks

Pain differentiated from angina pectoris by duration of longer than 30 minutes and lack of complete relief by rest or nitroglycerin

Typical presentation
- Anxious, restless, and diaphoretic.
- Cool and clammy skin.
- Bradycardia.
- Heart rhythm irregularities.
- Pump failure (e.g., hypotension, tachycardia, oliguria, cool extremities, peripheral cyanosis).
- Low-grade fever.
- S_4 gallop (S_3 gallop associated with heart failure).
- Pericardial friction rubs—occur frequently in the first days of myocardial infarction; usually are transient and intermittent; usually indicate a transmural infarction.

Differential Diagnosis

GERD (burning, epigastric pain, usually worse after eating)

Anxiety (generalized chest pain, usually coincides with anxiety symptoms)

Depression (similar to above)

Costochondral pain (patient usually able to localize pain; reproducible on palpation)

Pneumothorax (sudden chest pain, shortness of breath, localized tenderness)

Congestive heart failure (chest pain, shortness of breath, PND, peripheral edema)

Pneumonia (chest congestion, productive cough, fever/chills, aches)

Pericarditis (fever, precordial chest pain and tenderness, dry cough, dyspnea, palpitations)

Asthma (chest tightness, difficulty breathing, wheezing)

Aortic dissection (sudden pain, fatigue)

Diagnostic Tests

In the primary care setting, diagnostic tests are usually limited to ECG and measurement of cardiac enzyme levels. Further diagnostic testing would be ordered by a cardiologist or cardiac nurse practitioner.

Electrocardiographic findings: Evolutionary changes diagnostic of MI will be seen on serial tracings in approximately two thirds of clients with AMI, the remainder having only ST-segment and T-wave depression.

Classic pattern—Initial hyperacute T-wave peaking followed by ST-segment elevation, promptly following onset of ischemia or blood loss, in leads that represent this region.

Q waves develop as R wave is lost and are defined as those greater than 0.04 seconds in duration and 15% of total QRS height. The Q waves develop over hours to days.

ST-segment changes decrease toward base line and returns to normal with symmetrical T-wave inversion over subsequent days. (See Table 6–9.)

Isoenzyme Analysis

Creatine kinase (CK)

MM—muscle

BB—brain

MB—heart

Serum levels rise within 6–8 hours after onset of infarction.

Serum levels peak at 24 hours and return to normal at 48–96 hours.

Total CK rises following any form of muscle trauma, such as intramuscular injections or rhabdomyolysis, as well as hypothyroidism, renal failure, or stroke.

The MB isoenzyme of CK is currently the mainstay in the diagnosis of myocardial infarction:

Table 6–9   ECG Localization of Myocardial Infarction

Location	ECG Leads Involved	Probable Artery Involved
Anteroseptal	V_1-V_2	Proximal left anterior descending (LAD), septal perforators
Anteroapical	V_2-V_4	LAD or its branches
Anterolateral	V_4-V_6, I, aV_L	Mid-LAD or circumflex
Extensive anterior	V_1-V_6	Proximal LAD
High lateral	I, aV_L	Circumflex or first diagonal branch of LAD
Inferior	II, III, aV_F	Right coronary artery (RCA); less often circumflex or distal LAD
Posterior	Tall R, V_1, or mirror image V_1, V_2	Posterior descending
Right ventricular	V_1 and reversed chest leads RV_3, RV_4	RCA

It is nonspecific for heart muscle tissue; only minute amounts are found in noncardiac tissues. Its levels rise and peak slightly earlier than total CK levels and usually normalize in 36–72 hours.

Specificity of levels is accepted between 5% of total CK or 13 IU/ml is used.

Levels of lactate dehydrogenase (LDH) and its five isoenzymes rise within 24–48 hours of infarction, peak in 3–5 days, and persist for 7–10 days.

LDH may be present in other disorders, such as muscle, kidney, liver, brain, pancreas, and in hemorrhagic conditions. An LDH_1 level greater than that of LDH_2 is relatively specific for myocardial damage.

Measurement of LDH levels is helpful when the CK level is normal and the MI took place even 2–4 days previously.

Serum glutamic oxaloacetic transferase (SGOT) is another nonspecific marker for myocyte necrosis, peaking at 48–72 hours after infarction. Its usefulness is limited.

Cardiac troponin-T and troponin-I are proteins that regularly modulate the calcium-mediated interaction of actin and myosin in striated muscle tissue and are released after myocardial damage.

Elevation occurs 3 hours after infarction and peaks at 24 hours.

Levels remain elevated for 5–7 days.

Myosin light drains—detected within 6 hours after myocardial infarction. Remain elevated for 7 days.

Myoglobin appears and disappears in serum urine very early after infarction. Peaks at 3–10 hours.

Other laboratory abnormalities seen in MI:

Hyperglycemia (marked)/ketoacidosis.

Leukocytosis.

Serum lipids are altered and do not reflect true profile for weeks.

Chest x-ray examination (determines presence of pulmonary congestion; radiographic findings lag behind the clinical picture by up to 12 hours).

Other tests that may be done include radionuclide studies (usually done by the cardiologist), position-emission tomography, echocardiography, spine CT, and angiography.

Management/Treatment

Pharmacologic Management

THROMBOLYTIC AGENTS (USUALLY ADMINISTERED BY A PHYSICIAN)

Streptokinase and anisoylated plasminogen–streptokinase activator complex (anistreplase, also known as APSAC)

Recombinant single-chain tissue plasminogen activator

Double-chain-recombinant tissue plasminogen activator

Urokinase

Single chain urokinase plasminogen activator

CONTRAINDICATIONS FOR THROMBOLYTIC THERAPY

Absolute

Major trauma or surgery within past 2 months

History of cerebrovascular accident within past 6 months

History of intracranial tumor or neurosurgery

Active internal bleeding

Severe uncontrolled hypertension

Active peptic ulcer disease

Puncture of a noncompressible vessel

Relative

History of remote stroke or any cerebral pathology

History of recent transient ischemic attack

Prolonged (>10 minutes) or traumatic cardiopulmonary resuscitation

Impaired hemostasis

History of peptic ulcer disease

Hemorrhagic diabetic retinopathy

ADJUNCTIVE PHARMACOLOGIC THERAPY

β-Blockers: Reduce reinfarction rates, reduce mortality

Recommended doses: Timolol, 20 mg, propanolol, 180–240 mg, metoprolol, 200 mg, atenolol, 100 mg in divided doses

Antiplatelet drugs

Aspirin: Reduces mortality, reduces reinfarction rates

IIb/IIIa receptor agents: Monoclonal antibody, eptifibatide (Integrilin)

Nitrates: Used in the client with ischemia. Relieves coronary spasm by increasing collateral blood flow and reducing subendocardial ischemia by lowering end-diastolic pressure.

Calcium-channel blockade: Suggestion of lower reinfarction rate. Increases blood flow.

Inotropic drugs.

Digitalis.

IV inotropes: Dopamine, dobutamine, dopexamine, amrinone.

Magnesium: Some studies suggest increased survival rates when given early in clients with low magnesium levels.

Arterial vasodilators: Used for clients with CHF complicating AMI and those with severe hypertension.

IV agents: Nitroprusside, nitroglycerin.

ACE inhibitors: started within 24 hours of infarction, decreased mortality in all clients.

Nonpharmacologic Management

Low-fat, low-salt diet

Weight loss, if needed

Regular aerobic exercise

Decrease or ideally discontinue smoking

Client Education

Disease process and management information

Chest pain recognition

Use of 911

Encourage family members to obtain CPR certification

Medication information

Importance of lifestyle modification (Mortality rate is high.)

Follow-up

Depends on severity of patient symptoms.

Referral

There should be immediate consultation with a collaborating physician and referral to 911 or emergency medical system for any client in whom AMI is suspected.

PALPITATIONS

SIGNAL SYMPTOM ▶ rapid fluttering of heart

ICD-9 Codes	785.1	Palpitation (heart)
	306.2	Psychogenic

Palpitations present as a client's disquieting awareness of his or her own heartbeat>, which may be described as a pounding, racing, skipping, flopping, or fluttering sensation.

Most clients are unaware of their resting heartbeats. An increase in the stroke volume or contractility, a sudden change in rate or rhythm, or an unusual cardiac movement within the chest may cause a perceptible heartbeat (Driscoll et al., 1996).

Epidemiology

Atrial fibrillation is the most commonly encountered arrhythmia, with an incidence of approximately 2%. Other arrhythmias occur and can be problematic based on the symptoms exhibited by the client (Goroll et al., 2000).

Etiology

Isolated palpitations are usually the result of premature atrial and ventricular contractions followed by a long pause; the prolonged ventricular diastole results in an increased stroke volume, and a vigorous ejection of blood occurs on the next beat. This increase in stroke volume may be perceived as a pounding or forceful beat. A constant pounding may be felt at rest by clients with a hyperkinetic state, such as hyperthyroidism, fever, severe anemia, and anxiety. A large stroke volume can also be seen in valvular heart disease, such as aortic insufficiency.

Palpitations may be caused by excessive adrenergic stimulation—for example, anxiety, panic attacks, depression, hyperthyroidism, and rarely, pheochromocytoma.

Physiology and Pathophysiology

Palpitations may result from the mechanisms that cause cardiac arrhythmias: disorders of impulse formation or automaticity, abnormalities of impulse conduction, reentry, and triggered activity (Kopp & Wilber, 1992).

Clinical Manifestations

Subjective

History:

Nature of the palpitations (characteristics, mode of onset, mode of termination, precipitating factors, frequency, time of day, results of prior treatments)

Associated symptoms

Precipitating and aggravating factors

Ameliorating factors

Anxiety

Objective

Apical pulse (to determine regularity of rhythm)

Heart (for abnormal sounds)

Blood pressure (note changes such as elevation, marked postural changes, widened pulse pressure)

Jugular veins (for distention and cannon waves)

Extremities (for edema and calf tenderness)

Differential Diagnosis

Any of the following diagnoses can present with palpitations:

Anxiety (elicited via patient history; coincides with other symptoms of anxiety)

Pain (elicited via patient history; may be reproducible with movement and/or palpation)

Fever (elevated temperature)

Fear (elicited via patient history; fearful, anxious affect)

Hypoxia (decreased pulse oximetry, abnormal blood gases, fatigue, weakness)

Hyperthyroidism/hypothyroidism (abnormal TSH and/or free T_4)

Hypotension (low blood pressure, fatigue, weakness, possible syncope)

MI (see "Myocardial Infarction")

Coronary artery disease (precordial chest pain, elevated lipids, coronary artery disease on angiography)

Chronic obstructive pulmonary disease (shortness of breath, distant breath sounds, possible wheezing; patients are usually thin and have hyperinflated chests)

Drug/substance-related (excessive use of stimulants, such as alcohol, caffeine, digoxin, nicotine, cocaine; elicited via patient history)

Mitral-valve prolapse (chest pain, shortness of breath, palpitations)

Vagal response (fatigue, palpitations, syncope)

Electrolyte imbalance (e.g., hypomagnesemia)

Anemia (fatigue, weakness, abnormal CBC)

Diagnostic Tests

ECG (to determine rate, rhythm)

Ambulatory electrocardiographic monitoring (to examine relationship between symptoms and rhythm disturbance)

Exercise stress testing (to assess palpations precipitated by exertion)

Electrophysiologic studies (if palpations lead to syncope or near-syncope episodes)

Laboratory studies (to help determine underlying cause)

Management/Treatment

Treatment of the underlying cause is essential.

Pharmacologic Management

Pharmacologic therapy depends on the etiology of the palpitations

ORAL ANTIARRHYTHMIC DRUGS

Procainamide, 500–1000 mg PO Q4–6H

Quinidine, 200–600 mg PO Q4–6H

B-BLOCKERS

Propranolol, 80–160 mg/day

Atenolol, 50–100 mg/day

Nadolol, 40–100 mg 1–2 times/day

Metoprolol, 50–100 mg 2–3 times/day

Verapamil, 40–160 mg PO Q8H

Correct any underlying disease

Nonpharmacologic Management

Try to eliminate caffeine from diet.

Cut down on, or ideally quit, smoking.

Cut down on or eliminate alcohol intake.

Exercise may be helpful.

If underlying cause is related to blood sugar, attempt tighter control of blood sugar levels.

Reassure the client that most dysrhythmias are not immediately life-threatening.

Stress reduction

Valsalva and carotid sinus massage can be taught to clients who are free of carotid disease.

Complementary/Alternative Therapies

Relaxation therapy

Meditation

Yoga

Tai chi

Client Education

Often includes reassurance that most dysrhythmias are not immediately life-threatening.

Educate regarding underlying disease process.

Give medication information.

Follow-up

If not a cardiac emergency, initial follow-up usually in 2–4 weeks.

When patient is stabilized, follow-up can be 3–6 months.

Referral

Immediately refer to 911 or emergency medical system and transfer to hospital if client has ventricular tachycardia.

Consulting physician or cardiologist if unable to detect or treat the cause, if client has new-onset atrial fibrillation or paroxysmal supraventricular tachycardia, or if ventricular rate goes below 40 beats per minute.

PERIPHERAL VASCULAR DISEASE

SIGNAL SYMPTOMS peripheral discoloration, pain

ICD-9 Code	443.9	Peripheral vascular disease

Peripheral vascular disease occurs when any blood vessel outside the heart (arteries and veins), including the lymph vessels, experiences a disturbance in blood flow, interrupting the systemic circulation and its normal functioning.

Epidemiology

Peripheral vascular disease (PVD) is most related to atherosclerosis (AS).

More than 70 million Americans are affected by cardiovascular disease.

Other disease states, such as diabetes and hypertension, contribute to PVD.

Etiology

Includes arterial and venous disease, and can cause chronic disability.

10% of clients older than age 65 show evidence of PVD; most related to atherosclerosis.

Non aging, gender, and genetic factors.

Reversible risk factors include smoking, hypertension, and obesity.

Hyperlipidemia (hypercholesterolemia and hypertriglyceridemia); may be a secondary problem to uncontrolled diabetes, hypothyroidism, uremia, hypoproteinemia, or liver disease.

Other causes include the use of certain drugs, dietary or genetic factors, hypertension, smoking, hyperglycemia, obesity, physical inactivity, and stress/personality type.

Physiology and Pathophysiology

The physiology and pathophysiology of PVD depends on the cause and the physiology and pathophysiology of the specific cause.

Arterial System

Arteriosclerosis

Arterial insufficiency (atherosclerotic and nonatherosclerotic)

Arteriosclerosis obliterans (ASO)

Aneurysm

Nonatherosclerotic arterial causes: Cystic medial necrosis, arterial inflammation, vasospastic disorders, fibromuscular dysplasia, trauma, infection, compression, compartment syndrome, congenital, hyperviscosity (Fahey, 1999)

Arterial inflammation: Thromboangiitis obliterans (Buerger's disease), arteritis

Venous System

Vasospastic: Raynaud's syndrome

Venous obstruction

Thromboembolic disease

Thrombophlebitis

Superficial thrombophlebitis

Acute deep vein thrombosis (DVT)

Varicose veins

Varicosities

Theoretical causes

Venous insufficiency

Chronic venous insufficiency

Combination

Ulcers

Lymph system

Lymphedema

Clinical Manifestations

Subjective

See Table 6–10 for clinical manifestations and treatment of PVD.

Objective

See Table 6–10.

Table 6–10 Clinical Manifestations, Diagnostic Tests, and Treatment: PVD

Peripheral Vascular Disease	Clinical Manifestations	Diagnostic Tests	Treatment
Arterial: Atherosclerotic			
Arteriosclerosis obliterans	Gradual onset, subtle symptoms. Stage I: Asymptomatic. Stage II: Intermittent claudication. Pain usually unilateral. Normal pulses may be diminished after exercise. Stage III: Pain at rest Pain is a continuous numbness and burning, relieved when limb is dependent. Pain is worse when limb is horizontal. Stage IV: Includes all of the above symptoms. Severe, intolerable pain without exertion. Pain rarely completely relieved. Extremity cold, clear demarcation of warmth to coolness. Color changes: red when dependent, pallor when elevated. No edema unless disease is severe. Hair loss, muscle atrophy, paresthesia, ulcers, gangrene distal to occlusion.	ABI Doppler Treadmill Arteriography	Pentoxifylline (Trental), 400 mg PO T.I.D. with meals. Papaverine (vasodilator), 150 mg PO B.I.D. —Controversial use Aspirin and dipyridamole may decrease the progression of the disease Prostaglandins (vasodilators and inhibitors of platelet aggregation) can improve claudica-tion, and pain and promote ulcer healing
Aneurysms	Abdominal aortic aneurysm. Awareness of a pulsating mass in the abdomen, with or without pain. Abdominal, back, groin, flank pain. Epigastric distress, constipation. Impotence. Palpable mass in umbilical region, left of midline. Bruits may be audible. Femoral pulses may be diminished. Rupture of abdominal aortic aneurysm.	Ultrasound CT scan Chest/ abdominal x-ray examination	Refer to XXX.

Table continued on following page.

Table 6–10 Clinical Manifestations, Diagnostic Tests, and Treatment: PVD (Continued)

Peripheral Vascular Disease	Clinical Manifestations	Diagnostic Tests	Treatment
	Abdominal pain with intense back and flank pain and possible scrotal pain. Pulsating abdominal mass. Shock, with systolic blood pressure <100, apical pulse >100. Ecchymosis of flank and perianal area. Lightheadedness, nausea. Red cells decreased, white cells increased. Thoracic aneurysm. Dysphasia, hoarseness. Neck vein distension with edema of head and arms. Chest pain.		
Arterial: Non-atherosclerotic (inflammatory)			
Thromboangiitis obliterans (Buerger's disease)	Pain may be severe and worse at night. Rubor (from dilated capillaries) plus cyanosis. Paroxysmal "electrical shock" pain indicative of ischemic neuropathy. Coldness, numbness, burning sensation in affected extremity. Intermittent claudication in arch of foot. Noted with poorly healing ulcers, especially in distal portions of digits.	Arteriography	Pentoxifylline (Trental) 400 mg PO TID— with meals. Papaverine (vasodilator) 150 mg po b.i.d. - controversial use Aspirin and dipyridamole may decrease the progression of the disease Prostaglandins (vasodilators and inhibitors of platelet aggregation) can improve claudication, pain and ulcer healing
Arteritis	Decreased peripheral pulses More severe in lower extremities, may have intermittent claudication and/or ischemic ulcerations	Erythrocyte sedimentation rate: Usually markedly elevated. Angiography. Biopsy.	High dose daily steroid treatment, gradually tapered over months. Monitor for relapse.
Arterial: Non-atherosclerotic (vasospasmic)			
Raynaud's syndrome	Episodes of abrupt progressive tricolor change of the fingers in response to cold,	CBC Sedimentation rate Urinolysis	Consult and refer Drug of choice is nifedipine SR, 30–90 mg QD

Table continued on following page.

Table 6–10   Clinical Manifestations, Diagnostic Tests, and Treatment: PVD (*Continued*)

Peripheral Vascular Disease	Clinical Manifestations	Diagnostic Tests	Treatment
	vibration, or stress: First white (pallor) from arteriospasm and resulting deficit in supply, then blue (cyanosis) due to slight relaxation of the spasm that allows a slow trickle of blood through the capillaries and increased O_2 extraction of hemoglobin. Finally, red (rubor) due to return of blood into the dilated capillary bed or reactive hyperemia. May be demonstrated by immersion of hands in water at 10–15°C.	Chemistry panel Serum protein electrophoresis Antinuclear antibody Chest x-ray examination ECG Doppler studies	Consider sympatholytic agents: Reserpine 0.25–0.75 mg PO QD Guanethidine, 10–50 mg PO QD α-adrenergic antagonists: Prazosin (Minipress), thymoxamine, phentolamine and, phenoxybenzamine. Vasodilators: Nitroglycerin, nitroprusside, niacin. Calcium-channel antagonists. Serotonin receptor antagonist Other drug options: ACE inhibitors, prostanoids, thyroid hormones.
Arterial: Acute occlusion	6-Ps. Pain or loss of sensory nerves secondary to ischemia. Paresthesias and loss of position sense (client unable to detect pressure or sense a pinprick; cannot tell if toes are flexed or extended). Poikilothermia (coldness). Paralysis. Pallor due to empty superficial veins and no capillary filling; can progress to a mottled, cyanotic, cold leg. Pulselessness.	Same as above	Refer if sudden pain, coldness, numbness, and pallor to affected limb. Thrombolytic therapy and anticoagulation with heparin is started Analgesia: If conservative therapy does not improve color, temperature, or pain in 4 hr, institute embolectomy with anticoagulation . If thrombolytic therapy is successful in dissolving the thrombus, interventional therapy may be needed to prevent recurrence: Surgical bypass, and percutaneous transluminal angioplasty.

Table continued on following page.

Table 6–10 Clinical Manifestations, Diagnostic Tests, and Treatment: PVD (*Continued*)

Peripheral Vascular Disease	Clinical Manifestations	Diagnostic Tests	Treatment
Venous: obstructive			
Superficial thrombo-phlebitis	Tender, indurated, red, visible, palpable cord along vein and/or ovoid nodules in the skin.	History Physical examination	Consult with collaborating physician for initial therapy. Heat, most compresses. Elevate limb. NSAIDs for pain. Bed rest with bath-room privileges for 3–5 days. Follow-up in 24–48 hr, and then in 1 wk.
Deep venous thrombo-phlebitis	Increased muscle turgor and tenderness over affected vein. Possible superficial venous distention. Deep muscle tenderness, increased warmth in affected limb. Occasionally fever. Positive Homan's sign. Cyanosis of occlusion. Unilateral edema distal to occlusion.	Doppler ultra-sonography Venous duplex scanning (gold standard) Plethysmog-raphy	Acute phase: Heparin IV, 1.5–2.5× control prothrombin time Coumadin therapy: (intermation normalize ratio 2.0–3.0) Bed rest 5–7 days with leg elevated Warm, moist compresses to extremity Compression hose
Venous: Valvular			
Varicose veins	Aggravated by prolonged standing Tortuous, dilated, superficial vessels (greater and lesser saphenous veins) Heaviness and fatigue in legs Diffuse calf aching without exercise Elevation of legs produces rapid relief of symptoms Affected limb may be edematous	Doppler ultra-sonography Venogram	Weight loss, if obese. Elevate legs at intervals throughout the day. Avoid long standing Support hose daily. Avoid restrictive clothes especially at waist and groin. Consult surgeon if severe. Sclerotherapy injection with compression is an option.
Chronic venous insufficiency	May be unilateral or bilateral Edema progresses from distal to proximal. Tiredness or heaviness after prolonged standing or sitting. Hemosiderin staining (bronzing) of skin.	Doppler ultra-sonography Venogram	Decrease edema: 4–6 rest periods throughout the day, compression hose Correct dryness with emollients or moisturizing lotions and remove scales.

Table continued on following page.

Table 6–10 Clinical Manifestations, Diagnostic Tests, and Treatment: PVD (*Continued*)

Peripheral Vascular Disease	Clinical Manifestations	Diagnostic Tests	Treatment
	Scaly skin with cutaneous atrophy. Skin warm with normal color when elevated, cyanotic when dependent for prolonged periods. Usually a history of deep vein thrombosis.		-Topical corticosteroids to reduce inflammation and itching -Antibiotics for systemic infection or cellulitis
Lymphatic			
Lymphedema	Dull, heavy sensation No actual pain Elevation of the limb and rest in bed cause a reduction in, but not disappearance of, edema Skin becomes roughened. Edema is nonpitting.	Isotopic lymphography, Lymphangiography, Phlebography	Treat underlying problem

ANKLE-BRACHIAL INDEX (ABI)

The ABI is calculated as the ankle pressure divided by the brachial pressure. Normally ankle systolic pressure exceeds arm systolic pressure. Ankle pressure does not begin to change until the diameter of the artery is reduced by at least 50%. The ABI normally does not fall after exercise.

ABI >1.0:   Normal (no disease

ABI 0.9–1.0:   Minimal or no symptoms

ABI 0.5–0.9   Claudication

ABI 0.3–0.5   Ischemic rest pain

ABI <0.3   Gangrene

Differential Diagnosis

Any of the following diagnoses can cause signs and symptoms of PVD; differentiation is usually done via diagnostic testing.

Intermittent claudication: ASO, thromboangiitis obliterans, Takayasu's arteritis, arterial embolism, chronic pernio (chilblain), popliteal entrapment, fibromuscular dysplasia, aortic dissection, ergotamine toxicity, aortic coarctation (thoracic, abdominal), cystic adventitial disease of the popliteal artery, atheromatous emboli, lumbar canal stenosis and lumbar disk disease, degenerative joint disease of the hip and back (Krajewski & Olin, 1991).

Leg ulcers: Arterial ulcers, Martorell's ulcer (hypertension), venous ulcers, neuropathic/diabetic ulcers, drug user, sickle-cell anemia, vasculitis (arteritis), infection, trauma, pressure ulcer, IV or skin popping extravasation of IV fluid (Fitzpatrick et al., 1997)

Management/Treatment

See Table 6–10. The goals are to limit progression of the disease; improve blood flow to the affected limb; relieve pain; prevent and treat tissue damage, wound infection, ulceration, and gangrene; and prevent amputation.

Client Education

Educate client and family on disease and disease process.

Encourage health promotion: Identify and reduce modifiable risk factors, such as hyperlipidemia, obesity, sedentary lifestyle, stress, smoking, hypertension, diabetes, prolonged sitting or standing, oral-contraceptive use, pregnancy, autoimmune or connective-tissue disorders, trauma.

Encourage smoking cessation, low-fat, low-cholesterol diet, exercise.

Teach client how to perform proper foot care.

Follow-up

As indicated by client's condition.

Referral

Refer to vascular specialist if client has diminished functional ability or is unresponsive to therapy; immediate emergency referral if client experiences sudden pain, coldness, numbness, pallor, and/or decreased or absent pulses to affected limb.

PHLEBITIS/VENOUS THROMBOPHLEBITIS

SIGNAL SYMPTOMS▶ localized pain, warmth, tenderness

ICD-9 Codes	451.9	Phlebitis, NOS location
	997.2	Phlebitis, postoperative
	451.0	Thrombophlebitis, superficial leg
	451.2	Thrombophlebitis, deep leg
	453.9	Thrombosis NOS

Phlebitis is inflammation of a vein.

Venous thrombosis, thrombophlebitis, and deep vein thrombosis (DVT) although they do not represent identical pathology, are often used interchangeably.

Thrombophlebitis is inflammation of the walls of the veins in conjunction with formation of a thrombus or clot, (phlebothrombosis).

Thrombosis: formation, development, or existence of a blood coot within the vascular system.

Epidemiology

In the United States deep vein thrombosis develops in about 2 million people per year.

The incidence appears to be increased after general anesthesia that lasts longer than 30 minutes and with the age of the client.

Etiology

Virchow's triad: Venous stasis, vascular injury, and hypercoagulability.

Trauma—damage to vessel endothelium.

Surgery.

Infection.

Previous DVT.

Accidental trauma.

Immobility.

Cardiac or vascular disorder (varicose veins).

Pregnancy.

Obesity.

Dehydration.

Clotting abnormalities (cancer, polycythemia vera, sickle-cell anemia, oral-contraceptive use, estrogen-replacement therapy, antithrombin III deficiency, protein C deficiency, lupus, increased blood viscosity).

Sometimes etiology is unknown.

Physiology and Pathophysiology

Basically, phlebitis is an inflammatory reaction to some irritant, obstruction, or infection.

Coagulation cascade can be triggered by intrinsic or extrinsic pathways:

Intrinsic—activated by contact with factor XII.

Extrinsic—Activated by exposure of blood to tissue thromboplastin (which is released following tissue damage).

Clinical Manifestations

Thrombophlebitis

SUBJECTIVE

Localized pain/tenderness.

Area feels warm or hot.

OBJECTIVE

Pain with palpation along the course of the vein.

Localized inflammatory erythema.

Surface skin may or may not feel warm/hot.

Deep Vein Thrombosis

SUBJECTIVE

May be asymptomatic; one third of clients have no symptoms.

Localized pain/tenderness.

Pain may be more diffuse and intense.

Pain is worse with motion, walking, or dependency.

Swelling.

OBJECTIVE

Pain with manipulation (positive Homan's sign; however, this sign is nonspecific and insensitive, resulting in false positive results in 50% of cases and false negative results in 30%) (Dipiro, 1999).

May be warm or hot to touch.

Possible inflammatory erythema.

May have palpable cord.

May display a dusky cyanosis if extensive DVT.

Engorged or prominent superficial veins.

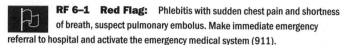

RF 6–1   Red Flag: Phlebitis with sudden chest pain and shortness of breath, suspect pulmonary embolus. Make immediate emergency referral to hospital and activate the emergency medical system (911).

Differential Diagnosis

Differential diagnosis of the clinical features of DVT

Pain and/or tenderness: Muscle strain or trauma, muscle tear, direct muscle or leg trauma, spontaneous muscle hematoma, arterial insufficiency, neurogenic pain, ruptured Baker's cyst, arthritis of knee or ankle joint or Achilles tendinitis, varicose veins, pregnancy, oral-contraceptive use.

Leg swelling: Compression of iliac vein, postphlebitic syndrome, leg immobilization or inflammation, lymphedema, lipedema, self-induced edema

Diagnostic Tests

Doppler flow study (most commonly ordered first, to rule out a blood clot)

Contrast venography (a contrast study of peripheral or central veins)

Duplex ultrasound (to determine the presence, amount, and location of plaques)

Management/Treatment

Pharmacologic Management

Low-molecular-weight heparin: This new kind of heparin, enoxaparin (Lovenox), is being used prophylactically for clients undergoing total hip replacements.

Thrombolytic agents: Drugs such as streptokinase, urokinase, and tissue plasminogen activator can rapidly dissolve a DVT.

Ancrod (Arvin): When available, this investigational IV drug may be used in emergencies for a client who has a documented case of heparin-induced thrombocytopenia or for a client who has an allergic reaction to heparin.

Nonpharmacologic Management

PREVENTIVE MEASURES

Active

    Exercise (dorsiflexion of feet)—Prevents stasis by promoting venous valve and muscle action.

    Deep breathing, using a spirometer when necessary—Increases venous return because of decrease in intrathoracic pressure during inspiration.

    Early ambulation—Prevents stasis by increasing blood flow.

Proper body alignment—Prevents pressure, vessel injury, and stasis when client is walking, sitting, and lying in bed.

Passive

Leg elevation by raising the foot of the bed—Increases blood flow velocity and promotes venous return.

Continuous passive motion devices—Increase muscle and venous valve action.

Elastic support stockings—Increase blood flow velocity, reduce venous stasis, and reduce venous distention.

Intermittent pneumatic compression—Increases blood flow velocity, reduces venous stasis, and stimulates fibrinolytic activity.

INVASIVE PROCEDURES/SURGERY

Filters: Easily inserted in the vena cava; these devices effectively filter out clots and are usually trouble-free.

Thrombectomy: Procedure in which the thrombus is surgically removed from the vessel.

Client Education

Educate about disease and disease process.

Give complete medication information (especially important if client is taking warfarin [Coumadin]); for example, wear a medical-alert bracelet and carry a warfarin ID card, and avoid aspirin or any preparation that contains aspirin (such as some cold medications) unless approved by health-care provider.

Teach how to minimize risks (preventive measures).

Inform when and how to contact health-care provider.

Follow-up

If patient is taking anticoagulants, follow-up will be weekly to monthly for 3–6 months

Referral

Refer to collaborating physician or vascular specialist for initial treatment or if client is unresponsive to therapy.

PULMONARY EDEMA

SIGNAL SYMPTOMS ▶ cough, dyspnea

ICD-9 Codes	518.4	Acute
	428.1	With heart disease or failure
	514	Chemical
	508.1	Radiation
	993.1	High altitude
	994.1	Near-drowning

Pulmonary edema is the life-threatening, acute development of alveolar lung edema; it is most often due to an elevation of hydrostatic pressure in the pulmonary capillaries (left heart failure, mitral stenosis) or increased permeability of the pulmonary alveolar-capillary membrane.

Epidemiology

An estimated 4.8 million Americans are affected.

Of those classified by the New York Heart Association as class IV, the mortality is approximately 50% in 2 years.

Etiology

Pulmonary edema associated with heart failure occurs when left atrial pressure is markedly elevated, with subsequent transudation of fluid into the alveoli (Kloner, 1995).

Typical causes of cardiogenic pulmonary edema include AMI or severe ischemia, exacerbation of chronic heart failure, acute overload of the left ventricular valve (valvular regurgitation or ventricular septal defect) and mitral stenosis (Tierney et al., 2001).

Noncardiac causes of pulmonary edema include decreased plasma oncotic pressure; hypoalbuminemia due to renal hepatic disease, nutritional causes, and protein-losing enteropathy; altered alveolar capillary membrane permeability (adult respiratory distress syndrome); lymphatic insufficiency; narcotic overdose; high-altitude pulmonary edema; neurogenic– subarachnoid hemorrhage; central nervous system trauma; eclampsia; and effects of cardiopulmonary bypass, cardioversion, or anesthesia.

Physiology and Pathophysiology

Pulmonary edema results from the failure of any number of homeostatic mechanisms. The most common cause of pulmonary edema is an increase in pulmonary capillary hydrostatic pressure because of left ventricular failure. Two other homeostatic pressures are oncotic and osmotic pressure in the vascular compartment. This results in disruption in the alveolar epithelium, interstitial lymph flow, and interstitial pulmonary pressure.

Clinical Manifestations

Subjective

Acute onset

Persistent cough

Tachycardia, diaphoresis, cyanosis

Dyspnea (worsening at rest)

Objective

Pulmonary crackles, rhonchi, expiratory wheezing

Differential Diagnosis

Cardiac etiologies (see "Chest Pain," "Myocardial Infarction," "Coronary Artery Disease")

Fluid overload (possible electrolyte disturbances)

Drug reaction (review per patient history)

Adult respiratory distress syndrome (dyspnea, tachypnea, tachycardia,
diaphoresis, changes in level of consciousness)
Pneumonitis (chest congestion, productive cough, fever/chills, aches)

Diagnostic Tests

Arterial blood-gas measurement (to rule out arterial hypoxemia)
Chest x-ray examination (to rule out pulmonary vascular distribution,
blurriness of vascular outlines, increased interstitial markings,
characteristic butterfly pattern of distribution of alveolar edema; possible
enlarged heart size)
Echocardiography (evaluates left ventricular function)
Cardiac catheterization (pulmonary capillary wedge pressure usually
elevated over 25 mm Hg, cardiac output normal or decreased; in
noncardiogenic pulmonary edema wedge pressure may be normal or even
low.)
Ventilation/perfusion scan (V/Q scan) (Figure 6–2)

Management/Treatment

Pharmacologic Management

Oxygen: By mask to obtain a PO_2 greater than 60 mm Hg. If respiratory
distress is severe, endotracheal intubation and mechanical ventilation
may be necessary.
Morphine sulfate: Initial dose of 4–8 mg IV; repeat every 2 to 4 hours
(Tierney et al., 2001).
IV diuretics: Furosemide, 40 mg, or bumetanide, 1 mg or higher, if client
has been receiving long-term diuretic therapy.

Nonpharmacologic Management

Reassurance
Positioning (sitting with legs dangling)

Complementary/Alternative Therapies

Relaxation therapy

Client Education

Educate regarding disease process
Identify worsening signs and symptoms
Possibly recommend low-sodium diet
Weigh regularly

Follow-up

Depends on severity of symptoms, and whether client is treated as an inpatient or
outpatient. Follow-up may be weekly to monthly; if stabilized, follow-up can be
longer.

Referral

Immediate activation of emergency medical system (911) for hospitalization,
and referral to cardiologist/pulmonologist.

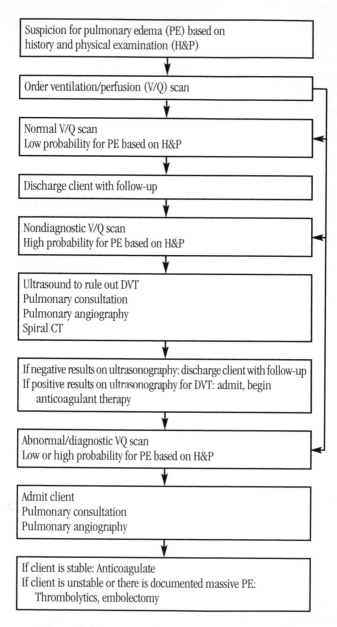

Suspicion for pulmonary edema (PE) based on history and physical examination (H&P)

↓

Order ventilation/perfusion (V/Q) scan

↓

Normal V/Q scan
Low probability for PE based on H&P

↓

Discharge client with follow-up

↓

Nondiagnostic V/Q scan
High probability for PE based on H&P

↓

Ultrasound to rule out DVT
Pulmonary consultation
Pulmonary angiography
Spiral CT

↓

If negative results on ultrasonography: discharge client with follow-up
If positive results on ultrasonography for DVT: admit, begin
    anticoagulant therapy

↓

Abnormal/diagnostic VQ scan
Low or high probability for PE based on H&P

↓

Admit client
Pulmonary consultation
Pulmonary angiography

↓

If client is stable: Anticoagulate
If client is unstable or there is documented massive PE:
    Thrombolytics, embolectomy

Figure 6–2 Diagnosis and Treatment of Pulmonary Edema

VALVULAR DISORDERS: MITRAL-VALVE PROLAPSE

SIGNAL SYMPTOMS shortness of breath, palpitations

ICD-9 Code	424.0	Mitral-valve prolapse

Mitral-valve prolapse (MVP) is a redundance of the mitral valve with degeneration and elongation of chordae tendineae.

Valvular heart disease is anything pertaining to, or affecting the nature of, the valve. See Table 6–11 for a summary of common valvular heart disorders.

Epidemiology

Affects approximately 5% of young adults.

More common in women.

Etiology

Causes include rheumatic fever, ischemic heart disease, atrial septal defect, and Marfan's syndrome; also may be idiopathic or familial.

Physiology and Pathophysiology

MVP results from redundant mitral-valve tissue with myxedematous degeneration and elongated chordae tendineae.

Complications may include arrhythmias (supraventricular tachycardia, ventricular tachycardia), left ventricular failure (with severe MVP), and rarely, systemic emboli from platelet fibrin deposits.

Clinical Manifestations

Subjective

Usually asymptomatic; client may present with atypical chest pain.

Objective

Mid or late systolic click followed by late systolic murmur (murmur exaggerated by Valsalva maneuver, reduced by squatting and isometric exercise)

 CP 6–3   Clinical Pearl: Auscultation

The harshness of the murmur generally may not determine the severity of the lesion.

Aortic murmurs generally radiate cephalad.

Mitral murmurs generally radiate to the left axillary region.

Differential Diagnosis

Benign arrhythmias/malignant dysrhythmias (determined via ECG)

Gastroestophageal reflux (burning epigastric pain, usually worse after eating)

Ischemic heart disease (see "Coronary Artery Disease")

Table 6–11   Valvular Heart Disorders

Mitral Stenosis
ICD code: 394.0

Etiology
  Most cases of mitral stenosis are rheumatic, although 50% of clients do not have a history compatible with rheumatic fever. In most cases of rheumatic fever symptoms develop over a 10-year period. Some clients will remain symptom-free until the stenosis progresses to a moderately severe state.

Clinical manifestations
  Atrial fibrillation
  Diastolic murmur

Diagnostic tests
  ECG (nonspecific, left atrial enlargement, right-axis deviation, right ventricular hypertrophy, atrial fibrillation)
  Echocardiography (most diagnostic; shows stenosis)
  Chest x-ray examination (left atrial enlargement: elevated main-stem bronchus and double cardiac density, prominent left heart border, pulmonary vascular redistribution, Kerley B lines, prominence of right ventricle and pulmonary artery)

Management
  Mild to moderate stenosis: No activity restriction
  Severe stenosis
    Avoid risk of precipitating symptoms
    Mild symptoms
      Begin mild diuretic—Hydrochlorothiazide, 50–100 mg/day.
      No-added-salt diet.
      Digitalis is of no added benefit unless atrial fibrillation is present.
      Avoid extreme exertion or emotional upset.
      Long-term warfarin therapy indicated in client with mitral stenosis and with atrial fibrillation.
  Severe symptoms: Immediate referral to cardiology.

Mitral Regurgitation
ICD code: 424.0

Etiology
  Rheumatic fever
  Mitral-valve prolapse
  Calicification of mitral valve

Clinical Manifestations
  Many patients are asymptomatic for years
  Any clinical manifestations usually have slow onset, but include:
    Dyspnea.
    Fatigue.
    Pansystolic murmur.

Diagnostic tests
  ECG
  Echocardiography

Management
  Asymptomatic
    Requires no restriction of activity
  Onset of dyspnea and fatigue
    Begin mild diuretic—hydrochlorothiazide, 50–100 mg/day.
    No-added-salt diet.
  Refractory congestive heart failure prior to surgery may be treated with vasodilator therapy, particularly ACE inhibitors (captopril, 25–50 mg TID)
  Long-term anticoagulation is indicated in clients with mitral regurgitation and atrial fibrillation.

Table continued on following page.

Table 6–11   Valvular Heart Disorders (*Continued*)

Mitral-valve Prolapse
ICD code: 424.0

Etiology
Mitral-valve prolapse may be structural—i.e., based on a specific structural abnormality of the valve or physiologic, in which concomitant physiologic circumstances are the source of the prolapse.
Structural changes include myxomatous generation, ruptured chordae tendineae, ruptured papillary muscle, Marfan syndrome, rheumatic fever, infective endocarditis, collagen vascular disease.
Physiologic changes include prolapse being influenced by the Valsalva maneuver, atrial septal defect, hyperthyroidism, emphysema, and hypertrophic cardiomyopathy.

Clinical manifestations
Symptoms vary, but some clients have palpitations, atypical chest pain, orthostatic dizziness, near-syncope, cold extremities, throbbing headaches, and neurasthenia. They may also report tachydysrhythmia, orthostatic hypotension, and peripheral vasoconstriction.
Late-systolic murmur

Diagnostic tests
ECG
Echocardiography

Management
Mitral-valve prolapse continues to be controversial with regard to prophylaxis.
The American Heart Association suggests endocarditis prophylaxis for those who have evidence of mitral insufficiency; other authorities suggest prophylaxis for all clients with mitral-valve prolapse. However, recent studies suggest that no prophylaxis is necessary if the valves prolapse without leaking (Dajani, 1997; Thornton, 2000). That is, a systolic click may be heard, but no murmur is present and no Doppler-demonstrated mitral regurgitation is present (Dajani, 1997). Prophylaxis is indicated if a murmur is present with audible clicks, and leaking is present as evidenced by Doppler.

American Heart Association Bacterial Endcarditis Prophylaxis (1997)*
Prophylactic regimens for dental, oral, respiratory tract, or esophageal procedures. (Follow-up dose no longer recommended.) Total children's dose should not exceed adult dose.
273 Standard general prophylaxis for clients at risk:
Amoxicillin, 2 g (children, 50 mg/kg) given orally 1 hour before procedure.
274 Unable to take oral medications:
Ampicillin, 2 g (children, 50 mg/kg) given IM or IV 30 minutes before procedure.
275 Clients allergic to amoxicillin/ampicillin/penicillin:
Clindamycin: Adults, 600 mg (children, 20 mg/kg) given orally 1 hour before procedure.
OR
Cephalexin or cefadroxil: Adults, 2 g (children, 50 mg/kg) orally 1 hour before procedure.
OR
Azithromycin or clarithromycin: Adults, 500 mg (children, 5 mg/kg) orally 1 hour before procedure.
276 Clients allergic to amoxicillin/ampicillin/penicillin who are unable to take oral medications.
Clindamycin: Adults, 600 mg (children, 20 mg/kg) IV within 30 minutes before procedure.
OR
Cefazolin: Adults: 1 g (children, 25 mg/kg) IM or IV within 30 minutes before procedure.
**Adapted from:* American Heart Association by the Committee on Rheumatic Fever, Endocarditis, and Kawasaki Disease (1997). Prevention of bacterial endocarditis. *JAMA, 277,* 1794–1801.

Aortic Stenosis
ICD code: 747.22

Etiology
Aortic valvular stenosis may follow rheumatic fever, but is more commonly caused by progressive valvular calcification on a congenitally bicuspid valve, or in the elderly, a result of aging.
There are three major varieties of adult valvular aortic stenosis: Rheumatic, senile-calcific or degenerative, and congenital bicuspid aortic valve. Clients 20 to 30 years of age may have the murmur, but symptoms may not develop until the sixth decade of life.
Table continued on following page.

Table 6–11   Valvular Heart Disorders (*Continued*)

Approximately 25% of clients over 65 years of age and 35% of those over 70 years of age have evidence of aortic stenosis, with 2%–3% exhibiting hemodynamically significant stenosis (Dipiro, 1999). Degenerative changes of the aortic valve are three to four times more common in men than in women. There is also a higher predisposition in clients with hypertension and those who smoke.

Clinical manifestations
    Midsystolic murmur

Diagnostic tests
    ECG (left ventricular hypertrophy)
    Chest x-ray examination (normal or enlarged silhouette, calcification of aortic valve, dilatation and calcification of the ascending aorta)
    Echocardiography
    Cardiac catheterization (definitive diagnosis; gradient is measured and valve area calculated: valve area below 0.8 cm^2 indicates severe stenosis)

Management
    Asymptomatic clients do not require restriction of activity
    Onset of angina, effort syncope, or congestive heart failure dictates prompt referral to cardiologist.
    Because calcification of the valve may advance rapidly, clients should have careful longitudinal care and regular follow-up

Aortic regurgitation (aortic insufficiency)
ICD code: 424.1

Etiology
    Rheumatic aortic regurgitation has become less common since antibiotics have become available. Nonrheumatic causes are frequent and are the major cause of isolated aortic regurgitation. These include congenitally bicuspid valve, infective endocarditis, and hypertension. Aortic regurgitation may also develop as a result of aortic root diseases such as cystic medial necrosis (Marfan's syndrome), aortic dissection, Reiter's syndrome, ankylosing spondylitis, and syphilis (Kloner, 1995).

Clinical manifestations
    The client is usually asymptomatic until middle age, and presents with symptoms of left heart failure or chest pain. As the valve deformity increases, large amounts of regurgitant blood flow occurs, resulting in diastolic blood pressure drop, and left ventricular dilatation.
    Exertional dyspnea and fatigue are the most common symptoms. Paroxysmal nocturnal dyspnea can also occur in addition to pulmonary edema. Chest pain may occur, but it is less commonly associated with coronary artery disease and syncope than seen in aortic stenosis.
    The major physical findings on examination relate to a widened arterial peak pressure. The pulse has a rapid rise and fall (Corrigan's water-hammer pulse), with an elevated systolic and low diastolic pressure, due to the large stroke volume and rapid diastolic runoff back into the left ventricle, respectively. De Musset sign is a head bobbing with each systole. Palpation of the carotid reveals a bisferious or double-peaked quality. These peripheral signs may be absent in acute cases or advanced cases with severe left ventricular failure.
    Diastolic murmur

Diagnostic tests
    ECG (moderate to severe left ventricular hypertrophy)
    Chest x-ray examination (cardiomegaly, left ventricular prominence)

Management
    No activity restriction in young client with mild regurgitation
    Clients with worsening left ventricular function with strain pattern on ECG, increasing heart size by radiography, falling ejection fraction, and increased left ventricular end-diastolic dimension should be referred to cardiology (Goroll, 1995).
    Onset of mild symptoms of dyspnea and fatigue with left ventricular dysfunction can be treated with a mild diuretic program (hydrochlorothiazide, 50–100 mg), digitalis, or afterload reduction.
    Clients with dyspnea prompted by minimal exertion, orthopnea, or paroxysmal nocturnal dyspnea require immediate referral (Goroll, 1995).

Table continued on following page.

Table 6–11 Valvular Heart Disorders (*Continued*)

Triscupid Stenosis

| ICD code: 397.0 | Tricuspid stenosis or regurgitation, rheumatic |
| 424.2 | Tricuspid stenosis or regurgitation, nonrheumatic |

Etiology
Tricuspid stenosis is usually rheumatic in origin.

Clinical manifestations
The usual client presents with symptoms of "right heart failure." Symptoms such as ascites, hepatomegaly, and dependent edema may all be symptoms of this lesion.

Diagnostic tests
ECG
Echocardiography

Management
If severe, surgical treatment is needed to replace valve.

Triscupid Regurgitation

| ICD code: 397.0 | Tricuspid stenosis or regurgitation, rheumatic |
| 424.2 | Tricuspid stenosis or regurgitation, nonrheumatic |

Etiology
Tricuspid regurgitation may occur in a variety of associated conditions. The most common is right ventricular overload resulting from left ventricular failure. Often associated with pulmonary hypertension.

Clinical manifestations
Pansystolic murmur
Severe right ventricular failure (hepatomegaly, jugular venous distention, edema)

Diagnostic tests
ECG
Echocardiography

Management
Diuretic therapy.
If severe, surgical treatment is needed to replace valve

Adapted from: American heart (1997). Prevention of bacterial endocarditis. Association by the Committee on Rheumatic Fever, Endocarditis, and Kawasaki Disease *JAMA,* 277;1794–1801.

Congenital heart disease (per patient history)
Valvular heart disease (determined via echocardiography)
Thyroid disease (determined via TSH and free T_4)
Pneumonitis (chest congestion, productive cough, fever/chills, aches)
Anxiety disorder (see "Anxiety")

Diagnostic Tests

Chemistry panel (to rule out metabolic derangement)
Thyroid studies (to rule out thyrotoxicosis)
CBC (to rule out anemia)
Chest x-ray examination (to rule out pulmonary abnormality)
ECG (to establish normal base line if client has chest pain)
Echocardiography (shows posterior displacement of posterior, occasionally anterior, mitral-valve leaflet late in systole)

Management/Treatment

The major goals of therapy in valvular heart disease are to preserve exercise capacity, lifestyle, and life expectancy and to minimize the chances of endocarditis and systemic embolization.

Pharmacologic Management
Prophylaxis for infective endocarditis as indicated
Anticoagulation for clients with history of embolization

Nonpharmacologic Management
Reassurance and education if client is asymptomatic
Valve replacement if client has severe murmur/disease

Client Education
Nature of disease; treatment plan

Follow-up
As indicated

Referral
Refer to physician as indicated, or for pharmacologic evaluation

REFERENCES

General
Dipiro, J.T., et al. (1999). Pharmacotherapy: A pathophysiologic approach (4th ed.). Stamford, CT: Appleton & Lange.

Driscoll, V., Bope, E., Smith & Carter, B. (1996). *The family practice desk reference*. St. Louis: Mosby.

Fauci, A.S., Braunwald, E., Isselbacher, K.J., et al. (2001). *Harrison's principles of internal medicine* (15th ed.). New York: McGraw-Hill.

Fenstermacher, K. & Hudson, B.T. (2000). *Practice guidelines for family nurse practitioners* (2nd ed.). Philadelphia: Harcourt Health.

Fox, J.A. (1997). *Primary health care of children*. St. Louis: Mosby Yearbook.

Goroll, A.H., May, L.A. & Mulley, A.G. (2000). *Primary care medicine* (5th ed.). Philadelphia: Lippincott Williams & Wilkins.

Hoole, Axalla J., et al. (1999). *Patient care guidelines for nurse practitioners* (5th ed.). Philadelphia: Lippincott Williams & Wilkins.

Noble, J. (2001). Textbook of primary care medicine (3rd ed.). St. Louis: Mosby Yearbook.

Pender, N. (1996) *Health promotion in nursing practice*. Stamford, CT: Appleton & Lange.

Price, S.A. & Wilson, L.M. (1997). *Pathophysiology: Clinical concepts of disease processes* (5th ed.) St. Louis: Mosby Yearbook.

Seller, R.H. (1999). *Differential diagnosis of common complaints* (4th ed.). Philadelphia: Harcourt Health.

Tierney, L.M., McPhee, S.J., Pappadakis, M.A. (2001). *Current medical diagnosis & treatment 2001*. Stamford, CT: Appleton & Lange.

Anemia
Herbert, V., Bigaouette, J. (1997). Call for endorsement of a petition to the Food and Drug Administration to always add vitamin B-12 to any folate fortification or supplement. *American Journal of Clinical Nutrition, 65,* 572–573.

Himes, J., Walker, S., Williams, S., Bennett, F., Grantham-McGregor, S. (1997). A method to estimate prevalence of iron deficiency and iron-deficiency anemia in adolescent Jamaican girls. *American Journal of Clinical Nutrition, 65,* 831–836.

Tickle, M. (1997). Folic acid and food fortification: Implications for the primary care practitioner. *Nurse Practitioner, 22*(3), 105–114.

Angina Pectoris

Birdwell, B., Herbers, J.E. & Kroenke, K. (1993). Evaluating chest pain: The patient's presentation style alters the physicians diagnostic approach. *Archives of Internal Medicine, 153,* 1991–1995.

Diamond G.A. & Forrester, J.S. (1979). Analysis of probability as an aid in the clinical diagnosis of coronary artery disease. *New England Journal of Medicine, 300,* 1350–1357.

Kopp, D.E., & Wilber, D.J. (1992). Palpitations and arrhythmias: Separating the benign from the dangerous. *Postgraduate Medicine 91*(1), 241–244, 247–248, 251.

Simons, G.R., Eisenstein, E.L., Shaw, L.J., Mark, D.B., & Pritchett, E.L.C. (1997). Cost effectiveness of inpatient initiation of antiarrhythmic therapy for supraventricular tachycardias. *American Journal of Cardiology, 80,* 1551–1557.

Arrhythmias

Taylor, R.D., Asinger, R.W. (1998, August). Atrial fibrillation: Clinical clues, keys to the work-up. *Consultant, 38,* 1983–1988.

Chest Pain

Birdwell, B., Herbers, J.E., & Kroenke, K. (1993). Evaluating chest pain: The patient's presentation style alters the physicians diagnostic approach. *Archives of Internal Medicine, 153,* 1991–1995.

Diamond, G.A., & Forrester, J.S. (1979). Analysis of probability as an aid in the clinical diagnosis of coronary artery disease. *New England Journal of Medicine, 300,* 1350–1357.

Simons, G.R., Eisenstein, E.L., Shaw, L.J., Mark, D.B., & Pritchett, E.L.C. (1997). Cost effectiveness of inpatient initiation of antiarrhythmic therapy for supraventricular tachycardias. *American Journal of Cardiology, 80,* 1551–1557.

Coronary Artery Disease

Cardiovascular disorders (2000). Atlanta: Centers for Disease Control & Prevention. National Center for Chronic Disease Prevention & Health Promotion.

Heart Failure

American Heart Association (1994). NYHA Functional Capacity Classifications, excerpted from 1994 revisions to Classification of Functional Capacity and Objective Assessment of Patients with Diseases of the Heart. AHA Medical Scientific Statement. *Nomenclature & Criteria for Diagnosis of Diseases of the Heart and Great Vessels.* (9th ed.). Boston: Little Brown.

Connolly, K. (2000, July). New directions in heart failure management. *Nurse Practitioner, 23,* 27–28, 31–34.

Frolich, E.D., & Zusman, R.M. (1997, Fall). Fine-tuning of antihypertensive therapy: When monotherapy fails: Effective use of combination therapy. *Patient Care,* 1–21.

Levy, D., Larson, M.G., Ramachandran, S.V., Kannel, W.B., & Kalon, K.L. (1996). The progression from hypertension to congestive heart failure. *JAMA, 275,* 1557–1561.

Joint National Committee on Prevention, Detection, Evaluation, and Treatment of High Blood Pressure (1997). The Sixth Report of the Joint National Committee on Prevention, Detection, Evaluation, and Treatment of High Blood Pressure. *Archives of Internal Medicine, 157,* 2413–2446.

Saltmarsh, N. (Ed.) (1997). *Congestive heart failure: The disease state management resource.* Atlanta: American Health Consultants.

Sonnenblick, E.H., & Lejemtel, T.H. (1993). Heart failure: Its progression and its therapy. *Hospital Practice, 9,* 121–130.

U.S. Department of Health and Human Services (1997). Put prevention into practice—Blood pressure. *Journal of American Academy of Nurse Practitioners, 12,* 27–32.

Heart Murmurs

Campbell, C. (1995). Primary care for women, comprehensive cardiovascular assessment. *Journal of Nurse-Midwifery, 40*(2), 137–149. (Includes the tools necessary for basic primary care assessment and evaluation of the cardiovascular system in women.)

Katz, J., Krafft, P., Kelly F. (1996). Assessing a murmur, saving a life: Current trends in the management of hypertrophic cardiomyopathy. *Nurse Practitioner. 21*(11), 62–74.

Yakowich Moody, L. (1997). Pediatric cardiovascular assessment and referral in the primary care setting. *22*(1), 120–134.

Hypertension

American Heart Association (June 9, 1998). *High blood pressure,* available at http://www.american heart.org/heart_and_stroke.A_Z_.

Cardiovascular disorders (1993). Atlanta: Centers for Disease Control and Prevention—National Center for Chronic Disease Prevention and Health Promotion.

Fine-tuning antihypertension therapy (Fall, 1997). *Patient Care: The Practice Journal for Primary Care Physicians.* Montvale, NJ: Medical Economics Company.

Joint National Committee on Prevention, Detection, Evaluation, and Treatment of High Blood Pressure (1997). The Sixth Report of the Joint National Committee on Prevention, Detection, Evaluation, and Treatment of High Blood Pressure. *Archives of Internal Medicine, 157,* 2413–2446.

Loggie, J.M.H. & Sardegna, K.M. (1997). Latest standards for hypertension in teens. *Pediatrics, 3,* 121–135.

National High Blood Pressure Education Program Working Group on Hypertension Control in Children and Adolescents (1996). A Working Group Report on High Blood Pressure in Children and Adolescents from the National High Blood Pressure Education Program. *Pediatrics, 98,* 649–658.

Rosner, B., Prineas, R.J., Loggie, J.M.H., et al. (1997). Blood pressure nomograms for children and adolescents by height, sex, and age in the United States. *Journal of Pediatrics, 98,* 649–658.

Lipid Disorders

Amsterdam, E.A., & Deedwania, P.C. (1998). A prospective on hyperlipidemia: Concepts of management in the prevention of coronary artery disease. *American Journal of Medicine, 105,* 215–221.

Lamarche, B., Tchernof, A., Moojani, S., et al. Small, dense, low-density lipoprotein particles as a predictor of the risk of ischemic heart disease in men. *Circulation, 95,* 69–75.

Mandelbaum-Schmid, J. (July/August 1998). Beyond cholesterol. *Health,* pp. 95–101.

Myocardial Infarction

Kloner, R.A. (1995). *The guide to cardiology.* Greenwich, CT: Le Jacq.

Marino, P.L. (1998). *The ICU book.* Baltimore: Lippincott Williams & Wilkins.

Rivello, R.J., & Hoekstra, J.W. (1998, October). Thrombolytic therapy, how best to use in acute MI. *Consultant,* 2365–2375.

Palpitations

Birdwell, B., Herbers, J.E., & Kroenke, K. (1993). Evaluating chest pain: The patient's presentation alters the physicians diagnostic approach. *Archives of Internal Medicine, 153,* 1991–1995.

Diamond, G.A., & Forrester, J.S. (1979). Analysis of probability as an aid in the clinical diagnosis of coronary artery disease. *New England Journal of Medicine, 300,* 1350–1357.

Kopp, D.E., & Wilber, D.J. (1992). Palpitations and arrhythmias: Separating the benign from the dangerous. *Postgraduate Medicine 91*(1), 241–244, 247–248, 251.

Peripheral Vascular Disease

Ague, A.M.R. (1991). Grant's atlas of anatomy (9th ed.). Baltimore: Williams & Wilkins.

Barr, D.M. (1996). The Unna's boot as a treatment for venous ulcers. *Nurse Practitioner, 21*(7), 55–74.

Bergan, J.J., & Goldman, M.P. (1993). *Varicose veins and telangiectasias.* St. Louis: Quality Medical.

Bullock, B.L. (1996). Alterations in systemic circulation. In B.L. Bullock & P.P. Rosendahl (Eds.), *Pathophysiology: Adaptations and alterations in function* (4th ed.). Philadelphia: Lippincott Williams & Wilkins.

Calabrese, L.H., & Clough, J.D. (1991). Systemic vasculitis. In J.R. Young, R.A. Graor, J.W. Olin, & J.R. Bartholomew (Eds.), *Peripheral vascular diseases.* St. Louis: Mosby Yearbook.

Collins, R.D. (1995). *Algorithmic diagnosis of symptoms and signs: Cost effective approach.* New York: Igaku Shoin.

Dennison, P.D., & Black, J.M. (1993). Nursing care of clients with peripheral vascular disorders. In J.M. Black & E. Mataassarin-Jacobs (Eds.), *Luckman and Sorensen's medical-surgical nursing: A psychophysiologic approach.* Philadelphia: Harcourt Health Sciences.

Fahey, V.A. (1999). *Vascular nursing* (3rd ed.). Philadelphia: Harcourt Health Sciences.

Fitzpatrick, T.B., Johnson, R.A., Wolff, K., Polano, M.D., & Suarmond, D. (1997). *Color atlas and synopsis of clinical dermatology: Common and serious diseases* (3rd ed.). New York: McGraw-Hill.

Harris, A.H. (1996). Managing vascular leg ulcers, part 1: Assessment. *American Journal of Nursing, 96*(1), 38–44.

Katsung, B.G. (1998). *Basic and clinical pharmacology.* Stamford, CT: Appleton & Lange.

Krajewski, L.P., & Olin, J.W. (1991). Atherosclerosis of the aorta and lower extremity arteries. In J.R. Young, R.A. Graor, J.W. Olin, & J.R. Bartholomew (Eds.), *Peripheral vascular diseases* (pp. 179–200). St. Louis: Mosby.

Ting, M. (1991). Wound healing and peripheral vascular disease. *Critical Care Nursing Clinics of North America, 3,* 515–523.

Young, J.R., Graor, R.A., Olin, J.W., & Bartholomew, J.R. (1996). *Peripheral vascular diseases* (2nd ed.). St. Louis: Mosby Yearbook.

Phlebitis

Lees, A. (1995). Thromboembolic complications in children and adolescents: Who is at risk? *Journal of Pediatric Health Care. 9,* 222–224.

Livesley, J. (1996). Peripheral IV therapy in children. *Pediatric-Nursing, 8*(6), 29–35.

Stonehouse, J., & Butcher, J. (1996). Phlebitis associated with peripheral cannulae. *Professional-Nurse, 12*(1), 51–54.

Villani, C., Johnson, D., & Burke, C. (1995). Bilateral suppurative thrombophlebitis due to *Staphylococcus aureus. Heart & Lung, 7,* 342–344.

Valvular Disorders

Marks, A.R., Choong, C.Y., Sanfilippo, A.J., et al. (1989). Identification of high-risk and low-risk subgroups of patients with mitral-valve prolapse. *New England Journal of Medicine, 320,* 1031–1036.

Thornton, S.E. (2000). Valvular heart disease. *Journal of American Academy of Nurse Practitioners, 5*(12), 179–184.

RESOURCES

General

American Heart Association
> National Center
> 7272 Greenville Ave.
> Dallas, TX 75231-4596
> Telephone: 1-800-242-8721
> www.amhrt.org

American Society of Hypertension
> 515 Madison Ave.
> Suite 1212
> New York, NY 10022
> Telephone: 212-644-0650
> Fax: 212-644-0658
> ash@ash-us.org

Centers for Disease Control and Prevention
> National Center for Chronic Disease Prevention and Health Promotion
> Mail Stop K-13
> 4770 Buford Hwy. N.E.
> Atlanta, GA 30341-3717
> Telephone: 770-488-5080

Cleveland Clinic
> www.clevelandclinic.org/heartcenter/

Mayo Clinic
> www.mayo.edu/MayoHome.html

Minneapolis Heart Institute Foundation
> 920 East 28th St.
> Suite 100
> Minneapolis, MN 55407
> Telephone: 612-863-3833 or 877-800-2729
> Fax: 612-863-3801
> www.mplsheartfoundation.org

National Heart, Lung, and Blood Institute Information Center
> P.O. Box 30105
> Bethesda, MD 20824-0105
> Telephone: 301-251-1222
> www.nhlbi.nih.gov

WomenHeart
> 1718 M St., #330
> Washington, DC 20036
> Telephone: 202-736-1770
> www.womenheart.org

Chapter 7

GASTROINTESTINAL DISORDERS

ANAL FISSURES

SIGNAL SYMPTOMS▶ rectal pain exacerbated by defecation

ICD-9 Code	565.0	Anal fissure

Anal fissures are linear tears of the epithelium in the anal canal; they usually appear below the dentate. Most anal fissures are posterior.

Epidemiology
Very common cause of rectal bleeding

Etiology
Trauma caused by constipation, passage of hard or large-caliber stools, and spasm of the internal sphincter; may also result from anal intercourse or objects inserted into the anal canal.

Other causes include irritable bowel disease, syphilis, tuberculosis, leukemia, and cancer.

Physiology and Pathophysiology
The anal canal is approximately 3 to 4 cm in length. The anus and rectum converge at a line called the dentate. Cells distal to the dentate line (anus) are squamous epithelium, whereas those proximal (rectum) are columnar epithelium. Circular muscles and muscularis propria create the inner layer of muscles, and striated muscles compose the external sphincters.

Anal fissures occur with a disruption of the epithelial lining within the anal canal. The squamous tissue will epithelialize if the causative factors are eliminated.

Clinical Manifestations

Subjective
Painful bowel movements
Rectal bleeding (bright red blood [BRB])
Constipation or diarrhea
Anorectal pain
Stool incontinence

Objective

Rectal examination reveals a tear or split in the anal canal.

 CP 7–1 Clinical Pearl: The examination may be very difficult because of the pain involved, so use 2% lidocaine.

Frank BRB on examination glove.

May have hard stool in rectal vault.

Perianal abscess may be found on palpation.

Differential Diagnosis

Hemorrhoids (episodic bleeding on passing stools, pruritus, mass)

Pruritus ani (rectal itching—a symptom of underlying cause e.g., hemorrhoids, fissure, condylomata)

Anorectal abscess (pain, possible discharge—an infected anal gland tracks along various places and results in focal abscess)

Anorectal fistulas (communication between epithelialized viscera, periodic discharge occasionally filled with blood)

Rectocele (rectal protrusion through the posterior vaginal wall)

Anal papillae (small nipple-shaped projections)

Malignant conditions (squamous carcinoma, Bowen's disease, Paget's disease, malignant melanoma)

Diagnostic Tests

Anoscopy (for fissure visualization)

Flexible sigmoidoscopy or colonoscopy (if bleeding is persistent, or client has anemia, change in bowel habits, or a family history of colon cancer)

Management/Treatment

Symptomatic treatment; if constipation or diarrhea present, correct these conditions.

Pharmacologic Management

Topical analgesics for comfort. Xylocaine (2.5%) apply every 3–4 hours PRN. May need hydrocortisone suppositories or creams. Anusol HC suppository BID 7–14 days.

Nonpharmacologic Management

Sitz baths BID/TID for 15 to 20 minutes in lukewarm water

Surgery for chronic anal fissures

Client Education

Advise client that fissures may take 6–8 weeks to heal; immunocompromised clients may take longer to heal.

Follow-up

2–4 weeks or sooner if symptoms worsen

Referral

Refer to gastroenterologist for flexible-sigmoidoscopy or colonoscopy

Referral to surgeon may also be necessary

APPENDICITIS

SIGNAL SYMPTOMS ▶ periumbilical then right-lower-quadrant (RLQ) abdominal pain, lessened with flexion of right thigh

ICD-9 Code	541.0	Appendicitis

Appendicitis is an inflammation of the appendix.

Epidemiology

Most common acute surgical condition of the abdomen.

Predominant age, 10–30.

Incidence in males is greater than that in females (3:2). After age 30, the incidence is equal in the two genders.

The incidence in the total population is 10 in 1 million.

Etiology

Mucosal ulceration with immunologic response of inflammation may be the cause.

Physiology and Pathophysiology

Fecal obstruction may also occur. Luminal bacteria begin to multiply, invading the appendix. Given enough time, gangrene and perforation may result.

Clinical Manifestations

Subjective

Abdominal pain in the periumbical and RLQ regions, although location of abdominal pain may be at other anatomical sites.

Anorexia.

Nausea, vomiting.

Urge to defecate, yet defecation does not relieve pain.

Fever.

The sequence of symptoms 99% of time is anorexia, then abdominal pain, then vomiting.

Objective

Tenderness on palpation at the site of appendix (varies). With retrocecal or pelvic appendix, tenderness will be elicited on rectal or pelvic examination, respectively.

Positive iliopsoas test—Push down over lower part of right thigh as person tries to hold leg up; a positive response is pain.

Obturator test—Lift right leg, flex at hip and 90 degrees at knee, hold ankle and rotate leg internally and externally; a positive response is pain.

Rovsing's sign—Pain in RLQ when palpating for rebound tenderness of left lower quadrant (LLQ tenderness is not necessary for diagnosis.

Normal to slight temperature increase, with a high fever (suspect perforation).

Cutaneous hyperesthesia.

Increase WBC with left shift.

Differential Diagnosis

The causes of an acute abdomen are numerous, and careful attention to the eight characteristics of symptoms is prudent: location, timing, associated symptoms, alleviating symptoms, quality of pain, severity of pain, onset, and duration.

Pelvic inflammatory disease, ectopic pregnancy, endometriosis, ruptured ovarian cyst (female clients)

Cholecystitis (right-upper-quadrant [RUQ] pain, radiates to back or shoulder, attacks 1–6 hr after meals)

Pancreatitis (epigastric abdominal pain amylase, can radiate to back; nausea and vomiting; flank discoloration increased amylase)

Diverticulitis, Meckel's diverticulitis (in younger clients presenting with gastrointestinal bleeding, half will have this)

Bowel obstruction, intestinal ischemia, mesenteric lymphadenitis

Renal calculi, pyelonephritis (back pain, hematuria, fever, costo-vertebral angle tenderness)

Gastroenteritis (see p 330)

Irritable bowel disease (see p 346)

Perforated ulcer (see p 352)

Diagnostic Tests

Clinical judgment should guide the diagnosis.

White-cell count (leukocytosis 10,000–18,000 with a shift to the left; if leukocytosis >18,000, suspect perforation or ruptured appendix).

Erythrocyte sedimentation rate (ESR) (possible elevation).

Choice of diagnostic procedures is very controversial, but includes ultrasonography of the abdomen, abdominal x-ray examination, and spiral computed tomography (possibly most popular at this time).

Management/Treatment

RF 7–1   Red Flag: If appendicitis is highly suspected through concurring clinical findings, client needs to be NPO, an IV line needs to be established for fluid replacement, and immediate consultation with a physician and a referral to a surgeon should take place.

Refer to surgeon for appendectomy.

Client Education

Disease process, explaining most individuals respond very well after surgery

Infection precautions, especially after surgery

Wound care

Slowly returning to physical activity

Follow-up

As indicated

Referral

Refer immediately to physician and surgeon

ASCARIASIS

SIGNAL SYMPTOMS abdominal pain, distention, wheezing, dyspnea

ICD-9 Code	127.0	Ascariasis

Ascaris lumbricoides (nematode), also referred to as roundworm, is a helminthic infection in the small bowel.

Epidemiology

Worldwide, about 1 billion persons infected by contaminated food; in North America approximately 4 million cases per year.

Higher prevalence in tropical countries and recent immigrants to the United States.

Most common in children (preschool, elementary-school ages).

Etiology

Consumption of infective eggs from raw fruits and vegetables contaminated by poorly treated sewage-fertilizer or infected food handlers.

Physiology and Pathophysiology

Ascaris lumbricoides eggs release larvae, which results in an early pulmonary phase caused by larval migration; this progresses to a later phase in the small bowel. The larvae sustain themselves in the jejunum, then migrate into the intestinal wall to the bloodstream and lymphatics, with ultimate progression to the lungs. The larvae ascend through the pulmonary system and are reswallowed and reintroduced into the intestines.

Clinical Manifestations

Subjective

Client reports wheezing, cough, dyspnea, abdominal pain, distention, nausea, vomiting, and fever.

Objective

Live passage of worms in stool, mouth, and/or nose

Differential Diagnosis

Pneumonia (nasal flaring, grunting, rust-colored/purulent sputum, fever, chills)

Acute appendicitis (see p 317)

Diagnostic Tests

Stool sample for ova and parasites (O&P) (*Ascaris lumbricoides* eggs found on fecal smear)

Chest x-ray examination (pulmonary ascariasis may reveal pulmonary infiltrate)

Sputum or gastric aspirate (pulmonary ascariasis may reveal blood eosinophilia)

Management/Treatment

Pharmacologic Management

Pyrantel pamoate, 11 mg/kg for one-dose maximum.
OR
Mebendazole, 100 mg PO QD for 3 days (>2 years old to adult).
Intestinal obstruction present—piperazine citrate, 75 mg/kg per day
   (maximum, 3.5 g) for 2 days; makes worms flaccid and easier to pass.

Client Education

Practice good personal hygiene
Engage in excellent handwashing routine
Wash all fruits/vegetables before eating

Follow-up

As indicated if symptoms persist or worsen

Referral

No referral is necessary. Consult with physician for treatment plan if indicated.

CHOLECYSTITIS

SIGNAL SYMPTOMS pain that may radiate to back especially right
after fatty meals

ICD-9 Code	574.0	Cholecystitis

Cholecystitis is inflammation of the gallbladder. It is usually caused by obstruction of the cystic duct by a gallstone. *Cholelithiasis* refers to the appearance of gallstones within the gallbladder or the cystic duct. *Choledocholithiasis* refers to common-bile-duct stones.

Epidemiology

Affects more women than men (approximately 2:1)
Most frequent in 5th and 6th decade
Incidence increases with increased body-mass index

Etiology

Risk factors include female gender, parity, obesity, rapid weight loss,
   advancing age, family history, American Indian heritage, gallbladder
   stasis syndromes, medications (fibrates, estrogens, anabolic steroids,
   octreotide), hypertriglyceridemia and low high-density lipoprotein
   cholesterol level, inborn errors of bile salt synthesis, and spinal cord
   injury (Stein et al., 1998, p 2223).

Physiology and Pathophysiology

The gallbladder becomes inflamed as a result of cystic-duct obstruction by a gallstone. The initial obstruction causes an inflammatory response with eventual bacterial invasion.

Clinical Manifestations

Subjective

History of previous "attacks" lasting 1 to 4 days.

Reports of RUQ pain that may radiate to the back between the scapula or to the right shoulder; pain occurs right after meals (especially after heavy or fatty meals).

Loss of appetite.

Nausea and vomiting; regurgitation of bitter fluid.

Fever.

Objective

Positive Murphy's sign (tenderness to palpation of the RUQ)

Distended gallbladder (felt in about one third of clients)

Jaundice (choledocholithiasis)

High fever and chills if septic

Differential Diagnosis

Pleurisy (dyspnea, stabbing pain, spasm of chest on affected side)

Perforated duodenal ulcer (tachycardia, tachypnea, abdomen diffusely tender, signs and symptoms of peritonitis)

Appendicitis (see p 317)

Ectopic pregnancy (pelvic pain, amenorrhea followed by irregular vaginal bleeding, abdominal tenderness, shoulder pain)

Perforated colon (pneumoperitoneum, diffuse abdominal tenderness, pain in right or left side of abdomen)

Splenic rupture (evaluate for Epstein–Barr virus)

Pancreatitis

Hepatitis (prodromal phase—anorexia, nausea, vomiting, malaise, upper respiratory infection, easily fatigued, fever, mild abdominal pain. Icteric phase—5–10 days after initial symptoms notice jaundice, dark urine)

Diagnostic Tests

Complete blood count (CBC) with differential (if CBC shows leukocytosis, obtain liver-function tests, bilirubin, alkaline phosphate, amylase, lipase (lipase increased with choledocholithiasis or stone passage through the common bile duct).

Ultrasound of the abdomen (very sensitive; 97% of stones more than 3 mm in diameter are visualized). If ultrasound is negative; consider hepatobiliary iminodiacetic acid scan with cholecystokinin for gallbladder functioning (ejection fraction <35% with reproduction of pain is a positive result).

Endoscopic retrograde cholangiopancreatography if retained common-bile-duct stones.

Management/Treatment

Refer to surgeon for cholecystectomy

Symptomatic management (e.g., analgesics)

Client Education
Disease process
Infection precautions, especially after surgery
Wound care
Low-fat diet, weight loss, if needed

Follow-up
It is important to note that approximately 50% of clients with a cholecystectomy will return to the office with same symptoms. The differential diagnoses need to be thoroughly reviewed.

Referral
Refer to surgeon or gastroenterologist

CONSTIPATION

SIGNAL SYMPTOM decreased frequency of passing stools—normal 3–5 times/week

ICD-9 Codes	564.0	Constipation
	787.99	Gas/bloating

Infrequent defecation and defecatory straining provide guidelines to defining constipation, as do consistency, frequency, and stool passage. At least 25% of clients who report hard stools, defecation two times or less per week, and/or difficulty in stool evacuation have constipation.

Constipation may be a result of functional, organic, or idiopathic causes, or may result from certain medications.

Epidemiology
Approximately 2.5 million office visits per year, affecting an estimated 4 million people a year
Most common gastrointestinal (GI) symptom
Higher at extremes of life (infants and children and elderly)

Etiology
Functional: Irritable bowel syndrome (IBS), decrease in or lack of dietary fiber, lack of physical activity, restraining urge to defecate when it arises, travel.
Organic: Endocrine disorders (diabetes, hypothyroidism, pregnancy), neurologic disorders (multiple sclerosis, spinal cord injury, Hirschsprung's disease), structural defects (obstruction, neoplasm), myogenic disorder (scleroderma), metabolic disorder (hypercalcemia, dehydration).
Idiopathic: Cause unknown.
Medications: Most common include calcium-channel blockers, antipsychotics, antidepressants, antacids, iron supplements, opiates, antispasmodics, anticonvulsants and over-the-counter cold remedies.

Physiology and Pathophysiology

Fecal water content, fecal flow, motility, and urge contribute to the maintenance of bowel movements. When the fecal water content is decreased, fecal flow is obstructed, an alteration in motility occurs, or altered fecal urge occurs, constipation results.

Clinical Manifestations

Subjective

Onset, duration, associated symptoms. Passage of hard and/or pelletlike stool, tenesmus, abdominal pain (be alert to other causes though), distention, gas/bloating, decrease in frequency of stools, but if consistency of stool is soft, then frequency of stool is not such a problem. Warning signs with constipation are blood in stool, nausea and vomiting, moderate to severe abdominal pain.

Objective

Abdominal examination: Soft abdomen; bowel sounds present; nontender (stool in the bowel may produce some mild discomfort); no rebound tenderness, guarding, or rigidity; no organomegaly.

Rectal examination (assess sphincter tone, presence of stool in the rectal vault or impaction, test stool for occult blood): Without masses, but may have hard, pellet-like stool; normal anal canal/verge; stool negative for occult blood (Hemoccult test negative).

 CP 7–2 Clinical Pearl: Remember the cause may be functional, organic, or idiopathic, or medication-related. Examination should be comprehensive.

Differential Diagnosis

Encopresis (stool incontinence after age 4).

The following are pathophysiologic considerations with constipation: neuromuscular (peripheral neuropathy [clients with diabetes], Parkinson's disease, cerebrovascular accident, scleroderma, amyloidosis, multiple sclerosis, spinal cord injury, Hirschsprung's disease).

Endocrine (hyperthyroidism, diabetes).

Metabolic (dehydration, hypercalcemia, hypokalemia).

Structural (anal fissure, hemorrhoids, colorectal cancer, diverticular disease, rectal prolapse, rectocele, intussusception, strictures from inflammatory bowel disease (IBD), ischemia, radiation therapy).

Diagnostic Tests

Stool for occult blood (Hemoccult)

Flexible sigmoidoscopy (for recent onset, unless warning signs [Hemoccult test positive, bleeding per rectum, change in bowel habits] present, then consider barium study or colonoscopy)

Plain films (to determine retention, obstruction, megacolon, volvulus, lesions; consider radiopaque marker study for transit time)

Management/Treatment

Uncomplicated, simple constipation with no organic cause, or idiopathic constipation, is a challenging medical condition; clients need continued encouragement to improve on simple lifestyle habits first (diet, fluids, exercise). Pharmaceutical agents are added when cause is certain and therapy with dietary fiber and fiber supplements fails.

Pharmacologic Management

Fiber supplement: Psyllium; begin with 1 tablespoon daily and increase fluid intake.

Osmotic agents: Miralax, 1 tablespoon BID; may increase or decrease dosage.

Other: Tap-water enemas and laxatives (use sparingly as they create dependency and can cause melanosis coli).

Senna concentrate (Senekot) may be substituted for or used alternately with stool softeners.

Nonpharmacologic Management

Diet (increase dietary fiber to 30 g/day; increase fluids, especially water and fruit juices, and not milk).

Exercise.

Toilet training: Advise client on responding to urge to defecate and making time to defecate each day.

For children, sit on toilet at least BID for 10 minutes, preferably on waking and after meals.

Client Education

Increase fluids, at least eight 8-oz glasses of water daily or 2–3 L/day or 30% increase above current level.

Exercise aerobically at least three times per week for 30 minutes each.

Follow-up

6–8 weeks after therapy or sooner if condition worsens or if there is no response to treatment, then as indicated

Referral

Consult with physician for constipation etiology that is unclear or secondary to myogenic, neurogenic, endocrine, metabolic, or structural cause.

Consult with physician for idiopathic constipation

DIARRHEA

SIGNAL SYMPTOMS ▶ loose stools and blood/mucous, abdominal pain

SIGNAL SYMPTOMS ▶ frequent stools, abdominal pain, weight loss, tenesmus, flatus

ICD-9 Codes	787.91	Acute diarrhea
	558.9	Chronic diarrhea

Normal stool volume per day is 100–180 g and contains 60%–80% water. Diarrhea is defined as more than 150–300 g/day of stool (Goroll, 2000, pg 408), which creates an increase in frequency, weight, and water (70%–90%). Acute diarrhea is diarrhea of less than 3 weeks' duration; chronic diarrhea is diarrhea greater than 3 weeks' duration.

Epidemiology

20% of acute care cases for children <2 years old
Cause of 8 per 1000 hospitalizations for children <1 year old
Acute diarrhea responsible for 500 deaths per year in United States for children 1–4 years old

Etiology

Acute diarrhea: Usually infectious (most common cause of acute diarrhea), medication-induced, and self-limiting
Chronic diarrhea: IBD, IBS, malabsorption (lactose intolerance, celiac sprue), lymphocytic colitis, medications, and systemic or infectious causes

Physiology and Pathophysiology

Diarrhea may be classified in three categories: increased motility, osmotic, and/or secretory:

Increased motility diarrhea is caused by reduced stool presence in the intestinal mucosa and increased transit time.

Osmotic diarrhea is caused by nonabsorbable osmotic agents such as carbohydrate malabsorption (most common cause), magnesium-containing laxatives and antacids, and cathartic solutions. This type of diarrhea usually subsides with fasting.

Secretory diarrhea is caused by an infectious process, inflammation, hormones, malabsorption, or stimulant laxatives. It has a greater stool volume, and does not subside with a 24-hour fast, except with fatty acid malabsorption. The client is at risk for electrolyte imbalance.

Clinical Manifestations

When differentiating the type of diarrhea determine if source is large or small bowel. In large-bowel diarrhea, the stools are very frequent (more than eight per day), loose, and in small amounts. In small bowel diarrhea the stools are less frequent (four to six per day), in larger amounts, and associated with postprandial, periumbilical, or RLQ quadrant pain. History should include questions about recent travel, new medications or recent antibiotic use, and other family members with diarrhea.

Subjective
See Table 7–1.

Objective
See Table 7–1.

Table 7–1 Clinical Manifestations of Diarrhea: Clues to Diagnosis

Clinical Manifestations	Clues	Possible Diagnoses
History	Family history of diarrhea	IBD, congenital absorption defect, celiac sprue
	Recent use of antibiotics	*Clostridium difficile* colitis
	Recent travel to mountainous area	*Giardia* infestation
	Employment in day-care center	*Shigella* species, *Giardial lamblia*, or *Cryptosporidum* infection
Subjective	Diarrhea alternating with constipation	IBS, diabetic autonomic neuropathy, intermittent bowel obstruction, OTC use of laxatives/antidiarrheals
	Diarrhea with excessive flatus	Carbohydrate malabsorption
	Diarrhea: large volume	Small bowel or proximal colon disease
	Diarrhea: small volume	Distal colon or rectal disease
	Stools: bloody	Inflammatory, infectious, or neoplasic conditions
	Stools: oily or greasy-looking	Fat malabsorption (pancreatic insufficiency)
	Fever	IBD, lymphohoma, Whipple's disease, hyperthryoidism, infectious diseases
	Weight loss	IBD, malabsorption, malignancy
	Flushing	Hyperthyroidism, carcinoid syndrome, pheochromocytoma, pancreatic cholera, systemic mastocytosis
Objective	Postural hypotension	Diabetic diarrhea, Addison's disease
	Cutaneous erythema	Glucagonoma syndrome, systemic mastocytosis
	Cutaneous hyperpigmentation	Whipple's disease, sprue, Addison's disease, systemic mastocytosis
	Dermatitis herpetiformis	Celiac sprue
	Pyoderma gangrenosum	IBD
	Oral ulcers	IBD, celiac sprue
	Neuropathy	Diabetes, amyloidosis
	Lymphadenopathy	Small bowel lmphoma. Whipple's disease, AIDS, metastatic cancer
	Arthritis	IBD, Whipple's disease, enteritis due infection with *Salmonella*, *Shigella*, *Yersinia*, and *Campylobacter* species, collagen vascular disease, collagenous colitis, gonococcal proctitis
	Atheroscelerosis	Mesenteric ischemia, ischemic colitis

Adapted from: P.F. Enstrom, Diagnosis and Management of Bowel Diseases, 1999, p. 21–22.

Differential Diagnosis

Acute diarrhea:
 Medications: Laxatives, antacids, colchicine, neomycin
 Foods: Lactose, dietetic foods
 Infections: Usually viral
Chronic diarrhea:
 Intestinal infection (parasitosis, bacterial, mycobacterial, fungal)
Intestinal inflammation (ulcerative colitis, Crohn's disease, sprue, collag-
  enous colitis, radiation enteritis):
  Malabsorption (generalized, carbohydrate, bile acid)
  Secretory (hormone-secreting tumor, colorectal villous tumor, idiopathic)
  Altered motility (dumping syndrome, diabetes, hyperthyroidism, IBS)
  Other (drugs, factitious, fecal impaction)

Diagnostic Tests

Stool (microscopic examination for white cells, red cells; culture for enteric
  pathogens [ova and parasites, fat, meat fibers], pH, sodium, potassium);
  24–72 hr stool collection may be indicated for chronic diarrhea).
CBC and serum chemistries (may be indicated for chronic diarrhea)
Flexible sigmoidoscopy with biopsy (may be indicated for acute diarrhea
  that continues despite treatment or for chronic diarrhea).
Small bowel x-ray examination, barium enema examination, or
  abdominal ultrasonography may be indicated, depending on the cause.

Management/Treatment

The client's symptoms should be treated as well as the underlying cause. For
management of specific causes, see the specific condition. If the diarrhea is
caused by medication use, stop the offending agent.

Pharmacologic Management

INFECTIOUS DIARRHEA NEEDING ANTIBIOTICS

Escherichia coli infection: Ciprofloxacin (Cipro) 500 mg BID for 5days.
  Infants and children: TMP/SMX, 8 mg TMP/kg/day in two divided doses
  for 7–10 days
Shigella infection: TMP/SMX BID for 3 days
  Infants and children: TMP/SMX, 8 mg TMP/kg/day in two divided doses
  for 5 days
Salmonella infection (severe cases only): TMP/SMX BID for 7 days
  Infants and children: Indicated for children <1 year old who are at risk
  for bacteremia and patients who are immunosuppressed, have cardiac
  or valvular disease, lymphoproliferative diseases, sickle cell disease of
  hemolytic anemias—Use amoxicillin, 40 mg/kg/day in three divided
  doses for 7–10 days or TMP/SMX, 8 mg TMP/kg/day in four divided
  doses for 7–10 days
Campylobacter infection: Erythromycin, 500 mg BID for 5 days; cipro-
  floxin (Cipro), 500 mg BID for 5 days

Infants and children: Erythromycin, 40 mg/kg/day in three divided doses

Giardiasis infection: Metronidazole (Flagyl), 250 mg QID for 7days

Nonpharmacologic Management

Eat BRATS (bananas, rice, applesauce, toast, saltines) diet.

Eat lactose-free diet.

Stop sugar-free foods (those that contain sorbitol, mannitol).

Reduce fruit juices and fluids if patient consumes more than 2 L/day.

Decrease carbohydrates, "roughage" (high-fiber foods).

In acute diarrhea in infants and children, restore hydration with oral electrolyte maintenance solution (Pedialyte), not fruit juices, Kool-aid, or soda.

In chronic diarrhea in toddlers, decrease excessive intake of fruit juices and milk and increase fiber intake.

Rehydration plan (treatment for dehydration)

Mild—40–50 ml/kg of oral rehydration solution (ORS) over 4 hours (10 ml/kg/hr)

Moderate—60–100 ml/kg of ORS over 4–6 hours (20 ml/kg/hr)

Maintenance plan

Total volume 0–10 kg = 100 ml/kg/24 hr

10–20 kg = 1000 ml + 50 ml/kg for each kg over 10 kg/24 hr

>20 kg = 1500 ml + 20 ml/kg for each kg over 20 kg/24 hr

Replacement of fluids lost (if continued heavy losses)

10 ml/kg, or 4–8 oz of ORS for each diarrheal stool (1–1.5 times the amount of the stool)

Client Education

Practice good hygiene

Stay hydrated

Follow-up

As indicated; for acute, follow-up if diarrhea persists beyond 3 weeks.

Referral

Refer to gastroenterologist for chronic diarrhea; client will need flexible sigmoidoscopy or colonoscopy for biopsy.

DIVERTICULITIS

SIGNAL SYMPTOMS ▶ LLQ pain, intermittent cramping

ICD-9 Code	562.11	Diverticulitis

Diverticulitis is an inflammation of the diverticulum as a result of impaction of a fecalith.

Epidemiology

Common after age 50 years

Most common in Western cultures

Etiology

Probably low-fiber diet, genetics, constipation, seedy fruits and vegetables becoming stuck in diverticuli

Physiology and Pathophysiology

In the normal passage of stool through the colonic lumen, there is increased luminal pressure. Peristaltic waves occurring several times per day propel the stool toward the rectum. The muscularis of the intestines is composed of circular and longitudinal fibers.

Diverticulosis occurs as the increased luminal pressure through the narrowed sigmoid colon herniate weakened muscularis fibers. The existence of scattered, multiple diverticula is associated with colonic wall thickening and hypertrophy. Diverticulitis results from the impaction of diverticulum with a fecalith. Perforation, abscesses, and bleeding are complications of diverticulitis. Fistulization can occur with abscesses that erode through surrounding viscera. The most common is to the bladder. Peritonitis occurs with perforation.

Clinical Manifestations

Subjective

Recurrent history of diverticulitis
LLQ pain
Change in bowel habits; constipation commonly seen
Fever
Nausea (but no vomiting)
Passage of rectal blood and mucus

Objective

LLQ tenderness with possible palpable mass.
Rectal examination may reveal a tender mass, frank bleeding, and positive results on Hemoccult test.

Differential Diagnosis

Intestinal ischemia (sharp, excruciating pain)
Bowel obstruction (abdominal distention, vomiting, increased bowel sounds, RLQ or LLQ pain)
Intestinal arteriovenous malformation
IBD (LLQ pain, diarrhea with mucus, pain relieved with defecation)
Meckel's diverticulitis (painless rectal bleeding, anemia, lower abdominal pain)
Carcinoma, volvulus (twisting of bowel that produces intestinal obstruction)
Appendicitis (see p 317)

Diagnostic Tests

CBC with differential (leukocytosis will be present)
Urinalysis (risk of infection, kidney problems)

CT scan (shows inflamed pericolic fat, presence of diverticula, colonic wall thickening)

Abdominal ultrasound (shows colonic wall thickening, presence of diverticula)

Contrast enema (barium or gastrograffin) (shows diverticula, segmental sigmoid narrowing)

Colonoscopy/sigmoidoscopy (shows diverticula and peridiverticular inflammation or pus; there may also be resistance to passage of the scope because of stricturing or spasm)

Management/Treatment

Pharmacologic Management

Uncomplicated diverticulitis: Metronidazole (Flagyl), 250–500 mg QID for 10 days, with ciprofloxacin (Cipro), 500 mg BID for 10 days; or amoxicillin/clavulanate, 875/125 mg BID for 10 days

Nonpharmacologic Management

Diet: Clear liquids for several days

Client Education

Eat high-fiber diet

Use a bulking agent (psyllium)

Avoid constipation

Follow-up

As indicated if no resolution of symptoms or worsening of symptoms

Referral

Refer to gastroenterologist if client has complications of perforation, fistulas, peritonitis, or bleeding.

GASTROENTERITIS

SIGNAL SYMPTOMS ► crampy, diffuse abdominal pain relieved by vomiting or defecation

ICD-9 Code	558.9	Gastroenteritis

Gastroenteritis is the inflammation of the small bowel lining, and although gastroenteritis may suggest gastric inflammation, the gastric mucosa remains unchanged.

Epidemiology

30%–40% of cases of infectious diarrhea are gastroenteritis.

Gastroenteritis is the second most common cause for presentation to the health-care provider.

Etiology

Most common: Norwalk virus (40% group-related diarrhea, winter months, oral/fecal route) and rotavirus (50% of hospitalized clients, infants, and young children [antibody develops by 3 years of age]); others include astroviruses and enteric adenoviruses.

Physiology and Pathophysiology

The villus tip cells are destroyed when infected with the virus. Alterations in the small bowel's ability to absorb and digest results in malabsorption and secretion.

Clinical Manifestations

Subjective

Abdominal pain/cramping
Diarrhea
Nausea and vomiting
Weight loss, anorexia
Hematemesis
Diaphoresis
Myalgias, arthralgias
Fever, chills

Objective

Abdominal tenderness (no guarding)
Hyperactive bowel sounds

Differential Diagnosis

Viral or bacterial gastroenteritis (vomiting, watery diarrhea, bilious vomitus)
Food poisoning (vomiting, abdominal pain, diarrhea)
Parasitic infestation (parasite-dependent, possibly diarrhea, bloating, distention, flatulence)
Intussusception (episodic cyclic pain with vomiting/calm periods, mass in the RUQ, legs drawn up at time of pain, "currant jelly" stool later)
Appendicitis (see p 317)

Diagnostic Tests

Stool for O&P, enteric pathogens, culture, *Clostridium difficile*
CBC and blood chemistry (dehydration will cause abnormal results—normal/elevated red cells, white cells, hemoglobin and hematocrit, blood urea nitrogen, creatinine—in the young and elderly)
ESR (risk of irritable bowel)

Management/Treatment

Dehydration most common. Hospitalize infants and young children and the elderly
Usually very self-limiting illness; only supportive care necessary
See rehydration plan (p 328)

Pharmacologic Management

Most cases are viral, so only supportive care if necessary.
Promethazine HCl (Phenergan), 25–50 mg PO Q4–6H, may be helpful for nausea and vomiting.

For infants and children, promethazine HCl, 0.5 to 1 mg/kg per dose PR
Q6H, may be helpful for nausea and vomiting.

If infectious diarrhea is bacterial, treat as indicated in section on "Diarrhea."

Nonpharmacologic Management
Drink only clear liquids
Eat BRATS diet
Stay hydrated

Client Education
Instruct about good hygiene
Encourage fluids and rest
Instruct to avoid antidiarrheals

Follow-up
As indicated

Referral
Hospitalization if dehydration occurs

GASTROINTESTINAL CANCERS

SIGNAL SYMPTOMS ▶ gastric cancer, esophageal cancer, colon cancer

ICD-9 Codes	151.9	Gastric cancer
	150.9	Esophageal cancer
	153.9	Colon cancer

Gastric, esophageal, and colon cancers may arise as squamous-cell carcinomas
and adenocarcinomas.

Epidemiology

Gastric cancer: Third most common GI cancer in the United States; second
most common worldwide. It has a greater incidence in men than in
women (2:1). It usually occurs in people over 50 years of age, and has a
60% incidence over the age of 65.

Esophageal cancer: Incidence is greater in men than in women (3:1).

Colorectal cancer: Second leading cause of death in the United States;
lifetime risk of 6%; increased risk with each decade lived after age 50.

Etiology

Gastric cancer: Linked to salted foods, smoked fish, nitrosamines,
benzopyrene, atrophic gastritis, *Helicobacter pylori* infection

Esophageal cancer: Squamous-cell carcinoma from smoking, alcohol;
adenocarcinoma linked to Barrett's esophagus from gastroesophageal
reflux disease (GERD)

Colorectal cancer: Risk factors include first-degree relatives with colorectal
cancer; history of adenomatous polyps, IBD; familial adenomatous
polyposis; high-meat diet; low-fiber diet; constipation; and possibly
uterine, breast, and ovarian cancer

Physiology and Pathophysiology

Esophageal squamous-cell carcinoma occurs with epithelial dysplasia. In squamous-cell dysplasia the basal zone shows increased mitotic activity, increased nuclear size, and hyperchromatism, with resulting fungating, ulcerating, and infiltrative cell patterning (Stein, 1998, p 2024). Esophageal adenocarcinoma is a result of intestinal metaplasia in which the columnar epithelium replaces the squamous epithelial cells that normally line the esophagus.

In colorectal adenocarcinoma the basal cells of the bowel crypts are epithelial stem cells, which when stimulated overgrow the crypt to give rise to aberrant crypts and ultimately adenomatous polyps (Engstrom & Goosenberg, 1999, p 208). Two types of polyps are hyperplastic (always benign) and adenomatous. Adenomas are staged, as follows: tubular, mixed tubovillous, and villous adenomatous (most likely to become adenocarcinoma). As the size of the polyp increases, the risk of staging increases in severity.

Clinical Manifestations

See Table 7–2.

Table 7–2   Clinical Manifestations: Gastrointestinal Cancers

Clinical Manifestations	Gastric Cancer	Esophageal Cancer	Colorectal Cancer
Subjective	Weight loss Dysphagia Epigastrum, sub-sternal, or back pain Nausea/vomiting Hematemesis Melena Weight loss Frank GI Bleed	Dysphagia (primary complaint) Weight loss Reflux Nausea/vomiting Hematemesis Substernal pain that radiates to the back, cervical adenopathy Nausea/vomiting	Rectal bleeding, Hematochezia Melena Abdominal pain Weight loss Nausea/vomiting Change in bowel habits (with constipation or diarrhea) Change in caliber size of stool ("pencil-like' stool suggests a family history of colon cancer or history of polyps
Objective	Early Stage Normal exam although client may have microcytic-anemia or mega-blastic anemia Later Stages Weight loss apparent Anorexia Anemia Palpable abdominal mass Jaundice (with liver metastasis) Ascites Stool positive for blood (Hemoccult positive) Lymphadenopathy	Hyperkeratotic palms and soles Cervical-lymph-node enlargement	Palpable rectal mass Stool positive for blood (Hemoccult positive) Anemia Weight loss apparent

Diagnostic Tests

A high index of suspicion for gastrointestinal cancer should lead to an immediate consultation with and referral to a gastroenterologist.

Diagnostic Tests

Gastric cancer (upper GI swallow study; when achalasia or obstructing lesion is evident, refer for endoscopy and biopsy [Goroll, 2000, p 392])

Esophageal cancer (esophagography; when stenosis or intrinsic narrowing is evident, refer for endoscopy and biopsy [Goroll, 2000, p 392])

Colorectal cancer (refer for flexible sigmoidoscopy or colonoscopy)

Management/Treatment

Refer for management by surgical/oncology team

Referral

Refer to surgeon and oncologist

GASTROESOPHAGEAL REFLUX DISEASE

SIGNAL SYMPTOMS ▶ heartburn, regurgitation, dysphagia, waterbrash

| ICD-9 Code | 530.81 | Gastroesophageal reflux disease |

Gastroesophageal reflux disease (GERD) is the backward movement of gastric contents into the esophagus (Porth, 1998, p 722).

Epidemiology

60 million Americans periodically experience symptoms of GERD, 17.5 million daily.

A common occurrence in infants; resolves by age 12 months.

Etiology

Weak or incompetent lower esophageal sphincter (LES)

Impaired peristalsis

Abnormality in swallowing saliva (helps with acid neutrality)

Hiatal hernia

Certain foods, substances, hormones, or medications

Pregnancy

Obesity

Physiology and Pathophysiology

Three normal defenses prevent reflux from occurring: LES, esophageal clearance, and gastric emptying. When any of these defenses fails, reflux may occur. The resting LES pressure is mainly responsible for preventing reflux of gastric contents from reaching the esophageal mucosa. When resting LES pressure decreases, reflux of acid occurs.

Factors that contribute to reflux include transient LES relaxation, a low or hypotensive LES, and anatomic disruption of the sphincter, as with hiatal hernia. Individuals with reflux clear acid more slowly from the esophagus (Goroll, 2000, p 587).

Hydrochloric acid, produced by parietal cells found in the gastric mucosa, have receptors for acetylcholine, gastrin, and histamine. Occupation of acetylcholine and/or gastrin receptors release stored calcium, while histamine receptor occupation increases the level of cyclic adenosine monophosphate (cAMP). cAMP releases into the parietal cell. The combined effect of increased calcium and cAMP activates the hydrogen–potassium adenosine triphosphatase (H^+/K^+-ATPase) system or proton pump to produce hydrogen ions for the production of hydrochloric acid (Ault & Schmidt, 1998, pp 81–82).

Clinical Manifestations

The clinical manifestations listed below are for adults. For clinical manifestations for infants and children, see Age-Related Considerations 7–1.

Subjective

History of smoking

Diet including alcohol, caffeine, chocolate, peppermint, and fatty meals

Use of oral contraceptives or hormone-replacement therapy, β-adrenergic agents, calcium-channel blockers, diazepam, and barbiturates (all decrease LES tone, promoting reflux)

History of taking antacids throughout the day (>50 tablets week indicate significant reflux; history of taking antacids that suppress symptoms is the number one clue to diagnosis)

Heartburn 30–60 minutes after eating (worsens with bending over or at night)

Substernal burning that radiates to throat, back. or shoulder (high index of suspicion—cardiac cause until proven otherwise)

Regurgitation

Age-Related Considerations: Infants and Children with GERD

Subjective:

Excessive crying and irritability
Refusal to eat or feed
Recurring spitting up and/or vomiting
Coughing/choking,
Eructation
Sleep disturbances
Wheeze, stridor

Objective:

Abdominal and/or substernal pain
Chronic cough or noctural cough (may have asthma related to reflux)
Wheeze
Dyspnea
Assess for "hard skin" appearance; scleroderma affects the motility of the esophagus and must be considered, so evaluate for sclerodactyly, calcinosis, telangietctasia,
Palpate abdomen for masses
Perform rectal exam; test stool for occult blood (Hemoccult)

Waterbrash

Odynophagia (consider esophagitis)

Dysphagia (consider esophagitis)

Dyspeptic symptoms (early satiety, postprandial fullness, nausea and vomiting—symptoms related to gastroparesis)

Pulmonary symptoms (Wheezing, coughing, dyspnea; onset of asthma in the second to fifth decade of life with no history of childhood asthma or smoking may suggest reflux disease. Some clients with asthma respond to GERD therapy with a reduction in asthma symptoms.)

Ear, nose, and throat symptoms (ENT) (hoarseness, sore throat, globus, choking)

Objective

Examination usually unremarkable, although ENT or respiratory examination may have abnormalities with significant GERD.

Throat: Erythematous oropharynx, no exudate or lesions.

Mouth: Erythema, gingival inflammation from severe waterbrash.

Lungs: Expiratory wheeze, with cough, respiratory effort—dyspneic asthma induced from severe reflux of acid into the trachea and bronchi.

Differential Diagnosis

Esophagitis, Barrett's esophagus, esophageal spasm, esophageal dysmotility (scleroderma), esophageal cancer (Heartburn more than one time per week carries an eightfold increase in risk for esophageal adenocarcinoma [Lagergren, 1999.)

Acute coronary syndrome (Angina, dyspnea—cardiac cause is of high suspicion in clients with cardiac history, increased age, history of coronary artery disease, and abnormal cardiac examination.)

Rumination syndrome (habitual regurgitation of small amounts of undigested food)

Cholecystitis (RUQ pain, radiating to right infrascapular and/or midepigastric, nausea and vomiting)

Musculoskeletal inflammation of sternum (pain on palpation of sternum, movement)

Peptic ulcer disease (see p 352)

Diabetic gastroparesis (nausea, vomiting, history of diabetes)

Infections such as *Candida albicans,* cytomegalovirus, human papillomavirus (HPV)

Diagnostic Tests

Approach by symptoms

Endoscopy (indicated for long-standing history of heartburn)

24-hour pH monitoring (to help diagnose reflux)

Upper GI series and/or endoscopy (indicated if client has warning signs of significant pathology (see "Referral" p 338)

Management/Treatment

Primary goal is to stop symptoms.

Pharmacologic Management
See Table 7–3.

Nonpharmacologic Management
See Table 7–3.

Table 7–3   Management: GERD

Steps	Nonpharmacologic Management	Pharmacologic Management
Step 1	Diet Avoid large, high-fat meals, spicy and acidic foods, caffeine, and chocolate; limit alcohol intake Avoid eating 2–3 hours before bedtime Eat small, frequent low-fat meals For infants and children, thicken feedings by adding 1 tablespoon of rice cereal per ounce of formula Lifestyle management Stop smoking (if applicable) Lose weight (if applicable) Elevate head of bed 4–6 inches Avoid lying down after eating; for infants and children, keep in upright position during and at least 20 minutes after feeding Avoid tight-fitting clothing	Antacids OR over-the-counter histamine 2 (H2) blocker BID
Step 2	As above	-Continue step 1 medications -Start first line therapy with H2 blocker (cimetidine 400–800 mg BID [12 weeks maximum] or ranitidine 150 mg BID- TID or famotidine 20–40 mg BID or nizatidine 150 mg BID or 300 mg HS [12 weeks maximum]) OR prokinetic agent (metoclopramide 10–15mg QID or 20 mg prn [12 weeks maximum]) OR sucralfate 1g QID
Step 3	As above	-Continue Step 1 medications -Try high-dose H2 blocker (cimetidine 800mg TID or famotidine 160 mg q6hr maximum) OR H2 blocker with prokinetic agent OR proton pump inhibitor (PPI) (omeprazole 20mg QD [4–8 weeks maximum] or lansoprazole 15–30mg QD [8 week maximum])
Step 4	As above Consider surgery—Nissen fundoplication (stitching of the stomach around the distal esophagus preventing reflux)	-Continue Step 1 medications

Client Education

Educate about disease process

Incline head of bed 30–40 degrees

Avoid smoking

Instruct to cut down on alcohol, chocolate, caffeine, tomato, garlic, onion, and peppermint

Do not eat 3 hours before bedtime

If appropriate, prescribe weight loss

Instruct client to stop smoking

Follow-up

6–8 weeks after initiation of medications, or sooner if symptoms worsen or do not begin to resolve; then yearly if symptoms are under control

Referral

Refer to gastroenterologist if disorder does not respond to treatment with proton-pump inhibitor (PPI) or if there are warning signs such as dysphagia, odynophagia, nausea and vomiting, weight loss, early satiety, severe pulmonary symptoms, Hemoccult-positive stools, anemia, abnormal examination, >5-year history of heartburn or if the client is a candidate for surgery.

HEMORRHOIDS

ICD-9 Code	544.0	Hemorrhoids

Hemorrhoids are swellings of the venous hemorrhoidal plexus (inferior, middle, or superior hemorrhoidal veins); they may be classified as internal or external.

Epidemiology

5% of the U.S. population experiences hemorrhoids; the incidence increases with age.

Etiology

Debate continues on the cause of hemorrhoids. Some causes may include pregnancy, obesity, portal hypertension, excessive exercise, low-fiber diet, excessive straining, poor bowel hygiene, prolonged standing, and the lack of venous valves of the hemorrhoidal plexus.

Physiology and Pathophysiology

Internal hemorrhoids originate above the dentate line, are insensate, and are covered with mucosa.

Stage 1: Bleeding, pain, no prolapse

Stage 2: Bleeding, prolapse with defecation but spontaneously reducible

Stage 3: Bleeding, prolapse, and manually reducible

Stage 4: Bleeding, prolapse, irreducible

External hemorrhoids originate below the dentate line, are sensate, and are covered with epithelium.

Clinical Manifestations

Subjective

External: Bleeding (BRB) on toilet paper, stool surface, or toilet water; pain; pruritus

Internal: Bleeding (BRB) on toilet paper, toilet water, or stool surface; painless; fecal incontinence; possible prolapse

Objective

Do a rectal examination to test for occult blood; assess for rectal mass or sphincter tone

Perform anoscopy for visual inspection of hemorrhoid or other causes (anal fissure, abscess, thrombosed hemorrhoid)

Rectal bleeding is a warning sign

Differential Diagnosis

Anal fissure (see p 315)

Anorectal abscess (pain, possible discharge caused by an infected anal gland tract along various places, resulting in focal abscess)

Anorectal fistula (communication between epithelialized viscera, periodic discharge occasionally filled with blood)

Pilonidal disease (hair-containing cyst or sinus located in the midline over the coccyx or lower sacrum; when advanced has a palpable sinus tract—first diagnosed at ages 15–30, though congenital)

Rectocele (posterior protrusion through the vaginal wall composed of the rectum)

Thrombosed hemorrhoid (hemorrhoid containing clotted blood that becomes painful, swollen, shiny, and blue and itches and bleeds on defecation)

Pruritus ani (rectal itching; symptom of underlying cause such as hemorrhoids, fissure, condylomata)

Colorectal neoplasm or adenoma (painless, firm nodule—as grows becomes irregularly shaped [cauliflower] and is fixed and stone hard)

Diagnostic Tests

Stool for occult blood

CBC (with rectal bleeding to rule out anemia)

ESR (with diarrhea)

Flexible sigmoidoscopy, barium study, or colonoscopy (for rectal bleeding or Hemoccult-positive stool to rule out more significant pathology)

Management/Treatment

Pharmacologic Management

Analgesic hydrocortisone suppository for 7–14 days (following sitz bath)

Stool softener (e.g., Colace), as indicated

Mineral oil 2 tablespoons BID

Nonpharmacologic Management

Use sitz bath (lukewarm) for 15–20 min twice a day

Eat a high-fiber diet; keep stools soft

Avoid straining and prolonged sitting on toilet

Client Education

Keep stool soft, regular

Avoid straining

Avoid heavy lifting

Advise about importance of sitz bath in helping to shrink hemorrhoids

Follow-up

2–4 weeks, or sooner if there is increased pain or bleeding.

Referral

Refer to general surgeon if client has persistent hemorrhoidal bleeding or chronic prolapsing hemorrhoids for possible hemorrhoidal rubber band ligation, hemorrhoidectomy, sclerotherapy, infrared coagulation.

HERNIAS

ICD-9 Code	553.9	Hernia

Hernias are protrusions of the abdominal viscera through an abnormal opening in the muscle wall.

Epidemiology

Indirect inguinal—Most common; 60% of all hernias. More common in infants <1 year old and in males 16–20 years old

Direct inguinal—Less common; occurs most often in men >40; rare in women

Femoral—Least common; 4% of all hernias; more common in women

Umbilical—Very common in newborns and infants up to 1 year

Etiology

Congenital or acquired (pregnancy, obesity, chronic cough, ascites, trauma, straining, muscle atrophy, heavy lifting, asthma, bronchial disease, frequent stooping)

Physiology and Pathophysiology

A hernia is a defect in the normal musculofascial continuity of the abdominal wall that permits the egress of structures that do not normally pass through the parietes (Goroll, 1995, p 379). May occur as reducible (structure returns to abdominal cavity), irreducible or incarcerated (structure does not return to abdominal cavity), or strangulated (interrupted blood flow to structure that has herniated.)

Indirect inguinal hernia: Intestine passes through the internal inguinal ring to the inguinal canal or into the scrotum (scrotal hernia).

Direct inguinal hernia: Intestinal herniation through external inguinal ring; reducible when lying down.

Femoral hernia: Intestinal protrusion through femoral ring.

Umbilical hernia: A protrusion of the omentum or intestine through a weakness or incomplete closure in the umbilical ring (Jarvis, 2000, p 779)

Clinical Manifestations

Indirect Inguinal Hernia

Subjective: Pain with straining, feels bulging in groin area or scrotal pain and swelling (scrotal hernia)

Objective: Insert finger into inguinal canal if possible to palpate for bulge

Direct Inguinal Hernia

Subjective: Inguinal swelling without pain

Objective: Insert finger through inguinal canal and have client bear down; palpate for bulging

Femoral Hernia

Subjective: Severe pain

Objective: Palpable inguinal mass. These hernias may become strangulated. If there is severe pain, immediate refer to surgeon.

Umbilical Hernia

Subjective: Periumbilical pain, even severe; seen with infant crying.

Objective: With the client lying supine, have the client bear down; palpate for mass at umbilicus; can also palpate the umbilical ring to measure size.

Differential Diagnosis

Inguinal adenopathy (enlarged, palpable inguinal lymph nodes)

Abdominal lesion

Incarcerated hernia (hernia that cannot be reduced)

Strangulated hernia (blood supply of incarcerated contents is interrupted; gangrene may quickly ensue)

Diagnostic Tests

Abdominal ultrasonography

Abdominal computed tomographic (CT) scan

Management/Treatment

Refer to surgeon

Analgesics/narcotics for pain management

Client Education

Explain disease process

Give guidance in anticipation of surgery

Give infection precautions

Instruct about wound management

Follow-up

As indicated

Referral
Refer to general surgeon

HIATAL HERNIA AND ESOPHAGITIS

SIGNAL SYMPTOMS heartburn, regurgitation, dysphagia

ICD-9 Code	553.3	Hiatal hernia and esophagitis

Hiatal hernia is the protrusion of viscera through the diaphragm, creating a gastric pouch of the mediastinum. Esophagitis is synonymous with GERD and is a result of reflux disease, which causes inflammation of the esophagus.

Epidemiology

90% are sliding hiatal hernias. Most clients with Barrett's esophagus have hiatal hernias of approximately 3.52 cm (Cameron, 1999).

Etiology

GERD
Esophageal dysmotility
Weakening or incompetent LES
Pregnancy
Obesity
Medications (such as alendronate, aspirin, nonsteroidal antiinflammatory drugs [NSAIDs], doxycycline)
Infections (such as clients with acquired immunodeficiency syndrome, candidiasis, cytomegalovirus, HPV)

Physiology and Pathophysiology

Squamous basal cells, in acute phase, become edematous and necrotic beginning distally in the esophagus and progressing to erosions, hyperplasia, intestinal metaplagia, and then scarring. Complications of this process include bleeding, strictures, pulmonary symptoms, Barrett's esophagus, adenocarcinoma, and esophageal ulcers.

Clinical Manifestations

Subjective
Heartburn
Odynophagia
Regurgitation
Dysphagia

Objective
Generally results of examination are normal unless complications have occurred.

Differential Diagnosis

Cardiac disease (chest pain, dyspnea, nausea, vomiting)
Peptic ulcer disease (see p 352)

Rumination syndrome

Zenker's diverticulum (circumscribed herniation of mucous membrane of pharynx as it joins esophagus)

Schatzki's ring (mucosal ring at gastroesophageal junction)

Neoplasm

Cervical web (thin, transverse membranes of epithelium)

Esophageal spasm (uncoordinated contractions of esophagus associated with dysphagia; sensation of food sticking retrosternally)

Diagnostic Tests

Esophagography with 12-mm tablet for dysphagia

Consider upper GI series

Immediate referral to gastroenterology for endoscopy and biopsy

Management/Treatment

Pharmacologic Management

H_2-Blockers:

Famotidine (Pepcid), 40 mg PO BID

Ranitidine (Zantac), 150 mg PO BID

Nizatidine (Axid), 150 mg PO BID

Proton-pump inhibitors:

Rabeprazole (Aciphex), 20 mg PO QD

Lansoprazole (Prevacid), 30 mg PO QD

Pantoprazole (Protonix), 40 mg PO QD

Omeprazole (Prilosec), 20 mg PO QD

Nonpharmacologic Management

Same as for GERD

Client Education

Same as for GERD

Follow-up

6–8 weeks after initiation of therapy or if symptoms worsen or do not begin to resolve

Referral

Refer to gastroenterologist for follow-up and symptom management, or if refractory to therapy

INFLAMMATORY BOWEL DISEASE (Ulcerative Colitis, Crohn's Disease)

SIGNAL SYMPTOMS ▶ bloody stools, tender colon, abdominal pain, RLQ pain, diarrhea, weight loss, anorexia

ICD-9 Codes	558.9	Inflammatory bowel disease
	556.9	Ulcerative colitis
	555.9	(Regional enteritis, unspecified site) Crohn's disease

Inflammatory bowel disease (IBD) encompasses two distinct diseases, ulcerative colitis and Crohn's disease. Ulcerative colitis affects the intestinal mucosa from the rectum proximally. Crohn's disease is more insidious, affecting the entire alimentary tract (mouth to anus); it often causes fistulas and abscesses. In Crohn's disease, the terminal ileum is usually involved.

Epidemiology

20–200/100,000 persons in the United States; most are in their late teens to the third decade of life; incidence increases around the sixth decade of life

Etiology

Etiology is unclear; however, infectious, allergic, environmental, genetic (having a first-degree relative who is affected increases risk 10-fold), psychological, and autoimmune factors have been implicated as possible causes.

Smokers are at increased risk for Crohn's disease, while ulcerative colitis may be triggered with smoking cessation.

Physiology and Pathophysiology

Crohn's disease typically spares the rectum, appears as patchy, asymmetrical lesions, and affects the perianal region. This is a mouth to anus disease, but significant disease emerges as ileocolitis (45%), ileitis (30%), and colitis (15%). Transmural inflammation and deep ulcerations give rise to a cobblestone appearance and development of fissures and fistulas. Extraintestinal manifestations include renal calculi (oxalate stones), cholelithiasis, oral aphthous ulcers, arthralgias, clubbing, uveitis, conjunctivitis, and erythema nodosum.

Ulcerative colitis is a mucosal and submucosal inflammation that begins in the rectum and extends proximally. Neutrophils assail the intestinal lining, forming crypt abscesses.

Clinical Manifestations

Crohn's Disease

Subjective: Diarrhea with or without blood (most common), abdominal pain, fever, nausea and vomiting, weight loss, perianal pain

Objective: Assess for extraintestinal manifestations (renal calculi [oxalate stones], cholelithiasis, oral aphthous ulcers, arthralgias, clubbing, uveitis, conjunctivitis, erythema nodosum).

Ulcerative Colitis

Subjective: Bloody diarrhea with tenesmus (most common), rectal bleeding, abdominal pain or cramping, nausea and vomiting, weight loss, fever

Objective: Assess for extraintestinal manifestations (oral aphthous ulcers, erythema nodosum, arthropathy, ankylosing spondylitis, primary sclerosing cholangitis, bile-duct disease)

Differential Diagnosis

Differential between Crohn's disease and ulcerative colitis
Infectious diarrhea (see p 342)
Antibiotic-associated diarrhea (associated with ingestion of antibiotics)
Pseudomembranous colitis (diarrheal disease in hospitalized patients who
    receive antibiotics that cause overgrowth of anaerobic spore-forming
    toxins that produce *Clostridium difficile*)
IBS (see p 346)
Celiac sprue (pale, foul-smelling stool that floats; abdominal distention)
Intestinal ischemia (abrupt, severe abdominal pain)
Neoplasm
Radiation colitis (diarrhea, bleeding and ulceration of mucosa of intestines
    related to radiation)
Diverticulitis (see p 328)
Lymphoma

Diagnostic Tests

ESR (elevated in Crohn's disease and ulcerative colitis)
Radiologic studies (Crohn's disease: Shows transmural ulceration,
    thickened mucosa, cobblestoning, fistulae, strictures, and obstruction
    along GI tract. Ulcerative colitis: Shows narrow, lead-pipe appearance,
    superficial ulcerations, strictures, and absence of haustral markings in
    colon and rectum.)
Endoscopy (Crohn's disease: Shows skip lesions, aphthous ulcers,
    cobblestoning, and friable tissue. Ulcerative colitis: Shows rectal
    involvement, pseudopolyps, and friable tissue.)

Management/Treatment

Pharmacologic Management

CROHN'S DISEASE

5-Aminosalicylic acid: First-line agents; used to maintain remission
    Oral (mesalamine)
    Topical (suppositories, enema): For distal disease
Sulfasalazine: First-line agent
Antibiotics (metronidazole, ciprofloxacin): Useful in inducing remission
Corticosteroids
    Oral (prednisone, budesonide): For disease not responsive to first-line
        agents; low doses used to maintain remission
    Topical (hydrocortisone suppositiories, Anucort HC, Anuprep HC): For
        distal disease
    IV (methylprednisolone): For severe disease
Immunomodulators
    Oral (azathioprine, methotrexate, mercaptopurine): For steroid-
        dependent/refractory disease

Oral or IV (cyclosporine): May induce remission, aids in closure of fistula

Antidiarrheals (atropine/diphenoxylate, loperamide, codeine, paregoric): Decreases frequency of stools in mild to moderate disease

Fish oil: May be useful in maintaining remission

Tricyclic antidepressants (amitriptyline, nortriptyline): Useful in treating abdominal pain

ULCERATIVE COLITIS

5-Aminosalicylic acid (mesalamine): Enema or oral

Corticosteroids

Nonpharmacologic Management

Increased risk for osteoporosis:

Prescribe calcium, 1200–1500 mg QD, and vitamin D (400 IU) QD

Nutritional management

May need iron, 325 mg BID/TID QD

May need folic acid, 1 mg QD

Client Education

Avoid aspirin/NSAIDs

Stress management

Follow-up

3 months, unless there is a flare-up or symptoms do not resolve

Referral

Refer to gastroenterologist for flexible sigmoidoscopy and colonoscopy, if client has fulminant colitis or toxic megacolon

May need surgical referral

IRRITABLE BOWEL SYNDROME

SIGNAL SYMPTOMS recurrent, intermittent dull crampy abdominal pain, watery malodorous stools

ICD-9 Code	654.1	Irritable bowel syndrome

Irritable bowel syndrome (IBS) is a biopsychosocial disorder that results from a combination of three interacting mechanisms: psychosocial factors, altered motility, and disordered sensory function of the intestine (Coulie and Camilleri, 1999). Various terms have been used to define and describe IBS, such as spastic colon, functional bowel disease, and colitis.

Epidemiology

Affects women more often than men, about 4 to 1; however, only about 10% of these people seek treatment.

Etiology

Psychosocial factors, including a history of abuse (e.g. sexual, physical, emotional)

Altered motility
Altered sensation

Physiology and Pathophysiology

Understanding the brain–gut connection offers the clearest explanation of IBS. Ninety-five percent of the serotonin receptors are in the gut and only 5% are in the brain. Interaction of the vagal nuclei along the brain–gut axis cause the various 5-hydroxytryptamine (2,3,4) receptor alteration with a resulting increase/decrease in motility and visceral hyperalgesia.

Clinical Manifestations

Subjective

Gas/bloating
Constipation (more predominant symptom in women)
Diarrhea
Alteration in bowel habits
Tenesmus
Abdominal pain
Feeling of incomplete evacuation, relief of pain on elimination
Psychosocial issues (may or may not be present)
Dyspepsia
Heartburn

Objective

Examination is mostly unremarkable, although abdomen is generally tender to palpation and stool may be palpated in the colon with clients who predominantly have constipation.
Rectal examination may reveal hard stool in the rectal vault; hemorrhoids and/or fissures may be present.

ROME CRITERIA

Three months or more of continuous or recurrent symptoms of:
(1) Abdominal pain that is relieved by defecation, and/or is associated with a change in the frequency of stool, and/or associated with a change in the consistency of the stool.
AND
(2) Two or more of the following on at least 25% of occasions or days:
Altered stool frequency (>3 movements/day or <3/week)
Altered stool form (lumpy and hard or loose and watery)
Altered stool passage (straining, urgency, tenesmus)
Passage of mucus
Bloating or feeling of abdominal distention (Vanner et al., 1999.)

Differential Diagnosis

Constipation predominant: Neurogenic causes (multiple sclerosis, diabetes), myogenic causes (scleroderma), hormonal causes (hypothyroidism)

Diarrhea predominant: IBD, lactase deficiency or intolerance, infectious
   diarrhea, medications (especially laxatives), celiac sprue
Structural causes: Cancer, diverticular disease, strictures from IBD,
   radiation therapy, rectoceles, intussusception, hemorrhoids, fissures
Medication-induced alteration in bowel habits

Diagnostic Tests

Stool for occult blood (Hemoccult); if diarrhea predominant, test for O&P,
   Giardia, C. difficile, white cells
Choice of blood studies depends on possible cause and may include CBC,
   thyroid studies, ESR, cytidine monophosphate, lactose-H_2 breath test
Colonoscopy or flexible sigmoidoscopy with barium enema

Management/Treatment

Pharmacologic Management

Constipation predominant
Bulk agents (psyllium)
Hyperosmolar agents (polyethylene glycol electrolyte solution [Golytely,
   Miralax])
Laxatives: Saline, lubricant, emollient, or stimulant (use caution with
   stimulant laxatives such as bisacodyl because dependency may develop)
Diarrhea predominant
Bulking agents (loperamide, diphenoxylate)
For symptoms of abdominal pain, gas and bloating
Antispasmodics, simethicone

Nonpharmacologic Management

Constipation predominant
High-fiber diet (30g daily) and increased fluids

Client Education

Role of fiber
Diet journal helpful
Stress management (therapy/counseling may be helpful for some)
Pain management (referral to pain specialist if needed)

Follow-up

With any pharmacologic therapy, 4–6 weeks, then as needed

Referral

Refer to gastroenterologist for flexible-sigmoidoscopy or colonoscopy
Refer to psychologist for evaluation for moderate to severe disease

NAUSEA AND VOMITING

ICD-9 Codes	787.2	Nausea
	787.2	Vomiting
	787.01	Nausea and vomiting

Nausea can be defined as an unpleasant sensation, usually felt in the upper abdomen, associated with the desire to vomit (Stein et al., 1998). *Vomiting* is defined as the forceful expulsion of gastric contents out of the mouth (Stein et al., 1998). Nausea and vomiting may be classified as acute (<1 week duration) or chronic (>1 week).

Epidemiology

Some studies suggest this may be the number one reason people present to primary care, while others suggest it is second to upper respiratory tract infections

Etiology

Organic and functional causes include infections, pregnancy, increased intracranial pressure, medications, intoxication, visceral pain, metabolic, bowel obstruction, psychiatric, trauma, neurologic, neoplasm, bulimia, pyloric stenosis, appendicitis, vestibular disease, and withdrawal.

Physiology and Pathophysiology

Altered autonomic activity, usually parasympathetic, occurs when the noxious stimulus causes nausea. Motility within the duodenum and small bowel is altered, causing gastric slowing. There is also skin pallor, an increase in respirations and salivation, and possibly vagal stimulation, which causes a decreased heart rate and decreased blood pressure. Vomiting occurs when the vomiting reflex is stimulated within the medulla. Two mechanisms are triggered, the vomiting center and the chemoreceptor trigger zone (CTZ). The vomiting center is primarily responsible for vomiting via afferent inducement from the alimentary tract. The CTZ receives stimuli from efferent pathways (phrenic, visceral, spinal). Communication from the CTZ to the vomiting center will induce vomiting.

Clinical Manifestations

Subjective
Nausea
Vomiting
Ask about associated symptoms, when the nausea and vomiting occur, last menstrual period, recent travel, etc. to help determine the cause.

Objective
Assess composition of emesis to help determine the cause (e.g., check for BRB, blood clots, coffee-grounds appearance, bile acid, food, etc.)
Assess for signs of dehydration (e.g., orthostatic hypotension, increased heart rate, poor skin turgor, dry mucous membranes, neuromuscular weakness)
Assess abdomen for epigastric tenderness, hyperactive bowel sounds

Differential Diagnosis (nausea and vomiting can be present with any of these diagnoses)

Central nervous system disorders
Esophageal disease

Gastrointestinal diseases
Gastrointestinal neuropathy
Gastrointestinal myopathy
Medications
Systemic disorders
Pregnancy (morning sickness, hyperemesis gravidarum)
Psychogenic disorders

Diagnostic Tests

As indicated by suspected differential diagnosis

Management/Treatment

Pharmacologic Management

May need IV hydration
Antiemetics:
Promethazine (Phenergan), 12.5–25mg PO/IM/PR Q6–8H PRN
Infants and children: 0.5–1 mg/kg PR Q6H
Prochlorperazine (Compazine), 5–10 mg PO/IM TID/QID, 25 mg PR
BID, 5–10 mg IV (maximum, 40 mg/day)

Nonpharmacologic Management

Push fluids, if self-limiting
Prescribe BRATS diet
Instruct patient to rest
Advise about nutritional restitution
Alleviate medical complications
Address psychosocial factors
Use a multidisciplinary approach
See rehydration plan for dehydration (p 328)

Client Education

Good hygiene
Reassurance about disease management

Follow-up

Follow-up is necessary if persists beyond 3–4 days in adults, 24 hours in infants/
children/elderly

Referral

Clients with chronic symptoms, and those who are dehydrated; will need hospitalization.

PANCREATITIS, ACUTE

SIGNAL SYMPTOMS ▶ severe LLQ pain with radiation to back, nausea
and vomiting

| ICD-9 Code | 577.0 | Acute pancreatitis |

Pancreatitis is the glandular inflammation of the pancreatic parenchyma extending from mild edematous disease to severe necrotizing disease.

Epidemiology

Seen in up to 9.5% of alcoholics
Seen also with biliary tract disease

Etiology

Ethanol or gallstones accounts for approximately 90% of all cases in the United States; causes of the remaining 10% include hypertriglyceridemia, medications (furosemide, thiazides, estrogen, azathioprine, tetracycline, sulfonamides, corticosteroids, procainamide, ethacrynic acid, phenformin), trauma, postoperative pancreatitis, pancreas divisum, pancreatic cancer, duodenal disease, infectious, and idiopathic

Physiology and Pathophysiology

The pathogenesis of pancreatitis is triggered by the causative agent, resulting in inflammation, edema, and necrosis. Autodigestion of the pancreas is the final stage; the enzymes culpable are trypsin, chymotrypsin, elastase, and phospholipase A.

Clinical Manifestations

Subjective

Severe abdominal pain in the left upper quadrant and/or epigastrium with radiation to the back
Nausea and vomiting
Low-grade fever

Objective

Severe abdominal tenderness, especially over epigastric area
May be accompanied by guarding, but without rigidity or rebound tenderness
Tachycardia
Pain on deep inspiration

Differential Diagnosis

Appendicitis (see p 317)
Diverticulitis (see p 328)
Cholecystitis/lithiasis (see p 320)
Renal calculi (dysuria, back pain, fever, hematuria)
Pyelonephritis (sudden onset of fever, shaking, chills, back pain, fatigue, diarrhea, marked tenderness on deep abdominal palpation and/or percussion to affected flank)
Inflammatory bowel disease (see p 343)
Irritable bowel syndrome (see p 346)
Gastroenteritis (crampy, diffuse abdominal pain relieved by vomiting or defecation)
Hepatitis (see p 000)

Constipation (decreased frequency of stooling—normal, 3–5 times/week)

Pelvic inflammatory disease (lower abdominal pain, cervical motion tenderness [CMT], unilateral/bilateral adnexal tenderness, temperature above 101°F, abnormal cervical/vaginal discharge)

Ectopic pregnancy (localized or diffuse colicky or dull pain, shoulder pain, rebound tenderness/guarding if ruptured, amenorrhea, abnormal vaginal bleeding)

Peptic ulcer disease (see below)

Diagnostic Tests

Amylase (will be increased first day of active symptoms, then return to normal in 3–7 days)

C-reactive protein (will increase)

Serum calcium (will decrease)

Hematocrit (as high as 50%–55%)

Lipase (will be increased first day of active symptoms, then return to normal in 3–7 days)

Abdominal ultrasonography (gold standard for gallstones)

Abdominal CT scan (definitive diagnosis of pancreatitis)

Management/Treatment

Pharmacologic Management

Analgesic management (usually narcotics)

IV hydration/NPO

Nonpharmacologic Management

Low-fat diet

No alcohol

Client Education

Disease process

Importance of avoiding alcohol

Follow-up

As indicated

Referral

Refer to gastroenterologist; client will need hospitalization; increase in serum amylase and lipase, along with symptoms will necessitate immediate referral for hospitalization.

ULCER DISEASE (Peptic Ulcer Disease, Duodenal Ulcer Disease)

SIGNAL SYMPTOMS for peptic ulcer: Gnawing, burning epigastric pain 1–3 hours after meals, relieved with food and/or antacids. For duodenal ulcer: Gnawing burning epigastric pain not associated with meals.

ICD-9 Codes	531.3	Acute peptic ulcer
	532.30	Acute duodenal ulcer

Ulcers are defects in the GI mucosa that extend through the submucosa into the muscle layer. Most cases represent an imbalance between acid, pepsin, and other potentially damaging agents and factors that act to protect mucosal integrity (Kelly, 1997, p 684).

Epidemiology

Lifetime risk, 5%–10%; annual prevalence, 1.8%; 350,000 new cases each year (in the United States). The incidence is equal in men and women. Increased risk with use of NSAIDs, smoking, *Helicobacter pylori* infection, type O blood, and dependent personality types (Kelly, 1997).

Etiology

Duodenal ulcers: *H. pylori* most common (80%–85%), use of NSAIDs (10%–30%); Zollinger–Ellison syndrome (3%–5%) Crohn's disease (1%) Ulcer disease: Tobacco use exacerbates disease.

Physiology and Pathophysiology:

Factors responsible for maintaining gastrointestinal mucosal integrity include mucus production (barrier), bicarbonate secretion (neutralization), specialized acid-resistant surface membrane, blood flow to mucosa, and prostaglandin production. Mucosa may be damaged when increased gastric acid secretion overwhelms normal mucosal protection (Zollinger–Ellison syndrome—gastrin-secreting tumor). Pepsin is often overlooked as a hostile agent. The precursor of pepsin is pepsinogen, which is produced chiefly by the cells in the gastric glands of the fundus. Pepsin is activated at pH lower than 4.0 and inactivated at pH higher than 6.0 (reducing or neutralizing stomach acid controls pepsin activation). Prostaglandins maintain mucosal blood flow and stimulate bicarbonate and mucus secretion; with use of NSAIDs this function is inhibited. *H. pylori,* a gram-negative rod found in the antrum injures the gastric mucosa through virulent proteases, urases, and cytotoxins, and increases gastrin secretion. Most duodenal ulcers are attributable to *H. pylori.*

Clinical Manifestations

Gastric Ulcers

Subjective: Burning, gnawing epigastric pain with possible radiation to back; pain aggravated by meals; weight loss

Duodenal Ulcers

Subjective: Burning, gnawing epigastric pain with possible radiation to back; pain not affected by meals

Perforated Ulcer

Subjective: Severe pain with radiation to back

Active Ulcer

Subjective: Nausea, vomiting, hematemesis and/or hematochezia

Differential Diagnosis

Gastric cancer (vague epigastric discomfort, anorexia, weight loss, unexplained iron deficiency anemia; many cases asymptomatic)

Cholelithiasis (nonlocalized abdominal discomfort, eructation and intolerance to certain foods, possibly severe abdominal pain)

Cholycystitis (acute: RUQ pain, nausea, vomiting, eructation and flatulence; chronic: pain at night after a fatty meal)

Pancreatitis (severe abdominal pain radiating to the back, fever, anorexia, nausea and vomiting; possibly jaundice if common bile duct obstructed)

Pancreatic cancer (anorexia, flatulence, weakness, dramatic weight loss, jaundice, pruritus, recent onset of diabetes, clay-colored stools)

Irritable bowel syndrome (diarrhea, pain in lower abdomen relieved by defecation)

Nonulcer dyspepsia (epigastric discomfort, postprandial fullness, early satiety, anorexia, belching, nausea, heartburn, vomiting, bloating, borborygmi, dysphagia, and abdominal burning)

Crohn's disease (frequent attacks of diarrhea, severe abdominal pain, nausea, fever, chills, weakness, anorexia and weight loss)

Angina (chest pain)

Anxiety, depression (various behaviors possibly indicating underlying psychosocial issues)

Diagnostic Tests

Serum *H. pylori* antibody test (for *H. pylori* infection; does not diagnose ulcer disease)

Gastroscopy (if acute nonperforated ulcer disease is suspected)

Upright, abdominal x-ray examination (if perforated ulcer disease is suspected; upper GI series and esophagogastroduodenoscopy contraindicated)

Endoscopy (definite diagnosis with accuracy >95%)

Serum gastrin (increased with Zollinger–Ellison syndrome)

Management/Treatment

Pharmacologic Management

Treat *H. pylori*

Stop use of aspirin and NSAIDs

Three-drug regimen:

Amoxicillin or tetracycline, 500 mg QID

AND

Metronidazole, 250 mg QID

AND

Bismuth subsalicylate (Pepto-Bismol), 2 tablets QID for 7–14 days

OR

Metronidazole, 500 mg BID

AND

Omeprazole, 20 mg BID
AND
Clarithromycin, 250 mg BID for 7–14 days
Two-drug regimen:
Clarithromycin, 500 mg TID
AND
Omeprazole, 40 mg QD (or 20 mg BID) for 14 days

Nonpharmacologic Management
Smoking cessation

Client Education
Caution about use of aspirin or NSAIDs
Instruct to stop smoking
May need maintenance dose of H_2-blockers/proton pump inhibitors, 8–12 weeks

Follow-up
1 month after pharmacologic initiation or sooner if symptoms persist or worsen

Referral
Refer to gastroenterologist if symptoms persist and/or for endoscopy.

REFERENCES

General
Behrman, R.E., Kliegman, R.M, & Arvin, A.M. (1996). *Textbook of pediatrics* (15th ed.). Philadelphia: Saunders.

Burns, C.E., Brady, M.A., Dunn, A.M., & Starr, N.B. (2000). *Pediatric primary care* (2nd ed.). Philadelphia: Saunders.

Dipro, J.T. (1997). *Pharmacotherapy: A pathophysiologic approach.* (3rd ed.) Stamford, CT: Appleton-Lange.

Dunphy, L.M., & Winland-Brown, J.E. (2001). *Primary care: The art and science of advanced practice nursing.* Philadelphia: F.A. Davis

Engstrom, P.F., & Goosenberg, E.B (1999). Diagnosis and management of bowel diseases. Philadelphia: Professional Communications.

Fenstermacher, K., & Hudson, B. T. (1997). *Practice guidelines for family nurse practitioners.* Philadelphia: Saunders.

Goroll, A.H., May, L.A., & Mulley, A.G. (1995). Primary care medicine: Office evaluation and management of the adult patient. Philadelphia: Lippincott.

Greene, H. L., Johnson, W. P., & Lemcke, D. (1998). *Decision making in medicine: An algorithmic approach.* (2nd ed.). St. Louis: Mosby.

Hicks, T.C., & Stamos, M.J. (1998, September). Practical approaches to common anorectal problems. *Patient Care Nurse Practitioner,* pp. 39–48.

Jarvis, C. (2000). Physical examination and health assessment (3rd ed.). Philadelphia: Saunders.

Kelly, W.N. (1997). Textbook of internal medicine (3rd ed.). Philadelphia: Lippincott-Raven.

Lagergren, J. Bergstrom, A. Lindgren, A. (1999). Symptomatic gastroesophageal reflux as a risk factor for esophageal adenocarcinoma. New England Journal of Medicine (340):825.

Porth, C.M. (1998). *Pathophysiology* (5th ed.). Philadelphia: Lippincott-Raven.

Stein, J.H., Eisenber, J.M., Hutton, J.J., Klippel, J.H., Kohler, P.O., LaRusso, N.F., O'Rourke, R.A., Reynolds, H.Y., Samuels, M.A., Sande, M.A., & Zvaifler, N.J. (1998). *Internal medicine* (5th ed.). St. Louis: Mosby.

Constipation

Schaeffer D.C., & Cheskin, L.J. (1998). Constipation in the elderly. *American Family Physician, 58:* 907–914.

Diarrhea

Fine, K.D., & Schiller, L.R. (1999). AGA technical review on the evaluation and management of chronic diarrhea. *Gastroenterology, 116,* 1464–1486.

Gastroesophageal Reflux Disease

Ault, D.L., & Schmidt, D. (1998). Diagnosis and management of gastroesophageal reflux in infants and children. *Nurse Practitioner, 23*(6): 78–100.

Claussen, J.R. (1999). Gastroesophageal reflux disease: A rational approach to management. *Clinician Reviews, 9*(6): 69–87.

Gastrointestinal Cancers

Held-Warmkessel, J. (1998, July). Colon cancer: Prevention and detection strategies. *Advance for Nurse Practitioners,* pp. 42–45.

Hiatal Hernia and Esophagitis

Cameron, A.J. (1999). Barrett's esophagus: Prevalence and size of hiatal hernia. *American Journal of Gastroenterology, 94:* 2054–2058.

Inflammatory Bowel Disorders

Botoman, W., Bonner, G.F., & Botoman, D.A. (1998). Management of inflammatory bowel disease. *American Family Physician, 57,* 57–68.

Norton, B.A. (1998, September). Crohn's disease: A review of medical, surgical and nutritional management. *Advance for Nurse Practitioners,* pp. 42–50.

Irritable Bowel Syndrome

Carlson, E. (1998). Irritable bowel syndrome. *Nurse Practitioner, 23:* 82–91.

Coulie, B., & Camilleri, M. (1999, November/December). Irritable bowel syndrome: Epidemiology, mechanism, and management. *Clinical Perspectives in Gastroenterology,* pp 329–338.

Vanner, S.J., Depew, W. T., Paterson, W.G., DaCosta, L.R., Groll, A.G., Simon, J.B., & Djurfeldt, M. (1999). Predictive value of the Rome criteria for diagnosing the irritable bowel syndrome. *American Journal of Gastroenterology, 94,* 2912–2917.

Ulcer Disease

Aronson, B. (1998). Update on peptic ulcer disease. *American Journal of Nursing, 98:* 41–46.

Fay, M., & Jaffe, P.E. (1996). Diagnostic and treatment guidelines for *Helicobacter pylori*. *Nurse Practitioner, 21*(7): 28–35.

Salcedo, J.A., & Al-Kawas, F. (1998). Treatment of *Helicobacter pylori* infection. *Archives of Internal Medicine, 158,* 842–851.

Practitioners, 5(12), 179–184.

Chapter 8

RENAL AND
GENITOURINARY SYSTEM

BENIGN PROSTATIC HYPERTROPHY

SIGNAL SYMPTOMS urinary frequency, weak stream

ICD-9 Codes	600	Benign prostatic hypertrophy
	599.6	Urinary obstruction, unspecified

Benign prostatic hypertrophy (BPH) is a nonmalignant condition in which an enlarged prostate compresses the urethra, causing increased urinary frequency with a weak stream.

Epidemiology

Rarely seen in men under 40 years of age.
Affects 50% of men over 50 years of age.
At least 90% of men between 70–90 years have symptoms of BPH.

Etiology

Exact etiology is unknown.
Thought to be due to the effect of the aging process on testosterone production.
May be due to increasing levels of estrogen as men age.
May be an autoimmune response.

Physiology and Pathophysiology

Histologic hyperplasia, which occurs in response to changing hormone levels in aging men, causes noncancerous enlargement of the prostate, which exerts an inward pressure, thus increasing resistance to urine flow.

Clinical Manifestations

Subjective

Weak stream
Straining to void
Hesitancy
Intermittency
Incomplete emptying
Dribbling

Frequency/urgency

Nocturia

American Urological Association Symptom Index Questionnaire score >7

Also include in history:

Complete health history

History of urinary tract infections (UTIs)

Over-the-counter medications (some of which can impair contractility of bladder and cause resistance to outflow of urine)

Objective

Prostate enlarged, firm, symmetrical

Median sulcus not identifiable

Possible distended bladder

Differential Diagnosis

Prostate cancer (elevated prostate-specific antigen [PSA] and enlarged prostate)

Urethral stricture (diagnosed using intravenous pyelography [IVP] and/or x-ray examination of the kidney, ureters, and bladder)

Neurogenic bladder (dysfunction of the bladder secondary to lesion of the nervous system)

Interstitial cystitis (diagnosed via history, cystoscopy, and bladder distention)

Diagnostic Tests

Urinalysis (UA) test (to rule out UTI and hematuria)

Blood urea nitrogen (BUN)/creatinine (to assess kidney status)

Table 8–1 Management: Benign Prostatic Hypertrophy

Symptomology	Management
Mild	-Monitor on an annual basis (physical examination with digital rectal exam and PSA) -Limit fluids, esp. in evening -Avoid decongestants -Refrain from full bladder -Avoid caffeine/alcohol

Moderate	***Pharmacologic Management***
	 —Finasteride (Proscar) 5 mg PO QD
	 (Side effects: impotence, decreased libido, ejaculate volume)
	 —Alpha-1 blockers:
	   Doxazosin (Cardura) 1–8 mg PO QD
	   Terazosin (Hytrin) 1–10 mg PO qhs
	   Tamsulosin (Flomax) 0.4–0.8 mg PO QD
	   (Side effects: dizziness, hypotension, edema, nausea, nasal congestion, priapism [rare])
	 Complementary/Alternative Therapies
	 —Saw palmetto 1–2g of ground, dried fruit QD OR 80 mg of extract

Severe	-Refer to urologist for further testing and treatment, and possible surgery -Transurethral resection of the prostate (TURP) (Side effects: diminished/absent ejaculation, impotence (<5%), urinary incontinence and hematuria)

PSA (to rule out prostate disease) [*Note:* Measuring PSA is worthless without a prostate examination.] Norms for PSA: Age 40–50, ≤2.5 ng/ml, 51–60, ≤3.5 ng/ml, over 60, ≤4 ng/ml.

Management/Treatment
See Table 8–1.

Referral
Refer to urologist if symptoms are severe, complications occur, or surgery is warranted

CYSTITIS

SIGNAL SYMPTOMS dysuria, frequency, urinary urgency

ICD-9 Codes	595	Cystitis
	595.1	Acute cystitis
	595.2	Chronic cystitis

Cystitis is an infection of one or more structures in the urinary tract, including the bladder, urethra, or renal pelvis/kidneys. Along with the symptoms of infection, there is also bacteria in the urine.

UTIs are classified as:

Upper: Acute or chronic pyelonephritis, renal or perirenal abscess
Lower: Cystitis, urethritis, or prostatitis
Uncomplicated: Upper or lower UTI, with no complicating factors
Complicated: Upper or lower UTI, with complicating factors (anatomic, functional or pharmacologic) that predispose a client to persistent and/or recurrent infection or treatment failure [e.g., elderly men, indwelling catheters, chronic diseases, pregnancy] [see Table 8–2])

Epidemiology
Women are disproportionately affected.
40% of women report having a UTI in their lives.
20% of women will experience recurrent infections.
Risk of UTIs is higher in women with diabetes.
Occur in up to 5% of young girls; only 1%–2% of young boys.
99% of UTIs in men are attributable to prostatitis.
By age 65, the incidence rate in men is similar to that in women.
In the United States, UTIs account for over 7 million office visits, and over 1 million hospitalizations per year; annual costs exceed $1 billion.

Etiology
Infection occurs when microorganisms, usually bacteria (most commonly from the digestive tract), adhere to the opening of the urethra, multiply, and ascend the urinary tract.
See Table 8–3.

Table 8–2 Bladder Cancer

Epidemiology	Bladder cancer is the second most common urologic malignancy, after prostate cancer Affects over 50,000 Americans per year and causes over 10,000 deaths per year
Risk Factors	Cigarette smoking Occupational exposure
Signs and Symptoms	Painless hematuria (either gross or microscopic) Urinary frequency and/or urgency Mild suprapubic pain NOTE: Often asymptomatic
Diagnostic Tests:	X-rays (radiologic testing) Ultrasound Cystoscopy IVP Transuretral resection/biopsy
Management:	Surgery (radical cystectomy) Chemotherapy Radiation

The shorter urethra in women makes the ascension of bacteria more likely, especially during and after intercourse.

If normal defense mechanisms (normal urine flow to expel bacteria, protective mucin coating of bladder, low pH, and lactobacillus colonization of vaginal mucosa) are altered, infection can occur.

Host factors also play a role:

Presence of reflux
Obstruction
Anatomical abnormalities
Constipation
Trauma
Poor hygiene

Table 8–3 Incidence of Bacterial Pathogens in Urinary Tract Infections

Uncomplicated Infections	E. coli (75%–90%) Staphylococcus saprophyticus (10%) Proteus mirabilis (5%) Klebsiella pneumoniae (4%) Enterobacter species (1%) Beta-hemolytic streptococcus ($<$1%)
Complicated Infections	E. coli (35%) Enterococcus faccalis (16%) Proteus mirabilis (13%) Staphylococcus epidermidis (12%) Klebsiella pneumoniae (7%) Pseudomonas (5%) Staphylococcus aureus (4%) Enterobacter species (3%) Others (5%)

Infrequent/dysfunctional voiding
Irritants
Sexual activity/diaphragm use
Benign postmenopausal
Diabetes
Catheterization
Anal intercourse
Vaginal intercourse with females with bacterial vaginosis

Physiology and Pathophysiology

The bladder is normally resistant to invading organisms. More specifically, the lining of the bladder is composed of mucin-producing cells, which maintain the integrity of the lining and prevent inflammation and damage. The urine, which is acidic, also helps to prevent infection.

There are three different routes by which bacteria enter the genitourinary system: (1) ascending infection (most common), (2) hematogenous spread (bacteremia), and (3) direct extension (enterovesical fistula).

Clinical Manifestations

Subjective

Dysuria: Pain, burning on urination
Frequency: Having to urinate frequently
Urgency: Feeling of having to urinate
Occasional gross hematuria
Suprapubic pain or pressure
Flank pain
Dribbling
Incontinence
Low back or abdominal pain
Cloudy, foul-smelling urine
Fullness in rectum (males)

Objective

Low-grade fever, or fever may be absent
Slight lower abdominal/suprapubic tenderness
Possibly vaginal erythema, edema, irritation, and/or discharge
No costovertebral angle (CVA) tenderness
Normal bowel signs

For age-related subjective and objective clinical manifestations in addition to the above, see Age-Related Considerations 8–1.

Differential Diagnosis

Adults

Urethritis (involvement of urethra only; urine is clear)
Pyelonephritis (higher urinary tract involvement, fever and chills, nausea and vomiting)

Age-Related Considerations: Symptoms of Cystitis

Age-Group	Subjective Symptoms	Objective Symptoms
Pediatric	**Infants** Malaise, irritability, difficulty feeding, fever, vomiting/diarrhea, strong odor of urine, dribbling **Toddlers** Abdominal/flank pain, foul smelling urine, altered voiding pattern, fever, vomiting/diarrhea **Pre-schoolers** Abdominal/flank pain, vomiting, fever, dysuria, fever, enuresis **Adolescents** "Classic" dysuria, frequency, urgency, fever, abdominal/flank tenderness, CVA	Obstructive signs: -Midline, low-abdominal distention or pain -Suprapubic tenderness Flank pain
Elderly	Confusion, lethargy, irritability	—

Asymptomatic bacteriuria (common in pregnancy: no symptoms, but urine is abnormal)

Interstitial cystitis (marked frequency with clear urine)

Renal calculi (often red cells [RBCs] present; diagnosed with IVP or spiral computed tomography [CT] scan)

Vaginitis/vulvovaginitis (other organisms present, verified by culture)

Prostatitis (tender, boggy prostate; prostatic secretions have organisms present)

BPH (no bacteria present; prostate enlarged)

Children:

Meatal stenosis (difficulty initiating urine; weak stream, dribbling)

Mechanical (confirmed by IVP or cystoscopy)

Foreign body (confirmed by x-ray examination, IVP, or ultrasonography)

Urethritis (involvement of urethra only; urine is clear)

Vesicoureteral reflux (confirmed by cystoscopy)

Sexual abuse (usually other factors/symptoms present)

Appendicitis (abdominal pain, complete blood count [CBC] reveals increased white-cell [WBC] count with left shift; confirmed by abdominal x-ray examination or ultrasonography)

Diagnostic Tests

Urine tests (see Table 8–4)

Collection

Clean-catch specimen

Straight catheterization

Suprapubic aspiration of bladder (infants)

Types

Dipstick (macroscopic)

Examination (microscopic)

Table 8–4 Urine Test: Abnormal Findings Seen with Urinary Tract Infections

Test Component	Abnormal Findings Seen with Urinary Tract Infections
Color	Often dark, with foul smell, with possible gross hematuria
Specific Gravity	<1.005 and >1.030. If too dilute, may give false reading
pH	Usually <4.5. If high, may be associated with urea stone forming Klebsiella
Nitrites	Confirms presence of bacteria that converts nitrates to nitrites; negative does not rule out UTI
Protein	1–2+ with lower UTI 3–4+ needs special attention related to kidney damage
Leukocyte esterase (WBCs)	Detect pyuria (75%–90% sensitivity; 65%–85% specificity)
Glucose	If positive, bacteria rapidly multiply
Blood	Not specific for UTI, but can be positive
Microscopic	WBCs >2–5/high power field
	RBCs >2–3/high power field
	WBC casts >2/high power field
	RBC casts >2/high power field

Culture and sensitivity

Bacterial identification and antibiotic susceptibilities

Not necessary in uncomplicated adult UTIs

Crucial in recurrent or relapse UTIs

Beneficial in children and males

Traditionally, 100,000 colony-forming units (CFU) of bacteria per milliliter or urine was diagnostic; now as few as 100 CFU per milliliter of urine can have a high positive predictive value for UTIs (especially in women)

Other diagnostic tests

CBC, electrolytes, BUN/creatinine (to rule out systemic involvement)

Renal ultrasonography, IVP, CT scan (to rule out structural abnormalities)

Cystoscopy, voiding cystourethrogram (invasive) (to rule out other bladder abnormalities)

Management/Treatment

The goals of treatment are to eradicate the infection, to find and correct an anatomical or functional abnormality, and to prevent recurrence. The pharmacologic choices vary according to age, sex, and symptoms of the client.

Pharmacologic Management

Common medications used to treat UTIs:

Ampillicin (Principen): Low cost, but increasingly resistant

TMP/SMX (Bactrim/Septra): Low cost; high rate of allergies

Cephalexin (Keflex/Keftab): Used during pregnancy

Third-generation cephalosporins: Higher cost, but useful with resistant organisms

Nitrofurantoin (Macrobid/Macrodantin): Useful when patient is allergic to sulfa drugs; good in pregnancy

Table 8–5   Common Drug Treatment Regimens: Urinary Tract Infections

Management	Regimen	Drug/Dosage
Acute Infections	One Day Dosing *Advantages:* low cost, low side effects, high compliance *Disadvantages:* high failure rate, will not treat suspected pyelonephritis	TMP-SMZ (Bactrim/Septra) DS 2-3 tabs Amoxicillin (Amoxil/Trimox) 3 grams Norfloxacin (Noroxin) 800 mg Fosfomycin tromethamine (Monurol) 3 gram sachet
	Three Day Dosing *Advantages:* decreased cost, decreased side effects, high efficacy *Disadvantages:* twice the side effects of single day dosing	TMP-SMZ (Bactrim/Septra) DS, 1 PO BID for 3 days Nitrofurantoin (Macrodantin/ MacroBID) 50–100 mg PO BID-QID for 3 days
	Seven-Day Dosing *Advantages:* Only 5% failure rates *Disadvantages:* Increased cost, increased side effects, decreased compliance	TMP-SMZ (Bactrim/Septra) DS, 1 PO BID for 7 days Nitrofurantoin (Macrodantin/ MacroBID) 50–100 mg PO BID-QID for 7 days
Recurrent Infections	Continuous Prophylaxis	TMP-SMZ (Bactrim/Septra) SS, 1/2 tablet PO qhs
	Post-Coital	TMP-SMZ (Bactrim/Septra) SS, 1 tablet PO post intercourse
Special Populations	Pregnant Clients	DO NOT use Bactrim Ampicillin (Principen) 250–500 mg PO QID for 7–10 days Amoxicillin (Amoxil/Trimox) 250 mg PO tid for 7–10 days Amoxicillin + Clavulantate (Augmentin) 250 mg PO QID for 7–10 days (useful for resistant strains) Cephalexin (Keflex) 250 mg PO QID for 10 days Nitrofurantoin (Macrodantin/ MacroBID) 100 mg PO QID for 10 days Fosfomycin (Monurol) 3g sachet PO once
	Pediatric Clients	TMP-SMZ (Bactrim/Septra) 8–40 mg/kg/24 hours in 2 divided doses × 10 days Amoxicillin (Amoxil/Trimox) 40 mg/kg/24 hours in 3 divided doses for 10 days Cefixime (Suprax) 100 mg/5cc, 4–8 mg/kg QD for 10 days Tylenol 10–15 mg/kg Q4 hours PRN fever, discomfort

COMMON DERMATOLOGIC DISORDERS

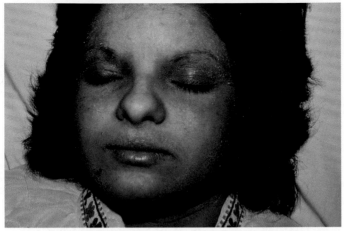

Plate 1. Atopic dermatitis. Red to reddish-brown, slightly scaly, poorly circumscribed maculopapular lesions, possibly with lichenification. It is extremely pruritic, leading patients to scratch and thereby predisposing them to infection. The lesions are often symmetrically distributed.

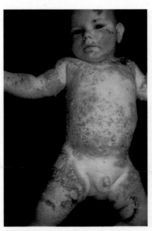

Plate 2. Atopic dermatitis in a child. Red to reddish-brown, slighty scaly, poorly circumscribed maculopapular lesions, possibly with lichenification. It is extremely pruritic, leading patients to scratch and thereby predisposing them to infection. In children under 4 years old, it is most common in the antecubital and popliteal spaces, thighs, neck, and hands.

See Credits section at the end of Chapter 1 for credit information.

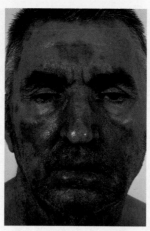

Plate 3. Seborrheic dermatitis. Poorly circumscribed, flat, red macular lesions with a greasy scale. Discrete papules may be seen. Secondary infection may occur. Usually symmetrically distributed and can be generalized. Most commonly occurs on the scalp, eyebrows, eyelids, area behind the ears, cheeks, beard area, anterior chest, axillae, and groin.

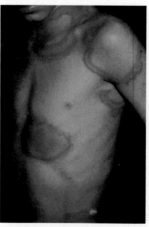

Plate 4. Urticaria. Erythematous, sharply circumscribed, flat macules and papules surrounded by pale halos. Size can vary, and may cover large areas. Extremely pruritic. Usually occurs after exposure to allergens, especially drugs, food preservatives, fish, nuts, eggs, and berries. Other causes include insect bites, acute infections, and physical factors such as heat and cold. Lesions last less than 24 hours.

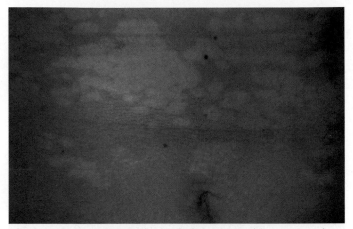

Plate 5. Tinea versicolor. Flat to slightly elevated brown papules and plaques that scale when rubbed. Area may be hypopigmented. May be slightly pruritic. Most commonly appears on the upper trunk, sholders, neck, and proximal arms and occasionally on the face.

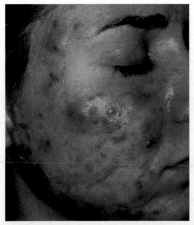

Plate 6. Acne. Pustules, papules, open comedones (blackheads), closed comedones (whiteheads), occasional cysts, and scarring. Occurs on the face, especially the forehead and cheeks, and on the chest, neck, and back. Most common in adolescents and young adults, but can occur throughout adult life. May flare up in response to some drugs, such as corticosteroids, anabolic steroids, and anitconvulsants. May also occur premenstrually and in women who use oily cosmetics.

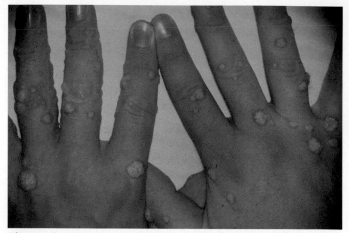

Plate 7. Common warts. Discrete, raised, hypopigmented, or pink lesions with an irregular, scaly surface. May occur singly or in groups anywhere on the body. When pared, they produce fine bleeding points.

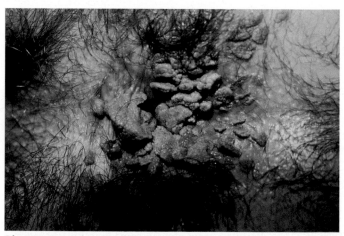

Plate 8. Genital warts. White or pink, slightly hyperpigmented papules with a highly irregular, scaly surface. Occur in the genital area. Early lesions may be flat and pink.

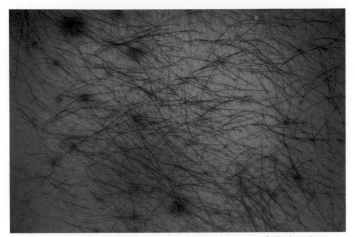

Plate 9. Folliculitis. Small red papules in the hair follicles that may become pustular. Occurs in hairy areas, especially the face, neck, scalp, chest, and back.

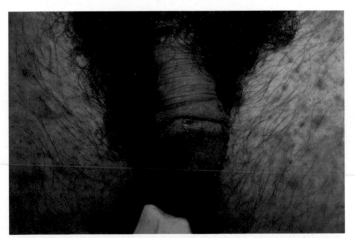

Plate 10. Scabies. Small, hivelike, excoriated, and sometimes purpuric papules that are extremely pruritic. Indurated nodules may occur, especially on the genitalia. Often occurs on the hands, arms, axillae, groin, and toes.

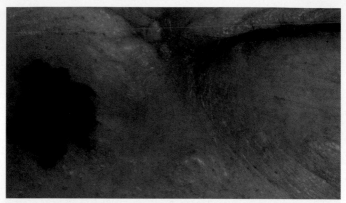

Plate 11. Malignant melanoma. Blue, black, or brown variegated, flat lesions that often have areas of white and red pigmentation. The borders become irregular, and there may be notches. The skin surface may be irregular under magnification. Most common in areas exposed to the sun.

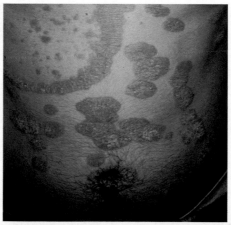

Plate 12. Psoriasis. Sharply circumscribed red papules and plaques with a powdery white scale. Tiny bleeding points may appear after removal of scale. Size varies, and pustules may occur around the periphery of the lesion. Pitting and dystrophy of nails are common. May occur anywhere on the body.

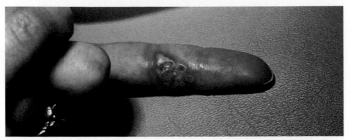

Plate 13. Herpes simplex. Begins as erythematous papules and plaques that develop into grouped, umbilicated vesicles on an erythematous base. Progresses to pustular and crusty lesions. Can occur anywhere, but most often appears around the mouth and genitals.

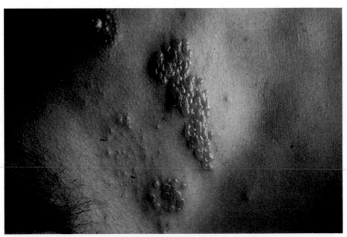

Plate 14. Herpes zoster. Umbilicated vesicles arising in groups of erythematous papules or urticarial plaques after 2 or 3 days. May become hemorrhagic. Crusting occurs rapidly, and scarring is common. Distribution follows a nerve path. The thorax, cervical area, trigeminal nerve area, and lumbosacral area are most commonly affected.

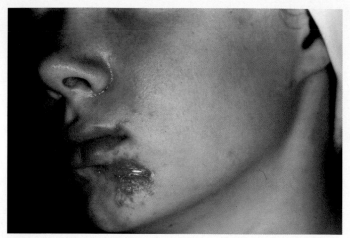

Plate 15. Bullous impetigo. Beginning as red macules, lesions progress to bullae with thin, easily broken roofs. Progression proceeds rapidly to weeping erosions that develop a tightly adherent honey-colored crust. Most commonly appear around the mouth and nose, but can occur anywhere. Very contagious.

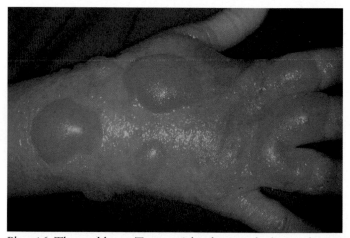

Plate 16. Thermal burn. Tense vesicles that may be hemorrhagic. Caused by heat, sunlight, x-rays, or extreme cold. Usually very painful.

Quinolones: Useful in recurrent infection, and in men (prostatitis); not for
   use in children
Acetaminophen (Tylenol), 650 mg Q4–6H PRN, for pain and fever
Phenazopyridine (Pyridium), 100–200 mg Q8H for 3 days for bladder
   spasms and discomfort (drug turns urine orange)
See Table 8–5.

Client Education

Finish all of medication, even if feeling better.
Wash genital area with water and no soap.
Avoid bubble baths, vaginal sprays, and douches
Wipe from front to back.
Avoid constipation.
Drink at least eight 8-oz glasses of water per day.
Avoid excessive use of alcohol, tea, coffee, and/or carbonated beverages.
Urinate at least every 3–4 hours, before bed, and after intercourse.
Wear cotton underwear.
Postmenopausal females may benefit from an estradiol vaginal cream.
Cranberry juice is slightly effective, but need to drink 1500–4000 ml per day.

Follow-up

Urine examination (dipstick) in 48–72 hours:
   If sterile, continue treatment.
   If not sterile or no clinical improvement, identify organism and change
      to broad-spectrum antibiotic.
Urine culture should be obtained 3–4 days after finishing antibiotics.

Referral

Refer to urologist for the following:
   Recurrent UTIs—within 2 weeks of prior infection, or three or more
      episodes per year
   Patients with diabetes
   Painless hematuria that is not cleared with first round of antibiotics
   Pediatric males with first UTI
   Pediatric females with second UTI
   Pediatric patients with gross hematuria

ENURESIS

SIGNAL SYMPTOM ▶ bed-wetting

ICD-9 Codes	307.6	Enuresis
	788.3	Incontinence NOS

Enuresis is the involuntary or unintentional discharge of urine after the age by
which bladder control should have been established (usually 5 years). Noctur-

nal enuresis is the most common form; diurnal (daytime) enuresis, after age 5 is uncommon, and can be associated with different physiologic mechanisms and conditions.

Primary enuresis occurs in a child who has never been dry at night for longer than a week; more than 90% of all cases of enuresis.

Secondary enuresis occurs in a child who has been dry at night for a prolonged period and subsequently loses bladder control.

Epidemiology

5–7 million children in United States are affected.

Boys are affected twice as often as girls.

15%–20% of children will have some degree of bed-wetting at age 5 years.

5% of children have enuresis at age 10 years.

1% will have enuresis at age 15 years.

Family history is significant: One parent with enuresis results in 44% occurrence in offspring; two parents results in 77% occurrence.

Etiology

Widely debated, poorly misunderstood

Primary enuresis:

Immature development of bladder with resultant small capacity

Immature arousal mechanism for non–rapid-eye-movement sleep

Secondary enuresis:

Neurogenic bladder

Spinal cord abnormalities

UTIs

Presence of posterior urethral valve in boys, or ectopic ureter in girls

Developmental delays

Diabetes mellitus or diabetes insipidus

Psychological problems, such as regression after birth of sibling

Physiology and Pathophysiology

Normal developmental milestones of urinary control:

Birth to 6 months: Bladder emptying is frequent, day and night; uninhibited reflex action.

6–12 months: Bladder emptying is less frequent; central nervous system (CNS) inhibition of reflex action.

1–2 years: Child consciously perceives bladder fullness; CNS inhibition of bladder contractions, and micturition increases.

3–5 years: Child has developed ability to inhibit the need to void voluntarily and unconsciously.

Bladder control is achieved earlier by girls than boys.

Clinical Manifestations

Subjective

A thorough history is essential. History alone often provides sufficient information for accurate assessment and initiation of appropriate treatment. Among the questions to ask are:

Has the child ever been dry?

What is the daytime voiding pattern?

How does the child sleep?

How frequently does the child wet the bed?

When does it occur? (day vs. night)

What do the parents do about it?

Is there a history of bed-wetting in the family?

Any family history of diabetes?

How does the child feel about it?

Any reports of urgency, pain, or burning?

Any new events in the family? (new baby, death of family member, divorce/separation of parents, school problems, loss of pet)

SUBJECTIVE DIFFERENTIATION

Primary enuresis:

Bed-wetting has persisted (since before toilet training)

Dysuria absent

Hematuria absent

Secondary enuresis:

Onset of bed-wetting is acute, after previous period of continence.

Dysuria present, with related UTI.

Hematuria rare; may exist with concurrent UTI or other infection.

Objective

Complete physical and neurologic examination is needed.

Examination generally shows no obvious abnormalities (in primary nocturnal enuresis)

Possible abnormalities:

Constant dribbling

Genitalia with external anomalies

Rectal sphincter tone abnormal

Sacral dimpling (spinal abnormalities)

Abdominal masses (enlarged kidneys)

Differential Diagnosis

UTI or cystitis (urinalysis abnormal; refer to "Cystitis")

Diabetes mellitus (glucose in urine; abnormally high fasting blood glucose)

Diabetes insipidus (inability to concentrate urine, hypernatremia)

Glomerulonephritis (presence of infection)

Pyelonephritis (presence of infection)
Urethritis (external involvement only)
Stress incontinence (structural abnormalities)

Diagnostic Tests

UA test and culture (to rule out infection)
X-ray examination (to rule out structural abnormalities)

Management/Treatment

Before any treatment is attempted, the child must want to be dry, and
parents must be willing to be involved in treatment.
Psychological issues should be resolved first.
Reassure parents that their child is not lazy.
Educate parents and child about origins of enuresis.
Educate parents not to be too aggressive and about the need to be patient.
Discuss various treatment options, side effects of medications, and
importance of commitment to treatment choice.
See Table 8–6.

Table 8–6   Management: Enuresis

Management	Methodology
Non-Pharmacologic	
-Behavioral Therapy	Involve child in treatment plan Restrict fluids after dinner Have child void before bed Avoid bladder irritants (caffeine, carbonated beverages) esp. before bed Make a chart to record bladder capacity and wet/dry nights Reinforce child's pride Provide encouragement for dry nights Do NOT punish child for regression or failures
-Alarm Systems	Most successful therapy Requires commitment from parents and child Alarm system sewn into pajamas or to a pad in the bed Alarm sounds when wetting is detected; child must then get out of bed, change clothes and empty bladder before returning to bed Process is repeated each time alarm sounds
Pharmacologic	
-Desmopressin acetate (DDAVP) (antidiuretic hormone that decreases urine production)	20 mcg at bedtime initially (one spray (10 mcg) per nostril Can be increased 10mcg/nostril every HS every 2 weeks to maximum of 40mcg Side effects: headache, rhinitis, nasal congestion, flushing
-Imipramine (Tofranil) (anticholinergic effect on bladder)	Initially 15–25 mg qhs Increase to maximum of 50 mg in children < 12 years; 75 mg in children > 12 years Continue treatment 6–8 weeks, then taper over 4–6 weeks to avoid relapse Side effects: dry mouth, blurred vision, sleep disturbances, mood swings

Referral

Refer to urologist if voiding dysfunction exists, child's disorder is not responsive to treatment, or child has recurrent infections.

Refer to psychology or psychiatrist if psychological distress exists or continues.

INTERSTITIAL CYSTITIS

SIGNAL SYMPTOMS ▶ urinary frequency without infection

ICD-9 Codes	599.0	Cystitis
	595.1	Interstitial cystitis

Interstitial cystitis is an inflammatory condition of the bladder of unknown etiology, causing symptoms of chronic cystitis, with sterile urine and no pyuria.

Epidemiology

Affects approximately 500,000 persons in the United States.

90% of patients afflicted are women.

Men with prostatalgia may actually have interstitial cystitis.

Patients suffer for an average of 4.5 years before they are correctly diagnosed.

15% of patients are of Jewish origin.

Etiology

Unknown; in the past, was thought to be a psychiatric disorder.

Physiology and Pathophysiology

The current theory hypothesizes that an alteration in the glycosaminoglycan layer of the bladder occurs, possibly secondarily to a previous UTI, which allows solutes in the urine to provoke an inflammatory response.

Clinical Manifestations

Subjective

Marked urinary frequency (at least eight times a day for 9 months)

Nocturia

Dyspareunia

Pelvic pain

Possible hematuria

Objective

Possible suprapubic tenderness.

UA usually negative.

Hematuria possibly present.

Symptom criteria for interstitial cystitis (Hanno, 1994)

Symptoms of suprapubic pain with nocturia and frequency at least eight times a day for at least 9 months

Patient older than age 18 years

Bladder capacity less than 350 ml and urge to void if distended with 150 ml of urine

No recent (within past 3 months) diagnosis of bacterial cystitis or prostatitis

No alternative explanation for the patient's syndrome (e.g., tubercular cystitis, radiation cystitis, tumors of the genitourinary tract, chemical cystitis, or active genital herpes or vaginitis)

Differential Diagnosis

Cystitis (dysuria, frequency with infection present; cystoscopy and bladder distention are normal; refer to "Cystitis")

Neurogenic bladder (dysfunction of the bladder secondary to nervous system lesion)

Diagnostic Tests

Cystoscopy (to rule out lower urinary tract disorders)

Bladder biopsies (to rule out carcinoma)

Management/Treatment

Treatment is aimed at relieving symptoms and improving function; no known curative therapy.

Pharmacologic Management

ORAL THERAPY

Pentosan polysulfate sodium (Elmiron), 300 mg PO QD

Amitriptyline (Elavil), 25 mg PO QHS, increasing 25 mg every 2–4 weeks, up to 150 mg

Hydroxyzine (Atarax), 25–50 mg PO QHS.

Nifedipine (extend release) (Adalat CC/Procardia XL), 30 mg QD, increasing to 60 mg per day

Cimetidine (Tagamet), 200 mg PO TID

INTRAVESICAL THERAPY

Intravesical dimethylsulfoxide (Rimso-50) instilled into the bladder for up to 8 weeks to reduce pain and inflammation

Nonpharmacologic Management

Hydrodistention to provide symptom relief via sensory denervation

Surgery for severe cases

Client Education

Disease process

Medication and side effects

Referral

Refer to urologist for initial diagnosis and management plan

Refer to psychotherapist, if indicated, because this condition is frustrating for patients, and depression or anxiety is common

PROSTATITIS

ICD-9 Codes	601.0	Prostatitis, acute
	601.1	Prostatitis, chronic

Prostatitis is the inflammation or infection of the prostate gland. There are four basic types of prostatitis:

Acute bacterial
Chronic bacterial
Nonbacterial
Prostatodynia (no infection or inflammation present)

Epidemiology

Comprise 25% of primary care visits by men.
Most common cause of UTIs in men.
Most common type is nonbacterial (eight times more common than bacterial).
Chronic prostatitis is more common in elderly men, and more difficult to treat.

Etiology

Gram-negative organisms (most common)
  Escherichia coli
  Klebsiella pneumoniae
  Proteus mirabilis
  Enterobacter faecalis
  Streptococcus faecalis
Other possible causes
  Neisseria gonorrhoeae
  Trichomonas vaginalis
Nonbacterial causes
  Gardnerella vaginalis
  Chlamydia trachomatis
  Trichomonas vaginalis
  Ureaplasma urealyticum

Physiology and Pathophysiology

The infection results from ascension of organized, colonized bacteria from the lower urethra to the prostate. Increases in intraurethral pressure (due to intercourse) can also result in bacterial deposition into the prostate.

Clinical Manifestations

Subjective
See Table 8–7.
  Also include in your history:
  Sexual history (and history of sexual partners)
  Contraceptive practices

Urethral/penile discharge, itching
Hematuria
Weight loss

Objective

See Table 8–7.

Differential Diagnosis

Prostatalgia (prostate pain without infection or inflammation)
UTI/cystitis (dysuria, frequency; refer to "Cystitis")
Urethritis (external involvement)
Pyelonephritis (systemic involvement; prostate normal)
Outlet obstruction (structural abnormalities)
BPH (enlarged prostate, weak stream, no infection present)
Prostate cancer (asymmetrical, firm, painless mass on prostate; elevated
PSA) (see Table 8–8)

Table 8–7   Clinical Manifestations: Prostatitis

Clinical Manifestations	Acute Prostatitis	Chronic Prostatitis	Non-Bacterial Prostatitis
Subjective			
Urination	Frequency Urgency Dysuria Nocturia >2x	Dribbling Hesitancy	Frequency Urgency Dysuria
Urinary Stream	Difficulty initiating urine stream Decreased force of stream and amount of urine	Loss of stream volume and force Hematuria	–
Pain	Low back pain Suprapubic pain	Painful ejaculation	Mild perineal pain
Other	Fever, chills Malaise, arthralgias	Can have uncommon presentation; may present with recurrent UTIs rather than prostatic symptoms	Discharge common No systemic illness
Objective			
Urine	Hematuria Pyuria Presence of bacteria	–	Presence of WBCs, but NO bacteria in urine
Prostate exam	Boggy, tender, enlarged prostate	Prostate slightly irregular (asymmetrical) to normal Possibly tender	Prostate mildly tender, normal
Other	Fever	–	–

Table 8–8   Prostate Cancer

Epidemiology	-Prostate Cancer is most common type of cancer among American men, and the second leading cause of death (after lung cancer) -The risk of developing Prostate Cancer increases with age, however the cause remains unknown -Possible causes/links include: Positive family history High fat/low fiber diets Testosterone levels -African American men have a slightly increased risk.
Clinical Manifestations	Weak, interrupted flow of urine Urinary frequency Blood in the urine Inability to urinate Urine flow that is difficult to stop Dysuria Persistent back, pelvic pain
Diagnostic Tests	Diagnosis is done by -digital rectal examination (DRE) AND -prostate-specific antigen (PSA) Age-Specific PSA Reference Ranges Age 40–49—normal range 0–2.5 Age 50–59—normal range 0–3.5 Age 60–69—normal range 0–4.5 Age 70–79—normal range 0–6.5
Management	-Referral to a urologist to confirm the diagnosis of prostate cancer and to stage the tumor according to the Gleason scale -Surgery (radical prostatectomy) and/or radiation -Hormones are also used for treatment

Diagnostic Tests

Expressed Prostatic Secretion (EPS) Examination

Examine for WBCs

Technique:

VB1 (first voided urine): Initial void of 5–10 ml.

VB2 (second voided/midstream urine): 50–100 ml of urine collected midstream (after ~100 ml).

EPS: Massage prostate from each lateral lobe to midline; milk urethra to produce secretion.

VB3 (third voided urine after EPS): Follow-up void of 5–10 ml.

Results:

Prostatitis: If EPS >10 WBCs per high power field

Bacterial prostatitis: If 10-fold increase in bacteria growth of EPS and VB3

Nonbacterial prostatitis: If WBCs in EPS and VB3, but no growth of bacteria

Probable cystitis: If culture growth in VB1 and VB2, but not in EPS or VB3

Management/Treatment

Pharmacologic Management

Discontinue all over-the-counter medications with anticholinergic properties

Acute or chronic prostatitis

TMP/SMX (Bactrim/Septra), DS PO BID for 4 weeks
Ciprofloxacin (Cipro), 500 mg PO BID for 4–6 weeks
Norfloxacin (Noroxin), 400 mg PO BID for 4–6 weeks
Nonbacterial prostatitis
Tetracycline (Achromycin/Sumycin), 500 mg PO QID for 7–10 days
Doxycycline (Doryx/Monodox) 100 mg PO BID for 2 weeks
TMP/SMX (Bactrim/Septra), DS PO BID for 2 weeks

Nonpharmacologic Management
Bedrest
Sitz baths
No alcohol or caffeine

Referral
Refer to urologist if:

Man is over 50 years of age (further work-up of BPH)
Unable to treat chronic prostatitis infection (difficult to cure)
Mass is felt on prostate
Elevated PSA with concurrent abnormal prostate examination

PYELONEPHRITIS

SIGNAL SYMPTOMS ▶ UTI symptoms, back pain, fever

ICD-9 Codes		
	590.1	Acute pyelonephritis
	590.10	Acute pyelonephritis without lesion of medullary necrosis
	590.0	Chronic pyelonephritis

Pyelonephritis is a kidney infection, usually from bacteria, that spreads from the bladder.

Epidemiology
20% of community-acquired bacteremias are from pyelonephritis.
Incidence rate of 16 per 100,000.
100,000 people are hospitalized per year (mostly women).
Nosocomial rate is 73 per 100,000.

Etiology
Mainly bacterial infection of the renal pelvis, calyces, and nephron.
Causative agents:

E. coli—most common causative agent (80–90%)
Proteus and *Klebsiella* (4%–10%)
Staphylococcus aureus and *Candida albicans* (3%–10%)
Pseudomonas/Providencia (1%)—common in immunocompromised patients
Mycobacterium tuberculosis (<1%)
Torulopsis glabrata (<1%)—common in patients with diabetes
Vesicoureteral reflux may lead to pyelonephritis.

Use of a catheter or cystoscope or surgery on urinary tract may also cause infection.

Conditions such as prostate enlargement or kidney stones, which prevent efficient flow of urine, may also cause pyelonephritis.

Often misdiagnosed in children as gastroenteritis (vague symptoms)

Physiology and Pathophysiology

Infection and inflammation cause the kidneys to become enlarged.

Inflammatory process destroys parenchymal tissue, particularly in the cortex.

Arteries, arterioles, and glomeruli restrict the infection from becoming systemic.

Clinical Manifestations

Subjective

ADULTS

Acute onset (may occur with UTI or soon after)

Dysuria, frequency, and urgency may or may not be present

Shaking chills/fever

Flank, abdominal, or low back pain

Malaise

Headache

Blood in urine

Nausea and vomiting

CHILDREN

See Age-Related Considerations 8–2.

Objective

ADULTS

Usually fever or 101°F or greater

Patient appears sick, dehydrated

CVA tenderness

Abdominal tenderness on deep palpation of involved flank area

Vomiting

CHILDREN

See Age-Related Considerations 8–2

Differential Diagnosis

Adults

Cystitis (dysuria, frequency, with usually no systemic involvement; refer to "Cystitis")

Urethritis (external involvement only)

Vaginitis (verified via vaginal culture)

Acute abdominal disorder (no urine symptoms on UA, negative dipstick and culture)

A		Age-Related Considerations: Clinical Manifestations and Differential Diagnosis of Pyelonephritis in Children
Clinical Manifestations	Subjective	Failure to thrive (esp. in infants) Fever of unknown origin Irritability Strong odor to urine Abdominal pain Nausea/vomiting Enuresis Dysuria, frequency, urgency
	Objective	Fever > 101°F CVA tenderness Possible hematuria Possible hypertension
Differential Diagnosis		Urethritis (external involvement only) Vaginitis (verified via culture) Viral cystitis (no bacteria present) Foreign body (diagnosed via x-ray or IVP) Reflux (diagnosed via cystoscopy) Sexual Abuse (usually other symptoms present concurrently) Dysfunctional voiding Appendicitis (increased WBC count and rebound tenderness) Pelvic abscess PID (cervical motion tenderness, "angry" cervix and positive cultures)

Cervicitis/salpingitis (lower abdominal pain verified by culture, possible fever)

Renal calculi (hematuria and low back pain, diagnosed via IVP or CT scan)

Asymptomatic bacteria (no symptoms)

Appendicitis (right-lower-quadrant pain, elevated WBC count, rebound tenderness)

BPH (enlarged prostate, weak stream, no infection present)

Chlamydia/Mycoplasma (genital discharge verified by culture)

Children

See Age-Related Considerations 8–2

Diagnostic Tests

Microbiologic (features generally mimic cystitis)

UA test dipstick (indicates positive leukocyte esterase, nitrites, and blood)

Urine culture of 100,000 CFU per milliliter of urine

Blood culture are positive in up to 20% of women

Other:

Possible x-ray examination, IVP, ultrasonography, or CT scan to detect abnormalities in kidney, ureters, and/or bladder

Management/Treatment

Outpatient management
No high fever
No complicating factors
Consider hospitalization
Pregnant women
Infants <6 months with symptoms
Clients with fever >103°F
Clients with hypotension, respiratory distress, refractory nausea and
vomiting and unable to keep fluids down
Clients with co-morbidities such as diabetes mellitus

Pharmacologic Management

ANTIBIOTICS

Broad-spectrum antibiotics are needed. (*Note:* Avoid fluoroquinoline use in children.)

TMP/SMX (Bactrim/Septra), DS PO BID for 14 days
Ciprofloxacin (Cipro), 500 mg PO BID for 14 days
Levofloxacin (Levaquin), 250 mg PO QD for 14 days
Ofloxacin (Floxin), 400 mg PO BID for 14 days
Cefixime (Suprax), 400 mg PO QD for 14 days

OTHER MEDICATIONS

Phenazopyridine (Pyridium), 100–200 mg PO Q8H PRN for bladder
spasms
Acetaminophen (Tylenol), 650 mg Q4–6 H PRN for pain and fever

Client Education

Stress the importance of drinking fluids.
Instruct to take all antibiotics prescribed.
Tell patient to urinate at least every 3–4 hours.
Discuss common causes.
If no improvement in 24 hours, consider hospitalization and/or referral.

Follow-up

Follow-up with office visit in 24 hours to check hydration status and
symptoms.
Recheck urine in 3 days after initiation of antibiotics; untreated kidney
infection can lead to permanent scarring and/or damage.

Referral

Refer to urologist for initial occurrence for:

Pregnant women
Toxic clients
Diabetics
Elderly
Recurrence in children

RENAL CALCULI

SIGNAL SYMPTOMS ▶ hematuria, back pain

ICD-9 Code	592.0	Calculus of kidney

Renal calculi occurs when stones (of differing etiology) form in the urinary tract, causing pain, obstruction, and occasionally, infection.

Epidemiology

Age: 30–50 years
Calcium stones: Incidence greater in men than in women
Struvite stones: Incidence greater in women than in men

Etiology

Four different types of stones:

Calcium stones (80%)—Due to many causes (hypercalciuria, hyperpara-thyroidism)
Uric acid stones (5%)—Due to excessive uric acid production (e.g., gout), excessive fluid loss, and/or low urinary volume
Cystic stones (2%)—Occur in children; defect in filtration of cystine
Struvite stones—Due to highly alkaline urine, which is usually secondary to bacteria that cause splitting of urea

Physiology and Pathophysiology

Renal calculi form either by decreased urinary volume or by increases in the excretion of calcium, oxalate, uric acid, cystine, or xanthine in the urine.

Clinical Manifestations

Subjective

Severe, intermittent back pain

Table 8–9   Renal Cancer

Epidemiology	-Kidney cancer is the 10th most common cancer in the US -Affects 40,000 Americans per year, and more than 10,000 will die from it annually -Risk factors: —Cigarette smoking —Industrial exposure to carcinogens —Obesity —High protein diet
Clinical Manifestations	-Renal triad —Palpable flank mass —Hematuria —Pain -Other: weight loss, fever, fatigue, anemia, hypertension, cough, bone fractures
Diagnostic Tests	-CT scan -Ultrasound -MRI
Management	-Surgery—complete or nephron-sparing surgery

Pain may radiate to groin and/or testicles.
Gross hematuria.
Nausea and vomiting.
Abdominal distention.
(See Table 8–9.)

Objective
Restlessness
CVA tenderness
Tenderness with deep palpation of abdomen
No fever, unless secondary UTI
No guarding or rebound of abdomen

Differential Diagnosis
Back strain (positive musculoskeletal findings; UA and IVP normal)
Lumbar disk pain (positive musculoskeletal findings with possible
    neurologic component; UA and IVP normal)
Gastroenteritis (gastrointestinal symptoms [nausea, vomiting, diarrhea];
    UA and IVP normal)
Acute appendicitis (increased WBC count; right-lower-quadrant abdominal
    pain with rebound tenderness)
Colitis (possible bloody diarrhea; UA and IVP normal)
Peptic ulcer disease (abdominal pain, Hemoccult-positive; positive
    esophagogastroduodenoscopy)
Cholecystitis (right upper quadrant pain, positive Murphy's sign)

Diagnostic Tests
UA:
    Microscopic or gross hematuria
    Presence of crystals
    pH: acidic (uric acid or cystine stones); alkaline (struvite stones)
IVP or plain x-ray examination (to determine location of stone)

Management/Treatment
Generally management is on an outpatient basis, unless there is severe pain,
nausea, vomiting, or concurrent infection.

Pharmacologic Management
Pain management
Over-the-counter nonsteroidal antiinflammatory drugs (ibuprofen)
Narcotics (Lorcet, Tylenol #3, Vicodin, Percocet)

Nonpharmacologic Management
Push PO fluids
Strain urine to collect stone for analysis
Surgery (rare)

Client Education
Dietary changes

Referral

Refer to urologist if pain and symptoms persist longer than 2 weeks.

URINARY INCONTINENCE

SIGNAL SYMPTOMS ▶ difficulty maintaining urinary control

ICD-9 Codes	596.51	Bladder hyperactivity
	596.59	Detrusor instability
	625.6	Stress incontinence, female
	788.30	Incontinence NOS
	788.31	Urge incontinence
	788.32	Stress incontinence, male
	788.33	Mixed incontinence, female and male
	788.34	Incontinence without sensory awareness
	788.37	Continuous leakage

Urinary incontinence is the inability to stop urine leakage. There are several different types of incontinence:

Urge incontinence is the involuntary loss of urine, preceded by a strong urge to void whether or not the bladder is full.

Stress incontinence is the involuntary loss of urine with coughing, sneezing, laughing, or exercise.

Overflow incontinence is the loss of urine associated with overdistention of the bladder.

Mixed incontinence is when patients experience several different types of incontinence.

Epidemiology

Affects approximately 13 million Americans
Affects 10%–25% of women 15–64 years old
Elderly commonly affected

Etiology

Urge incontinence is caused by detrusor instability or detrusor hyperreflexia, both of which increase with aging.

Stress incontinence is when the intravesical pressure exceeds maximum urethral pressure and urethral hypermobility allows for the loss of urine. Another possible cause is intrinsic urethral sphincteric deficiency

Overflow incontinence is caused by overdistention of the bladder.

Mixed incontinence has mixed etiologies.

Physiology and Pathophysiology
Clinical Manifestations

Subjective

History: Include incontinence history, voiding diaries, medication review, and good review of systems (including ability to self-toilet)
(See Table 8–10.)

Table 8–10   Clinical Manifestations: Urinary Incontinence

Type	Clinical Manifestations
Urge Incontinence	Sudden urge to urinate Gets up frequently during the night to urinate Often does not reach the bathroom in time Urinates often; e.g. every 2 hours May wet the bed at night
Stress Incontinence	Leaks urine with coughing, sneezing, laughing and even exercising Uses bathroom frequently to avoid accidents May have urine leakage first thing in the morning
Overflow Incontinence	Gets up frequently during the night to urinate Weak, dribbling stream with minimal force Urinate small amounts May feel urge to urinate, but cannot
Mixed Incontinence	Mixed symptoms, which may make diagnosis difficult

Objective

Physical examination: include neurologic examination and genital examination, the cotton swab test
(See Table 8–10.)

Differential Diagnosis

Urge incontinence (see above definition)
Stress incontinence (see above definition)
Overflow incontinence (see above definition)
Delirium/confused state (review patient history and rule out acute infectious process)
Urinary tract infection (dysuria, frequency; refer to "Cystitis")
Atrophic urethritis or vaginitis (external involvement)

Diagnostic Tests

Urodynamics (to determine normal bladder sensations, pressure, and function)
Cystoscopy (to rule out lower-urinary-tract disorders)

Management/Treatment

Pharmacologic Management

(*Note:* Anticholinergic medications can cause dry mouth, confusion, blurred vision, and constipation.)

URGE INCONTINENCE

Tolterodine tartrate (Detrol), 2 mg BID
Oxybutynin chloride (Ditropan XL), 5 mg QD
Hyoscyamine (Urised/Levsin), 0.375 mg BID
Dicyclomine (Bentyl), 10–20 mg QID
Imipramine (Tofranil), 10–75 mg QHS

Nonpharmacologic Management

URGE INCONTINENCE:

Use absorbent undergarment products
Keep fixed or flexible voiding schedules
Utilize bladder retraining
Use bladder biofeedback
Monitor diet (avoid caffeine, spicy/acidic foods)

STRESS INCONTINENCE

Kegel or pelvic floor muscle exercises (must be done for at least 2–3 months before effective)
Biofeedback (and the use of weighted vaginal cones/devices)
Occlusive devices
Collagen implants
Surgery

Client Education

Discuss prescription and over-the-counter medications
Advise patient to maintain bowel regularity (avoid constipation by increasing fiber)
Advise patient to maintain a healthy weight
Advise patient to avoid smoking cigarettes

Referral

Refer to urologist, especially if complicated

REFERENCES

Benign Prostatic Hypertrophy

Mosier, W.A., Schymanski, T.J., & Walgren, K.D. (1998). Benign prostatic hyperplasia: Focusing on primary care. *Clinician Reviews, 8*(7), 55–75.

Pfeiffer, G.M., & Giacomarra, M. (1999). Benign prostatic hyperplasia. *Advance for Nurse Practitioners, 7*(4), 31–36.

Roberts, R.G. (1999). Evaluation of dysuria in men. *American Family Physician, 60*(3), 86–872.

Cystitis

Ahmed, S.M., & Swedlund, S.K. (1998). Evaluation and treatment of urinary tract infections in children. *American Family Physician, 57*(7), 1573–1582.

Armitage, K.B., Bologna, R.A., Horbach, N.S., & Whitmore, K.E. (1999). Best approaches to recurrent UTI. *Patient Care, 33*(11), 38–66.

Buttaro, T.M., Trybulski, J., Bailey, P.P., & Sandberg-Cook, J. (1999). *Primary care: A collaborative practice.* St. Louis: Mosby.

Delzell, J.E., & Lefevre, M.L. (2000). Urinary tract infection during pregnancy. *American Family Physician, 61*(3), 713–721.

Hellerstein, S. (1998). Urinary tract infections in children: Why they occur and how to prevent them. *American Family Physician, 57*(10), 2440–2446.

Kurowski, K. (2000). Bacterial cystitis in women: A primary care approach. *Women's Health in Primary Care, 3*(8), 554–565.

Kurowski, K. (1998). The woman with dysuria. *American Family Physician, 57*(9), 2155–2164.

Mulholland, S.G. (1999). UTI in women: How best to treat acute and recurrent infections. *Consultant, 39,* 1457–1464.

Orenstein, R., & Wong, E.S. (1999). Urinary tract infections in adults. *American Family Physician, 59,* 1225–1234.

Ross, J.H., & Kay, R. (1999). Pediatric urinary tract Infection and reflux. *American Family Physician, 59,* 1472–1480.

Enuresis

Cendron, M. (1999). Primary nocturnal enuresis. *American Family Physician, 59,* 1205–1216.

Lawrence, P.R. (1999). Nocturnal enuresis in children: Treatment is a family matter. *Advance for Nurse Practitioners, 7*(2), 41–96.

Mosier, W.A. (1998). Update on childhood enuresis. *Clinical Advisor, 1*(4), 32–34.

Interstitial Cystitis

Hanno, PM (1994). Diagnosis of interstitial cystitis. *Urology Clinics of North America, 21*(1), 63–66.

Kurowski, K. (1998). The woman with dysuria. *American Family Physician, 57*(9), 2155–2164.

Prostate Cancer

American Cancer Society. *Facts on Prostate Cancer* (brochure). Atlanta.

Cookson, M.S., & Smith, J.A. (2000). PSA testing: Update on diagnostic tools. *Consultant, 40*(4), 670–676.

Cotter, V. (1998). Prostate cancer: Examining the risks and benefits of screenings. *Advance for Nurse Practitioner, 8*(7), 51–53.

Goolsby, M.J. (1998). Screening, diagnosis and management of prostate cancer: Improving primary care outcomes. *Nurse Practitioner, 23*(3), 11–41.

Naitah, J., Zeiner, R.I., & Dekernion, J.B. (1998). Diagnosis and treatment of prostate cancer. *American Family Physician, 57*(7), 1531–1539, 1541–1542, 1545–1547.

Prostatitis

Armitage, K.B., Nickel, J.C., & Shoskes, D. (2000). Helping patients cope with Chronic prostatitis. *Patient Care, 34*(8), 22–32.

Buttaro, T.M., Trybulski, J., Bailey, P.P., & Sandberg-Cook, J. (1999). *Primary care: A collaborative practice.* St. Louis: Mosby.

Donovan, D.A., & Nicholas, P.K. (1997). Prostatitis: Diagnosis and treatment in primary care. *Nurse Practitioner, 22*(4), 144–156.

Steverner, J.J., & Easley, S.K. (2000). Treatment of prostatitis. *American Family Physician, 61*(10), 3015–3022.

Renal Calculi

Goldfarb, D.S., & Coe, F.L. (1999). Prevention of recurrent nephrolithiasis. *American Family Physician, 60*(8), 2269–2276.

Renal Cancer

Blutte, M.L., Droller, M.J., & Strup, S.E. (2000). Contemporary management of bladder cancer. *Patient Care, 34*(7), 72–90.

Thaller, T.R., & Wang, L.P. (1999). Evaluation of asymptomatic microscopic hematuria in adults. *American Family Physician, 60*(4), 1143–1152.

Urinary Incontinence

Bruskewitz, R.C., Ruoff, G.E., & Chancellor, M.B. (1999). Ending the silence about urinary incontinence: New treatment options for bladder control disorders. *Consultant, 39*(5), S3–S24.

Czarapata, B.J. (2000). Managing urinary incontinence. *Patient Care for the Nurse Practitioner, 2*(4), 37–47.

Culligan, P.J., & Sand, P.K. (1998). Involuntary urine loss in women: Help for a hidden problem. *Patient Care, 33*(20), 141–162.

Jay, J., & Staskin, D. (1998). Urinary incontinence: Strategies for effective diagnosis and management. *Advance for Nurse Practitioners, 8*(10), 32–37.

Winkler, H.A., & Sand, P.K. (1998). Stress incontinence: Options for conservative treatment. *Women's Health in Primary Care, 1*(3), 279–294.

RESOURCES

General

American Foundation for Urologic Disease
1120 N. Charles St., Ste. 401
Baltimore, MD 21201
Telephone: (800) 242-2383

American Urological Association
Telephone: (877) DRY-LIFE

Bladder Health Council
c/o American Foundation for Urologic Disease
300 W. Pratt St., Ste. 401
Baltimore, MD 21201
Telephone: (800) 242-2383

National Bladder Foundation
Telephone: (877) BLADDER or (877) 252-3337

National Kidney Foundation
Fax: (212) 779-0068
Web site: http://www.kidney.org

Enuresis

National Enuresis Society
7777 Forest Lane, Ste. C-737
Dallas, TX 75230-2518
Telephone: (800) NES-8080
Web site: http://www.peds.umn.edu/centers/nes

Interstitial Cystitis

The Interstitial Cystitis Association
P.O. Box 1553
Madison Square Station
New York, NY 10159-1553
Telephone: (212) 979-6057 or (800) HELP-ICA

Prostatitis/Prostate Cancer

American Cancer Society
Telephone: (800) 227-2345

Prostate Health Council/American Foundation for Urologic Disease
    1128 N. Charles Street, Ste. 401
    Baltimore, MD 21201
    Telephone: (800) 242-2383

Prostatitis Foundation
    1063 30th St., Box 8
    Smithshire, IL 61478
    Telephone: (888) 891-4200
    Fax: (309) 325-7184
    Web site: http://www.prostate.org

Urinary Incontinence

National Association for Continence
    Telephone: (800) 252-3337

Simons Foundation for Continence
    Telephone: (800) 237-4666

ALZA Corporation
    Telephone: (888) DXL 1-A-DAY
    Web site: http://www.ditropanxl.com

Chapter 9

REPRODUCTIVE SYSTEM

AMENORRHEA

SIGNAL SYMPTOM ▶ absence of menstruation

ICD-9 Code	626.0	Absence of menstruation

Primary amenorrhea is the absence of menses by age 16 or the absence of menses after age 14 when normal growth and signs of secondary sexual characteristics are present. Secondary amenorrhea is the absence of menses for three cycles or 6 months in a female client with previously normal menses.

Epidemiology

Secondary amenorrhea has a prevalence rate of 3%–4% in the U.S. population, not including pregnancy. Incidence is higher in particular subgroups such as college students (stress) and athletes (3%–5% and 5%–60%, respectively). Primary amenorrhea is less common (0.3%).

Etiology

Primary Amenorrhea

Uterovaginal abnormalities
Imperforate hymen
Agenesis of the uterus and vagina
Turner's syndrome
Constitutional delay

Secondary Amenorrhea

PHYSIOLOGICAL

Pregnancy and lactation
Corpus luteal cyst
Menopause

HYPOTHALAMIC DYSFUNCTION (CAUSING ESTROGEN PRODUCTION TO BE INADEQUATE
AND A FAILURE OF LUTEINIZING HORMONE [LH] SURGE)

Emotional stress
Strenuous exercise
Anorexia nervosa

Severe dieting
Chronic illness
Low body mass index

HYPERPROLACTINEMIA

Medications:
    Phenothiazines
    Butyrophenones
    Thioxanthenes
    Methyldopa
    Reserpine
    Metoclopramide
    Meclizine
    Cimetidine
    Amitriptyline
    Imipramine
    Steroids
    Danazol
    Methamphetamine/cocaine abuse
    Corticotropin-releasing hormone–releasing factor analogs
    Temporary post–birth-control-pill amenorrhea (usually resolves in 6 months)

OTHER CAUSES

Chemotherapy or pelvic irradiation
Uncontrolled endocrinopathies
Prolactinoma (pituitary prolactin-secreting tumors)
Nipple stimulation
Chest wall trauma
Prolonged elevation in thyroid-stimulating hormone

OVARIAN FAILURE

Anovulation
Premature menopause
Hypothyroidism
Polycystic ovaries (polycystic ovarian disease [PCOs])

UTEROVAGINAL ABNORMALITIES

Asherman's syndrome (intrauterine adhesions)

Physiology and Pathophysiology

In normal individuals, the mean age of onset of menarche is 13.3 years, with a range of 11–17. Ninety percent of healthy teenagers begin menses by age 16 years.

Clinical Manifestations

Subjective

    Nausea, fatigue, breast tenderness, and urinary frequency (may represent symptoms of early pregnancy).

Symptoms of ovarian failure, including hot flashes, vaginal dryness, and dyspareunia.

Emotional lability (may be evident in clients with anorexia, ovarian failure, and pregnancy).

Objective

Missed menses.

Radical changes in eating behavior, weight or exercise habits (may be present with hypothalamic dysfunction, and may also be evident in the presence of a chronic illness).

Galactorrhea, headaches, and visual changes (may be prolactinoma).

Abnormal reflexes (may be related to thyroid disease and/or hypothalamic dysfunction).

Hirsutism, acne and oily skin (may be seen with PCOs).

Atrophic vaginal mucosa (accompanies ovarian failure).

Absence of breast and pubic hair development in clients over age 14 (uterovaginal abnormalities implicated).

Imperforate hymen may be one visible anomaly on examination.

Differential Diagnosis

Any of these diagnoses may present with amenorrhea and they should be ruled out if appropriate.

Pregnancy and lactation

Emotional stress, strenuous exercise, anorexia nervosa, or severe dieting

Chronic illness

Endocrinopathies

Hyperprolactinemia

Menopause

Anovulation

Polycystic ovaries

Asherman's syndrome or other uterine abnormalities

Diagnostic Tests

Pregnancy test (to rule out pregnancy)

TSH level (may be hypothyroid)

Serum prolactin (if elevated, perform magnetic resonance imaging [MRI] of anterior pituitary)

Progesterone challenge (if pregnant, hypothyroidism and pituitary tumor ruled out)

Follicle-stimulating hormone (FSH) and LH levels

Hysteroscopy

Management/Treatment

Restore menses. Hypothalamic dysfunction resolves when secretion of gonadotropin-releasing hormone (GnRH) decreases.

Primary Amenorrhea

Refer to pediatric endocrinologist.

Secondary Amenorrhea

Step 1: Rule out pregnancy.

Step 2: Check TSH. Treat if needed.

Check serum prolactin. If elevated perform MRI of anterior pituitary.

Step 3: Perform progesterone challenge:

If positive, anovulation.

If negative, give estrogen and progesterone. If no response to combined hormones, indicates uterine or outflow abnormality, therefore refer to gynecologist. If positive response to combined hormones, indicates hypoestrogenic amenorrhea.

Step 4: Check FSH and LH. If elevated, indicates gonadal failure; if normal or low, perform MRI of sella turcica; if normal, indicates hypothalamic amenorrhea.

Step 5: Perform hysteroscopy to determine uterine anomalies.

Hyperprolactinemia

Resolved when the stimulus is corrected or when suppressive medication is used. Bromocriptine (Parlodel) inhibits the secretion of prolactin as long as the medication is taken. It re-establishes fertility and normal menses. Start at 2.5 mg at bedtime to avoid side effects. Increase to twice daily. If prolactin levels not normalized, increase to 2.5–5.0 mg every 4 hours until normal prolactin level obtained. Menses normally return 6–12 weeks after prolactin level normalizes.

Medroxyprogesterone acetate (Provera): 10 mg/day for 10 days each month to induce menses if fertility is not desired, and if client cannot tolerate bromocriptine.

Hypothalamic Dysfunction

Provide estrogen supplementation until normal hormonal function returns to protect against bone loss. This may be achieved with oral contraceptive pills (OCPs) or combination estrogen/progestin therapy.

For exercise-induced amenorrhea, decrease training by 3–5%.

Anorexia-induced amenorrhea requires a multidisciplinary referral.

Discourage smoking and encourage adequate calcium intake to prevent bone loss.

Ovarian Failure

Clomiphene citrate (Clomid) to induce ovulation.

Hormone treatment options are the same as for clients with estrogen deficiency.

Weight loss in clients with PCOS to help slow down estrogen production.

Exercise.

Uterovaginal Abnormalities

Refer to gynecologist. Asherman's syndrome is treated by curettage or hysteroscopy and hormone-replacement therapy (HRT).

Congenital anomalies may require reconstructive surgery.

Client Education
Amenorrhea does not necessarily protect a client from becoming pregnant.

Follow-up
Reevaluate every few months to ascertain if further testing is needed.

Periodic discontinuation of hormone replacement in clients with anovulation and hypothalamic amenorrhea is recommended to determine if ovulation and menses resume spontaneously, whether pregnancy is desired, or whether alternative birth control is preferable.

Referral
Refer to pediatric endocrinologist for primary amenorrhea.

Refer to gynecologist or endocrinologist if indicated.

In the case of PCOS and desired fertility refer to obstetrician–gynecologist/infertility specialist.

Refer to endocrinologist or neurosurgeon for macroprolactinomas.

BREAST CANCER

SIGNAL SYMPTOMS ▶ breast pain, mass

ICD-9 Codes	174	Malignant neoplasm of female breast
	174.0	Nipple and areola
	174.1	Central portion
	174.2	Upper-inner quadrant
	174.3	Lower-inner quadrant
	174.4	Upper-outer quadrant
	174.5	Lower-outer quadrant
	174.6	Axillary tail
	174.9	Unspecified
	233.0	Carcinoma in situ of breast
	611.71	Mastodynia
	611.72	Breast lump/mass

Breast cancer is a malignant neoplasm of the breast.

Epidemiology
Breast cancer is second only to lung cancer as cause of cancer deaths in all women; however, it is the leading cause of cancer deaths in premenopausal women (estimated that 1 in 28 women will die from breast cancer).

Most common cancer in American women (32% of all cancers in this population).

Risk of developing breast cancer increases with age (at age 40, risk is 1 in 217; at 70, 1 in 14; at 90, 1 in 8).

Three of four breast cancers are found in postmenopausal women.

White women (highest rate overall) and African-American women (highest incidence under age 50; overall, highest death rate) have breast cancer incidence and death rates higher than those of other races and ethnic groups.

Breast cancer mortality has declined at an average of 1.8% per year because of improved breast cancer treatments and mammogram screening. (See Table 9–1.)

Etiology

Severity of breast cancer at time of diagnosis increases with age
See Risk Factors 9–1.

Physiology and Pathophysiology

Ductal carcinoma in situ: Within the ductal system; microcalcifications found on mammography; may grow for years; frequently nonpalpable.

Infiltrating ductal carcinoma: Breaks through duct walls; accounts for 75% of cancers).

Lobular carcinoma in situ: Terminal ducts of the lobules.

Infiltrating lobular carcinoma: Uncommon, accounts for only 5%–10% of breast tumors.

Inflammatory breast carcinoma: Lymph vessels in the skin of the breast are blocked by the cancer cells, causing the breast to become red,

Table 9–1 Breast Cancer in Men

Incidence is 1% of that in women

Because breast cancer is rarely suspected in men, it more often progresses to an advanced stage. Also, since men have little breast tissue, cancers do not need to grow very far before they spread beyond the breast. On the other hand, because men have less breast tissue than women, it is easier to feel small masses in their breasts and cancers tend to be slightly smaller in men when they are first found

Mean age at diagnosis is 65, but breast cancer can strike men of all ages

Most breast lumps in men are due to gynecomastia and not cancer

Infiltrating ductal cancer is the most common tumor type found in men

Lymph node involvement is similar to that found in female breast cancer

Risk Factors:

Known risk factors: aging, radiation exposure, estrogen administration (such as used for prostate cancer), and diseases associated with hyperestrogenism (e.g., Klinefelter's syndrome or severe liver disease such as cirrhosis), men who have a number of female relatives with breast cancer or who are from families in which the BRCA2 mutation on chromosome 13q has been identified.

Possible risk factors: alcohol consumption (greater than 2 drinks per day for women, amount not yet quantified for men), adult obesity, sedentary life-style

Clinical Manifestations:

Signs and symptoms: lump or swelling, skin dimpling or puckering, nipple retraction, redness or scaling of the nipple or breast skin, discharge from a nipple

Diagnostic Tests

Diagnostic mammograms are used for men with signs/symptoms of breast cancer

Management/Treatment

Treatment for men is the same as for women, although orchidectomy may be indicated and breast-conserving surgery is rarely used.

The TNM staging system for male breast cancer is identical to the staging system for female breast cancer.

At the same stage of cancer, the prognosis for men is identical to that for women

Resources

The American Cancer Society Male Breast Cancer Resource Center

National Cancer Institute

RF 9–1 Risk Factors: *Breast Cancer*

- Increasing age—most influential risk factor (77% of new cases and 84% of breast cancer deaths occur in women aged 50 and older)
- Family history of breast or ovarian cancer, especially first degree relatives (this includes male relatives) or any breast cancer in any relative that is early in onset or bilateral.
- Personal history of previous breast biopsy (fibrocystic changes, benign conditions of atypia or hyperplasia)
- Personal history of previous breast cancer
- Mutated BRCA-1 and BRCA-2 genes together account for 3–10% of all cases of breast cancer and the risk for breast cancer in women with either of these mutated genes is 80% to 85% by age 70 (women with BRCA1 also have a 44% risk of ovarian cancer by age 70). Ashkenzai Jewish descendants are at higher risk for carrying these mutated genes
- Women age 45 or older who have at least 75% dense tissue on a mammogram (not only does dense breast tissue make it more difficult to see tumors, it is related to an increased chance of developing breast cancer in older women)
- Nulliparous or having first full-term pregnancy after age 30
- Not breast feeding (however, data are inconsistent on the effect of lactation on breast cancer risk)
- Length of exposure to estrogens: early menarche (<12 years), late menopause (>55 years)
  Hormone replacement therapy (HRT) (estrogen only or estrogen-plus-progestin for more than 5–10 years—increased risk seems to disappear 5–10 years after HRT is discontinued)
  Oral contraceptives (Ocs) (may increase risk by 16%, increased risk disappears 10 years after OC is discontinued; however, having a first degree relative with breast cancer and have ever used the earlier, stronger formulations of OCs may put a women at high risk)
- Chest radiation at age 30 or younger for conditions such as Hodgkin's disease
- Consumption of 2 or more alcoholic drinks per day (2 drinks per day may increase breast cancer risk by 25%; in general, there is a linear correlation between increase in breast cancer incidence and alcohol consumption and this exists regardless of the type of alcoholic beverage consumed)
- Altered estrogen metabolism due to: high fat diet (however there is new research that low-fat diets do not decrease breast cancer risk), obesity (primarily central obesity and obesity after menopause), physical inactivity
- Cigarette smoke exposure in adolescence
- Augmentation mammoplasty (breast implants), stress, caffeine, coffee, underarm shaving and antiperspirant use, and cigarette smoking as an adult do not appear to increase the risk of breast cancer.
- Breast reduction surgery appears to reduce breast cancer risk in proportion to the amount of tissue removed

swollen, warm with an peau d'orange appearance. Nipple retracts and/
or has a discharge. In addition, axillary and supraclavicular lymphadenopathy may be present. Rapid cancer growth and metastasis are
common.

Clinical Manifestations

Subjective

Palpable lump (upper outer quadrant most frequent site, 85% are painless)

Nipple discharge (only in 2% of breast cancers), nipple retraction, and/or irritation

Skin edema, redness, heat, tenderness, and/or dimpling

Enlarged and/or tender axillary, supraclavicular, and/or infraclavicular lymph nodes

Objective

Fixed, poorly defined, usually painless mass (any breast mass in a postmenopausal woman should be assumed to be cancer (85% of breast masses in women 55 years and older are malignant; best time to examine questionable mass or thickening is days 3–10 of menstrual cycle)

Spontaneous (not self-induced) nipple discharge, irritation, retraction; dimpled breast skin (peau d'orange); nodal involvement—axillary, supraclavicular; skin retraction (Cooper ligament retraction)

Differential Diagnosis

Fibrocystic breast (presence of single or multiple cysts palpable in the breasts)

Fibroadenoma (benign tumor, nontender, encapsulated, round, movable, and firm)

Abscess (cavity containing pus and surrounded by inflamed tissue)

Rupture of implanted breast augmentation device

Mastitis (inflammatory condition of breast—pain, swelling, redness, axillary lymphadenopathy)

Thrombosis of a superficial vein

Intraductal papilloma (benign epithelial neoplasm characterized by branching or lobular tumor)

Diagnostic Tests

Diagnostic mammography

Ultrasonography (distinguishes between cystic and solid mass) especially if patient <30 years old

MRI (to stage and identify multifocal or multicentric involvement)

Biopsy:

Fine-needle aspiration (FNA) and core needle biopsy

Image-guided biopsy

Excisional/surgical biopsy

Stereotactic biopsy

Sentinel node mapping

Lung, liver, bone scans

Hormone receptor assays (to determine presence of estrogen receptors)

Microscopic examination of nipple discharge

(See Table 9–2.)

Table 9–2 Triple Diagnosis of a Solid Breast Mass

"Triple diagnosis" of a solid breast mass:

If the clinical breast exam, mammogram, and fine needle aspiration (FNA) biopsy results are benign (may also want a negative diagnostic ultrasound), with 99% accuracy can consider the lesion benign and the client should be offered the choice between open biopsy or follow-up visits at 3 month intervals. However, if anyone of the above is questionable, should have open biopsy performed.

Breast cancer that is undiagnosed or misdiagnosed accounts for the largest number of malpractice claims, the largest number of paid claims, and the highest overall litigation expenses. 75% of these suits involve a patient less that 45 years of age, a false-negative mammogram, and a self-discovered breast mass.

Management/Treatment

Stage of disease determines treatment (see Table 9–3).

Pharmacologic Management

HORMONAL THERAPY

Used for estrogen-receptor-positive tumors; side effects include hot flashes and other menopausal symptoms.

Tamoxifen (Nolvadex): An estrogen antagonist in the breast; resistance to tamoxifen generally develops 2 to 5 years into the course of the treatment; increased risk of blood clots and endometrial cancer.

Letrozole (Femara) and anastrozole (Arimidex): Newer drugs; true antiestrogens, significantly inhibit estrogen productions, no estrogenic side effects such as increased risk of endometrial cancer; work as well if not better than tamoxifen; also approved for initial therapy of metastatic breast cancer.

CHEMOTHERAPY

Used for estrogen-receptor-negative tumors.

Nonpharmacologic Management

SURGICAL OPTIONS

Lumpectomy: Removal of the lump usually followed by 6 weeks of radiation

Partial mastectomy: Removal of one fourth or more of breast, followed by 6–7 weeks of external-beam radiation therapy

Simple or total mastectomy: Removal of entire breast but not of axillary lymph nodes or chest wall muscles under the breast

Modified radical mastectomy: Removal of entire breast and some of the axillary lymph nodes

Radical mastectomy: Removal of entire breast, axillary lymph nodes, and underlying chest wall muscles

Radiation after lumpectomy or mastectomy

Ovarian ablation (removal of ovaries): Used in premenopausal women with estrogen-receptor-positive tumors

Bone marrow transplantation plus high doses of chemotherapy: Under study for patients with metastatic breast cancer.

Table 9–3   Stage of breast cancer at time of diagnosis and survival rate at 5 years

Stage at Initial Diagnosis	Percent diagnosed at Each Stage	Five-year Survival Rate
In situ	15%	97%
Locally invasive	52%	97%
Regional metastasis	27%	76%
Distant metastasis	3%	20%
Not staged	3%	Not applicable

Complementary/Alternative Therapies

DIET

Diets high in vegetables and in proteins from poultry and dairy products may increase survival of breast cancer; however, diets that are merely low-fat do not appear to increase survival rates.

HERBAL REMEDIES

Phragmites communis (reed herb)—Active ingredients include vitamins A, C, B$_1$, and B$_2$—in Oriental medicine it is used for breast cancer

Melilotus officinalis (sweet clover)—Used for lymphedema (has diuretic properties and improves lymphatic kinetics); monitor liver enzyme levels; steep 1 to 2 teaspoonfuls in boiling water, strain after 5–10 minutes.

Ginger root—Used for appetite stimulation and queasiness

HOMEOPATHY

Scrophularia nodosa (Figwort)—For lymphedema; 15–20 drops TID

ACUPUNCTURE

Used for nausea, pain, stress relief

Few side effects

AROMATHERAPY

Used for anxiety, insomnia, nausea, pain

Precautions/contraindications: Skin allergies, asthma

MAGNET THERAPY

Used for muscle, nerve, and joint pain

Contraindications: Cardiac pacemakers, defibrillators, thrombocytopenia, bleeding disorders, anticoagulant therapy

MASSAGE THERAPY

Used for pain (including postoperative), stress, complications of lymphedema

Precautions/contraindications: Do not massage any tumor/metastatic sites, rash, unhealed wound, anticoagulant therapy, thrombocytopenia

MEDITATION

Used for hypertension, chronic pain, stress

THERAPEUTIC TOUCH

Used for pain and to increase sense of well-being

YOGA

Used for hypertension, stress, and to increase flexibility and improve breathing
Precautions/contraindications: Yoga positions following back injury or
   surgery

Client Education

BREAST SELF-EXAMINATION

Premenopausal—1 week after menses
Postmenopausal—Same date each month

PREVENTIVE MEASURES

Avoidance of alcohol, radiation exposure
Increased physical activity and prevention of obesity to alter estrogen
   metabolism

PHARMACOLOGIC THERAPIES

Currently two selective estrogen-receptor modulators—tamoxifen (Nolvadex) and raloxifene (Evista)—are being studied in trials to evaluate benefits,
including ability to prevent breast cancer. Tamoxifen was approved by the FDA
in 1998 for reduction of breast cancer risk.

DIET

Diets that include daily intake of fruits, green and yellow vegetables, soy-
beans, and soy products have been associated with a protective effect against
breast cancer. Beta-carotene (e.g., carrots, tomatoes, citrus fruits, spinach) may
provide protection against cancer due to its antioxidant properties, which inhibit
factors in the early stages of cancer.

Phytoestrogens (isoflavones such as soy, garbanzo beans, and legumes, and
lignans such as whole-grain cereal, onions, carrots, pears, cherries, apples, and
olive and linseed oils) have been associated with decreased incidence of breast
cancer; those who consume Asian diets have a low breast cancer rate, such diets
usually contain 40–80 mg of isoflavones per day.

EXERCISE

Aerobic exercise immediately after high-dose chemotherapy is safe, partially
prevents loss of physical conditioning, and may decrease toxic side effects of the
therapy.

Do not breast-feed with breast cancer—lactation promotes elevated prolactin
levels, which may in turn promote the breast cancer.

Early detection is important (See Table 9–4).

Follow-up

As indicated by diagnosis and treatment. (See Table 9–4 for screening guidelines.)

Referral

Refer to oncologist.

**Table 9–4   Early Detection and Breast Cancer Screening
Guidelines**

Early Detection
Women's Health and Cancer Rights Act
  Signed into law 10/21/98
  Contains new protections for breast cancer patients who elect breast reconstruction with
    a mastectomy
  For questions/concerns re this law, contact Department of Labor's hotline (202) 219-
    8776 or your State Insurance Commissioner's office

The National Breast and Cervical Cancer Early Detection Program (NBCCEDP)
  Established by the Breast and Cervical Cancer Mortality Prevention Act of 1990
  Provides free breast and cervical cancer screening and follow-up diagnostic services to
    underserved women
  Services were extended by the Breast and Cervical Cancer Prevention and Treatment Act
    of 2000, which gives states the option to provide medical assistance through Medicaid
    to eligible women who were screened for and found to have breast or cervical cancer,
    including precancerous conditions, through the NBCCEDP
  For further information call 1-888-842-6355, or contact www.cdc.gov/cancer/nbccedp

Breast Cancer Screening Guidelines

Age	Test	U.S. Preventive Task Force	American Cancer Society	National Cancer Institute
20–39	Self-Breast Exam	No recommendation	Monthly	No recommendation
	Clinical Breast Exam	Annually starting at age 35 for high-risk women only	Every 3 years	Every 3 years
	Screening Mammogram	No recommendation	Baseline mammogram between ages 35–40	No recommendation
40–49	Self-Breast Exam	No recommendation	Monthly	No recommendation
	Clinical Breast Exam	Annually	Annually	Annually
	Screening Mammogram	No recommendation	Every 1 year	Every 1–2 years
50+	Self-Breast Exam	No recommendation	Monthly	No recommendation
	Clinical Breast Exam	Annually (age 50–69)	Annually	Annually
	Screening Mammogram	Every 1–2 years (age 50–69)	Annually	Annually

Other Considerations
  Women who are at an increased risk of breast cancer should be considered for screening
    mammograms before age 40 or for screening on an annual basis. For example, if a first
    or second degree family member has or had breast cancer, starting annual mammo-
    grams at an age 10 years younger than the age that relative's cancer was diagnosed
    should be considered.
  Mammograms are not contraindicated for women who are breast-feeding, but it is recom-
    mended that they express their breast milk before getting a mammogram.
  For women who do not perform self-breast exam, annual clinical breast exams may be
    appropriate at any age

CERVICAL CANCER/ABNORMAL PAPANICOLAOU (Pap) SMEAR

SIGNAL SYMPTOM▶ abnormal vaginal bleeding

ICD-9 Codes	180.9	Cervical malignancy
	219.0	Benign cervical neoplasm
	233.1	Cervical carcinoma in situ
	622.1	Cervical dysplasia

Cervical cancer is a progressive neoplasm of the uterine cervix.

Epidemiology

Annually, 15,000 women will be diagnosed with cervical cancer.
4000–5000 will die as a result of this disease.
Third most common type of gynecologic cancer (after uterine and ovarian).
Rare in adolescence; average age at diagnosis of invasive cervical cancer, 50–55 years.
Average age at diagnosis of carcinoma in situ of the cervix, 25–35 years.
5-year survival rates (direct relationship between survival and stage of disease at time of diagnosis).
   Nearly 100% for preinvasive cervical cancer
   91% for early invasive cervical cancer
   13% for metastasis at time of diagnosis
   70% for all stages of cervical cancer combined
African-American women have a cervical cancer death rate twice the national average; the rate for Hispanic and Native American women is above the national average.
Of those with newly diagnosed invasive cervical cancer, 60%–80% have not had a Pap smear in the past 5 years, some have never had a Pap smear.

Etiology

Cause of cervical cancer is unknown; however, there are several risk factors (see Risk Factors 9–2).

Physiology and Pathophysiology

Metaplasia

Benign cell growth or repair, normal transformation process from columnar to squamous epithelium

Dysplasia

Precancerous lesions that are not full thickness of the cervical epithelium
Preinvasive malignancies
   Classified as stage 0 cervical cancer
   Carcinoma in situ (CIS)—Precancerous lesions that are the full thickness of the cervical epithelium, but do not penetrate the basement membrane

RF 9–2 Risk Factors: *Cervical Cancer*

- Human papillomavirus (HPV) infection (associated with 80% of cervical cancers)
- History of other sexually transmitted diseases (STDs) (past infection with Chlamydia trachomatis, especially serotypes G, I, and D, has been associated with cervical squamous cell carcinoma)
- More than 2 lifetime sexual partners (some sources cite more than one partner, others only cite "multiple" partners)
- High-risk sexual partner (heterosexual or homosexual; has history of multiple partners; has condyloma or a history of genital warts; has had intercourse with a woman who has abnormal Paps, genital warts, or developed cervical cancer)
- Early age of first intercourse (depending on source, before age 17, 18, or 20)
- Unprotected sex at any age
- History of prior lower genital tract neoplasia
- Greater than 3 years since last Pap
- A prior abnormal Pap
- Contraceptive hormones (associations have been with long-term oral contraceptive use, e.g., greater than 5 years; oral contraceptives can cause eversion of columnar epithelium, which is more susceptible to inflammation than squamous epithelium; may be related to folic acid deficiency; may be related to presence of HPV since the cells of HPV lesions have a significantly greater number of estrogen and progesterone receptors than normal cervical cells)
- Smoking—appears to enhance the progression from HPV to dysplasia; tobacco byproducts, such as nicotine and cotinine, have been found in cervical mucus, it is believed these byproducts may damage cervical cellular DNA; may cause cervical immunosuppression; estimates range from 2 to 7-fold increased risk of getting cervical cancer)
- Diet poor in fruits and vegetables may be linked to increased risk of cervical cancer (there is evidence that folate and beta carotene deficiencies may contribute to the development of dysplasia)
- Immunosuppression (HIV, organ transplant, chronic use of steroids, chemotherapy; in these women cervical disease may be more severe and prolonged)
- Poor women are at greater risk—this may be due to lack of regular health care, including Pap tests, and to poor nutrition
- High parity (however, pregnancy itself is not a risk factor, nor does pregnancy impact the course of the disease)
- Radiation exposure
- Diethylstilbestrol (DES) in utero exposure (DES is a nonsteroidal estrogen)
- Oral contraceptive in utero exposure—no evidence at this time, however, given documented effect of DES exposure, would be prudent to carefully monitor women who have had in utero exposure to OCs.
- Possible genetic predisposition to cervical tumors

Cervical adenocarcinoma in situ—Precursor to invasive adenocarcinoma of the cervix

Classification systems for cervical-cell abnormalities (See Table 9–5.)

Malignancies

Squamous-cell carcinoma—85%–90% of all cervical cancers; usually occurs in the transformation zone and is preceded by cervical dysplasia and CIS.

Table 9–5   Cervical Cancer: Classification Systems

Classification Systems	Description
Class System (outdated)	Range from Class 0 (Pap specimen unsatisfactory for evaluation) to Class 5 (carcinoma)
Cervical intraepithelial neoplasia (CIN) System (classifies squamous cell abnormalities	CIN 1—mild dysplasia CIN 2—moderate dysplasia CIN 3—severe dysplasia to carcinoma in situ
Bethesda System (classifies squamous and glandular cell abnormalities; current standard for Pap smears)	*Adequacy of Specimens* Satisfactory for evaluation Satisfactory for evaluation but limited Unsatisfactory for evaluation *General Categorization* Within normal limits Benign cellular changes (see descriptive diagnosis) Epithelial cell abnormalities (see descriptive diagnosis)
	Descriptive Diagnoses Benign Cellular Changes Infection (Trichomonas vaginalis, Candida species, predominance of coccobacilli/Actinomyces species, Herpes simplex virus, other) Reactive changes associated with i(includes typical repair), atrophic vaginitis, radiation, IUD, other Epithelial Cell Abnormalities -Squamous Cell ASCUS: Atypical squamous cells of undetermined significance LGSIL: Low-grade squamous intraepithelial lesions HGSIL: High-grade squamous intraepithelial lesions AGUS: Atypical glandular cells of undetermined significance; high risk for cervical and other gynecologic pathology Squamous Cell Carcinoma -Glandular Cell Endometrial cells, cytologically benign AGUS Endocervical adenocarcinoma Endometrial adenocarcinoma Extrauterine adenocarcinoma Adenocarcinoma, not otherwise specified
National Cancer Institute	Stage 0—CIS; treatment options include LEEP, laser therapy, conization, cryotherapy; 5-year survival rate:100%
	Stage IA -Limited to cervix; microscopiclesions only; treatment options inlcude total hysterectomy conization, radical hysterectomy, intracavitary radiation alone; 5-year survival rate:95+%
	Stage IB—Limited to cervix, clinical lesions; treatment options include radiation therapy, radical hysterectomy and bilateral pelvic lympadenectomy, same plus postoperative total pelvic irradiation and chemotherapy; 5-year survival rate:85%-90% Stage IIA—Carcinoma extended to no more than upper 2/3rds of vagina; treatment options include radiation therapy, radical hysterectomy and pelvic lympadenectomy, Same plus postoperative total pelvic irradiation plus chemotherapy, radiation therapy and chemotherapy; 5-year survival rate:80%-90% Stage IIB—Parametrial involvement; treatment options include radiation therapy and chemotherapy; 5-year survival rate:65%

Table continued on following page.

Table 9–5   Cervical Cancer: Classification Systems (*Continued*)

Classification Systems	Description
	Stage IIIA—Carcinoma extended to lower third of vagina; treatment options include radiation therapy and chemotherapy; 5-year survival rate:40%
	Stage IIIB—Carcinoma extended to pelvic wall and/or blocks urine flow to the bladder; treatment options include radiation therapy and chemotherapy; 5-year survival rate:40%
	Stage IVA—Carcinoma spread to adjacent organs; treatment options include radiation therapy and chemotherapy; 5-year survival rate:<20%
	Stage IVB—Carcinoma spread to distant organs; treatment options include chemotherapy and palliative irradiation therapy; 5-year survival rate:<20%
	Recurrent cervical cancer—Postoperative recurrence treatment options include radiation therapy and chemotherapy, palliative chemotherapy

Adenocarcinoma—10%–15% of all cervical cancers.

Mixed or adenosquamous carcinoma—Features of both types of cervical cancer.

What has been described as rapidly progressive cervical cancer is considered by some to actually be prior inadequate screening of endocervical cells

Human papillomavirus (HPV) infection

Whether HPV leads to cancer appears to be dependent on initial immune response to the virus plus a continued high viral load.

High-risk/oncogenic HPV types are 16 and 18.

High viral loads of oncogenic HPV types are predictive of persistent or progressive dysplasia and can precede diagnosis of CIS by 10 years.

Most visible raised bumpy genital warts are caused by types 6 and 11 and are considered low-risk viruses.

Clinical Manifestations

Subjective

Cervical dysplasias/preinvasive stages are usually asymptomatic.

Invasive cervical cancer.

Abnormal vaginal bleeding is the most significant symptom (most commonly postcoital, intermenstrual spotting, or postmenopause; may also see spotting immediately following menses or douching).

Persistent vaginal discharge (most commonly serosanguineous or purulent; pale, watery, pink, or brown discharges have also been reported).

Dyspareunia

Advanced invasive cervical cancer.

Persistent aching pelvic, lower back pain, or leg pain (tumor against nerve).

Weight loss, severe fatigue, anorexia, urinary frequency, urgency, hematuria
Rectal bleeding, urine or feces loss from the vagina (through a fistula
from the bladder or rectum)

Objective

Dyplasia and precancerous conditions:

Cervix may appear normal or may be irregular, enlarged, firm, irritated,
or inflamed and/or may bleed easily. (Do not use term *friable* as this
term medically and legally means "cancer.")

Invasive cervical cancer:

Cervix may appear normal or have erosion, ulcer, lesion, and/or tumor
(exocervix may appear normal if the tumor lies in the endocervix, but
will feel indurated and tumor may protrude from the os on palpation).
Serosanguineous or purulent strong-smelling discharge.
Possible induration of parametria and uterosacral ligaments.
Pap smear (it is a screening test, not a diagnostic tool) (see Table 9–6).

Table 9–6   Pap Smears

Pap smears are performed for detection of squamous and endocervical glandular dypsplasias
and malignancies

Frequency

American Cancer Society (ACS) recommends starting annual testing at age 18 or when the
client become sexually active, whichever occurs first

Premenopausal and postmenopausal women with intact uterus:

Annual Paps

ACS recommends that if a woman has 3 annual negative Paps in a row, the provider
may wish to do Paps less often, such as every 2 to 3 years.

Posthysterectomy Pap smears may be done every 3–5 years (or omitted altogether) unless
one of the following conditions is met according to ACOG recommendations:

1. The cervix is present.
2. There is a history of a significant abnormality detected on a previous Pap test.
3. The hysterectomy was part of the treatment for gynecologic cancer.
4. The patient has risk factors for vaginal cancer:
    a. Older age, half of all women affected with vaginal cancer are older than 60 years,
       with most between 60 and 70 years old.
    b. Exposure to diethylstilbestrol (DES) as a fetus.
5. History of cervical cancer.
6. History of cervical precancerous conditions.
7. HPV infection.
8. Vaginal adenosis.
9. Vaginal irritation.
10. Uterine prolapse.
11. Smoker.

In women who have had hysterectomies and have any of the above conditions, Pap testing
should be performed annually. And regardless of whether a Pap test is included, pelvic
examinations should be performed as part of health care in all women.

Post cancer treatment, with or without a cervix: Paps every 3 months for 2 years after comple-
tion of treatment and then every 6 months thereafter

Tips for Improving Pap Smear Collection

Collection devices:

ThinPrep test: Spatula plus cytobrush or the broom-type sampling device plus cytobrush
are significantly better for collection of endocervical cells than use of the broom alone.

Conventional smear: extended-tip spatula plus cytobrush better than Ayre's spatula
(without the extended tip) plus cytobrush for collection of endocervical cells

Table continued on following page.

Table 9–6   Pap Smears (*Continued*)

Use spatula first, then the endocervical brush, there will be less obscuring of cells by blood and therefore a better quality smear

Signs/symptoms of vaginal or cervical infection present—have client return for Pap after infection is resolved; since inflammatory changes can produce false positive Paps, if a woman is unlikely or unable to return, then remove any discharge carefully with saline-soaked cotton swab before obtaining Pap smear

Pregnant women—brush may be used but should be careful not to disrupt mucous plug

Multiparous or obese women (redundant vaginal tissue)—for better visualization of cervix, use large Graves' speculum and a condom with the tip cut off, slide the condom over the speculum, this will retract vaginal walls

Women with in utero exposure to DES—upper 2/3rd of the vagina should also be sampled with the spatula in a circumferential manner

Cervical bleeding due to Pap done on friable cervix—management options: pressure with cotton swab, silver nitrate stick, Monsel's Solution

Interpretation and Management of Papanicolaou Smears

Reported Findings	Etiology	Management
Adequacy of Specimen		
Satisfactory for evaluation; Class 1	—	No other S/S—routine Paps
Satisfactory but limited	50%–75% of cells are obscured	High-risk women: repeat Pap; Low-risk women: repeat Pap in 1 year
Unsatisfactory for evaluation; Class 0	Too few cells and/or 75% of cells obscured by blood, or inflammation (any exogenous hormone use, intercourse, douching, tampon use)	Repeat Pap Try to resolve any inflammation before repeating Pap
No endocervical cells	Os sampling is questionable	High-risk women: repeat Pap; Low-risk women: repeat Pap in 1 year Postmenopausal women: endocervical cells not normally found in smears of these: women, repeat Pap in 1 year
Benign Cellular Changes		
Infection	—	Treat infection; HIV positive: repeat Pap in 3 to 5 months High-risk woman: repeat Pap in 6 months; Low-risk woman: repeat Pap in 1 year
Reactive changes; Class 2	Inflammation, atrophy, radiation, IUD, chemicals (e.g., douching preparations, spermicides), chemotherapy, DES effect, treatment for cervical dysplasia, hormonal changes, pregnancy, abortion, miscarriage	Treat inflammation if symptomatic Post-menopausal women: treat with estrogen (Premarin) vaginal cream (1g vaginally QD for 4 weeks or QOD for 6 weeks), then repeat Pap; second Pap normal: routine Paps; second Pap abnormal: colposcopy

Table continued on following page.

Table 9–6 Pap Smears (*Continued*)

Reported Findings	Etiology	Management
Squamous Cell Abnormalities		
ASCUS; Class 2; atypia	Unable to determine whether abnormality is benign cellular change or dysplasia; Pap smear may have been air dried rather than fixed immediately	Treat any infection that may be present; if severe inflammation is also reported, try treating with metronidazole 500 mg po BID × 7 days before doing repeat Pap Post-menopausal women: see reactive changes; High-risk women: colposcopy Low-risk women: repeat Pap in 3 months; second Pap normal: repeat Pap in 1 year; second Pap abnormal: colposcopy (another approach, irregardless of risk—repeat Pap Q 4–6 months × 3–colposcopy for any ASCUS or higher grade lesion)
LGSIL; mild dysplasia; CIN 1; HPV lesions (condylomatous atypia, koilocytic atypia); Class 2/Class 3	Majority are reactive atypia or due to HPV	Offer HIV testing Colposcopy For 1 year after colposcopy: Paps Q3 months, colposcopy Q 6 months No reoccurrence: high-risk women: Paps Q6 months; low-risk women: annual Paps
HGSIL; moderate or severe dysplasia; CIN II; CIN III; CIS; Class3/Class 4	Long term usage of depot-medroxyprogesterone (Depo-Provera) may cause changes that mimic HGSIL	Offer HIV testing Colposcopy and ECC; No matter the findings of the colposcopy: minimally should have annual Pap for rest of life
Squamous cell carcinoma; Class 5	—	Colposcopy to establish diagnosis and start staging; Referral to gynecologist or gynecologic oncologist
Glandular Cell Abnormalities		
Endometrial cells	—	Premenopausal women with cells out of phase with menstrual cycle and/or abnormal uterine bleeding and postmenopausal women: endometrial biopsy
AGUS; Class 2	Infection; endometriosis; endometrial hyperplasia; premalignant or malignant lesion of the endocervix or endometrium	Colposcopy; In middle-aged and older women: consider endometrial biopsy

Table continued on following page.

Table 9–6   Pap Smears (*Continued*)

Reported Findings	Etiology	Management
AIS; Endocervical adeno-carcinoma; Endometrial carcinoma; Class 5	–	Colposcopy to establish diagnosis and start staging; referral to gynecologist or gynecologic oncologist
Miscellaneous		
Hyperkeratosis, parakeratosis, dyskeratosis	Abnormal keratinization; may be benign (due to cervical cap, diaphragm, or infection) or may be LGSIL (HPV-associated change)	Treat any infection; repeat Pap in 6 months; second Pap positive, repeat Pap again in another 6 months or colposcopy

Differential Diagnosis

Abnormal vaginal bleeding
Cervical polyps (small tumorlike projection from surface of cervix)
Cervical ulceration (syphilis, chancroid, herpes)
Chronic cervicitis (inflammation of cervix)

Diagnostic Tests

Human chorionic gonadotropin test
Colposcopy with directed biopsies
Other forms of cervical biopsy
    Endocervical curettage (ECC)
    Cone biopsy (indications for cone biopsy = HGSIL and subsequent
        colposcopy results unsatisfactory, finding of dysplasia with ECC,
        significant discrepancy between Pap smear and biopsy results, any
        suspicion of invasive carcinoma)
Proctoscopy (to determine if the cancer has spread to the rectum)
Cystoscopy (to determine if the cancer has spread to the bladder and urethra)
Chest x-ray examination (to determine if the cancer has spread to the lungs)
Computed tomography (CT) scan (to determine if the cancer has spread to
    pelvic and para-aortic lymph nodes)
MRI (to determine if the cancer has spread to lymph nodes and/or organs
    near the cervix)
Intravenous urography (also known as intravenous pyelography, or IVP)
    (to determine if the cancer has spread to the pelvic lymph nodes by
    detecting abnormalities of the urinary tract)

Management/Treatment

Pharmacologic Management

Chemotherapy
    Most common agent used for cervical cancer is cisplatin (Platinol) given
        IV.

Used when cancer has metastasized and other forms of treatment would be ineffective; chemotherapy may cause infertility.

National Cancer Institute recommends that women with cervical cancer requiring radiation therapy also receive concurrent cisplatin-based chemotherapy.

Cisplatin plus radiation is considered by many to be the standard of treatment for women with locally advanced cervical cancer.

Discontinue OCP use.

Nonpharmacologic Management

Based on colposcopy findings.

HPV—No treatment.

CIN 1—Serial colposcopy or Pap smears alternating with colposcopy or cryotherapy.

CIN 2/3—See section on surgical treatment of dysplasia.

Discrepancy between Pap cytology and biopsy histology (especially when biopsy shows less severity than Pap smear).

A one-grade difference in findings is acceptable (e.g., Pap = CIN 2, biopsy = CIN 3).

Repeat colposcopy or conization for any significant discrepancy that cannot be explained (cryotherapy or laser cone are not appropriate since no specimen is then available to rule out invasive carcinoma).

Inadequate colposcopy or positive ECC—Cone biopsy.

SURGICAL TREATMENT OF DYSPLASIA

Cryotherapy—Freezing cells, which are then shed in a heavy, watery discharge for 2–4 weeks; for treatment only of small areas of mild or moderate dysplasia that does not enter the cervical os.

Loop electrical excision procedure/large loop excision of the transformation zone—Electrically heated fine wire loop to remove abnormal tissue; treatment-of-choice for CIN 3 and CIS lesions

Cold knife cone biopsy—Conventional surgery; removal of cone-shaped piece of cervix; preferred method when lesions are extensive

Laser cone—Colposcopy-directed laser vaporizes cells

SURGICAL TREATMENT OF CERVICAL CANCER

Cone biopsy—Considered only for clients with stage I cancer who desire a subsequent pregnancy

Hysterectomy—Lowest cancer recurrence rate of any treatment

Pelvic exenteration—Removal of all reproductive organs and adjacent tissues such as bladder, rectum, and part of colon; used when prior treatment is unsuccessful

RADIATION THERAPY FOR CERVICAL CANCER

External therapy is done first for several weeks, then intracavitary radiation is done via capsules or implants; may be used in combination with chemotherapy (see above); may cause infertility, vaginal scarring, and increased risk of cancer at a later date in adjacent tissues.

Complementary/Alternative Therapies

Folic acid (1 mg/day), beta-carotene (15 mg/day), and vitamin C supplementation (controversial); folic acid supplementation is especially recommended if client continues use of OCPs.

See complementary and alternative therapies under "Breast Cancer."

Client Education

REGULAR PAP SMEARS

Scheduling Pap smear: Best is at least 5 days after menses stops; do not use tampons, birth-control foams, jellies, or other vaginal creams, or douche 2–3 days prior to the examination.

MEASURES TO PREVENT CERVICAL CANCER

Prevent precancerous lesions

Beta-carotene (e.g., carrots, tomatoes, citrus fruits, spinach) may provide protection against cancer due to antioxidant properties; research suggests that low levels of vitamin A (retinol) may contribute to SILs in human immunodeficiency virus (HIV)–positive women via a synergistic interaction with HPV.

Avoid risk factors (e.g., use condoms, do not smoke, avoid multiple sexual partners).

Follow-up

Set up a system to track clients with abnormal Pap smears; more than one reminder may be necessary.

Referral

Refer to gynecologist or gynecologic oncologist.

CONTRACEPTION

SIGNAL SYMPTOMS none

ICD-9 Codes	V25.09	Family planning, advice
	V61.9	Family planning, problem

Contraception is the temporary or permanent prevention of pregnancy; it includes a variety of methods and practices.

Epidemiology

Contraception targets 41 million women in the United States between the ages of 15 and 44.

Two thirds of American females have at least one unplanned pregnancy (49% of all pregnancies in the United States are unintended).

26.5% of all pregnancies will end in elective abortion.

90% of pregnancies in adolescents aged 15–19 years are unintentional.

Three million females do not use birth control because of actual or imagined side effects.

Unintended pregnancies occur because contraceptives are not used, are used inconsistently, or are used improperly.

58% of females report using a method of birth control during the month of conception.

Etiology

Prevention of pregnancy.

At risk are those who have lost partners, women who believe they are protected either immediately after giving birth or while nursing, women with irregular menses (perimenopausal), and rape victims.

Physiology and Pathophysiology

Female fertility is cyclic and relatively constant. The average menstrual cycle lasts 28–30 days and is divided into the follicular phase and the luteal phase. The first day of menstrual flow is day 1 of the cycle. The luteal phase is the time interval between ovulation and the first day of menses; it averages 12–17 days. A woman is most likely to conceive if sperm are present in the reproductive tract when ovulation occurs. The cycle days of fertility are the 3 days before ovulation, with a 20% probability of pregnancy if the woman has intercourse on any one of these days. The next most fertile day is the day of ovulation, with the probability of pregnancy of 15%. On other cycle days, the probability of pregnancy is 0%–10%.

Pharmacologic contraceptive management is targeted to suppression of ovulation, disruption of the corpus luteum, alteration of the luteal phase, alteration of cervical mucus, suppression of pituitary hormone secretion, immobilization of sperm, or prevention of a fertilized ovum.

Clinical Manifestations

Subjective

No symptoms of pregnancy

Objective

Normal menstrual cycle
No physical signs of pregnancy

Differential Diagnosis

Pregnancy

Diagnostic Tests

Females

Negative pregnancy test (qualitative or quantitative)
Screening for sexually transmitted disease (STD)

Males

Semen analysis after vasectomy showing no sperm (requires up to 15 ejaculations before aspermia is present for three consecutive studies).

Management and Treatment

Goals are to provide an effective, reversible method of birth control, with minimal risks of adverse effects from estrogen and progestin, and to provide treat-

Table 9–7   Contraception: Pharmacologic Management

Types

Combined Oral Contraceptives (OCs)

Reversible contraceptives which suppress ovulation by inhibiting gonadotropins. All OC's have different doses of estrogen and five types of progestin (except the progestin-only pills). Biphasic and triphasic OCs deliver different amounts of hormone throughout the menstrual cycle (chosen to mimic the natural hormone production of the client). Low-dose pill may be used initially (alter the dose as needed). Failure rate for the ideal user is 0.1% for the combined pill, and 0.5% for the progestin-only pill. (Actual failure rates are 2–3% for both pills).

Depo-Provera

Depo-medroxyprogesterone acetate injection 150 mg IM every three months is indicated when estrogen-containing OCs are contraindicated, client has difficulty with barrier method compliance, or for females older than age 35 years who smoke. It should be administered by the fifth day of menses in non-postpartum clients, and the fifth day postpartum in non-nursing mothers. Pregnancy test before initial administration strongly recommended.

MPA/E2C (Lunelle)

Monthly contraceptive injection is a combined hormonal contraceptive option, which contains medroxyprogesterone acetate and estradiol cypionate (similar to hormones used in OCs). Estradiol cypionate converts to 17-beta-estradiol to promote a monthly cycle and medroxyprogesterone acetate prevents ovulation.

Contraceptive Patch

A reversible method of contraception. Patch releases continuous systemic dose of ethinyl estradiol 20 μg and norelgestromix 150 μg (Low androgenicity) Apply weekly for 3 weeks Apply same day of each week, 4th week is patch free.

Intrauterine Device (IUD)

Immobilizes sperm, prevents implantation of the fertilized ovum, and removes the blastocyst from the endometrium. The contraceptive action of all IUD's is mainly in the uterine cavity. Ovulation is not affected. It is thought to be spermicidal. Both IUD's available are T-shaped, and have fine nylon tails than hang through the cervix. The ParaGard T380A (10 year duration) has copper wound around the base, and the minera (5 year duration) is infused with progesterone

Mifepristone (RU-486)

19-norsteroid that acts as a progesterone antagonist and blocks proesterone receptor sites in the decidua, inducing bleeding in pregnant women within a few days. It also sensitizes the uterus to prostaglandins that are given after the antagonist. It is used for pregnancy termination up to 9 weeks gestation. A single 600mg oral dose of mifepristone is given, followed by 400mcg misoprostol within 36–48 hours. Vaginal bleeding is then experienced within 4 hours of taking second drug. The combination is 80%-95% effective.

Contraindications

Absolute: Thromboembolic disorders; cerebrovascular disease; ischemic heart disease; smoke and over age 35; known or suspected carcinoma of breast, endometrium or known estrogen-dependent neoplasia; known or suspected pregnancy; undiagnosed or abnormal vaginal bleeding; hepatic carcinoma or adenoma

Relative: Hypertension, migraine or vascular headaches, uterine leioma, epilepsy, diabetes mellitus, gallbladder disease, obstructive jaundice, elective surgery, sickle cell disease or trait

Vaginal Ring (NuvaRing)

A low-dose combination hormonal device. Releases an average continuous dose of 0.120 mg of etonogestrel and 0.0015mg of ethinyl estradiol. The flexible, transparent ring is placed in the vagina, where it remains for 21 consecutive days; it is then removed for 7 days and a new ring inserted at the end of this time, Precise placement is not critical because it is not a barrier type of contraceptive.

Contraindications to NuvaRing include those usually associated with the use of contraceptives. Women who use combination hormonal contraceptives, including THE NuvaRing, are strongly advised not to smoke. Adverse reactions reported include vaginitis, headache, upper-respiratory-tract infection, weight gain, and nausea.

Table continued on following page.

Table 9–7 Contraception: Pharmacologic Management (*Continued*)

As with other contraceptives, NuvaRing does not protect against HIV infection or other sexually transmitted diseases.

Client Education

OC's do not protect against STD or HIV transmission. Condom use recommended.

Keep a record of menses.

Start pill packet in the first day of the next menses, or the first Sunday after the next menses (a convenience of not having period on weekend). If no menses after one week, call health care provider and do a serum pregnancy test. Menses should occur during last 7 pills, usually within 2 days of starting the final 7 pills.

To prevent nausea, take pill at bedtime with food.

Take one pill daily at the same time.

Complete the entire package.

If one pill missed, take it as soon as remembered. If 2 missed pills, take 2 tablets for the next 2 days. If more than 2 pills missed, notify health care provider. Continue taking the rest of the tablets and use additional method of protections such as condoms.

When pregnancy desired, discontinue 3 months before trying.

Notify health care provider if vision changes, chest pain, abdominal tenderness, numbness, weakness, leg pains, amenorrhea, jaundice, depression, right upper quadrant abdominal pain.

If taking antibiotics, use an additional form of contraceptive such as condoms.

---

ment with which the client can comply. In choosing a birth control method, theoretical efficacy rates, actual efficacy rates, safety concerns, financial costs, and individual client preferences and experiences must be considered.

Pharamacologic Management

See Table 9–7.

Nonpharmacologic Management

See Table 9–8.

Client Education

No perfect method of birth control exists.

The correct use of any birth control method does not guarantee protection against pregnancy (20% of females who experience an unplanned pregnancy used their method of birth control properly).

Educate on proper use of method selected.

Advise client about availability of emergency postcoital contraception (EC) (see Table 9–9).

Follow-up

Annual Pap smears

STD screening

Pelvic examinations

Fasting chemistry evaluations and breast examinations recommended for all women of childbearing age

Referral

Refer to gynecologist for female surgical contraceptive methods.

Refer to general surgeon for male surgical contraception.

Table 9–8 Contraception: Nonpharmacologic Management

Method	Advantages	Disadvantages	Client Education
Abstinence	Free	No preparation or protection for unplanned sex.	Total avoidance of sexual intercourse
Rhythm	Free	Theoretical failure 2–10% Actual failure rate 20% with basal body temperature and mucus monitoring. 47% failure if calendar method used alone.	Abstinence required about 17 days of each cycle. Not to be used in females nursing, nearing menopause, or with irregular cycles.
Withdrawal (coitus interruptus)	Free	No protection from STD's. Interruption of the sexual cycle can diminish pleasure. Failure rate is approximately 4% if used ideally, and has an actual rate of 18%.	Fluid from penis must be wiped off before intercourse, and intercourse should not be repeated. Not recommended if either partner cannot exercise control.
Barrier Methods: Condoms (Male and Female)	Inexpensive No prescription or office visit needed Provide STD protection Female condoms can be inserted before intercourse	Possible breakage Possible latex allergy to either partner May be considered cumbersome or have altered sensation for male. The ring on the female condom may be uncomfortable Ideal failure rates are 2%, and 12% for actual use.	*Condoms:* Use water-based lubricants. Check for holes before usage. Leave space in tip for semen reservoir. Withdraw from vagina before penis becomes flaccid to avoid accidental removal of condom. Use a spermicide to increase effectiveness and protect against STD's. *Female condom* Use a new condom before each coitus event. Insert so that the ring is into the vagina and the outer rings lies against the vulva. Make certain the penis enters the inside of the sheath. Remove the condom after sex and take care not to spill semen contents
Barrier Methods: Cervical Cap		May be difficult for some. Failure rate is 5% ideally, and 18% in reality	Absolute contraindications include HPV infection, atypia on smear, acute PID, cervicitis, vaginitis, and cervical biopsy or surgery within the previous 12 weeks
Barrier Methods: Diaphram	May insert up to 6 hours before intercourse	Failure rate is 3% ideally, and 18% actually Increased incidence of vaginal infection or UTI in some users	Check holes or wear by filling dome with water, and observe for leakage. Place a tablespoon of spermicidal gel or cream into the

Table continued on following page.

Table 9–8   Contraception: Nonpharmacologic Management (Continued)

Method	Advantages	Disadvantages	Client Education
			dome and line the entire rim of the device with it. Insert the diaphragm and check for proper placement and fit. Leave in at least 6 hours after coitus, then remove it and clean with mild soap and water If repeat coitus occurs before 6 hours, inset additional spermicidal cream or gel into the vagina and do not remove or displace the diaphragm. Leave the diaphragm in another additional 6 hours, then remove and clean
Barrier Methods: Vaginal Sponge *Not available in U.S. due to toxic shock syndrome but new sponge may be available soon.*	—	—	—
Barrier Methods: Spermicides	Inexpensive No prescription or office visit needed Provides some STD protection	High user failure. Potential allergic reaction to either partner. Women who use spermicides have ½ likelihood of cervical cancer as other sexually active women	The two most commonly used are nonoxynol 9 and octoxynol 9.
Surgical Contraception: Elective Abortion (intentionally induced expulsion of products of conception (POC) before the end of the 20th week when the fetus weighs less than 500g.	Low maternal complications rates, about 0.6% per 100,000, or less than 1% of all abortion cases No evidence of subsequent childbearing problems.	Possible complications include incomplete abortion, uterine perforation, hemorrhage, infection and cervical laceration. States may place restrictions on abortion services, waiting periods, and requirements for informed consent and parental notification.	Discuss religious, ethical, social and personal issues in non-judgemental manner with client Post-abortion may lead to feelings of fear, guilt, sadness and loss; best addressed before and after procedure

Table continued on following page.

Table 9–8   Contraception: Nonpharmacologic Management (Continued)

Method	Advantages	Disadvantages	Client Education
Surgical Contraception: Sterilization: Tubal Ligation	Reliable Diminished rate of PID	Requires outpatient surgical procedure Mortality rates are 3 deaths per 100,000 cases in the U.S.	Discuss permanent nature of procedure; reversal is not always successful After a tubal ligation, females report a change in menses, including menorrhagia and dysmenorrhea.
Surgical Contraception: Sterilization: Vasectomy	Reliable Office procedure, that takes about 20 minutes Mortality rate is 0% in the U.S. Theoretical failure rate is 0.15% and the actual rate is less than 3%	Mild swelling, bruising, and pain, which are common side effects	Discuss permanent nature of procedure; reversal is not always successful

Table 9–9   Emergency Postcoital Contraception

Emergency postcoital contraception (EC) may be used when birth control methods have failed, or when no birth control method has been used. It is not considered an abortifacient by medical and legal definition.

The pills for EC inhibit ovulation, disrupt the corpus luteum, shorten the luteal phase, suppress pituitary hormone secretion, and may make cervical mucus impenetrable. They may also suppress endometrial hormone receptors and their function or inhibit endometrial development necessary for implantation.

Clients who miss taking OC's should be offered EC. They may restart a pill pack after the second dose of EC, and use a backup method of birth control for the first 7 days of that cycle. EC will not protect from future unprotected intercourse.

Advantages:
    Simple to use and treatment is confidential.
    May be used more than once in the same cycle, and can be used as often as is needed.
    Oral contraceptives are not teratogenic, and therefore if EC fails, the risk of anomalies to the fetus is no greater than 2%–3% in any pregnancy.

Disadvantages:
    Must be taken within 72 hours of sexual exposure (more effective the sooner it is taken after unprotected intercourse).
    The most frequent side effects of estrogen-containing EC are nausea and vomiting. (Antiemetics should be recommended for all clients using EC).

Client Evaluation
    History of when unprotected intercourse occurred within the client's cycle. (After 72 hours the regimen may be less effective than 75–85%, but may still be worthwhile at approximately 60% effectiveness or less).
    Known last menses and previous menses.
    History of contraceptive use.
    Evaluate for absolute contraindications to use of estrogens. (If a history of thromboembolic disease, stroke, liver tumor, or breast cancer, consider progestin-only EC's).

Table continued on following page.

Table 9–9 Emergency Postcoital Contraception (*Continued*)

EC Treatment Regimen

EC

Take *one* of the following products in 2 doses, 12 hours apart:

Plan B–.75 mg levonorgestrel (in two doses of one pill each)

Preven Emergency Contraceptive Kit–Levonorgestrel 0.25 mg and ethinyl Estradiol 0.05 mg (in two doses of two pills each)

Alesse–5 pink tablets immediately, followed by 5 tablets 12 hours later

Nordette–4 light orange tablets immediately, followed by 4 tablets 12 hours later

Triphasil/Trilevlin–4 yellow tablets immediately followed by 4 tablets 12 hours later

Antiemetic:

Promethazine (Phenergan) 25mg orally

Dimenhydrinate (Dramamine) 50–100mg every 4–6 hours as needed

Cyclizine (Marazine) 50mg every 4–6 hours as needed

Trimethobenzamide (Tigan) 200mg suppository 3–4 times a day

Prochlorperazine (Compazine) 5–10mg PO 3–4 times/day

Client Education

Take estrogen-containing EC pills with food to minimize nausea.

Plan the second dose of estrogen-containing pills before bedtime to minimize nausea.

Provide a third dose of EC's in the event the client vomits within 1 hour after taking.

Inform the client of danger signs associated with estrogen-progestin combination OC's and the signs of ectopic pregnancy.

If no menses in 3–4 weeks, have client return for pregnancy test.

Menses depends on when hormones are taken during the cycle. (If EC's are taken during the follicular phase, menses may occur around day 21; if taken during ovulation, menses may return around day 26; if taken during the luteal phase, menses may occur around day 29).

If unplanned, undesired pregnancy, refer to a family planning center to review surgical options.

DYSMENORRHEA

SIGNAL SYMPTOM painful menses

ICD-9 Code	625.3	Dysmenorrhea

Dysmenorrhea is painful menstruation. Primary dysmenorrhea involves no identifiable pelvic pathology, but may include premenstrual syndrome and biopsychosocial factors. Secondary dysmenorrhea is painful menstruation characterized by pelvic pathology, including endometriosis, adenomyosis, and leiomyomas, pelvic inflammatory disease (PID), and intrauterine devices (IUDs). Congenital abnormalities may also cause secondary dysmenorrhea, including uterine polyps, cervical stenosis, a septate uterus, an imperforate hymen, or uterine adhesions.

Epidemiology

Primary Dysmenorrhea

The most frequently reported gynecologic symptom in the United States.

Affects approximately 50% of adult females.

About 10% of females are incapacitated for 1–3 days every month.

The rate of dysmenorrhea in parous women is one third that in nulliparous women.

Of those affected by primary dysmenorrhea, 35% are between 12 and 18 years of age.

Secondary Dysmenorrhea

Affects women most frequently between 30 and 40 years of age.

The prevalence varies with the underlying cause.

Dysmenorrhea due to endometriosis is most frequently found in nulliparous women between 25 and 50 years of age (rare in adolescent females).

Leiomyomas (fibroids) affect 25% of women over 30 years of age, and are the most common benign uterine tumors; they are more prevalent in African-American women.

Adenomyosis (when the endometrium invades the myometrium) is more common in multiparous women over the age of 40.

Etiology

Primary Dysmenorrhea

Elevated production of prostaglandins and other pain mediators in the uterus

Secondary Dysmenorrhea

Congenital abnormalities of the uterus or vagina

Cervical stenosis

Pelvic infection, adenomyosis, endometriosis, and pelvic tumors

Physiology and Pathophysiology

Primary dysmenorrhea is thought to be attributable principally to an increased prostaglandin production. The prostaglandins cause a hypersensitivity of the pain fibers to bradykinin and other noxious stimuli, increasing the pain. Endometrial levels of these prostaglandins are low in the proliferative phase of the menstrual cycle, but rise throughout the secretory phase and peak during menstruation.

Secondary dysmenorrhea as a result of endometriosis may be due to prostaglandin-secreting endometrial implants found on the ovaries, uterosacral ligaments, cul-de-sac, or elsewhere in the peritoneum. Leiomyomas consisting of bundles of smooth muscle are often associated with metrorrhagia and an excess production of prostaglandins. Dysmenorrhea caused by adenomyosis is poorly understood.

Clinical Manifestations

Subjective

Onset is usually within 12 months after menarche, and when ovulatory cycles begin.

Lower abdominal cramping up to 72 hours. If severe, the uterine pain may last 2–7 days.

50% suffer with nausea, vomiting, fatigue, diarrhea, low back pain, thigh pain, and headache.

Nervousness, dizziness, and syncope have been reported in severe cases.

With endometriosis, may begin a few days to 1 week before menses and may be present throughout the menstrual cycle.

Prolonged menses, dysmenorrhea, and a sensation of heavy pelvic pressure may occur in clients with leiomyoma.

Objective

No clinical signs may actually be present.

There may be a pelvic mass or uterine enlargement.

Adnexal and cervical motion tenderness may be present, which indicates infection.

Anemia may be present.

Differential Diagnosis

Pelvic infection (discharge, dyspareunia, odor)

Pregnancy (could be miscarriage)

Missed abortion or incomplete abortion (vaginal bleeding, cramping)

Ectopic pregnancy (one-sided lower abdominal pain with possible radiation to shoulder—may also be asymptomatic)

Endometriosis (chronic pelvic pain, dyspareunia, premenstrual spotting)

Urinary tract infection (dysuria, frequency, urgency)

Uterine or ovarian neoplasm

Diagnostic Tests

STD testing for chlamydia and gonorrhea

Urinalysis (to rule out bladder pathology)

Pelvic ultrasonography (for leiomyomas, cysts, or lesions)

Endometrial biopsy (to evaluate adenomyosis)

Hysterosalpingography (to identify if congenital uterine anomalies exist)

Laparoscopy (if endometriosis or adhesions are suspected)

Management and Treatment

Pharmacologic Management

Aspirin—2 tablets Q4H for a day or two before menstruation (because of antiprostaglandin activity)

Nonsteroidal antiinflammatory drugs (NSAIDs)—Begin with onset of menses

  Ibuprofen (Motrin), 400–800 mg initially, then 400 mg Q4H

  Naproxen sodium (Napralan), 550 mg PO immediately, then 275 Q6–8H

  Sulindac (Clinoril), 200 mg initially, then 200 mg BID

  Tolmetin (Tolectin), 400 mg initially, then 400 mg Q4H

Oral contraceptives (OCPs)—Suppress menstrual fluid and prostaglandin release by causing endometrial hypoplasia, effective in 60%–80% of clients. OCPs are especially useful for clients with dysmenorrhea who require contraception. If no improvement in dysmenorrhea after three cycles of OCPs, add an NSAID. Consider a referral for laparoscopy if this combination is not effective after 6 months.

Hydrocodone or tramadol—Useful for the management of severe pain.

Antibiotics—To treat PID, STDs.

OCPs or danazol—For endometriosis.

Nonpharmacologic Management

Remove IUDs that cause dysmenorrhea.

Surgery may be indicated for endometriosis.

Avoid alcohol and refined sugars, especially the week before symptoms are expected.

Avoid caffeine, it may increase uterine contractions and worsen pelvic pain.

Vitamin B complex is thought to reduce water retention and reduce stress, and it increases oxygen flow to the uterus and other reproductive organs.

Complementary/Alternative Therapies

Massage therapy.

Acupuncture.

Herbs used to minimize menstrual cramps include lemon balm, black hew, black cohosh, dong quai (dosage not available).

Primrose oil, 200 mg TID.

Vitamin B complex, 50 mg TID.

Relaxation techniques are helpful for the management of pain.

Client Education

Primary dysmenorrhea improves with age and parity.

Exercise is recommended to increase endorphins, raise the estrone:estradiol ratios that decrease endometrial proliferation, suppress prostaglandin release, and shunt blood away from the uterus, thereby decreasing pelvic congestion and pain.

Limit sodium-containing foods and increase water intake.

Heating pads and warm baths are helpful to decrease muscle spasms.

Support groups are suggested for clients with severe dysmenorrhea.

Follow-up

Once a well-tolerated medical regimen has been established to successfully reduce uterine pain, annual gynecologic examinations are recommended.

Referral

Refer to gynecologist.

Refer for secondary dysmenorrhea and treatment of the underlying condition.

ENDOMETRIOSIS

SIGNAL SYMPTOM recurrent abdominal and/or pelvic pain

ICD-9 Codes	617.0	Endometriosis of uterus
	617.1	Endometriosis of ovary
	617.2	Endometriosis of fallopian tube
	617.3	Endometriosis of pelvic peritoneum
	617.4	Endometriosis of rectovaginal septum and vagina
	617.5	Endometriosis of intestine
	617.8	Endometriosis, other specified sites (e.g., bladder, vulva)
	617.9	Endometriosis, unspecified site

Endometriosis is the nonmalignant growth of functioning endometrial tissue outside the uterus. It results in a chronic disease that is usually both painful and progressive.

Epidemiology

Occurs in women during childbearing years, with an estimated prevalence of 5%–10%; however, 5% of all cases occur in postmenopausal women, primarily in those on hormone-replacement therapy

Prevalence of 10%–15% in women aged 25–44

The average age at time of diagnosis is 25–30.

Infertility

Estimates of percentage of infertile women who have endometriosis range from 20% to 50%.

Women with endometriosis have a 50%–60% risk of infertility.

After completing hormonal or surgical treatment only 30% with severe disease and 50% of those with moderate disease will be able to conceive.

Japanese women have a rate twice that for Caucasians.

Women of Asian descent have a higher incidence than is seen in the general population.

Those with a first-degree relative with endometriosis are at 6 to 10 times greater risk of having it themselves and tend to have more severe symptoms and to manifest those symptoms earlier.

Lower incidence rate among poor women (may be related to their higher rates of PID, earlier marriage, and early and frequent childbearing).

Endometriosis is a major reason for hysterectomies.

Endometriosis is the third most frequent gynecologic cause for hospitalization.

Etiology

Unknown, probably multifaceted. Most widely accepted cause is retrograde menstruation.

Other possible or contributing causes include:

Transportation of endometrial cells via the lymphatic and circulatory systems

Accidental transportation during abdominal surgery

Exposure to environmental chemotoxins such as dioxin

Genetic factors (evidenced by familial occurrence)

 Increased exposure to menstruation

 Increased age

Menstrual cycles less than 27 days or menstrual flow greater than 7 days (twice as likely to develop endometriosis), heavy menstrual flow, delayed childbirth, few or no pregnancies.

IUDs cause an increase in menstrual flow and are associated with a three times greater risk for endometriosis.

Oral contraceptives tend to decrease menstrual flow and are associated with a 50% decrease in the risk of endometriosis.

Severely retroverted (tipped backward) uterus,

Genital-tract anomalies (associated with endometriosis in adolescents).

Physiology and Pathophysiology

Endometriosis is steroid-responsive. Estrogen supports the growth of endometriotic lesions. Androgens and progestins promote atropy of the lesions. After menopause, symptoms usually abate. Because of steroid responsiveness, most endometrial implants can shed/bleed during menses, and because the shedding of ectopic tissue does not flow from the body as menstrual discharge, the ectopic site tends to become inflamed, which in turn may cause symptoms such as pain and the formation of fibrosis, adhesions, and scar tissue.

Ectopic endometrial lesions may occur in any organ system:

Most common sites are the ovaries (50%), fallopian tubes, peritoneum, uterine broad ligaments, and outer surface of the uterus.

Endometrioma—Endometrial cystic mass >2–3 cm located on an ovary; may be asymptomatic until ruptures; "chocolate cyst"—an endometrioma that is filled with old, brown-colored blood.

Gastrointestinal tract (bowel) is the most common site outside the reproductive tract.

Less common sites are the urinary tract and the external genitalia.

Rare sites are distant organs such as lungs, spleen, gallbladder, kidneys, and scar tissue (e.g., cesarean sections, appendectomies, and episiotomies).

Infertility may result from endometriosis due to:

Disruption of normal anatomy as a result of adhesions and scar tissue. Anovulation.

Antibodies formed against endometrial implants attack uterine lining and cause spontaneous abortions.

Protaglandin secretion due to young endometrial implants can cause spasms that may inhibit ovum transport and sperm mobility.

Clinical Manifestations

Subjective

Severity of symptoms do not always correlate with severity of disease. It is not uncommon to find an inverse relationship between the severity of symptoms and disease.

Chronic pelvic pain (dull, burning, stabbing, or grinding, localized or diffuse, may radiate to back, rectum, or thigh; may be midline pelvic pain)

Increasing dysmenorrhea (onset usually precedes menses and may continue after cessation of menses; for some women the most intense pain is associated with ovulation rather than menses)

Dyspareunia (usually positional, worse with deep penetration)

Premenstrual spotting (may be the most predictive of endometriosis)

Infertility (may be client's only symptom)

Acute pelvic pain (rupture of endometrioma)

Dysuria (presents as suprapubic pain during urination), urgency, urine retention, hematuria during menstruation (endometrial lesions located in urinary tract)

Dyschezia (painful defecation), tenesmus (sense of rectal fullness), rectal bleeding with menses, nausea, abdominal bloating/cramping, diarrhea, constipation, pain in lower back/rectum/umbilicus (endometrial lesions located in GI system)

Symptoms due to chronicity of the disease (fatigue, depression, insomnia, despair)

May also report history of allergies, chemical sensitivities, frequent yeast infections (associated with alterations in immune system functioning; women with endometriosis are twice as likely to report these symptoms)

Objective

Pelvic examination may be normal (normal findings are seen in 20%–30% of adolescents with endometriosis).

Tender masses or nodules palpated in the pelvic/sacral area (frequently at the uterosacral ligament and posterior vaginal fornix).

Induration of the rectovaginal septum.

Laterally deviated cervix.

Generalized pelvic tenderness.

Localization of tenderness generally corresponds to the site(s) of the implants.

Tender and/or enlarged adnexa (endometriomas) with decreased mobility.

Fixed (due to adhesions), retroverted uterus.

Pain on motion of pelvic structures just prior to and during menses.

Visualization of lesions (rare) in the vagina, or on the vulva or cervix.

Differential Diagnosis

Acute salpingo-oophoritis (inflammation of fallopian tube and associated ovary)

Psychogenic pain (functional pain with no organic cause)

Nerve entrapment (injury and/or inflammation of nerve caused by pressure from surrounding tissue)

Pelvic inflammatory disease (fever, foul vaginal discharge, pain in lower abdomen, dyspareunia, tenderness, and pain)

Ectopic pregnancy (one-sided lower abdominal pain with possible radiation to shoulder; may also be asymptomatic)

Uterine leiomyoma/fibroids (benign smooth-muscle tumor)

Ovarian cysts (lower abdominal pain, pelvic pain, dyspareunia)

Chronic salpingo-oophoritis (chronic inflammation of fallopian tubes and ovaries)

Prior acute salpingitis (20% suffer chronic pelvic pain)

Adenomyosis (severe dysmenorrhea and abnormal uterine bleeding)

Benign or malignant ovarian neoplasm (irregular vaginal bleeding, pain)

Irritable bowel syndrome (diarrhea and pain in lower abdomen relieved on defecation)

Hernias (protrusion of an organ through abnormal opening in muscle wall of cavity it surrounds; pain, bulging)

Interstitial cystitis (bladder wall becomes inflamed, ulcerated, and scarred causing frequent, painful urination)

Diagnostic Tests

Human chorionic gonadotropin test (pregnancy test).

Laparoscopy and biopsy are used for definitive diagnosis.

Pelvic ultrasonography.

Magnetic resonance imaging (for endometriomas but not routinely used because of high cost).

Elevated serum levels of cancer antigen 125 (is sensitive only to advanced endometriosis, and elevation is also seen in ovarian cancer, myomas, adenomyosis, ovarian cysts, pregnancy, menses, and acute PID).

Colonoscopy and biopsy.

Cystoscopy and biopsy.

Management/Treatment

Pharmacologic Management

Pharmacologic management is used only to manage pain or dyspareunia. It is not curative, nor does it restore fertility, and symptoms usually return when treatment is discontinued, until the woman reaches menopause. If pharmacologic treatment results in cessation of abnormal bleeding but inadequate pain relief, there may be a coexisting problem, most commonly abdominal-wall trigger points, hernias, interstitial cystitis, pelvic congestion, or irritable bowel syndrome

ANALGESICS

NSAIDs (block prostagladin synthesis)—Effective for 80% of women with mild to moderate pain associated with dysmenorrhea.

Narcotics (only if NSAIDs ineffective).

HORMONAL THERAPY (DECREASE ESTROGEN OR INCREASE ANDROGEN OR PROGESTIN)

OCPs

High-dose OCPs no longer recommended for treatment of endometriosis.

Combination low-dose estrogen and intermediate/high-dose progesterone (with low endometrial activity) monophasic OCPs are recommended for long term therapy: Aleese, Lo-Estrin, Lo-Ovral,

Ortho-Cept, Ortho-Novum 1/35, start on day 5 of menstrual cycle and take continuously for at least 6 to 9 months, preferably until shortly before conception is desired or until women reaches menopause.

If recurrence of symptoms or inadequate pain relief with OCPs, client's endometriosis may be particularly sensitive to estrogen—Change to progestin-only pill.

Progestins

Medroxyprogesterone acetate—Effective in controlling symptoms in mild to moderate cases; commonly used but no longer FDA-approved for this indication

Depo-Provera, 100 mg IM Q2 weeks for 2 months, then 200 mg IM every month for 4 months or 150 mg IM every 3 months; may be the best choice for adolescents who wish to delay childbearing; after discontinuation there is a 7–9 month delay in return of ovarian functioning and 10–22 month delay for fertility.

Provera, 10–30 mg daily for 3 to 6 months, need to use barrier contraception during therapy.

Norethindrone acetate (Aygestin): Adults, initially 5 mg QD for 2 weeks, then increase by 2.5 mg/day every 2 weeks up to 15 mg/day maintenance dose; continue for 6–9 months; may temporarily discontinue if breakthrough bleeding occurs.

Danazol (Danocrine)—Synthetic androgen with mild antiestrogenic and antiprogestational effects; start on first day of menses; 400 mg QD for mild endometriosis, 400 mg BID for moderate to severe disease. If no relief in 6 weeks increase the dose. Pregnancy category X (contraindicated) and not proven as a contraceptive, therefore use a barrier method while taking danazol.

Gonadotropin-releasing hormone (GnRH) agonists—Suppress ovarian function, resulting in a drug-induced menopause. Pregnancy category X and not proven as a contraceptive, therefore must use barrier method while on GnRH agonists.

Leuprolide acetate (Lupron Depot): >18 years, 3.75 mg IM once per month for up to 6 months.

Nafarelin (Synarel, 200 mg/spray)—Older than 18 years, start between days 2 and 4 of menstrual cycle, one spray in one nostril in morning and one spray in the other nostril in evening. If menstruation continues after 2 months, increase to one spray in each nostril morning and evening for up to 6 months.

Goserelin acetate (Zoladex SC implant)—Older than 18 years, one 3.6-mg implant into upper abdominal wall, implant every 28 days for up to 6 months.

GnRH agonist plus HRT—Conjugated estrogen/norethindrone acetate (Aygestin), 2.5 mg PO QD; effective pain relief with less bone loss and other hypoestrogenic side effects.

Nonpharmacologic Management

Wait-and-see conservative approach (NSAIDS used for pain)

For perimenopausal or infertile clients with mild endometriosis and mild symptoms

Surgery

Major indications for surgery: endometriomas, significant pelvic adhesions, rectovaginal endometriosis, ureteral or intestinal occlusion with deep wall involvement, fallopian-tube obstruction, intractable/incapacitating pain not responsive to other forms of treatment.

Presurgery treatment of GnRH for 3 months is often used to reduce pelvic vascularity and inflammation, size and activity of endometriotic implants, diameter of ovarian cysts, and thickness of cyst walls.

Conservative surgery (laparoscopy or laparotomy; for moderate to severe cases when future fertility is desired; microscopic endometrial implants are often missed and disease usually recurs).

Laser surgery (60% pregnancy success rate; best chance to conceive is within first year after surgery).

Electrocautery.

Adhesion formation after surgery is common; less of a risk with laparoscopy than with laparotomy.

Hysterectomy with bilateral salpingo-oophorectomy (curative; up to 30% recurrence of symptoms if only one ovary is removed; for moderate to severe cases when future fertility is not desired. After surgery, if low-dose estrogen-replacement therapy is used to treat the side effects of hypoestrogenism, progestin therapy must be also added to avoid endometrial hyperplasia and possible cancer in any residual endometrial tissue).

Presacral neurectomy (for management of midline abdominal pain).

Laparoscopic uterosacral nerve ablation (for pain management).

Complementary/Alternative Therapies

Essential fatty acids (evening primrose, fish oil; antiinflammatory effect that may reduce dysmenorrhea)

Stress management/relaxation techniques (lessen effects of stress on immune and hormonal systems and increase ability to cope)

Yoga (may lessen dysmenorrhea, pelvic congestion, low back pain)

Exercise (may lessen dysmenorrhea, pelvic congestion, low back pain)

Client Education

Complications of endometriosis include infertility and increased risk of spontaneous abortion.

Follow-up

As needed

Referral

Refer to gynecologist.

Refer to reproductive endocrinologist (for treatment of infertility).

Refer to professional mental health counseling for marital, sexual, and coping problems related to endometriosis.

EPIDIDYMITIS

SIGNAL SYMPTOMS scrotal heaviness, dysuria, unilaterail pain

ICD-9 Codes	604.0	Epididymitis, with abscess
	098.0	Epididymitis, acute
	098.2	Epididymitis, chronic (2 months or more)
	098.0	Epididymitis, gonococcal

Epididymitis is an inflammatory condition of the epididymis.

Epidemiology

1 man in 1000 is affected annually in the United States.

Accounts for over 600,000 medical visits per year.

Etiology

Bacterial infection (primarily *Escherichia coli* and *Pseudomonas*).

STD (gonorrhea, syphilis, or *Chlamydia trachomatis*).

Tuberculosis (TB) epididymitis (may be presenting feature of genitourinary TB).

Infrequently caused by distant infection from teeth, ears, or skin (travels to the epididymis through the blood).

Direct trauma to the epididymis.

Instrumentation (cystoscopy or bladder catheterization).

In the pediatric client, an abnormally positioned ureter (may empty into a seminal vesicle and cause recurrent epididymitis).

Viral orchitis with epididymitis (most often due to mumps or varicella virus).

Bladder-outlet obstruction (due to benign prostatic hypertrophy or urethral strictures).

Amiodarone-induced epididymitis (due to concentration of drug in the epididymis).

Physiology and Pathophysiology

Epididymitis often occurs as a result of an STD or bacterial infection in the urethra, which ascends from the urethra in a retrograde manner through the ejaculatory ducts and vas deferens to the epididymis. In older men, the infection often begins in the bladder and is a result of bladder-outlet obstruction. Traumatic epididymitis is a noninfectious inflammatory condition that usually occurs within a few days after a blow to the testes when they are forcefully compressed against the pubic bones.

Clinical Manifestations

Subjective

Scrotal pain increasing over hours to days (initially felt in the groin or lower abdomen)

Scrotal heaviness common (but not specific)

Relief of discomfort with elevation of the scrotum when recumbent

Abdominal pain

Dysuria

Objective

Erythema, edema, and tenderness (scrotum, epididymis, and inguinal area)

Febrile (not necessary to confirm diagnosis)

Urethral discharge

Urinary tract infection

STD

Enlarged, tender, or palpable prostate mass (prostate boggy with acute prostatitis)

Parotid swelling (mumps orchitis)

Confirmed TB infection

Differential Diagnosis

Testicular torsion (axial rotation of spermatic cord cuts off blood supply to testes, epididymis and other structures)

Testicular cancer (epididymitis may be a presenting sign)

Hydrocele, spermatocele, epididymal cyst (generalized edema)

Abdominal aortic aneurysm, ureteral colic, rectocecal appendix, retroperitoneal cancer, and prostatitis (an extrascrotal source indicated by pain in the absence of scrotal pathology)

Masses, hernias, or varices in the scrotum (may also cause pain)

Diagnostic Tests

Complete blood count (CBC; elevated white-cell [WBC] count and a possible shift to the left, but most often normal)

Urinalysis and culture (presence of WBCs, and possible bacteria if the process originated as a lower urinary tract infection).

Blood cultures (to determine if systemically ill; positive results prove bacterial infection)

STD screening (to rule out possible bacterial cause; urethral smear)

Digital rectal examination (enlarged prostate; use caution in case of acute bacterial prostatitis)

Ultrasonography is the gold standard (to detect scrotal abscess or complications of epididymitis, or bacterial orchitis; ultrasonography of scrotum shows increased blood flow to affected side)

Management and Treatment

Pharmacologic Management

PAIN MANAGEMENT

Drug of choice: Ibuprofen (Motrin), 400–800 mg TID for 7–10 days.

Alternative: Acetaminophen (Tylenol), 650 mg TID for 7 days.

Early in the disease process, a block with bupivacaine (given by urologist) may decrease or prevent severe discomfort.

BACTERIAL INFECTION MANAGEMENT

Begin antibiotics before culture results are obtained, then change as appropriate.

STD: For a suspected STD (unconfirmed)—Doxycycline (Vibramycin), 200 mg PO loading dose. Follow with doxycycline (Vibramycin), 100 mg BID for 14 days.

Chlamydia infection: Azithromycin (Zithromax), 1–2 g PO, single dose, or doxycycline (Vibramycin), 100 mg PO BID for 7 days.

Gonorrhea: Ceftriaxone (Rocephin), 250 mg IM single dose, plus doxycycline, 100 mg BID for 10 days; alternative: ofloxacin (Floxin), 300 mg PO BID for 10 days.

Bacterial infection from bladder, prostate, or infection spread by the blood: Ciprofloxacin (Cipro), 500 mg PO BID for 10 days, OR trimethoprim/sulfamethoxazole DS (TMP/SMX) BID for 10 days. (Epididymitis due to chronic bacterial prostatitis, continue therapy for 6–10 weeks.)

TB epididymo-orchitis triple therapy: Rifampin, 450 mg QD for 2 months, then 900 mg QD for 2 months; isoniazid, 300 mg QD for 2 months, then 600 mg QD for 2 months; and pyrazinamide, 25 mg/kg/day for 2 months only. (Pyridoxine replacement also recommended.)

Nonpharmacologic Management

Bedrest (for severe pain only, and not always required).

Scrotal support or jock strap (to relieve pain in spermatic cord until edema subsides).

Cold compress to scrotum for 24 hours; then warm compresses and or sitz baths to decrease edema and inflammation.

Chronic epididymitis may be relieved with epididymectomy (25% of men with chronic epididymitis will continue to suffer from scrotal pain).

Complementary/Alternative Therapies

Dysuria, prostatitis: Saw palmetto (no standardized dose) (may cause aggravation of underlying bacterial infection)

Drink 8–10 glasses of water per day (dilution of urine may decrease symptoms of dysuria)

Client Education

Complete entire course of medication. If treated insufficiently, complications include chronic epididymitis and sterility.

Avoid heavy lifting, straining with stool, or sexual intercourse during the acute phase.

Recovery may last up to 4 weeks.

Pain should decrease over 2 weeks (swelling should decrease over 4 weeks).

Advise client to have sexual partner examined (if causative organism is related to STD).

Testicular self-examination.

In clients with human immunodeficiency virus, infections and/or inflammatory process will likely take longer to heal.

Follow-up

Until all signs of infection have been resolved

Referral

Refer to urologist immediately in cases of suspected torsion, if varicocele does not deflate when lying down, if pain persists, or if disorder is associated with infertility.

Refer to urologist or general surgeon if there is a suspicion of carcinoma or if inflammation has not resolved within 3 weeks and the testes can be palpated as normal.

ERECTILE DYSFUNCTION

SIGNAL SYMPTOM ▶ inability to develop or maintain an erection

ICD-9 Codes	607.84.1.1	Erectile dysfunction, organic origin
	302.1	Erectile dysfunction, sexual disorders
	302.7	Erectile dysfunction, psychosocial dysfunction

Erectile dysfunction (ED) is the inability to develop or maintain an erection sufficient for satisfying sexual intercourse. It may be described as dissatisfaction with the size, rigidity, or duration of an erection.

Epidemiology

Affects about 30 million men in the United States; often unreported.

Transient ED occurs in about half of adult males (may not be dysfunctional).

ED occurs more frequently in older men (but can occur in younger men as well).

Prevalence: 5% of men 40 years old, 10% in men in their 60s, 15% in their 70s, and 30%–40% in their 80s.

Etiology

End-organ dysfunction is more frequent with advancing age (age-related decrease in testosterone levels may lead to a decrease in erectile tone).

Neurogenic and vascular end-organ dysfunctions occur more frequently in the presence of other disease states.

Risk factors are similar to those for coronary artery disease (diabetes mellitus, hyperlipidemia, hypertension, hypothyroidism, chronic renal failure, smoking, obesity, alcohol abuse, and lack of exercise).

Etiology of ED is often multifactorial:

Neurogenic (pelvic trauma or surgery, spina bifida, intervertebral disk lesion, stroke, and multiple sclerosis).

Medication-induced: Antihypertensives (diuretics, vasodilators, central sympatholytics, ganglion blockers, β-blockers, ACE inhibitors [enalapril], calcium-channel blockers [nifedipine], antidepressants (tricyclics, monoamine oxidase inhibitors), tranquilizers (phenothiazines, thiozanthines), anticholinergics (atropine, propantheline, diphenhydramine), luteinizing-hormone–releasing hormone analogs, antiandrogens, anxiolytics (benzodiazepines), psychotropics (alcohol, marijuana, amphetamines, barbiturates, nicotine, opiates), miscellaneous (cimetidine, clofibrate, digoxin, estrogens, indomethacin, others)

Endocrinologic (hypothyroidism, hypogonadism, and hyperprolactinemia) (recognized causes of endocrine-related ED).

Psychogenic (depression, stress and anxiety, relationship difficulties, personal beliefs regarding sexual intercourse, which influence sexual function).

Vasculogenic.

Anatomic abnormality.

Physiology and Pathophysiology

The pathology of ED is related to the underlying etiology. Neuropathy and vasculopathy as seen in diabetes contribute to neuronal anoxia and a decreased perfusion of the erectile apparatus. Atherosclerosis contributes to obstruction of the arteries that serve the cavernosa and results in inadequate tissue pressures for erection. Hypertension and hyperlipidemia contribute to microthrombus trauma and ischemia of the erectile apparatus. An age-related decrease in testosterone may result in decreased tone of the erectile tissues.

Clinical Manifestations

Subjective

Inability to develop or maintain an erection sufficient for penetration

A reduction of erectile size and rigidity

Inability to achieve or maintain an erection

Lack of sexual desire

Rapid detumescence (flaccid)

Objective

Evidence of endocrine or other disease, such as a palpable thyroid, gynecomastia, testicular atrophy, reduced body hair, malformed penis, peripheral vascular disease, neuropathy

Differential Diagnosis

Endocrine (low or high thyroxine, low testosterone, high prolactin, diabetes, high estrogen effect, renal failure, zinc deficiency)

Neurologic (neurologic damage, such as with diabetes or hypertension)

Vascular (arterial insufficiency, cavernosal insufficiency, venous insufficiency)

Psychological (depression, schizophrenia, relationship disorders, personality disorders, anxiety)

Structural

Diagnostic Tests

CBC, fasting chemistry panel, lipid panel, thyroid-function tests urinalysis, serum prolactin level, testosterone level, prostate specific antigen (evidence of underlying causes).

Functional Tests

Injection of papaverine into the penis by urologist (to assess vascular function)

Concurrent ultrasonography (to give a precise measurement of blood flow into the penis)

Nocturnal penile monitoring (Rigi-scan) (measures the erections that occur normally during rapid eye movement sleep)

Psychiatric tests (depression, anxiety, alcoholism screening)

Pelvic angiography (in the presence of pelvic trauma)

Management and Treatment

Treatment is based on the cause of ED and the importance of the problem to the client; encourage client involvement in the selection of therapy, and establish a working relationship with the client and sexual partner (to avoid or reduce misinformation).

Pharmacologic Management:

Hormone therapy (if testosterone level low):

Testosterone (Androderm) transdermal patch, 2.5–5.0 μg QD

Testosterone gel (Androgel), 1.0% to upper extremities daily

Methyltestosterone capsules, 10–50 mg QD

Sildenafil (Viagra), 25–100 mg 0.5 to 4 hours before sexual activity once daily.

Vasomax, Spontane (undergoing clinical trials and testing).

Alprostadil (MUSE) urethral suppository, 125 to 250 mg; maximum, two suppositories a day.

Penile injections: A small needle is used to inject a drug directly into the penis prior to intercourse. Either prostaglandin E_1 (Caverject) or a combination of vasoactive compounds (papaverine, phentolamine, and prostaglandin) are used.

Nonpharmacologic Management

Vacuum erection device: A device used to pull blood into the penis. A constricting band is placed at the base of the penis to allow the erection to be maintained for about 20 minutes.

Semi-rigid penile implants:

Inflatable penile prosthesis: A reservoir and pump are attached to the implant, which is surgically placed into the penis. When the pump placed in the scrotum is compressed, fluid from the reservoir fills the implant, causing the penis to become erect. Once implanted, it is not usually possible to change to other treatment options.

Complementary/Alternative Therapies

Yohimbine (long considered an aphrodisiac; dose not consistent)

Sex therapy

Client Education

Eat a low-fat, low-cholesterol diet.

Exercise routinely.

Avoid tobacco products.

Keep alcohol consumption to a minimum.

Avoid activities that could cause penile or groin injuries.

Advise client and partner to read: Masters and Johnson (1970).

Follow-up

Meet monthly with client and, if possible, sexual partner as required for treatment.

Referral

Refer to sex or family therapist/counseling to help speed recovery and prevent future problems.

Refer to psychologist if organic disease, such as depression, is present.

Refer to urologist for initial consultation to confirm the physical findings and to initiate the appropriate therapy; primary health-care practitioner may then co-manage the client's progress.

FIBROCYSTIC BREAST DISEASE

SIGNAL SYMPTOMS breast pain, thick/lumpy breasts

| ICD-9 Codes | 610.0 | Solitary cyst of breast |
| | 610.1 | Cystic breast, fibrocystic breast |

Fibrocystic breast disease is the result of benign cystic and fibrous connective-tissue changes in the breast, occurring in response to endogenous hormone stimulation (primarily estrogen). Also known as cystic disease, chronic cystic mastitis, and mammary dysplasia.

Epidemiology

50%–90% of all women have fibrocystic breast changes at some point in their lives.

Most commonly occurs during childbearing ages.

Found in approximately 10% of those less than 21 years of age.

May occur in postmenopausal women using HRT.

Etiology

Exact etiology unknown, but appears to be secondary to excess estrogen, breast tissue response to monthly fluctuations in estrogen and progesterone levels, and extra sensitivity of breast tissue to estrogen.

Fibrocystic breast disease may be a symptom of vitamin E deficiency.

Associated with caffeine intake (controversial).

In general, does not increase breast cancer risk; however, there is a slight (1.5 to 2 times) increase in risk if epithelial hyperplasia/proliferative breast disease (such as ductal or lobular hyperplasia) is present, or a moderate (4 to 5 times) increase in risk if the epithelial hyperplasia is atypical.

Physiology and Pathophysiology

Fibrocystic breast disease is a physiologic change, not an actual disease. The changes associated with fibrocystic breast disease include:

Fibrosis (e.g., a prominence of fibrous tissue).

Cysts, which start as accumulations of fluid in breast glands, are influenced by hormonal changes; pain/discomfort related to the presence of cysts is due to the surrounding breast tissue being stretched as the cyst(s) enlarges just before the commencement of menses.

Epithelial hyperplasia (overgrowth of cells that line ducts or lobules), duct ectasia, and sclerosing adenosis (enlarged lobules that contain more glands than usual and that are distorted by fibrous tissue).

Clinical Manifestations

Subjective

Usually bilateral (may also present as unilateral) breast tenderness, pain, ache, or feeling of breast fullness or heaviness, especially just before onset of menses (approximately 7– 14 days prior to menses)

Breast masses that become tender and vary in size throughout the menstrual cycle (smallest and least tender at end of menses)

May present with breast pain or tenderness throughout entire menstrual cycle

Report of thick and/or lumpy breasts

Objective

Cysts:

Typically round or elliptical, soft or fluctuant, movable tender lumps.

No associated breast dimpling or nipple retraction.

Often multiple in number; upper outer quadrant and axillary tail most common sites.

Transillumination allows light to pass through the lump.

Not present in all women with fibrocystic changes.

Fibrosis:

Rubbery, firm, or hard to the touch lumps or areas of thickening.

Commonly found in outer quadrants (may be seen in older and postmenopausal women as a ridge that may be felt on the underside of the breasts).

White or clear nipple discharge may be present but usually is not.

Palpable axillary lymph nodes (seen in 20%); clavicular nodes not palpable.

Differential Diagnosis

See Differential Diagnosis in section on "Breast Cancer."

When presented with only breast pain, also consider costochondritis, respiratory infection, and cardiac causes.

Pregnancy (recent onset of breast swelling and tenderness).

Diagnostic Tests

Asymmetric areas of nodulation: In women under age 35—
ultrasonography; in women older than 35—mammography, but may
also want to consider ultrasonography

Ultrasonography (see section on "Breast Cancer"; distinguishes between
cystic and solid mass; used to evaluate palpable lesions, especially in
women under age 30)

Fine-needle aspiration (see section on "Breast Cancer"; used especially if
there is a dominant mass; confirms diagnosis of cysts and also drains
cyst)

Diagnostic mammography (for any masses)

Biopsy (persistent lumps or any dominant lump)

Management/Treatment

Pharmacologic Management

Mild analgesics such as aspirin are first-line treatment if measures
discussed under "Complementary/Alternative Therapies" and "Client
Education" are not effective.

Other drugs for treatment of breast pain, but should be considered for use
only in cases of severe, activity-limiting pain.

Danazol (Danocrine), 100 to 200 mg PO in two divided doses daily,
continuously for 2 to 6 months

Tamoxifen (Nolvadex)—An antiestrogen used for severe symptoms

Bromocriptine (Parlodel)—Inhibits pituitary prolactin

Diuretics—To decrease fluid retention and thereby decrease breast swelling;
however, research to date finds no difference between diuretics and placebos.

OCPs (low to intermediate estrogenic activity)—Concept is that OCPs decrease
ovarian production of estradiol and regulate progestins, which antagonize
estrogen and prolactin stimulation of breast tissue (see Table 9–10).

Nonpharmacologic Management

Fine-needle aspiration (drains cyst, reducing the pressure; however, fluid
may return, requiring subsequent aspirations)

Subcutaneous mastectomy (controversial; often results in failure to
alleviate symptoms and in complications)

Prophylactic bilateral total mastectomy (controversial; to be considered
only in those with fibrocystic breast changes who also have a considerable
family history of breast cancer, or in those in whom the fibrocystic
changes are progressive or are unresponsive to treatment and produce
constant pain that is no longer tolerable)

Complementary/Alternative Therapies

Natural progesterone cream—Controversial; should not be used in
conjunction with synthetic progestins such as Provera because they
compete for same receptor-binding sites.

Vitamin E—To decrease breast tenderness/pain; controversial; 150–600 IU
oral supplementation daily.

Table 9–10 Oral Contraceptives for Fibrocystic Breast Disease

Before prescribing oral contraceptives (OCs) be sure to evaluate client for absolute and relative contraindications to OC usage.

If client has breast pain or masses while on OCs and

-no edema is present, change to OCs with less estrogen and progestin and also rule-out malignancy

-edema is present, change to OCs containing less estrogen or containing progestins with less androgenic activity; if the pain continues or masses do not decrease in size within one month after changing OC, discontinue OCs until rule-out malignancy

Type (Estrogen/ Progestin)	Oral Contraceptive	Estrogen Dose	Activity
Combination Monophasic	Alesse Loestrin 1/20 Loestrin 1.5/30	20 mcg ethinyl estradiol 20 mcg ethinyl estradiol 30 mcg ethinyl estradiol	Endometrial: Low Progestational: Intermediate/ High Androgenic: Intermediate/ High
	Levlen Lo-Ovral Nordette	30 mcg ethinyl estradiol	Endometrial: Intermediate Progestational: Intermediate Androgenic: Intermediate
	Desogen Ortho-Cept	30 mcg ethinyl estradiol	Endometrial: Intermediate Progestational: Intermediate/ High Androgenic: Low
	Demulen 1/35	35 mcg ethinyl estradiol	Endometrial: Low Progestational: High Androgenic: Low
Combination Triphasic	Tri-Levlen Triphasil	32 mcg ethinyl estradiol (average)	Endometrial: Intermediate Progestational: Low Androgenic: Intermediate
Combination Estrophasic	Estrostep	30 mcg ethinyl estradiol (average)	Endometrial: Low Progestational: Intermediate/ High Androgenic: Intermediate/ High
Progestin Only	Micronor Ovrette	No estrogen	Endometrial: Low Progestational: Low Androgenic: Low

Kelp—1500–2000 mg daily in divided doses; possible iodine deficiency related to fibrocystic breast disease.

Primrose oil (γ-linolenic acid)—1500 mg daily; some efficacy in reducing breast pain; may reduce breast lump size; side effects seen in less than 2% of women.

Poke root poultice to relieve breast inflammation.

Client Education

Reduce salt intake to reduce fluid retention and thereby reduce physiologic edema of the breasts and concomitant pain/discomfort.

Avoid caffeine and other methylxanthines found in coffee, tea, chocolate, many soft drinks, theophylline, and theobromine.

Use hot or cold compresses.

Wear bras that provide good support, especially for sleep.

Perform monthly breast self-examination.

Undergo mammography (if possible, schedule at end of menses when breasts are least tender).

Follow-up

For clients who are taking OCPs for fibrocystic breast changes: Physical examination every 3 months twice, then every 6 months.

For clients who are taking danazol: Lipid panel every 3 months until danazol is discontinued.

Referral

Refer to surgeon for biopsy.

INFERTILITY

SIGNAL SYMPTOM ▶ inability to conceive

ICD-9 Codes	Female infertility	614.6	Female infertility, associated with adhesions; peritubal
		628.0	Female infertility, anovulation
		617.0	Female infertility, endometritis
		256.4	Infertility, Stein–Levanthal syndrome
		628.2	Infertility, fallopian tube anomaly
		628.2	Infertility, tubal occlusion or block
ICD-9 Codes	Male infertility	606.0	Absolute infertility due to azoospermia; germinal cell aplasia; spermatogenic arrest
		606.8	Infertility due to drug therapy, infection, afferent duct obstruction, or systemic disease, extra-testicular cause

Infertility is the inability to conceive after 1 year of unprotected intercourse.

Epidemiology

An estimated 15%–17% of couples in the United States experience transient or permanent infertility. Of these, half will be unable to have a biologic child (Youngkin, 1995, pg 224).

10%–50% of involuntarily childless couples never seek professional help.

Etiology

More than one factor may contribute to infertility in 40% of infertile couples.

Combined male and female factors contribute to 30% of all infertile couples.

Physiologic infertility in men accounts for 20%–50% of all cases of infertility.

Male infertility may be secondary to chromosomal or structural defects or endocrine abnormalities of the hypothalamic–pituitary–testicular axis. Causes include:

Obstruction in the genital tract.

Varicoceles when accompanied by abnormal results of semen analysis.

Cryptorchidism.

Congenital absence of the vas deferens.

Systemic illness.

Erectile or ejaculatory dysfunction.

Inflammation, infection, injury, radiation, chemotherapy, heat, medication, and substance abuse may all affect spermatogenesis or motility.

Ovulation dysfunction in females contributes to 25% of cases of infertility. Causes may include:

Hypothalamic anovulation

Anatomic or congenital defects

Medication

Psychogenic trauma

Anorexia nervosa

Pituitary anovulation (tumor or ischemia)

Ovarian anovulation (premature ovarian failure, ovarian tumors, or ovarian dysgenesis)

Integrative anovulation (polycystic ovary syndrome).

Tubal factors contribute to 20% of cases of infertility; may be due to partial or total obstruction of tubes from salpingitis, or pelvic inflammatory disease. (STDs are the leading cause of preventable infertility.)

Endometriosis contributes to 5% of cases of infertility.

Infertility remains unexplained in about 28% of infertile couples.

The prognosis is more encouraging if the duration of infertility is less than 3 years, the female is under age 32 years, and the couple has previously conceived.

Physiology and Pathophysiology

The physiology and pathophysiology of infertility depends on the etiology, and may be due to multiple causes. In many cases, the reason for infertility may never be fully understood. Metabolic or endocrine conditions, pathologic conditions of the reproductive tracts, and other etiologies of infertility in general are thought to contribute in some way to a hostile or nonfavorable environment for fertility.

Clinical Manifestations

Inability to conceive after 12 months of unprotected intercourse.

Manifestations vary with the cause.

Differential Diagnosis

Any of these systems may be responsible for the infertility and should be investigated.

Genetic disorder

Structural disorder

Endocrine disorder

Infection

Antisperm antibody

Eating disorder (anorexia, bulimia)

Psychiatric disorder

Neoplasm

Drug ingestion

Diagnostic Tests

See Table 9–11.

Management/Treatment

Treat any existing bacterial infection.

Address any necessary lifestyle modifications, including nutritional status, folate supplementation, stress reduction, smoking, caffeine and alcohol intake, illicit drug use, and exposure to reproductive toxins.

Treatment plan should involve a full discussion regarding treatment options, including adoption, in vitro fertilization, intracytoplasmic sperm injection, and donor surrogacy should treatment be unsuccessful.

Treatment usually requires co-management with infertility specialist.

Pharmacologic Management

Pharmacologic management should be done in consultation with a gynecologist or infertility specialist.

If amenorrheic or oligomenorrheic, consider clomiphene treatment. Start with 50 mg PO daily on days 3–7 of the menstrual cycle; increase to 50 mg daily during the second and third cycles. Ovulation is expected 3–8 days after treatment ends.

Menotropin (Pergonal), 150 IU IM QD for 5 days; begin on cycle days 2–5 if treatment with clomiphene fails. Enhances corpus luteum production of progesterone).

Medroxyprogesterone (Provera; for hypothalamic disorder), 10 mg PO for 10 days.

Naltrexone, a chronic opiate agonist treatment; may be used for the induction of ovulation for women with hypothalamic ovarian failure (administered only by a fertility specialist).

Bromocriptine (Parlodel), 2.5–15 mg QD for increased prolactin secretion, often due to a pituitary adenoma.

Fertility specialists may also attempt a trial pulsatile administration of gonadotropin-releasing hormones to induce follicular development and ovulation and normalize luteal function.

Nonpharmacologic Management

Basal body temperatures to confirm if ovulation has occurred.

Assisted reproductive technologies: Gamete intrafallopian transfer, in vitro fertilization, intracytoplasmic sperm injection.

Table 9–11   Diagnostic Tests: Infertility

Test	Male	Female
General	CBC	CBC
	Chemistry panel	Chemistry panel, thryoid panel
	Urinalysis and culture if indicate	Urinalysis and culture if indicate
	STD, VDRL screening	STD, VDRL screening

Reproductive System	-Semen analysis (2–3 tests as needed)
	  Abstain 2 days; masturbate into sterile container; take to lab within 2 hours:
	Results:
	  Volume: 2–5 ml
	  Liquelaction: complete in 30 minutes.
	  Sperm count: 60–150 million/mL
	  Motility: >60%
	  Morphology: >60% normal forms
	  Oligospermia after 3 sperm analysis, obtain
	  LH, FSH, and serum testosterone.
	  If aspermia, consider testicular biopsy
		-Serum prolactin
		-Day #3 FSH/LH and Estradiol
		-Pap smear
		-Serum progesterone (done 5–7 days after ovulation; if serum level >3ng/ml, ovulation has occurred)

	-Postcoital Test (PCT) (Sims-Huhner)
	  Performed just prior to expectedovulation.
	  A couple refrains from intercourse 2 days prior to the test, and then has intercourse without lubricants 2–10 hours before the test.
	  A mucus sample is taken from the cervix, and microscopically assessed for quality of mucus and sperm motility. The smear should be clear, elastic, fern and should show 5–10 motile sperm.
		-Postcoital Test (PCT) (Sims-Huhner) (also known as the cevival mucus test)
		  Perform around estimated time of ovulation.
		  Determines the number and the condition of sperm and their ability to penetrate cervical mucus. (See description under male)

	-Testicular biopsy
	  If aspermia
		-Hysterosalpingography
		  Test for tubal patency, done 2–3 days after menses. May enhance fertility temporarily.
		-Laparoscopy
		  Allows examination of pelvic contents; performed if hysterosalpingography is unproductive
		-Endometrial biopsy
		  To determine if luteal phase defect, done 2–3 days before anticipated menses

Table continued on following page.

Table 9–11 Diagnostic Tests: Infertility (*Continued*)

Test	Male	Female
Other	-Reproductive Assessment Hair pattern distribution Genitalia Meatus size, location Prostate Scrotum -Neurologic examination Visual fields	-Reproductive Assessment Breast formation Galactorrhea Body fat distribution Hair pattern: virilization Pelvic examination -Neurologic examination Visual fields -Home Basal Body Temperature (BBT) Temperature for 5–10 minutes orally every day before arising for 3 months

Rarely, women may have antibodies to her partner's sperm. It may be helpful to have the man use a condom for at least 30 days, which is thought to decrease the sperm antibodies. After that, intercourse during ovulation without the use of a condom may lead to conception.

Complementary/Alternative Therapies

The following suggestions have not been supported by available scientific studies:

Selenium (deficiency thought to lead to decreased sperm count), 200–400 mg/day

Vitamin C (thought to be important in sperm production, and thought to keep sperm more motile and to prevent clumping of sperm): 2000–6000 μg per day

Vitamin E (thought to carry oxygen to the sex organs), 200–1000 IU/day

Zinc (thought to be important to help sexual organs function), 80 mg per day

Astragalus extract (thought to stimulate sperm motility)

Damiana, ginseng, sarsaparilla, saw palmetto, and yohimbine (thought to enhance sexual function)

Damiana, dong quai, ginseng, gotu kola, licorice root and wild yam root (noted for women)

Client Education

Research indicates a disparity between the actual cause of infertility, and the couples' perceived cause.

There is a tendency for self-blame for infertility.

The interval for intercourse should be about twice weekly.

Avoid lubricants (may act as spermicidal).

Avoid overuse of alcohol (may contribute to reduced sperm count and may interfere with implantation of the fertilized egg in females).

Do not smoke.

Eat a balanced diet.

Help couples determine their own endpoint and timeline for intervention.

Diminished ovarian reserve may be a significant problem, as many couples are prolonging family planning.

Infertility is stressful; stress management techniques or family counseling may be helpful.

If unexplained infertility has been identified after the appropriate treatment has failed, discuss with the couple adoption options, in vitro fertilization, surrogacy, or living without children.

Follow-up
As indicated

Referral

Refer to gynecologist or surgical gynecologist if client has endometriosis or tubal dysfunction.

Refer to infertility/endocrinology specialist if client has suspected endocrine disorder.

Refer for family counseling/support groups.

MENOPAUSE

SIGNAL SYMPTOM ▶ cessation of menstural activity

ICD-9 Codes	627.0	Premenopausal menorrhagia
	627.2	Menopausal, or female climacteric state
	627.4	Condition associated with artificial menopause

Menopause is the cessation of menstrual activity. It is defined as the permanent cessation of spontaneous menstruation caused by loss of ovarian function, diagnosed after no menses have occurred for 12 consecutive months. Late menopause is menopause at or after age 55.

Perimenopause reflects the signs of approaching menopause and a decline in ovarian function. It encompasses physiologic and symptomatic changes surrounding the transition from reproductive to nonreproductive functioning. Postmenopause is the period after menopause. (Knapp, 1999).

Epidemiology

Between 0.2% and 1% of primary care visits are for menopausal symptoms.

Affects approximately 40 million U.S. women.

The mean age of menopause is 51.4 years, and ranges from 41 to 59 years of age.

Unaffected by the age of menarche, race, parity, socioeconomic status, or mother's age at menopause.

Smokers may have an accelerated onset of menopause.

Etiology

All women will become postmenopausal as a result of the depletion of oocytes.

May be due to surgical removal of ovaries either due to disease or as a result of hysterectomy.

May be secondary to treatment of endometriosis with danazol or as a result of breast cancer treatment with antiestrogens or chemotherapy.

Physiology and Pathophysiology

The menstrual cycle involves the hypothalamus, pituitary gland, and ovaries. The hypothalamus secretes gonadotropin-releasing hormone, which then stimulates the pituitary gland to secrete luteinizing hormone (LH) and follicle-stimulating hormone (FSH). LH and FSH stimulate the ovarian follicle to produce estrogen and progesterone. With approaching menopause, the number of ovarian follicles decreases, estrogen levels decline, and the eggs do not respond to the gonadotropins with a rise in both FSH and LH. Estradiol, the main ovarian estrogen, declines at a rate that corresponds to the rise in FSH levels.

Many organs have specific receptors for particular circulating steroid. End-organ alterations occur as a result of declining or absent circulating estrogen levels:

Neuroendocrine: Hot flashes, hot flushes
Skin: Dryness, pruritus, wrinkles, facial hair, dry mouth, dry eyes
Skeleton: Osteoporosis
Vocal cords: Deeper voice
Breasts: Softer, smaller, droop
Heart: Coronary artery disease, increased lipids
Vulva: Atrophy
Vagina: Dyspareunia, vaginitis
Uterus: Prolapse
Bladder: Stress incontinence (Knapp, 1999)

Clinical Manifestations

Subjective

Hot flashes
Nervousness
Insomnia
Depression
Dyspareunia
Stress or urge urinary incontinence
Decreased libido

Objective

Cessation of menses
Vaginal atrophy
Skin atrophy
Osteoporosis
Atherosclerosis
Coronary artery disease

Differential Diagnosis

Pregnancy
Premenstrual syndrome
Perimenopause

Polycystic ovary syndrome

Pituitary adenoma (pituitary tumor composed of glandular epithelium; may cause excessive secretion by gland resulting in excess growth hormone)

Hypothalamic dysfunction (may be related to stress, depression, and anxiety and will lead to amenorrhea because of interruption of normal processes that stimulate ovulation and menstruation)

Asherman's syndrome (secondary amenorrhea caused by obliteration of the endometrial cavity by adhesions that form as a result of curettage of infection)

Thyroid dysfunction (hypothyroidism)

Connective-tissue disorder

Alcoholism, chemical dependency (addiction, diet deficiencies, stress)

Diagnostic Tests

Perimenopause

Menstrual cycles become irregular. Estrogen and androgen levels remain the same, but FSH and LH levels increase dramatically. Progesterone levels are variable.

FSH levels >10–25 indicate some ovarian resistance consistent with menopausal transition.

FSH levels >40 mIU/ml indicate ovarian failure.

LH level remains in the high normal range.

Saliva testing (measures the bioavailable free hormone molecules in the saliva)

Postmenopause

Amenorrhea, estrogen, and progesterone levels decrease; androgen levels decrease.

FSH level >100 mIU/ml indicates postmenopause.

LH and FSH peak 1–3 years after menopause and gradually decline thereafter.

Management and Treatment

Pharmacologic Management

HORMONE THERAPY

The objective of hormone therapy (HRT) is to restore the premenopausal hormonal environment pharmacologically by prescribing estrogen and progesterone.

There are two indications for HRT in perimenopausal and postmenopausal women: relief of vasomotor symptoms and prevention and treatment of osteoporosis and possibly cardiovascular disease. (The issue of whether HRT provides long term cardiovascular protection is very controversial at this time. The risk of cardiovascular incidence and breast cancers is known to increase with combined hormone replacement therapy (estrogen and progesterone).

Absolute contraindications to HT include estrogen-dependent neoplasia of the breast or endometrium, pregnancy, and abnormal vaginal bleeding. Relative contraindications include endometrial hyperplasia, history of thrombosis, diabetes mellitus, hypertension, cholelithiasis, and a family history of estrogen-dependent neoplasia of the breast or endometrium. (See Table 9–12.)

Target Organ Menopause Symptoms

Use the following measures in consultation with an endocrinologist.

General: Low-dose OCPs (for nonsmokers in early menopause who have normal serum lipid levels, do not smoke, and who have no absolute contraindications); Selective estrogen receptor modulators: Tamoxifen and raloxifene (provide estrogen-antagonist effect on breast tissue)

Hot flashes/flushes: Clonidine, 0.1mg PO once or twice daily.

Skin: Estrogen cream applied every night to face with added sunscreen in the morning may improve skin thickness, elasticity, firmness, and moisture.

Hirsutism: Spironolactone (Aldactone), 25mg four times daily or 50 mg twice daily may help decrease androgen production and block the effect of testosterone on hair follicles; cimetidine may provide antiandrogenic effect; dexamethasone, 0.5 mg every night to suppress adrenal hyperfunction.

Osteoporosis: Alendronate sodium (Fosamax), 10 mg every day or 70 mg once a week with 8 oz water (on empty stomach.); calcitonin, 50–100 U subcutaneously three times weekly (at bedtime to avoid nausea); calcitonin nasal spray (Miacalcin), 200 U, or 1 spray per day alternate nostrils.

Nonpharmacologic Management

FOR VASOMOTOR SYMPTOMS

Keep diary of symptoms such as hot flashes. Record timing, severity, food and beverage consumption, recognized stressors, and ambient temperature.

Examine diary for relationships that increase or decrease the hot flash. Eliminate known triggers.

Layer clothing, keep the ambient air cool, drink plenty of fluids, and refrain from excessive alcohol or caffeine intake.

Exercise may lower the incidence of hot flashes.

Relaxation, biofeedback, meditation, and guided imagery have been helpful to some.

Vitamin E, 800 IU daily until symptoms decrease, then 400 IU daily maintenance; bioflavanoids, 500–1000 mg/day; vitamin B complex, 50–100 mg/day; vitamin C, 500 to 3000 mg/day.

SKIN CHANGES

Increase fluids: Drink 8 glasses of water a day; take two teaspoons of oil by mouth per day in dietary intake.

Use mild soaps, natural oils, and sunscreens.

Table 9–12 Hormone Therapy: Menopause

General Considerations

No one product has been shown to be superior.

There is a high variation in medication absorption, which leads to variable individual responses.

Oral and skin patches improve bone density, suppress calcium excretion, and increase calcium absorption.

Oral products increase high-density lipoproteins (HDL), decrease low-density lipoproteins (LDL) better than transdermal preparations.

Transdermal products lower triglycerides; oral estrogen raises triglycerides.

Transdermal skin patches are better for clients with gall bladder disease, liver disease, diabetes, risk for thrombosis, and migraine sufferers.

Vaginal creams or rings are good when relief of urogenital symptoms is necessary. Must use progestogen for endometrial protection.

The lowest dose estrogen that provides relief is the best choice.

Standard menopausal hormone treatment includes the addition of a progestogen to offer protection against the risk of endometrial cancer.

Progestins used alone or in combination with estrogen therapy may increase LDL and decrease HDL levels, supporting a minimum progestin dose. Progestogens (progestins) are synthetic steroids with the same action as progesterone, and may be helpful in relieving vasomotor symptoms in postmenopausal clients, and may be used alone or in with estrogens. They are also useful for the client whom estrogen therapy is contraindicated, or experience intolerable side effects on estrogen therapy.

Evaluate why you are treating with HT, and reassess annually if treatment is effective.

Risks

Endometrial cancer:

4 to 8 fold increase in the risk of developing in users of unopposed estrogen. The increased risk persists for 10 years after discontinuing unopposed estrogen. Adding a progestin reduces risk to level equal to that of nonusers of estrogen.

Breast cancer:

No conclusive evidence has demonstrated an overall increased risk. Risk of breast cancer may increase with duration of use (research in progress).

Estrogen users who do develop breast cancer have been shown to have a decreased mortality over non-users.

Current doses of estrogen replacement therapy thought to protect against osteoporosis and possibly against cardiovascular disease are not currently associated with an increased risk of breast cancer.

Thromboembolic disease:

No increased risk for with oral estrogens.

Type	Drug/Dose	Comments
Estrogen Only	Premarin 0.625 to 1.25mg/day Estratab 1.25mg/day Estrace 1–2mg/day	Cyclic conjugated estrogen: 3 weeks on, one week off. Regimens of less than 0.625 mg daily may not be effective in preventing bone loss. Higher doses must be balanced against the still to be determined risk of endometrial and breast cancer
Synthetic conjugated Estrogen	Cerestin 0.625	
Continuous Conjugated Estrogen	Ethinyl estradiol: Estinyl 0.02 mg to 0.05 mg/day Estropipate: Ogen 0.625mg to 5.0mg/day Ortho-Est 0.75mg to 6.0mg/day	

Table continued on following page.

Table 9–12 Hormone Therapy: Menopause (*Continued*)

Type	Drug/Dose	Comments
Transdermal Estradiol Estrogen	Estraderm 0.05 mg/day or 0.1 Climara 0.05 mg/day or 0.1 Fempatch patch 0.025 Vivelle 0.0375, 0.05, 0.075, or 0.1 mg/day Alora patch 0.05, 0.075, 0.1 Estring vaginal ring 2 mg per 90 day	Transdermal patches provide prolonged blood levels with a limited effect on hepatic function with clotting and lipid abnormalities, relieves vasomotor symptoms and prevents osteoporosis. Permeable adhesive disks are applied to the skin every 3–4 days for 3 of every 4 weeks. Some clients will complain of skin irritation, which is managed by site rotation.
Intramuscular (IM) Injection of Estrogens	Estradiol valerate 10, 20, 40 mg/ml every month.	IM injections vary in absorption and metabolism, and require monthly injections.
Vaginal Therapy (Conjugated estrogens)	Premarin 0.625 to 0.3 mg/g on days 1–21 each month or continuous therapy on weekdays. Estropipate (Ogen) 1.5 mg/g on days 1–21 each month or continuous therapy on weekdays. Estrace 0.5, 1, 2	Daily administration of 1.2 to 2.4 grams is recommended on days 1–21 of each month, or continuous therapy on weekdays only.
Progestins	Norethindrone (Micronor) 0.35 or 0.7 mg daily. Nor QD Norethindrone 0.35 mg Norethindrone acetate 5 mg Medroxyprogesterone acetate (MPA) 5 to 10 mg orally every day. Prometrium 100–300 mg/day MPA Cycrin 2.5, 5, 10 mg MPA Provera 2.5, 5, 10 mg	Micronised oral progesterone formulations have overcome problems of poor absorption, but oral progesterone must be obtained from compounding pharmacists. Progesterone 4% creams and gels are also available, offering minimal systemic side effects with endometrial protection. For the client with an intact uterus progestin is prescribed for at least 10–12 days (day 14–25) of each calendar month: Continuous daily oral administration of both estrogen and progestin is another approach, which allows for eventual cessation of withdrawal bleeding experienced by many clients on cyclic therapy.
Combination of Estrogen and Progestin	Prempro 0.625, 1.25 conjugated equinine estrogen + 2.5 (MPA) Premphase 0.625 mg conjugated equine estrogens for 14 days and 0.625 mg conjugated equine estrogens and 5 mg MPA for 14 days Femhrt 5 ug (ethinly estradiol) + 1 mg (norethindrone) Combipatch 0.05 , 0.1 (estradiol) + 0.14 or 0.25 (norethindrone) (transdermal)	Protection against endometrial hyperplasia occurs when progestin is given for at least 10–12 days (days 14–25) of each calendar month. Continuous daily oral administration of both estrogen and progestin is the newest approach to HRT for the woman with an intact uterus.

Table continued on following page.

Table 9–12   Hormone Therapy: Menopause (Continued)

Type	Drug/Dose	Comments
Testosterone	Estratest 1.25 +2.5 Premarin + methyltestoste- rone 625 + 5, or 1.25 + 10 Testosterone propionate cream 2.5%/day-4%	Esterified estrogens with methyltestoste- rone or conjugated estrogens with methylestosterone may be used when when the client's primary concern is loss of liBIDo. Progestins must be added if a client has an intact uterus. Vulvar pruritis may respond better to a testosterone ointment or cream, which maintains thickness of the vulvar epi- thelium relieving dryness and itching.

VAGINAL DRYNESS

Natural oil to outer labia or water-based lubricant in vagina; avoid soap
on labia.

Avoid douching.

OSTEOPOROSIS PREVENTION

Weight-bearing exercise.

Avoid calcium-wasting triggers such as refined sugars, preservatives,
caffeine, alcohol, and fat and cigarettes; add whole grains, fresh fruits and
vegetables, legumes, etc.

Calcium, 1200–1500 mg a day; manganese, 15–20 mg per day; vitamin D,
250–600 mg per day; zinc, 15–50 mg/day; vitamin B_6, 50–200 mg/day;
folic acid, 400–800 mg/day; vitamin K, 150–500 mg/day.

Complementary/Alternative Therapies

Dong quai root, black cohosh, licorice root, red raspberry leaves, elder, squaw
vine, ginseng, ginger, or any combination herbal preparation for menopause

Soy products (phytoestrogens) such as soy, tempeh, miso, and soy milk

Client Education

Provide anticipatory guidance regarding the expected physiologic changes

Provide nutrition counseling, especially the reduction of dietary fats, and
increase dietary calcium or add a calcium supplement.

Encourage weight-bearing exercise for the prevention of osteoporosis.

Avoid tobacco products, and encourage minimum use of alcohol.

Promote stress reduction.

Review all risks, benefits, and side effects of HRT.

Discuss sexuality changes that commonly occur with menopause.

Follow-up

As indicated and as per age- and risk-related guidelines

Referral

Refer clients who have intermenstrual or postmenopausal bleeding to a gynecologist.

OVARIAN CANCER

SIGNAL SYMPTOMS ➤ vague reports of abdominal pain, weight gain/loss, pelvic pain

ICD-9 Code	239.5	Ovarian neoplasm

Ovarian cancer is a malignant neoplasm of the ovaries.

Epidemiology

Accounts for one third of all gynecologic cancers.

Accounts for only 4% of cancer in women, but is the fourth leading cause of death due to cancer (after lung, breast, and colorectal).

Rare during adolescence, but accounts for 60%–70% of all gynecologic neoplasms that occur during childhood and adolescence.

Lifetime risk for most women is about 1%; however, risk peaks when a women is in her 80s.

The risk for women with a history of ovarian, breast, endometrial, or colon cancer is close to 50%; the risk for women with a close relative who has had ovarian cancer is approximately 5%.

Known as "the silent killer" because the cancer is well established in the peritoneum (pelvic and abdominal organs) in 75% of the patients by the time of diagnosis, resulting in a 5-year survival rate of less than 20%.

After surgery and chemotherapy, 75% achieve complete remission; however, within 3 years most will have a recurrence of the disease.

If at the time of diagnosis, the cancer is limited to the ovaries, 5-year survival rate is 60%–70%.

Etiology

Not well understood.

Suppression of ovulation (e.g., pregnancy, lactation, OCP use) is correlated with reduced risk. This has led to two theories:

Uninterrupted ovulation causes chronic irritation to ovarian epithelium, potentially resulting in cancer.

Repeatedly elevated gonadotropin levels lead to cancer (such levels are suppressed during pregnancy and by OCPs and increased after menopause).

BRCA1 gene mutations, which are also linked to inherited breast cancer, are responsible for approximately 80% of these cases.

Protective factors:

Combination OCP use:

Protection believed to be greatest in nulliparous women.

Better protection the earlier in life OCPs are started.

Inverse relationship between decreased risk and length of time OCPs used; approximately 40% reduction in risk with use of OCPs for at least 3 years.

Decreased risk may last at least 10–20 years after discontinuing use of OCPs.

Exercise (may decrease ovarian cancer risk even after adjusting for all
other risk factors; decreased risk may be due to resulting decreased
incidence of obesity and/or to effects on various hormones)
Increasing number of pregnancies (whether or not reached full term)
Increasing duration of lactation
Possible decreased risk with tubal ligation and with hysterectomy
without removal of ovaries
Hysterectomy with bilateral oophorectomy (does not entirely eliminate
risk since ovarian cancer can still occur in the surrounding tissue that
is not removed)
See Risk Factors 9–3.

Physiology and Pathophysiology

Metastasis can result via the lymphatic system or via direct seeding of the
abdomen and pelvis.

Clinical Manifestations

Subjective

Reports of vague, persistent gastrointestinal pain: feeling of fullness, bloating,
diarrhea, indigestion, constipation, gas, abdominal pain, food intolerance,
abdominal distention (most common sign), weight gain or loss
Pelvic pressure or pain, pain during intercourse
Changes in bladder function: urgency, frequency, increased pressure
Fatigue
Backache

 RF 9–3 Risk Factors: *Ovarian Cancer*

- Age over 40, especially once postmenopausal (most significant risk factor)
- Those of northern European descent have a 40% higher risk than those of other
  racial/ethnic groups
- Talc is a possible risk factor when used in powders applied to the perineum, used
  in feminine hygiene sprays, or used on sanitary napkins, condoms, or for storing
  diaphragms
- Celibacy, nulliparity, few pregnancies, infertility (may be additional increased risk
  if received clomiphene citrate therapy to hyperstimulate the ovaries without
  achieving pregnancy)
- High dietary fat intake (primarily saturated fat; limited studies; results
  inconclusive)
- Other risk factors include repeated spontaneous abortion, endometriosis, prior
  mumps infection, previous irradiation of pelvic organs, exposure to chemical
  carcinogens such as asbestos.
- No known risk—smoking
- Controversial—risk related to menarche before age 12, late menopause, or first
  child after age 30

With advanced disease may have nausea and vomiting, anorexia, abnormal vaginal bleeding

Symptoms most commonly reported by adolescents: bladder/rectum/pelvic pain, menstrual irregularities, precocious puberty, virilization.

Objective

Palpable ovarian mass

Ability to detect mass may be limited due to obesity, uterine enlargement, and/or examiner experience.

Risk that enlarged ovaries are malignant is directly proportional to woman's age; usually the ovaries of postmenopausal women are not palpable.

In young girls, because of physiologic development, ovarian masses are more likely to be palpated over inguinal ligament or higher at suprapubic level.

Differential Diagnosis

Any condition that presents with reports of abdominal fullness, bloating, pain, or intestinal discomfort

Ovarian cysts (midcycle sharp abdominal pain, may be associated with bleeding or spotting)

Metaplastic ovarian tumors (abdominal fullness, pelvic pressure, low backache, early satiety, constipation, gas, intestinal obstruction, pleural effusion, intraabdominal mass)

Germ-cell tumor (majority benign)

Acute appendicitis (severe general abdominal pain that develops rapidly and usually becomes localized to the lower right quadrant)

Diagnostic Tests

Human chorionic gonadotropin test (increased values in quantitative serum human chorionic gonadotropin tests are found in pregnancy and ovarian tumors, while decreased values are found in ectopic pregnancy).

Transvaginal ultrasonography (TVS); preferred method.

Serum CA-125 tumor antigen level (for use with TVS; not recommended as lone screening tool due to high rate of false positive and false negative results; benign conditions such as endometriosis, pregnancy, pelvic inflammatory disease, and uterine fibroids can also elevate CA-125 levels).

Color Doppler imaging.

CT scanning.

Exploratory laparotomy for diagnosis and staging.

For premenarchal children and adolescents and postmenopausal women with a palpable ovarian mass, must do TVS and CA-125 tumor antigen blood test.

For women over 40 who report abdominal pressure, gastric symptoms, or changes in bowel or bladder function: TVS and serum CA-125 tumor antigen level; barium enema and proctosigmoidoscopy and gastrointestinal series to rule out primary colorectal and gastrointestinal cancers

Management/Treatment

Management depends on the stage, grade, size, and location of the tumor.

Pharmacologic Management

Chemotherapy used for metastatic disease and postoperatively for high-risk patients; combination drug therapy is more effective than single-drug therapy.

CA-125 can be used to measure response to chemotherapy.

Nonpharmacologic Management

Surgery (first-line treatment in most cases)

Usually a total hysterectomy and bilateral salpingo-oophorectomy with multiple biopsies.

Women with stage I/grade I tumors who want to preserve fertility may consider a unilateral oophorectomy, postponing removal of the uterus and other ovary.

Adjuvant radioactive therapy (effective when the diameter of the tumor is less than 2 cm; rarely used in the United States for ovarian cancer)

External abdominal and pelvic radiation

Intraperitoneal radiocolloid phosphorus-32 administered by catheter

Complementary/Alternative Therapies

Diets high in fruits and vegetables (especially green) have been associated with a protective effect against ovarian cancer; no specific dietary intakes have been associated with an increased risk of ovarian cancer.

Transdermal testosterone (150 mg/day) to improve sexual functioning and psychological well-being.

See "Complementary/Alternative Therapies" section under "Breast Cancer."

Client Education

Report changes in appetite, increased fatigue, and pain.

Eat small, frequent, low-fiber meals to help control nausea, vomiting, anorexia, and diarrhea.

High-dose chemotherapy—Aerobic exercise immediately after therapy is safe, partially prevents loss of physical conditioning, and may decrease toxic side effects of the therapy.

Follow-up

Schedule regular pelvic examinations and CA-125 tumor-marker blood tests.

Referral

Refer to gynecologic oncologist.

PELVIC INFLAMMATORY DISEASE

SIGNAL SYMPTOMS lower bilateral abdominal/pelvic pain, vaginal discharge, spotting, dyspareunia, dysuria

ICD-9 Code	614.9	Pelvic inflammatory disease

Pelvic inflammatory disease (PID) is an infection of the female upper genital tract.

Epidemiology

More than 1 million cases of PID occur in the United States annually; 1 in 7 women will have at least one episode of PID.

Approximately one third of those who have PID will have at least one more episode.

Sexually active adolescent females have the highest rate of PID; their risk is three times greater than that of women 25–29 years old.

Uncommon in postmenopausal women.

Second only to HIV as serious complication of STDs.

25% of those with PID (both symptomatic and asymptomatic) experience one or more long-term complications.

20%–25% of those with suspected PID must be hospitalized, with an average stay of 4.8 days.

Leading cause of preventable infertility; approximately 20% of those with PID become infertile; risk of infertility increases with each recurrent episode of PID.

50% of all ectopic pregnancies are attributable to PID; 6 to 10 times greater risk of tubal pregnancy.

Pregnant woman with PID are at high risk for preterm labor, fetal wastage, and maternal morbidity.

Etiology

Polymicrobial

80% of all PID is attributable to sexually transmitted organisms; *Neisseria gonorrhoeae* and *Chlamydia trachomatis* alone account for two thirds of all cases of PID.

See Risk Factors 9–4.

 RF 9–4 Risk Factors: *PID*

- Prior history of PID
- Multiple sex partners
- STD infection (up to 1/2 of those with an STD will develop symptomatic or asymptomatic PID)
- Vaginal douching (especially if douche one or more times per month; may flush micro-organisms into upper genital tract; may mask or reduce a discharge due to infection, thereby delaying health-care-seeking behaviors; may be due to resulting altered vaginal environment)
- Intrauterine device (IUD; small increased risk, primarily during the first month after insertion; controversial as to effectiveness of antibiotic prophylaxis at time of insertion to decrease risk; risk not significantly increased with monofilament tailstring; no increased risk in monogamous women)
- Instrumentation of the uterine cavity (e.g., endometrial biopsy, dilation and curettage)
- Cigarette smoking has been correlated with PID (unknown whether correlation due to associated lifestyle or to a pathophysiological change such as altered immune system)

Physiology and Pathophysiology

PID most commonly involves salpingitis. Endometritis, tubo-ovarian abscess, and oophoritis are also common. Pelvic peritonitis and/or inflammation of contiguous structures is less common

PID results from a vaginal and/or endocervical infection (usually chlamydial or gonorrheal), which ascends along contiguous mucosal surfaces to the uterus and fallopian tubes. It may subsequently drain into the ovaries. The exact mechanism is unknown.

The scarring and inflammation that results from PID causes tubal abnormalities that often result in chronic pelvic pain, dyspareunia, pelvic abscess, adhesive disease, infertility (due to tubal obstruction), and/or increased risk of tubal pregnancy (due to tubal ciliary dysfunction). Not being detected or treated and the delay between onset and treatment greatly increase scarring and its resultant risk of infertility and ectopic pregnancy.

Clinical Manifestations

Subjective

Wide variation in symptoms; may have subtle symptoms or be asymptomatic (high rate of asymptomatic PID in adolescents and in women with chlamydial infections)

Lower abdominal/pelvic pain, usually bilateral

Abnormal vaginal discharge

Abnormal spotting

Dyspareunia

Dysuria

Urinary frequency

Right-upper-quadrant abdominal tenderness (perihepatitis, Fitz-Hugh–Curtis syndrome)

Objective

Most important signs: Direct or rebound lower-abdominal tenderness, adnexal tenderness, cervical motion tenderness

Other signs: Oral temperature greater than 101°F, abnormal (particularly purulent) endocervical cervical discharge, cervicitis, right-upper-quadrant tenderness

Differential Diagnosis

Abnormal vaginal bleeding, cervicitis, vaginal discharge, pelvic pain (see "Differential Diagnosis" in section on "Cervical Cancer")

Appendicitis (severe general abdominal pain that develops rapidly and usually becomes localized to the lower right quadrant)

Ovarian cyst (midcycle sharp abdominal pain; may be associated with bleeding or spotting)

Ruptured ovarian cyst (sudden onset of pain midcycle)

Adnexal torsion (pain, bleeding)

Ectopic pregnancy (lower abdominal pain with possible referred shoulder pain on same side; bleeding; may be asymptomatic)

Septic incomplete abortion (systemic infection, pain, discharge)

Endometriosis

Pelvic adhesions (abdominal pain, nausea and vomiting, distention)

Urinary tract infection (frequency, dysuria, polyuria)

Gastrointestinal inflammation (diverticular abscess) or bleeding

Diagnostic Tests

Human chorionic gonadotropin (hCG; to rule out ectopic pregnancy, which are associated with impaired hCG production; urine hCG tests are positive in only 65% of ectopic pregnancies; decreased quantitative serum hCG levels are found in ectopic pregnancy)

Urinalysis (to rule out urinary tract infection)

CBC (elevated white-cell count is a nonspecific indication of infection)

Erythrocyte sedimentation rate or C-reactive protein (elevation in either test is a nonspecific indicator of possible infection)

Cervical cultures (to confirm gonorrhea or chlamydia)

Endometrial biopsy (to confirm endometritis; usually used only when signs and symptoms are questionable)

Laparoscopy (to diagnose salpingitis and pathogen; not useful to detect endometritis; may not detect subtle inflammation of the fallopian tubes; indicated when there is an unclear diagnosis because it provides a more definitive diagnosis, but it is more costly and is invasive)

TVS (to identify suspected pelvic masses)

Management/Treatment

Pharmacologic Management

See Centers for Disease Control and Prevention (CDC) guidelines (Table 9–13.)

Nonpharmacologic Management

Surgical intervention and/or additional diagnostic tests if no significant clinical improvement (reduced or resolved fever; reduced abdominal, adnexal, and cervical motion tenderness) within 3 days after initiating oral or parenteral therapy

Remove IUD

Screen for other STDs and HIV

Client Education

Counsel client to avoid sexual activity until cured (this includes both the woman and her sex partner).

Counsel on safe sex practices:

Use of male latex condoms will prevent transmission of gonorrhea and partially prevent transmission of chlamydia.

In general, barrier forms of contraception decrease risk of STDs and PID.

A diaphragm together with spermicide provide good protection against PID.

Follow-up

Within 72 hours for clients on outpatient oral or parenteral therapy.

4–6 weeks after therapy is completed, rescreen for chlamydia and gonor-

Table 9-13   CDC Guidelines: Management of PID

PID should be empirically treated if all the following are present:
  Sexually active young woman or others at risk for STDs
  Lower abdominal tenderness
  Adnexal tenderness
  Cervical motion tenderness
  No other cause for the signs/symptoms can be identified
Diagnosis of PID is supported by
  Elevated temperature, ESR, and C-reactive protein
  Cervical culture of N. gonorrheoeae or C. trachomatis
  Abnormal cervical or vaginal discharge
Definitive diagnosis of PID requires endometrial biopsy, TVS, or laparoscopy; but these
  procedures are warranted only in a few cases.
Criteria for immediate hospitalization:
  Pregnancy
  Insufficient clinical response to oral therapy
  Appendicitis and other surgical emergencies cannot be excluded
  Tubo-ovarian abscess
  Unable to understand, follow, or tolerate oral therapy
  Severe illness, nausea, vomiting, high fever
  Immunodeficiency
  Postmenopausal women (not CDC guideline, but recommended by others due to serious
    implications in this age group)
  Nulligravida adolescents (not CDC guideline, but recommended by Infectious Disease
    Society for Obstetrics and Gynecology to enhance monitoring, treatment, and client
    education in order to protect future fertility and health)
Any sex partners during the 60 days prior to the onset of symptoms should be examined and
  treated. Male sex partners should be treated for N. gonorrhoeae and C. trachomatis even if
  asymptomatic and regardless of pathogens cultured from the infected female client.
Recommended Treatment Regimens
Oral Regimens
  Ofloxacin (Floxin) 400 mg PO BID for 14 days, plus metronidazole (Flagyl) 500 mg PO BID
    for 14 days
  Or
  Ceftriaxone (Rocephin) 250 mg IM once, plus doxycycline (Vibramycin) 100 mg PO BID for
    14 days
  Or
  Cefoxitin (Mefoxin) 2 g IM once, plus probenecid 1 g PO concurrently once, plus
    doxycycline (Vibramycin) 100 mg PO BID for 14 days
Parenteral Regimens
  Cefotetan (Cefotan) 2 g IV Q12H, plus doxycycline (Vibramycin) 100 mg IV or PO Q12H
    (due to infusion pain, oral route is preferred)
  Or
  Cefoxitin (Mefoxin) 2 g IV Q6 hours, plus doxycycline (Vibramycin) 100 mg IV or PO Q12H
  Or
  Clindamycin (Cleocin) 900 mg IV Q8 hours, plus Gentamicin loading dose IV or IM
    (2mg/kg), followed by maintenance dose (1.5mg/kg) Q8 hours
  Discontinue parenteral therapy 24 hours after clinical improvement, then start doxy-
    cycline (Vibramycin) 100 mg PO BID or clindamycin (Cleocin) 450 mg PO QID for a
    total of 14 days

rhea; for high-risk clients, perform frequent testing for asymptomatic chlamydial infection.

Referral

Refer to physician or gynecologist if client meets criteria for hospitalization or oral therapy does not result in significant improvement within 72 hours.

POLYCYSTIC OVARY SYNDROME

SIGNAL SYMPTOM ▶ midcycle pain, sharp, may be associated with bleeding/spotting

ICD-9 Codes	256.4	Polycystic ovary syndrome/polycystic ovary disease/ Stein-Leventhal syndrome/polycystic ovaries
	620.2	Ovarian cyst

Polycystic ovary syndrome (PCOS), also known as polycystic ovary disease and Stein–Leventhal syndrome, is a complex endocrine disorder involving hypothalamus and pituitary dysfunction and characterized by excess serum androgens and anovulation.

Epidemiology

Considered the most common endocrine disorder in women of reproductive age.

PCOS occurs in 4%–10% of women of reproductive age; 75% of anovulatory infertility cases; 30%–40% of secondary cases amenorrhea; 80%–90% of cases of oligomenorrhea; and 80% of women with hirsutism.

Usually diagnosed during teen years and is progressive until menopause.

20% of women with PCOS are asymptomatic.

Etiology

Exact etiology is unknown.

Strong familial predisposition; possible autosomal transmission.

Related to imbalance of LH to FSH (FSH normal or suppressed, LH elevated).

Obesity increases insulin resistance and hyperandrogenism.

Increased risk of ovarian cancer (two to three times increased risk; greatest in non-obese and those who have not used OCPs), dysfunctional uterine bleeding (DUB), menometrorrhagia, endometrial cancer (due to chronic unopposed estrogen stimulation), breast cancer (possible increased risk), abnormal uterine bleeding, infertility, pregnancy loss (one third of all pregnancies of PCOS women result in spontaneous abortion), pregnancy complications (pre-eclampsia, gestational diabetes, premature labor, stillborn births, cesarean sections because of large infant), hirsutism, insulin resistance (>50%), type 2 diabetes mellitus (up to 40% by age 40), hypertension, dyslipidemia, premature cardiovascular disease, myocardial infarction (sevenfold increased risk)

Physiology and Pathophysiology

PCOS is believed to be an interaction of insulin abnormality and androgen biosynthesis dysfunction:

Hyperinsulinemia, independent of obesity, secondary to insulin resistance.

LH hypersecretion and relatively low FSH level cause ovaries to produce more androgens than estrogen, which in turn leads to an unfavorable environment for maturation of ovarian follicles and results in the failure of ova to develop and the formation of multiple cysts on the ovaries over an extended period of time (months to years) and anovulation.

Abnormal estrogenic pattern: Acyclical production of estrogen and estrone plus progesterone deficiency leads to episodic DUB/menometrorrhagia and endometrial hyperplasia with increased risk of endometrial cancer.

Initial onset is peripubertal, and the syndrome is progressive throughout the reproductive years.

Clinical Manifestations

Subjective

Infertility

Menses (70% report oligomenorrhea, amenorrhea, or DUB; of those reporting normal menses, up to one fifth are found to be anovulatory)

Hirsutism (70%; usually gradual onset in teens or early 20s)

Acne (70%; severe and/or persists into adulthood)

Obesity (40%–70%; waist:hip ratio usually >0.85)

Objective

Enlarged ovaries (bilateral, unilateral, or absent)

Hirsutism (some ethnic groups, such as Asians, do not present with hirsutism, even with significant hyperandrogenism)

Other signs of virilization (male-pattern alopecia, voice changes, clitoromegaly)

Dermatologic manifestations of insulin resistance such as acanthosis nigricans (increased pigmentation of the skin, usually on the neck), intertrigo (increased pigmentation of skin between the thighs), skin tags

Stretch marks (usually related to obesity)

Central obesity with increased waist:hip ratio (>40%)

Acanthosis nigricans (may be seen in those with obesity and especially in those with significant insulin resistance)

Differential Diagnosis

Hirsutism (ovarian tumors; adrenal causes such as congenital adrenal hyperplasia, Cushing's syndrome, and adrenal tumors, suggested by elevated levels of dehydroepiandrosterone sulfate [DHEAS]; drug-related causes such as cyclosporine [Sandimmune], danazol [Danocrine], phenytoin [Dilantin], glucocorticoids, minoxidil [Loniten], diazoxide [Hyperstate], and anabolic steroids; Mediterranean or East Indian heritage; perimenopausal; idiopathic in 50%)

Amenorrhea (pregnancy, lactation, emotional stress, strenuous exercise, anorexia nervosa, severe dieting, chronic illness, endocrinopathies, hyper-prolactinemia, menopause, Asherman's syndrome or other uterine abnor-malities, amenorrhea, pregnancy, lactation; see section on "Amenorrhea")

Anovulation/infertility

Anorexia nervosa, bulimia (low FSH and LH levels)

Rapid weight fluctuations or extreme physical exertion (normal FSH and LH levels)

Premature ovarian failure (high FSH and LH levels)

Progestational medications

Pituitary adenoma (elevated prolactin levels)

Thyroid dysfunction (hyperthyroidism or hypothyroidism)

Other causes include androgen excess, central nervous system infection, neoplasm, anosmia, congenital anomalies, psychiatric disorder; see section on "Infertility")

Obesity

Diagnostic Tests

The National Institutes of Health has proposed that the diagnosis of PCOS be based on hyperandrogenism (elevated levels of testosterone and DHEAS) and chronic anovulation (demonstrated on ultrasonography) after congenital adrenal hyperplasia, hyperprolactinemia, and androgen-secreting neoplasms have been excluded.

Human chorionic gonadotropin (hCG) test (urine and qualitative serum hCG are positive for pregnancy; increased values in quantitative serum hCG tests are positive for pregnancy and ovarian tumors)

Serum total and free testosterone (increased total levels seen in adrenal tumors, ovarian tumors, and idiopathic hirsutism; increased free levels seen in hirsutism, PCOS, and virilization; testosterone levels are highest in the morning)

Prolactin (may be mildly elevated in PCOS; if profoundly elevated must exclude other causes, including pituitary adenoma)

LH and FSH levels (LH levels elevated, no midcycle LH surge, LH:FSH ratio elevated, some consider a ratio of 3:1 as diagnostic; changes are seen in significant number of women with PCOS but are not necessary for diagnosis)

Fasting serum glucose

Management/Treatment

The main goals of therapy are symptom management and the treatment of obesity, dyslipidemia, and insulin resistance, taking into account the woman's desire for fertility.

Treat concurrent conditions (e.g., hirsutism, infertility, acne, alopecia) as indicated.

Pharmacologic Management

Low-dose combination OCPs (as preventive therapy for ovarian, endometrial cancer, and endometrial hyperplasia; increases HDL cholesterol; regulates irregular menses; controls acne and hirsutism [may take up to 6 months to see decrease in hirsutism]; avoid norgestrel and levonorgestrel because of their androgenic activity)

Agents to decrease insulin resistance, especially metformin (Glucophage), 500 mg BID (if client has diabetes mellitus or has significant insulin resistance; not approved by the FDA for treatment of PCOS, but has been found to restore ovulation within 4–6 months in a significant percentage of women with PCOS, including those with normal glucose function)

Medroxyprogesterone (Provera), 5–10 mg PO QD 10–14 days per month (to induce withdrawal bleeding and decrease risk of DUB and endometrial cancer; does not decrease hirsutism and other hyperandrogenic effects; for women who do not wish to conceive and not at risk for pregnancy)

Menopausal PCOS clients (no evidence that HRT is inappropriate, but little research has been done; because of risk factors, should use method that allows for regular shedding of the uterine lining); micronized progesterone (e.g., Prometrium) preferred over synthetic progestin (e.g., Provera); avoid androgenic progesterones (e.g., levonorgestrel) and testosterone replacement therapy (e.g., Estratest)

Nonpharmacologic Management

Weight loss/dietary modifications/exercise (15% decrease in body weight may restore ovulation and decrease hyperandrogenemia, improve insulin resistance, improve lipid profile by increasing HDL and lowering LDL cholesterol and triglycerides)

Counseling/psychological intervention (especially for adolescents for impact of hirsutism, acne, obesity, and infertility)

Laparoscopic ovarian cautery or laser vaporization (restoration of ovulation/fertility; potential postoperative complications such as adhesions)

Client Education

Advise client that as she ages and testosterone levels decrease, androgen-related effects do not automatically lessen; at menopause hirsutism and acne usually do not worsen, whereas the incidence of alopecia increases.

Possible increased risk of breast cancer; therefore, breast self-examinations, annual clinical examinations, and mammography are important.

Follow-up

Monitor lipid profiles every 3–5 years after early adulthood.
Monitor blood pressure annually.

Referral

Refer to reproductive endocrinologist.
Refer to dietician.

PREGNANCY

SIGNAL SYMPTOMS amenorrhea, uterine elargement

ICD-9 Codes	648.8.1	Pregnancy, complicated
	644.2.1	Pregnancy, premature delivery
	645.0	Pregnancy, postmaturity

Intrauterine pregnancy is the condition of carrying a fertilized embryo in the uterus.

Epidemiology

90% of the general population of women should be able to have a healthy pregnancy outcome.

The rate of cesarean section in the United States is about 25%.

Etiology

Favorable conditions for implantation of a fertilized egg into the womb.

Physiology and Pathophysiology

The physiologic, biochemical and anatomic changes during pregnancy are extensive. They are outlined in Table 9–14.

Clinical Manifestations

Subjective

Breast tenderness and enlargement
Fatigue
Urinary frequency
Nausea and vomiting
Fetal movements (quickening)

Objective

Amenorrhea
Uterine enlargement
Chadwick's sign (cervix becomes bluish)
Braxton–Hicks contractions
Goodell's sign (cervix softens)
Hegar's sign (uterus becomes globular in shape, softens, flexes easily over cervix)
Palpitation of fetal contours
Auscultation of fetal heart tones, palpation of fetal movements, ultrasound verification of gestation

Differential Diagnosis

Secondary amenorrhea
Ectopic pregnancy (vaginal bleeding, abdominal pain and syncope usually at 9–12 weeks of gestation)
Abdominal mass

Diagnostic Tests

hCG β-subunit (β-hCG) is detected by maternal serum and urine assays 8–10 days after fertilization or at 22–24 days of gestation
Abdominal ultrasonography: Usually done at 4–5 weeks of gestation

Management/Treatment

For management/treatment of common problems that occur during pregnancy, see Table 9–15.

General

Prenatal visits occur every 4 weeks through the 28th week, then every 2 weeks through the 36th week, then weekly until delivery.
Frequency of visits is determined by risk status of client.
Weight, blood pressure, fundal height, urine dipstick, and fetal heart rate should be measured at each visit.

Table 9–14   Physiologic Changes During Pregnancy

System	Changes
Cardiovascular	*Heart:* displaced upward, to the left with the apex moved laterally; size increases about 12% due to increased volume or hypertrophy *Cardiac output:* increases about 40% with a peak at 24 weeks gestation. *Blood pressure:* may decline slightly. *Other:* obstruction of the inferior vena cava, and pressure of the common iliac vein results in decreased blood return to the heart. This decreases cardiac output, decreases blood pressure, and causes edema in the lower extremities
Respiratory	*Respirations:* as the uterus enlarges, the diaphragm is elevated, the rib cage displaced. Abdominal muscles decreased tone causes respirations to be more diaphragmatic in nature. *Other:* early in pregnancy, capillary dilatation occurs throughout the respiratory tract leading to engorgement of the nasopharynx, larynx, trachea, and bronchi; the voice may change, and breathing made difficult.
Gastrointestinal	*Oral changes:* increased salivation due to nausea; alteration in oral pH may lead to dental caries; gums may become hypertrophic, swollen and tender due to increased estrogen levels during the first trimester *Stomach:* gastric acidity may increase or decrease; esophageal peristalsis is decreased, and contributes to complaints of reflux due to reduced emptying time and relaxation or dilation of the cardiac sphincter. Elevation of the stomach due to the enlarged uterus contributes to reflux, especially while supine. *Bowel:* large and small bowel are pushed up and laterally, the appendix is displaced superior in the right flank; increased levels of progesterone decrease gastric motility, food is retained in the GI tract longer, more water is absorbed, and constipation occurs. *Gallbladder:* hypotonia of the smooth muscle wall, slow and incomplete emptying, thickened bile, and stasis may lead to gallstone formation. *Liver:* increased serum alkaline phosphatase due to placental isoenzymes; decreased albumin/globulin ratio occurs normally in pregnancy.
Renal/Urinary	*Kidneys:* size increases 1–1.5 cm; renal pelvis dilates, ureters dilate and lengthen contributing to urinary stasis and infection. *Bladder:* displaced upward, and pressure from the uterus leads to frequency.
Hematologic	*Blood volume:* increases, with an average of 45%–50% at term. *Red blood cells:* (RBCs) mass increases 33%. Plasma volume increases, hematocrit falls until the end of second trimester when the RBC and plasma volume synchronizes. As RBC increases, so does the need for iron.
Metabolism	*Weight gain:* due to the uterus and its contents, increased breast tissue, blood and water volume; average weight gain is 12.5 kilograms. *Total body fat:* increases and varies with the total weight gain; plasma lipids increase, triglycerides, cholesterol and lipoproteins decrease after delivery.

First Prenatal Visit

DETERMINE ESTIMATED DATES OF CONFINEMENT (EDC)

Document first day of last menstrual cycle and first positive pregnancy test. Document date of first pelvic examination and estimated gestational age. Fundal height in centimeters is similar to the length of gestation from

20–30 weeks. Fetal heart tones are audible with Doppler fetoscope at 10–12 weeks. If dates are in question, ultrasonography during the first or second trimester is critical for determining EDC.

PHYSICAL EXAMINATION

Fetal heart tones.

Pelvic examination to document uterine size and the bony pelvis that includes the conjugate diameter.

Table 9–15 Management/Treatment of Common Problems of Pregnancy

Problem	Management/Treatment
Abdominal Pain	**Always evaluate.** Ectopic pregnancy should be ruled out. Pre-eclampsia should be ruled out if pain in the epigastrum or right upper quadrant. Placental abruption should be considered if pain is associated with vaginal bleeding, especially in late pregnancy. UTI should be considered, especially if symptomatic. Round ligament or broad ligament discomfort may be present with tension on these structures as the uterus increases.
Backaches:	A maternity girdle, low-heeled shoes, improved posture, and walking are helpful
Constipation	Encourage high fiber foods and limit refined carbohydrates, encourage adequate water intake and mild exercise.
Edema	Common in third trimester due to water and sodium retention and increase venous pressure. Consider preeclampsia if associated with hypertension or proteinuria. Benign edema responds to leg elevation.
Headaches	Common before week 20, usually benign. Acetaminophen is safe. Migraine patterns may change during pregnancy. Always consider pre-eclampsia, especially later pregnancy.
Heartburn	Frequent small meals, avoid lying flat. Antacids may be helpful, but are thought to impair absorption of iron.
Hemorrhoids	Sitz baths, topical anesthetics, stool softeners.
Medication Use	Medications considered safe: Antihistamines, acetaminophen (low dose), cephalosporins, erythromycin, meclizine low dose of 12.5-25 may be safe), penicillin, trimethoprim-sulfamathoxazole (safe in early pregnancy) Medications to avoid: Antiemetics, acetaminophen (avoid continuous high doses), diphenhydramine (Benadryl), metronidazole (contraindicated in first trimester), nitrofurantoin (use with caution in late pregnancy), promethazine, prochlorperazine, tetracycline, trimethobenzamide
Nausea and Vomiting	Usually starts at 6 weeks and disappears by week 16. If severe, seek medical care. May require fluid replacement. Reassure, eat small more frequent meals, avoid foods that worsen symptoms. Use of antiemetics is controversial. Vitamin B-6 supplement may be helpful (25–50 mg/day).
Vaginal Bleeding	Always investigate. Consider extrauterine pregnancy or spontaneous abortion in early pregnancy, or placenta previa or abruptio in late pregnancy.
Vaginal Discharge	Common in pregnancy, but infections should be ruled out.
Varicose Veins	Due to increased femoral pressure. Periodic resting and leg elevation is safe. Elastic stockings may be helpful.

Evaluate the ischial spine, shape of the sacrum, distance between the ischial tuberosities, and angle of the pubic arch.

<u>DIAGNOSTIC TESTS</u>

CBC
Blood type and Rh factor
Antibody screen
Syphilis serology
Test for hepatitis B surface antigen
Rubella titer
Urinalysis and culture
Pap smear
Cultures for *N. gonorrhoeae* and *C. trachomatis*
HIV counseling and testing (if not done during preconception care)

<u>CLIENT EDUCATION</u>

Discuss risk behaviors:

> Smoking has been associated with placenta previa and increased placental complications.
> Alcohol use is linked to fetal alcohol syndrome.
> Cocaine use is associated with spontaneous abortions, abruptio placentae, and early behavioral and environmental response alterations in the newborn.
> Opiates are linked to premature delivery and growth retardation and neonatal withdrawal symptoms.

Discuss nutrition and weight gain:

> Average 26–28 lb gain during pregnancy. A gain of less than 10 lb at 28 weeks is associated with complications.
> Usually requires 2400 kcal/day, and diet high in calcium, complex carbohydrates, 20% protein, 30% fat. A multivitamin and mineral supplement with 300 mg of iron and 1 mg of folic acid is recommended.

Encourage enrollment and participation in childbirth preparation classes.

Sexual intercourse: Only contraindicated if at risk for spontaneous abortion or premature labor.

Physical activity: Normal nonstrenuous levels may be maintained.

Discuss when to immediately contact health-care provider:

> Vaginal bleeding or fluids from the vagina
> Swelling of face and fingers
> Continuous headache
> Alteration of vision
> Abdominal pain
> Persistent vomiting
> Chills or fever
> Dysuria
> Change in frequency or intensity of fetal movements

First Trimester (0–14 weeks)

Offer early prenatal diagnostic studies to clients with genetic risks.

Chorionic villus sampling (CVS) may be done from 8 to 12 weeks of gestation.

Amniocentesis may be performed at 10–14 weeks.

Fetal heart tones heard at 10–12 weeks with Doppler ultrasonography.

Cervical β-streptococcus screening is recommended at first trimester and before delivery.

Second Trimester (14–28 weeks)

The fundal height roughly corresponds to the number of weeks of gestation.

Ultrasonographic dating of pregnancy is helpful.

Fetal heart tones heard at 17–20 weeks with a standard fetoscope.

Quickening is felt at 16–20 weeks.

Maternal serum α-fetoprotein screening is present between 15 and 20 weeks.

Standard amniocentesis may be performed at 16 weeks.

Screen all clients for gestational diabetes between 26 and 28 weeks. A glucose-tolerance test is standard to test for gestational diabetes.

Rh-negative clients should be given Rh_0 immune globulin at 28 weeks of gestation, or earlier if an event has exposed the client to fetal blood, such as early amniocentesis, CVS, or trauma. A repeat dose is given within 72 hours after delivery.

Third Trimester (28–36 weeks)

Hemoglobin and hematocrit at 28 weeks of gestation for anemia.

Preterm Labor (<36 Weeks of Gestation)

Occurs in 8%–10% of pregnancies, but is responsible for 60% of perinatal morbidity and mortality.

Risk factors include smoking, cervical incompetence, infections, multiple gestation, stress, and low socioeconomic status.

Early diagnosis is imperative to arrest preterm labor. Confirm by external monitoring and cervical examination.

Treat underlying cause of uterine irritability, such as urinary tract infection.

Rest and increased fluids are indicated.

Tocolytic therapy initiated in hospital is indicated.

Postdate Pregnancy (>42 Weeks)

Begin fetal assessments between 34 and 36 weeks of gestation, or sooner if pregnancy is high-risk.

At 41 weeks, begin daily fetal movement testing: Count 10 fetal movements each day and report to health-care provider if this does not occur in 12 hours.

Fetal heart rate testing: The nonstress test is noninvasive; it shows an accelerated fetal heart rate with movement. Three or more accelerations of >15 beats per minute, each lasting for 15 seconds in a 20-minute period is normal.

At 41–42 weeks, begin twice weekly contraction stress test (CST) and ultrasonography. The CST stimulates uterine contraction; requires three contractions in 10 minutes.

Amniotic fluid evaluation: Ultrasonography to estimate amniotic fluid volume, which directly measures placental function.

At 43 weeks, CST, ultrasonography, induction of labor.

Referral

Refer to obstetrician.

PREMENSTRUAL SYNDROME/ PREMENSTRUAL DYSPHORIC DISORDER

SIGNAL SYMPTOMS▶ irritability, tension, dysphoria, lability of mood

ICD-9 Code	625.4	Premenstrual dysphoric disorder

Premenstrual syndrome (PMS) and premenstrual dysphoric disorder (PMDD) are characterized by luteal-phase mood, behavioral, and physical symptoms that remit with the onset of menses or shortly thereafter. Women with PMS have two to four premenstrual symptoms that may be affective or somatic but do not cause significant functional impairment. Women with PMDD have at least five premenstrual symptoms, at least one of which is affective, and suffer functional impairment in domestic, occupational, or social domains and have a 2-month history of symptoms, primarily irritability and functional disability/inability.

Epidemiology

Actual prevalence not known.

Only ~10% of menstruating women have no premenstrural symptoms; as many as 75% experience mild to moderate PMS, and about 15% suffer from PMDD.

PMS may commence with menarche, while the onset of PMDD usually occurs in the mid-20s.

Affects clients of childbearing age and all ethnic groups.

PMS/PDD symptoms may worsen with age.

Many PMS/PMDD clients have a history of pre-eclampsia or postpartum mood disorders.

Cyclic symptoms of PMS/PMDD have been documented after menopause.

Etiology

True etiology is unknown; suggested causes include decreased progesterone levels, metabolic and endocrine disorders, disruption of the hypothalamic feedback mechanism, and preexisting psychiatric disorders.

Risk factors include maternal or familial tendency for PMS/PDD, pre-eclampsia during pregnancy, and midlife onset of symptoms

Physiology and Pathophysiology

PMS/PMDD is presumed to be hormonal because symptoms occur cyclically as levels of estrogen and progesterone decline and levels of prolactin elevate. A higher level of free serum testosterone has been implicated, because this has been found in some women who have PMS. Abnormalities of neurotransmitters have been suggested, such as aberrant platelet uptake of serotonin and altered norepinephrine function. The physical symptoms of weight gain and breast tenderness have been linked to an increase in renin–angiotensin and aldosterone. Altered sleep cycles, changes in melatonin secretion, vitamin and mineral deficiency, and dietary and behavioral abnormalities have also been suggested as causes of PMS or PMDD.

Clinical Manifestations

Subjective

One of the four core symptoms (irritability [most common symptom reported for PMDD], tension, dysphoria, and lability of mood) and at least five of the symptoms typically listed in a PMS diary

Symptoms must be of sufficient severity as to disrupt the daily life of a client (if the intensity of symptoms increases at least 30% in the 6 days before onset of menses and occurs for at least two menstrual cycles—three cycles is preferred)

Must also be a history of one or more of the predisposing factors:

Breast tenderness

Headaches

Backache

Decreased urinary frequency

Dizziness/syncope

Tingling of hands or feet, edema, new or exacerbation of old skin disorders

Vision changes

Abdominal bloating, nausea, vomiting, constipation, colic or alteration in appetite

Psychogenic manifestations, including sleep disturbance, mood swings, anxiety, anger and violent behavior, depression, difficulty concentrating, irritability, lethargy, and fatigue

Objective

Comprehensive physical examination findings are within normal limits.

Differential Diagnosis

Any of the following diagnoses may present with one or more of the subjective findings described above.

Thyroid dysfunction

Hyperprolactinemia

Depression

Dysthymia

Anxiety

Diabetes

Menopause

Dysmenorrhea

Menstrual migraine

Diagnostic Tests

The symptom diary is the essential test for PMS/PMDD and should be kept for a minimum of 2 months—3 is preferred.

Laboratory tests are not useful, except to rule out other causes.

Management and Treatment

Pharmacologic Management

Depression, sleep disturbance, and cognitive difficulty: Selective serotonin reuptake inhibitors (SSRIs), fluoxetine (Prozac), 20–60 mg daily, sertraline (Zoloft), 50 to 150 mg PO daily (Serafem for PMDD), 20 mg daily

For PMS symptoms that are below the threshold for PMDD (do not significantly impair functioning), luteal-phase or symptom-onset dosing of an SSRI may be appropriate.

Anxiety: Buspirone, 5–10 mg three times daily.

PMS primary physical symptoms may be controlled with between 100 and 1200 mg of calcium daily.

Pain: Acetaminophen and aspirin for simple general muscular pains or headaches.

Migraine headaches as part of PMS: May be treated approximately 1–10 days before menses; fenoprofen, 400 mg four times/day; naproxen sodium, 550 mg twice daily, or propranolol, 40–160 mg twice daily; and ergotamine suppository, 1–2 mg at bedtime are preventive measures. Treat with conventional abortive migraine therapy if needed.

Water retention related to elevated aldosterone and prolactin levels: Spironolactone (Aldactone), 25 mg four times daily, begin 3 days before the expected onset of symptoms and continue until the start of menses); bromocriptine mesylate (Parlodel), 1.25–2.5 mg twice daily, suppresses prolactin production and may be given throughout the menstrual cycle; danocrine, 200 mg daily, and attenuated androgen have been used if the above medications have been unsuccessful.

Other: OCPs and medroxyprogesterone have proved beneficial to some for reducing symptoms of PMS, especially if the client is under 40 years of age, does not smoke, and requires contraception (Ugarriza et al., 1998).

Nonpharmacologic Management

Nutrition/Diet

Low-sodium diet from midcycle to the onset of menses relieves symptoms associated with fluid retention, including bloating, weight gain, backache, and headache.

Avoid foods with nitrites, high-fat foods, salted butter or margarine, and high-sodium chips and canned foods.

Fresh foods high in potassium decrease aldosterone secretion, which may cause sodium retention and associated symptoms.

Eat three well-balanced meals consisting of higher protein and lower carbohydrates reduces hypoglycemia, which may lead to headaches, fainting, dizziness, and fatigue.

Avoid refined sugars and caffeine products.

Dietary supplements of vitamin B_6, magnesium, zinc, and vitamin C provide relief of symptoms.

Activity/Exercise

Increased activity/exercise increases endorphins, improves mental health through stress reduction and may improve altered sleep patterns.

Complementary/Alternative Therapies

Encourage client to take control of symptoms by eliminating adverse health habits, such as smoking or drinking alcohol.

Reduce negative emotions by developing cognitive restructuring and problem-solving skills, which may provide physical and emotional relief of symptoms.

Biofeedback, meditation, relaxation, yoga, and other forms of relaxation techniques have beneficial effects.

Aroma therapy has had some success in relieving or diminishing associated symptoms of PMS. As has hot baths scented with bergamot, rosemary, orange, and ylang ylang.

For affective symptoms related to altered levels of magnesium and vitamin B_6: Vitamin B_6, 200–800 mg daily.

L-tryptophan, 2 g three times a day from day 14 through day 3 of the menstrual cycle has been a helpful adjunct to antidepressant therapy.

For water retention related to elevated aldosterone and prolactin levels: Vitamin E, 400 mg twice daily.

For appetite changes related to increased insulin receptor sites: Vitamin supplements A, C, and E. Evening primrose oil, 1000 mg twice daily is also helpful.

Client Education

Educate clients about misinformation regarding PMS/PMDD. Provide information based on medical and research-based studies, and assist client to establish realistic expectations for symptom improvement.

Follow-up

Initially, see client every 3 months to make diagnosis and monitor treatment.

Referral

Refer to mental health counselor if indicated.

TESTICULAR CANCER

SIGNAL SYMPTOMS ▶ testicular mass, scrotal heaviness

ICD-9 Code	789.3	Testicular lump

Testicular cancer is a malignant intrascrotal mass.

Epidemiology

The third most frequently found tumor in men ages 20 to 34.

Affects 2–3 per 100,000 men each year.

An undescended testicle, even if surgically reduced has an increased risk of cancer that is 2.5–20 times greater than that of a male with a descended testicle.

Rare in African-Americans.

Etiology

Most testicular tumors are of germ-cell origin, such as a seminoma, embryonal-cell carcinoma, teratoma, and choriocarcinoma.

Some are of a mixed histology, containing more than one cell type (Porth, 1999, pg 1167).

Choriocarcinoma is the most aggressive testicular cancer, with a rapid spread to the lungs and other viscera.

Non–germ-cell tumors are often benign. Interstitial-cell (Leydig-cell) tumors are the most common. These tumors in prepubertal males may secrete androgens and estrogens and cause gynecomastia.

Sertoli-cell tumors are rare, and they metastasize only infrequently.

Physiology and Pathophysiology

Testicular tumors spread through both the vascular and the lymphatic systems, and they are predictable. The lymphatics of the left testicle drain to the left para-aortic retroperitoneal nodes, and the lymphatics of the right testicle drain to the inter-aortocaval group. The most common site of metastasis is in the lung.

Clinical Manifestations

Subjective

Testicular neoplasms are usually asymptomatic.

About 20% of those affected experience heaviness, or a unilateral discomfort is present.

Acute hemorrhage into the tumor may also occur, causing capsular distention.

Objective

Testicular neoplasms are usually firm to hard, nontender masses on the testicle that do not transilluminate.

A palpable left supraclavicular node or epigastric mass may be found.

May have an associated gynecomastia from chronic gonadotropin or estrogen secretion.

A hematoma that appears after minimal trauma should be considered a testicular tumor until proven otherwise.

The testicular tumor may be small, as with a choriocarcinoma, and it is not easily palpable through the thick, overlying tunica albuginea.

Differential Diagnosis

Hernia (protrusion of organ through abnormal opening in muscle wall of cavity it surrounds; pain, constipation, swelling)

Epididymitis (testes tender)

Intratesticular epidermoid cyst (diagnosed by ultrasonography of the scrotum)

Hydrocele (usually tender; confirmed by ultrasonography)

Hematoma

Spermatocele (cystic swelling, either of epididymis or of the testis; usually painless)

Syphilitic gumma (granuloma with tertiary syphilis; may be localized or diffuse on trunk, legs, and face and various internal organs, especially the liver)

Varicocele (swelling of spermatic cord that can cause pain, usually more painful in standing position and more common in left cord than right)

Diagnostic Tests

Tumor marker tests:

α-fetoprotein

hCG

Lactate dehydrogenase (may indicate tumor burden)

Plasma alkaline phosphatase (elevated with recurrent/disseminated seminomas)

Scrotal ultrasonography (to evaluate testicular mass for potential neoplasm)

Biopsy (to confirm neoplasm)

Chest x-ray examination, CT scan (for staging)

Management/Treatment

Testicular neoplasm is confirmed by orchiectomy. If an intratesticular lesion is found, the spermatic cord is ligated at the inguinal ring and the testis and coverings are removed. Treatment is based on the tumor type determined by histologic findings and by tumor staging, which includes tumor extent and vascular space tumor invasion.

For staging and management of testicular cancer, see Table 9–16.

Client Education

Testicular self-examination.

Duration of treatment and importance of follow-up appointments.

Relapse may occur, often within the first 2 years after diagnosis.

Follow-up

The American Urology Association recommends annual testicular examinations beginning at age 15, every 3 years from ages 20 to 40, and annual examinations thereafter.

Chest x-ray examinations and tumor-cell markers for 18–24 months are advised; CT scans of the chest and abdomen are also recommended.

Referral

Refer to urologist.

Table 9–16   Staging and Management: Testicular Cancer

Stage	Description	Treatment	Five-Year Survival Rate
	Seminomas		
I	Tumor confined to the testis	Radical orchiectomy 25–30 cGy of radiation to the retro-peritoneum	>95%
IB		Abdominal and mediastinal Irradiation Cisplatin-based chemotherapy is curative	
II	Nodal metastases		>95%
IIA	Limited nodal metastases	Radical orchiectomy 25–30 cGy of radiation to the retroperitoneum	
IIB	Bulky nodal metastases		
III	Tumor involving lymphatics above the diaphagm	Abdominal and mediastinal Irradiation Cisplatin-based chemotherapy is curative	75%
IV	Hematogenous metas-tasis		
	Nonseminomatous Germ Cell Tumors NSGCT)		
I and II		Inguinal orchiectomy and irradiation. Retroperitoneal lymph node dissection. Controversial, as only 25% have metastasis.	Close to 100%
II and higher		Primary chemotherapy with resection of residual tumor after chemotherapy. Continue chemotherapy until maximal shrinkage has occurred. Re-sect masses in other organs.	Exceed 90%

TESTICULAR TORSION

SIGNAL SYMPTOMS ➤ sudden and severe unilateral testicular pain

ICD-9 Codes	608.2	Testicular torsion

Testicular torsion is an acute scrotal condition caused by twisting of the testis and spermatic cord, resulting in acute ischemia. Intravaginal torsion occurs within the tunica vaginalis. Extravaginal torsion involves twisting of the testis, cord, and processus vaginalis and in undescended testes.

Epidemiology

The peak incidence of torsion of the testicular appendage is around age 10 years and occurs before puberty.

The risk for men by age 25 is 1 in 160; it is rare in men over age 30.

Etiology

Cause is spontaneous and not clearly understood; may include contraction of cremasteric muscles from cold, fright, or intercourse; alteration in testosterone level during nocturnal sex response; excessive exercise, straining, or attempts at reducing hernias; and inadequate, incomplete, or absent fixation of testis within scrotum.

Approximately 20% of clients report prior trauma; one third of clients have had prior testicular pain.

Physiology and Pathophysiology

Spontaneous testicular torsion is caused by a sudden twisting of the spermatic cord, when the testicular mesentery anchors the testes to the scrotal wall. Neonates can sustain torsion of the entire testicle and spermatic cord above the tunica vaginalis.

Clinical Manifestations

Subjective

Sudden and severe unilateral testicular pain; pain may be intermittent, reflecting spontaneous detorsion and retorsion.

Often associated with nausea, vomiting, and fever.

Torsion of the testicular appendage causes unilateral scrotal pain and swelling, perhaps less pronounced than testicular torsion.

Objective

Erythema of the testicle.

Fever.

Testes may be high in the scrotum with a transverse lie.

May have absence of cremasteric reflex.

Differential Diagnosis

Torsion may mimic epididymitis at onset of symptoms.

Incarcerated or strangulated inguinal hernia (inguinal pain, swelling).

Testicular tumor (painless lumps; may cause pain related to bleeding from rapid tumor growth and necrosis).

Hydrocele, spermatocele, epididymal cyst, or generalized edema.

Abdominal aortic aneurysm, ureteral colic, retrocecal appendix, retro-peritoneal cancer, and prostatitis.

Diagnostic Tests

Doppler ultrasonography (gold standard)

Urinalysis (can detect pyuria, bacteriuria, and hematuria to rule out bacterial etiology)

Urethral smear (helpful in detecting epididymitis)

Doppler stethoscope (will reveal reduced or absent blood flow with torsion and increased vascular perfusion with epididymitis)

Management/Treatment

Immediate urologic consultation and surgical referral is required.

Unless the possibility of testicular torsion has been eliminated by Doppler ultrasonography, emergency surgery is indicated because the testicle will die from total torsion 3 to 24 hours after onset.

Testicular viability is improved (70%–100%) if detorsion is accomplished within 10 hours; viability after 10–12 hours of ischemia is about 20%, and nearly 0% after 24 hours of ischemia (Burns, 1997, pg 1017).

In testicular torsion, bilateral orchidopexy is necessary because of the possibility of future contralateral testicular torsion, primarily because the bell clapper deformity normally occurs in both testicles. Orchiectomy of the nonviable testicle must be included.

Torsion of the testicular appendage is managed nonsurgically with analgesics and ice.

A local nerve block or excision of the twisted appendage may be indicated if swelling and pain are severe.

Client Education

There is a possibility of testicular atrophy in the salvaged testis, causing a depressed sperm count that results in infertility.

Follow-up

Postoperatively, monitor at 1–2 week intervals; then yearly visits until puberty to evaluate for atrophy (Fox, 1997).

Referral

Refer immediately to urologist and/or surgeon.

UTERINE/ENDOMETRIAL CANCER

SIGNAL SYMPTOM abnormal uterine bleeding

ICD-9 Codes	233.2	Uterine carcinoma
	236.0	Uterine neoplasm

Uterine cancer is a malignancy of the uterus; more than 95% are endometrial carcinomas (developing in the uterine lining); 2%–4% are uterine sarcomas (developing in the connective tissues of the uterus).

Epidemiology

Fourth most common cancer in women (after breast, lung, and colon cancers); accounts for 13% of all cancers in women.

Approximately 35,000 new cases and 6000 deaths annually.

Primarily seen in postmenopausal women (85% of those with uterine cancer are over age 50).

73% overall 5-year survival rate (86% for stage I, 66% for stage II, 44% for stage III, 16% for stage IV).

Etiology

See Risk Factors 9–5.

Recurrence (most common in high-risk women and in premenopausal women; 85% of recurrences occur within 3 years after treatment)

RF 9–5 Risk Factors: *Uterine/Endometrial Cancer*

■ Family history of endometrial cancer or colon cancer (especially hereditary nonpolyposis colon cancer)
■ Prior history of ovarian or breast cancer
■ Untreated endometrial hyperplasia (see sidebar)
■ Increased estrogen exposure
　Early menarche (before age 12)
　Late menopause (after age 50–52)
　Total lifetime span of menstruation (early menarche plus late menopause; greater risk than either one alone)
　Increased bleeding during perimenopause (4 times greater risk)
　Nulliparity
　Infertility
　Obesity, high caloric intake, and high animal fat intakes (depending on severity of obesity there is a 2 to 5 times greater risk; high animal fat consumption is believed by some to have a direct impact on estrogen metabolism)
　Tamoxifen (overall 1.5 increased risk, 2.0 increased risk if tamoxifen taken 2 to 5 years, 6.9 increased risk if taken for at least 5 years; risk does not decrease after discontinuation of tamoxifen)
　Estrogen replacement therapy (ERT; should not be used in women with an intact uterus)
　Ovarian disease such as polycystic ovaries and granulosa-theca cell tumors
■ Previous pelvic radiation
■ Age (risk increases with age)
■ Hypertension
■ Diabetes mellitus types I and II
■ Decreased risk/protective effect
　Decreased risk with use of hormonal contraceptives (estrogen/progesterone combination and progestin-only, including Norplant and Depo-Provera; linear correlation between length of use and decrease in risk; decreased risk believed to last for at least 10 years after discontinuation of the contraceptive)
　Combined hormone replacement therapy (no increased risk; those who have taken continuous combined HRT for only a few years may have a lower risk than those who have never used HRT)
　Decreased risk with smoking (greatest reduction in current smokers, obese smokers, and postmenopausal women; may be due to alterations in metabolism, aborption, or distribution of hormones)
　Reduced risk associated with high intake of vegetables, especially green vegetables
　Alcohol has a protective effect or no effect (research divided)
　High parity

Physiology and Pathophysiology

Endometrial carcinoma subtypes: Adenocarcinoma (75% of women with uterine cancer), papillary serous carcinoma (15%, poor prognosis), adenosquamous carcinoma (5%, poor prognosis), adenoacanthoma (less than 1%), clear-cell adenocarcinoma (3%, poor prognosis), undifferentiated carcinoma (1%, poor prognosis), and secretory adenocarcinoma

Sarcoma subtypes: Carcinosarcomas (most common sarcoma; also known as malignant mixed mesodermal tumors or malignant mixed Müllerian tumors); start in endometrium; have features of both sarcoma and carcinoma); leiomyosarcomas (develop in the muscular wall of the uterus); and endometrial stromal sarcomas (least common; develop in the stroma of the endometrium)

Staging (see Table 9–17)

Clinical Manifestations

Subjective

Abnormal uterine bleeding (80%–90%)

Postmenopausal bleeding (one third will have endometrial cancer; may have been preceded by vaginal discharge for several weeks or months)

Premenopausal recurrent metrorrhagia

Mucosanguineous discharge (10%)

Pelvic pain (10%, usually a sign of advanced disease)

Weight loss (usually a sign of advanced disease)

Table 9–17   Staging: Uterine/Endometrial Cancer

Stage	Endometrial Carcinoma	Uterine Sarcoma	Five-Year Survival Rate
I Limited to corpus uteri	IA: Limited to endometrium		Endometrial: 90% Sarcoma: 50%
	IB: spread less than halfway through myometrium		
	IC: Spread more than halfway through myometrium		
II Spread to cervix	IIA: Involves endocervical glands		Endometrial: 70%–85% Sarcoma: 20%
	IIB: Involves cervical stroma		
III Spread outside uterus but confined to pelvic area	IIIA: Spread to adnexa, uterine serosa (outer layer), or peritoneal fluid	IIIA: same	Endometrial: 50% Sarcoma: 10%
	IIIB: Vaginal metastases	IIIB: same	
	IIIC: Spread to pelvic and/or para-aortic lymph nodes	IIIC: same	
IV Spread to non-gynecological organs	IVA: Spread to mucosa of bladder and/or rectum	IVA: same	Endometrial: 10%–30% Sarcoma: 10%
	IVB: spread to groin lymph nodes and/or to distant organs	IVB: same	

Reference: American Cancer Society

Objective

Blood in the vaginal vault

Enlarged, soft uterus/pelvic mass (usually seen in advanced disease)

Pap smear (should not be used as a screening tool for endometrial cancer)

Benign endometrial cells or atypical squamous cells of undetermined significance (ASCUS) suggestive of endometrial cells

Premenopausal woman (especially if approaching menopause) with clinical presentation of abnormal vaginal bleeding or out of phase with menstrual cycle: Endometrial biopsy

Premenopausal woman who is asymptomatic: No further work-up

Postmenopausal woman: Endometrial biopsy (20% risk of carcinoma)

Endometrial carcinoma: Colposcopy to establish diagnosis and start staging; referral to gynecologic oncologist

Differential Diagnosis

Endometrial hyperplasia (abnormal vaginal bleeding, peak incidence in perimenopausal women at 50 years of age)

Leiomyomas (pelvic pressure, bloating, pelvic congestion, urinary frequency, dysmenorrhea, dyspareunia, menorrhagia)

Other genital cancers

Endocervical and endometrial polyps (red or pink growth; may be visible at cervical os or introitus; soft; few millimeters to fill vaginal vault; may have atypical Pap results)

Abnormal vaginal bleeding

Pelvic pain

Diagnostic Tests

CBC (to assess for anemia if client presents with prolonged bleeding)

hCG; urine and serum hCG tests are positive for pregnancy; urine hCG is positive in about 65% of ectopic pregnancies; increased values in quantitative serum hCG are found in pregnancy and ovarian tumors, while decreased values are found in ectopic pregnancy)

Endometrial biopsy (diagnostic in 90% of cases)

Dilation and curettage (can be performed when endometrial biopsy results are inadequate or inconclusive)

Transvaginal ultrasonography

Assessment of metastases

Serum CA-125 (elevated in some endometrial cancers; significant elevations suggest metastasis)

Cystoscopy (used if signs and symptoms suggest bladder involvement)

Proctoscopy (used if signs and symptoms suggest spread to the rectum)

CT scan

Chest x-ray examination (used if signs and symptoms suggest metastasis to lungs)

Management/Treatment

Pharmacologic Management

Hormonal therapy (for advanced or recurrent cancer)

Progesterone therapy results in remission for up to 2–3 years (especially of pulmonary, vaginal, and mediastinal metastases) in 35%–40%; experimental use of progesterone in early-stage uterine cancer for young women who want to have children; megestrol acetate (Megace), 10–80 mg PO QID for palliative treatment

Chemotherapy (for extensive disease; PO or IV; single drug or combination of drugs, including doxorubicin, cisplatin, and paclitaxel)

Nonpharmacologic Management

SURGICAL

Simple hysterectomy (removal of only the uterus; may be via abdomen or vagina)

Radical hysterectomy (removal of uterus, parametrium and uterosacral ligaments, and upper approximate 1 inch of vagina; may be via abdomen or vagina)

Abdominal hysterectomy with bilateral salpingo-oophorectomy

Abdominal pelvic node sampling/dissection at time of hysterectomy

Laparoscopic lymph node sampling

RADIOTHERAPY (POSTOPERATIVE; RARELY USED PREOPERATIVELY)

Brachytherapy (vaginal applicator; used when only upper third of vagina and/or the vaginal cuff need to treated)

External-beam radiation therapy

Complementary/Alternative Therapies

See "Complementary/Alternative Therapies" in section on "Breast Cancer."

Client Education

Aerobic exercise immediately after chemotherapy is safe, partially prevents loss of physical conditioning, and may decrease toxic side effects of the therapy.

Beta-carotene (e.g., carrots, tomatoes, citrus fruits, spinach) may provide protection against cancer because of its antioxidant properties, which inhibit factors in the early stages of cancer.

Follow-up

Pap smear every 2–3 months for first 3 years after treatment and every 6 months thereafter

Annual chest x-ray examination and mammography

Annual endometrial biopsies beginning at age 35 for women with family history of colon cancer

Periodic CA-125 in women who have upper vaginal stenosis due to radiation therapy

Referral

Refer to gynecologic oncologist.

VULVODYNIA

SIGNAL SYMPTOM ▶ vulvar pain

ICD-9 Code	625.9	Vulvodynia

Vulvodynia is a complex syndrome of chronic vulvar pain; it is also known as vulvar dysesthesia.

Epidemiology

Fourth most common condition associated with interstitial cystitis

Affects up to 15% of general gynecologic practice population

Average age of onset is 25, but range is from 2 to 91

Vast majority of those with vulvodynia are fair-skinned Caucasian women

Etiology

Unknown; may be result of multiple factors.

Subsets of vulvodynia include vulvar, dysesthetic vulvodynia, cyclic vulvovaginitis, vulvar dermatoses.

Other possible causes: High levels of oxalate crystals in urine, spasms/irritation of pelvic floor muscles.

No evidence caused by STDs or physical or sexual abuse or that it is a psychosomatic condition.

Physiology and Pathophysiology

Affected areas include the labia minora, clitoral glans, Skene's glands, Bartholin's glands, tissue surrounding the introitus, and hymen.

Pain often occurs in the absence of tissue injury; it may be initiated by mediators after lesions or trauma to the tissue. Complex interactions result in increased pain sensitization such as allodynia (light touch interpreted as pain) and hyperesthesia (increase, prolonged pain)

The essential differences between the four subsets are:

Primarily a consequence of dermatosis or infection: Cyclic vulvovaginitis (*Candida* infection) and vulvar dermatoses

Primarily due to other causes and differential by pain presentation: Dysesthetic vulvodynia (constant, unprovoked pain) and vulvar vestibulitis (pain provoked by attempted vaginal entry)

Clinical Manifestations

See Table 9–18.

Differential Diagnosis

Vestibular papillomatosis (widespread nipplelike growths)

Bartholin's duct cysts (cysts, dyspareunia)

Folliculitis, furuncles, and carbuncles (pain, swelling, discharge)

Table 9–18 Clinical Manifestations and Management: Vulvodynia

Vulvodynia	Clinical Manifestations	Management
Vulvar vestibulitis	**Subjective** Burning, dry, raw sensation localized in vuvlar vestibulum Entry dyspareunia Pain usually caused by external touch or pressure from tampon insertion, tight pants, bicycling, horseback riding Vaginismus **Objective** Positive swab test: vestibular point tenderness when touched with cotton swab Focal or diffuse vestibular erythema	-Intralesional interferon injection -Estradiol (Estrace) 0.01% vaginal cream (pea-sized amount) BID for 4 to 8 weeks
Dysesthetic vuvodynia	**Subjective** Non-cyclic unremitting pain which may radiate to anus, groin, down inner thighs Generalized/diffuse sensations of burning/irritation Pain may be sharp or have a deep aching quality Urethral or rectal discomfort Less dyspareunia and point tenderness **Objective** Vulva may appear normal No erythema Less or no point tenderness	-Tricyclic anTIDepressants: e.g., amitriptyline (Elavil), desipramine (Norpramin), and imipramine (Tofranil) 10mg hs, gradually increasing by 10mg weekly to 40–100mg daily for 4 to 6 months, then gradually decrease to minimum dosage necessary to control symptoms -Anticonvulsants: e.g., carbamazepine (Tegretol) and gabapentin (Neurontin) (if tricyclic therapy unsuccessful)
Cyclic vulvo-vaginitis	**Subjective** Itching, burning pain Some symptom-free days with pain flare up just before and during menses Pain exacerbation with intercourse, especially the following day History of frequent Candida infections and/or antibiotic therapy **Objective** Minimal vaginal discharge Erythema and edema variable Pelvic and colposcopoc examination findings usually normal	-Topical anti-fungal creams: e.g., clotrimazole (Gyne-Lotrimin) (OTC) insert one applicator full intravaginally, for 7 to 14 consecutive days; nystatin (Mycostatin) 100,000 U insert one vaginal tablet high into vagina daily or BID for 7 to 14 days -Oral antifungals For initial treatment: fluconazole (Diflucan) 150 mg weekly for 2 months, then twice monthly for 2 to 4 months For cyclic vulvovaginitis that does not respond to topical antifungal or is recurrent: fluconazole (Diflucan) 150 mg weekly, ketoconazole (Nizoral)100mg QD, itraconazole (Sporanox) 100mg qod; take for 6 months
Vulvar dermatoses	**Subjective** Significant itching, burning History of douching, topical medication use, especially steroids	-Underlying psoriasis, lichen planus, contact dermatitis, lichen simplex: hydrocortisone 2.5% ointment or triamcinolone 0.1% ointment one to four times daily short-term use only)

Table continued on following page.

Table 9–18   Clinical Manifestations and Mangement: Vulvodynia (*Continued*)

Vulvodynia	Clinical Manifestations	Management

	Objective
	  Erythema
	  Thick and/or scaly lesions
	  Erosions or ulcers related
	    to scratching
	  Blisters or ulcers not related
	    to scratching lesions on
	    other parts of body
		-Underlying lichen sclerosis: testoste-
		  rone priopionate 2% ointment
		  (controlled substance schedule
		  III); clobetasol propionate
		  (Temovate) 0.05% ointment BID
		-Underlying tinea cruris: terbinafine
		  hydrochloride (Lamisil) 1% cream
		  1 to 2 times daily until resolved

Diagnostic Tests

Diagnosis made by exclusion of other causes

Fungal cultures and KOH preparation for suspected cyclic vulvovaginitis

Biopsy of any lesions

Management/Treatment

No cure, treatments directed toward symptom relief.

Pharmacologic Management

See Table 9–18.

Nonpharmacologic Management

Nerve block

Laser surgery (removal of hypersensitive tissue; best for vulvar vestibulitis; high success rate; last resort)

Lidocaine (Xylocaine), 5% topical ointment (apply 10–15 minutes before intercourse)

Complementary/Alternative Therapies

Boric acid (600 mg in a gelatin capsule, per vagina once daily for 14 days)

Vitamin E oil several times a day or after every urination

Baking soda douche (1–2 teaspoons of baking soda in 1 pint warm water; gently douche 1–2 times weekly PRN)

Compresses: Colloidal oatmeal (Aveeno; 2 tablespoons in 1 quart of water, keep refrigerated, apply compress 3–4 times a day); tea bag (warmed, soaked tea bags); viola tricolor (Heartsease) (1.5 g with 1 cup of water); use sanitary pads to hold compresses in place.

Sitz baths: Tea (steep tea bags in warm water); viola tricolor (same as for compresses).

Low-oxalate diet (for cyclic vulvovaginitis and vulvar vestibulitis; to decrease acidity of urine, avoid all beans, beer, beets, berries, celery, chard, chocolate, eggplant, green peppers, some grapes, peanuts, rutabagas, spinach, squash, tofu).

Calcium citrate (Citracal), 200 mg/950 mg tablets, two tablets TID (for cyclic vulvovaginitis and vulvar vestibulitis; alkalizes urine).

Kegel exercises (strengthens pelvic muscles and may lessen vaginismus; consider physical therapy referral; biofeedback may be helpful in monitoring progress; for cyclic vulvovaginitis, vulvar vestibulitis, and dysesthetic vulvodynia).

Acupuncture.

Client Education

Underwear: Wear white 100% cotton underwear; do not wear pantyhose or tights; do not wear underwear at night, allow vulva area to air; washing underwear: put through second rinse cycle; do not use fabric softeners; use mild soap; try washing in baking soda; wash new underwear before wearing.

Sanitary pads and tampons: Use only 100% cotton.

Cleaning vulvar area: Rinse vulva with water frequently and after urination (sitz bath, squirt bottle, bidet); avoid frequent bathing with soaps (avoid perfumed soaps and any bubble baths or bath oils; try Neutrogena, Basis, Pears, and castile soap); dry skin gently (pat dry or use hair dryer on cool setting); avoid feminine deodorant products.

Sexual intercourse: Use lubricants at initiation of sexual activity (use pure almond oil, pure vegetable oil, Astroglide, Lubrin, Moistur-el, Replens, KY Jelly; avoid petroleum jelly, lanolin); avoid contraceptive devices and creams.

Remove wet bathing suit as soon as possible.

Avoid constipation and full bladder (pressure may affect vulva area).

Follow-up

As needed.

Referral

Refer to gynecologist and/or dermatologist as indicated.

VULVOVAGINAL INFECTIONS

SIGNAL SYMPTOM ▶ vaginal discharge, vulvar itching or irritation

ICD-9 Codes	112.1	Candidal vulvovaginitis (thick, white discharge, itching)
	131.01	Trichomonas vulvovaginitis (greenish-yellow discharge, itching, dysuria)
	616.60	Bacterial vulvovaginitis/vaginosis (white frothy discharge, itching, fishy odor)

Vulvovaginitis, or vaginitis, is usually characterized by a vaginal discharge, vulvar itching, and or vulvar irritation, and is due to infection, lack of estrogen, or external irritant.

Symptoms of candidal vulvovaginitis include thick white discharge, itching; symptoms of trichomonal vulvovaginitis include greenish-yellow discharge, itching, and dysuria. Symptoms of bacterial vulvovaginitis/vaginosis include white frothy discharge, itching, fishy odor.

Epidemiology

Vaginitis is the most common gynecologic problem.

Bacterial vaginosis (BV) accounts for 40%–50%, vulvovaginal candidiasis (VVC) for 20%–25%, and vaginal trichomoniasis for 15%–25% of all cases of vaginitis.

75% of all women will have VVC, 40%–45% will have more than one episode; <5% have recurrent VVC.

20% of women will have *Trichomonas* vaginalis during their reproductive years.

Etiology

The most common causes are *Candida albicans, Trichomonas vaginalis, Gardnerella vaginalis,* and anaerobic bacteria.

Other causes include lack of estrogen and external irritants.

Insufficiently treated or untreated bacterial vaginosis is associated with an increased risk of poor pregnancy outcomes (e.g., premature rupture of membranes, preterm labor, and preterm birth), PID, and vaginal cuff cellulitis after invasive procedures (e.g., endometrial biopsy, hysterectomy, placement of intrauterine contraceptive device, cesarean section, abortion, and uterine curettage).

Trichomoniasis is associated with an increased risk of adverse pregnancy outcomes, especially premature rupture of membranes and preterm birth.

Physiology and Pathophysiology

The predominant microbe in a healthy asymptomatic vagina is *Lactobacillus,* which maintains vaginal equilibrium by producing lactic acid (keeps pH at 3.8 to 4.2) and hydrogen peroxide (suppresses growth of anaerobic bacteria). BV results from a change in the vaginal ecosystem that causes an increase in non-lactobacillus and anaerobic bacteria. BV is labeled vaginosis rather than vaginitis because of the lack of inflammation, as evidenced by the lack of white cells in the discharge.

VVC also results from ecosystem changes, which are often triggered by diabetes mellitus, recent antibiotic therapy, corticosteroid use, or human immunodeficiency virus. Vaginal trichomoniasis is a protozoal infection, which is primarily sexually transmitted.

Clinical Manifestations

See Table 9–19.

Differential Diagnosis

Healthy, asymptomatic vagina (discharge is white to slate gray, no odor, pH 3.2 to 4.5)

Atrophic vaginitis (due to lack of estrogen; sparse brittle pubic hair; labia less prominent; vaginal mucosa without rugae and pale pink to white; thinned vaginal epithelium; pH usually 5.0–7.5; lactobacilli no longer dominant; vaginal discharge scant and gray in appearance; dyspareunia with spotting afterward; may have urinary incontinence and dysuria due to urine flowing over atrophic tissue)

Contact vulvovaginitis (due to external irritant; itching, and/or burning of vulva only, vagina is involved only if irritant is introduced into the vagina; vulva erythematous, excoriated, no discrete lesions; normal vaginal pH unless client has been douching)

Human papillomavirus vestibulitis (entry dyspareunia; itching, burning of vestibule and introitus with surrounding erythema that may be tender to touch; application of 5% acetic acid turns affected epithelium white)
Cytolytic vaginosis
Vulvar vestibulitis (severe point tenderness of the vulva or introital tissue)

Table 9–19 Clinical Manifestations and Management: Vulvovaginal Infections

Vulvovaginal Infection	Clinical Manifestations	Management
Bacterial Vaginosis	Subjective Foul or fishy smelling vaginal discharge (may increase before menses and after sexual intercourse) Increased vaginal discharge that is copious, then, gray-white ("spilled milk") appearance. Itching and burning are rare Objective Thin, homogenous, gray-white, adherent vaginal discharge	Pharmacologic Management (CDC Guidelines) Routine treatment of sex partners is not recommended Nonpregnant women (treatment of asymptomatic women is controversial; consider treatment prior to invasive procedures) Metronidazole 500 mg po BID times 7 days Or clindamycin cream 2%, one full applicator (5g) intravaginally qhs times 7 days Or metronidazole gel 0.75%, one full applicator (5g) intravaginally BID times 5 days Alternative regimens: metronidazole 2 g po in a single dose or clindamycin 300 mg po BID times 7 days Pregnant women high-risk for premature delivery (prior preterm birth), symptomatic or asymptomatic: metronidazole 250 mg po TID times 7 days (alternative regimens: metronidazole 2 g po once or clindamycin 300 mg po BID times 7 days) Low-risk for premature delivery and symptomatic same as for high-risk pregnant women plus additional alternative regimen of metronidazole gel 0.75% one full applicator (5g) intravaginally BID times 5 days Complementary/Alternative Therapies Garlic vaginal suppository (peeled garlic clove wrapped in unbleached gauze) overnight up to 6 nights Goldenseal douche (one tablespoon simmered in 3 cups water, strain and cool before using) Boric acid suppository ("00" gelatin capsule filled with 600 mg bolic acid powder) QD times 14 days Cranberry juice (unsweetened) 8 ounces QD Yogurt (with live cultures) soaked tampon, insert into vagina nightly (remove upon awakening) *Table continued on following page.*

Table 9–19   Clinical Manifestations and Management: Vulvovaginal Infections (Continued)

Vulvovaginal Infection	Clinical Manifestations	Management
Vulvovaginal Candidiasis	Subjective Erythema, pruritis, and swelling of external genitalia Objective Client may be taking antibiotics or Ocs Whitish yellow cottage cheese appearing discharge that is adherent to vaginal walls Musty odor	Pharmacologic Management (CDC Guidelines) No treatment for asymptomatic women Consider treatment of sex partners only if woman has recurrent infections Pregnant women: topical azole therapies only (butoconazole, clotrimazole, miconazole, terconazole for 7 days) Intravaginal regimens: butoconazole 2% cream 5 g times 3 days or clotrimazole 1% cream 5 g times 7–14 days or clotrimazole 100 mg vaginal tablet times 7 days or clotrimazole 100 mg vaginal tablet, 2 tablets times 3 days or clotrimazole 500 mg vaginal tablet once or miconazole 2% cream 5 g times 7 days or miconazole 200 mg vaginal tablet times 3 days or miconazole 100 mg vaginal suppository times 7 days or nystatin 100,000-unit vaginal tablet QD times 14 days (azole drugs are considered more effective than nystatin) or tioconazole 6.5% ointment 5 g once or terconazole 0.4% cream 5 g times 7 days or terconazole 0.8% cream 5 g times 3 days or terconazole 80 mg vaginal suppository times 3 days Oral regimen: fluconazole 150 mg tablet po once Complementary/Alternative Therapies Garlic as a beverage (blend with carrots), suppository (see under bacterial vaginosis above), or douche (garlic juice mixed with yogurt) Goldenseal tea Yogurt soaked tampon Tea tree oil (1 to 2 drops added to yogurt in which tampon is then soaked) Centaurea cyanus (Cornflower)—1 gram per cup—store protected from light
Trichimonas Vaginalis	Subjective Excessive, frothy, green-yellow, foul smelling vaginal discharge Pruritis (vulvar itching) Dysuria Symptoms increase during and after menses Dyspareunia May be asymptomatic	Pharmacologic Management (CDC Guidelines) Sex partner should be treated Metronidazole 2 g po once (alternative regimen: metronidazole 500 mg BID times 7 days) Complementary/Alternative Therapies None

Table continued on following page.

**Table 9–19   Clinical Manifestations and Management:
Vulvovaginal Infections (*Continued*)**

Vulvovaginal Infection	Clinical Manifestations	Management
	Objective Yellow-green, frothy, adherent discharge strawberry (punctate microhemorrhages) cervix that bleeds easily (25%) vaginal edema and erythema	

Diagnostic Tests

Bacterial Vaginosis
Vaginal pH test: pH >4.5
Potassium hydroxide preparation: positive "whiff" test results
Decreased lactobacilli
Clue cells (vaginal epithelial cells with stippled appearance due to the adherence of bacilli on their surfaces)
Gram stain
Vaginal culture not specific

Vulvovaginal Candidiasis
Potassium hydroxide preparation positive for hyphae
Gram stain positive for yeast or pseudohyphae
Vaginal culture

Trichimonas vaginalis
"Whiff" test may or may not yield positive results
pH >4.5 (75%)
Vaginal culture: *Trichomonas* on microscopic examination (50%–75%)

Management/Treatment
See Table 9–19.

Client Education
See "Client Education" in section on "Vulvodynia."

Follow-up
As indicated by response to treatment

Referral
Refer to gynecologist or infection-control specialist if condition does not respond to treatment.

REFERENCES

General
Beers, M., & Berkow, R. (Eds.) (2000). *Merck manual of diagnosis and therapy* (18th ed.). Whitehouse Station, NJ: Merck.

Conn, H.F, & Rakel, R.E. (Eds.) (2000). *Conn's current therapy*. Philadelphia, Harcourt Health Sciences.

CPT 2000. (1999) *Current procedural terminology* (4th ed.). Chicago: American Medical Association.

Dickey, R. (1998). *Managing contraceptive pill patients* (9th ed.). Durant, OK: EMIS.

Dunphy, L., & Winland-Brown, J. (2001). *Primary care: The art and science of advanced practice nursing*. Philadelphia: F.A. Davis

Goroll, A., & Mulley, A. (2000). *Primary care medicine: Office evaluation and management of the adult patient.* (4th ed.). Philadelphia: Lippincott Williams & Wilkins

Hoekelman, R., Adam, H., Nelson, N., Weitzman, M., & Wilson, M. (2001). *Primary pediatrics care*. St. Louis: Mosby-YearBook.

Koda-Kimble, M., &Young, L. (2001) *Applied therapeutics: The clinical use of drugs.* (7th ed.). Philadelphia; Lippincott Williams & Wilkins.

Noble, J.H., et al. (Eds.) (2001). *Textbook of primary care medicine* (3rd ed.). St. Louis: Mosby-YearBook.

Nurse practitioner's drug handbook (3rd ed.) (2000). Springhouse, PA: Springhouse.

Physician ICD-CM-9 (1999). Medicode, (vol. 1&2) (5th ed.) Salt Lake City, UT: Medicode.

Wynne, A., Woo, T., &Millard, M. (2002). *Pharmacotherapeutics for nurse practitioner prescribers*. Philadelphia: F.A. Davis.

Youngkin, E.Q., & Davis, S.D., (1998) Women's Health: A Primary Care Clinical Guide. Stamford: Appleton & Lange.

Amenorrhea

Lesser, C. (1999, March). Ovarian decline in the later reproductive years: Assessing ovarian reserve. *Advance for Nurse Practitioners,* pp. 36–44.

Breast Cancer

Alexander, W. (1999). ASCO and ACOG update: Breast cancer screening and prevention. *Oncology Issues, 14*(4), 13, 27–28.

Brinton, L., Lubin, J., Burich, M., Colton, T., Brown, L., & Hoover, R. (2000). Breast cancer following augmentation mammoplasty. *Cancer Causes Control, 11*(9), 819–827.

Brinton, L., Persson, I., Boice, J., McLaughlin, J., & Fraumeni, J. (2001). Breast cancer risk in relation to amount of tissue removed during breast reduction operations in Sweden. *Cancer, 91*(3), 478–483.

Cain, S. (2000). Breast cancer genetics and the role of tamoxifen in prevention. *Journal of the American Academy of Nurse Practitioners, 12*(1), 21–32.

Fountain, M. (2000). Do I have breast cancer? *Nurse Practitioner, 25*(4), 10.

Grabick, D., Hartman, L. Cerhan, J., Vierkant, R., Therneau, R., Varchon, C., Olson, J., Couch, F., Anderson, K., Pankratz, S., & Sellers, T. (2000). Risk of breast cancer with oral contraceptive use in women with a family history of breast cancer. *JAMA, 284,* 1791–1798.

Huang, Z., Willett, W., Colditz, G., Hunter, D., Manson, J., Rosner, B., Speizer, F., & Hankinson, S. (1999). Waist circumference, waist:hip ratio, and risk of breast cancer in the Nurses' Health Study. *American Journal of Epidemiology, 150,* 1316–1324.

Kavanagh, A., Mitchell, H., & Giles, G. (2000). Hormone replacement therapy and accuracy of mammographic screening. *Lancet, 355,* 270–274.

Keller, C., Fullerton, J., & Mobley, C. (1999). Supplemental and complementary alternatives to hormone replacement therapy. *Journal of the American Academy of Nurse Practitioners, 11*(5), 187–198.

Meister, K. (2000). *Chemoprevention of breast cancer*. New York: American Council on Science and Health.

Moore, K., & Schmais, L. (2000). The ABCs of complementary and alternative therapies and cancer treatment. *Oncology Issues, 15*(6), 20–22.

Morrow, M. (2000). The evaluation of common breast problems. *American Family Physician, 61*(8), 2371–2390.

Norris, J., Paige, L. Christensen, D., Chang, C., Huacani, M., Fan, D., Hamilton, P., Fowlkes, D., & McDonnell, D. (1999). Peptide antagonists of the human estrogen receptor. *Science, 285,* 744–746.

Protheroe, D., et al (1999). Stressful life events and difficulties and onset of breast cancer: Case-control study. *BMJ, 319,* 1027–1030.

Reddy, P., & Chow, M. (2000). Safety and efficacy of antiestrogens for prevention of breast cancer. *American Journal of Health-System Pharmacy, 57*(14), 1315–1322.

Rutter, C., Mandelson, M., Laya, M., & Taplin, S. (2001). Changes in breast density associated with initiation, discontinuation, and continuing use of hormone replacement therapy. *JAMA, 285,* 171–176.

Smith-Warner, S., Speigelman, D., Yaun, S., Adami, H., Beeson, W., van den Brandt, P., Folsom, A., Fraser, G., Freudenheim, J., Goldbohm, A., Graham, S., Miller, A., Potter, J., Rohan, T., Speizer, F., Toniolo, P., Willett, W., Wolk, A., Zeleniuch-Jacquot, A., & Hunter, D. (2001). Intake of fruits and vegetables and risk of breast cancer. *JAMA, 285,* 769–776.

Storm, H., & Olsen, J. (1999). Risk of breast cancer in offspring of male breast-cancer patients. *Lancet, 353,* 209–212.

Stowe, A. (1999). Diagnostic work-up of breast cancer in females. *Journal of the American Academy of Nurse Practitioners, 11*(2), 71–80.

Cervical Cancer/Abnormal Pap Smear

American Thoracic Society (2000). Diagnostic standards and classification of tuberculosis in adults and children. *American Journal of Respiratory and Critical Care Medicine, 161,* 1376–1395.

Anttila, T., Saikku, P., Koskela, P., Bloigu, A., Dillner, J., Ikaheimo, I., Jellum, E., Lehtinen, M., Lenner, P., Hakulinen, T., Narvanen, A., Pukkala, E., Thoresen, S., Youngman, L., & Paavonen, J. (2001). Serotypes of *Chlamydia trachomatis* and risk for development of cervical squamous cell carcinoma. *JAMA, 285,* 47–51.

Apgar, B., & Brotzman, G. (1999). HPV testing in the evaluation of the minimally abnormal Papanicolaou smear. *American Family Physician, 59*(10), 2794–2803.

Bailey, J., Kavanagh, J., Owen, C., McLean, K., & Skinner, C. (2000). Lesbians and cervical screening. *British Journal of General Practice, 50,* 481–482.

Bristow, R., & Montz, F. (2000). Workup of the abnormal pap test. *Clinical Cornerstone, 3*(1), 12–24.

Canavan, T., & Doshi, N. (2000). Cervical cancer. *American Family Physician, 61,* 1369–1382.

Cullins, V., Dominguez, L., Guberski, T., Secor, R., & Wysocki, S. (1999). Treating vaginitis. *Nurse Practitioner, 24*(10), 46–63

Ellerbrock, T., Chiasson, M., Bush, T., Sun, X., Sawo, D., Brudney, K., & Wright, T. (2000). Incidence of cervical squamous intraepithelial lesions in HIV-infected women. *JAMA, 283,* 1031–1037.

French, A., Kirstein, L., Massad, S., Semba, R., Minkoff, H., Landesman, S., Palefsky, J., Young, M., Anastos, K., & Cohen, M. (2000). Association of vitamin A deficiency with cervical squamous intraepithelial lesions in human immunodeficiency virus-infected women. *Journal of Infectious Diseases, 182,* 1084–1089.

Goodman, A. (2000). Abnormal genital tract bleeding. *Clinical Cornerstone, 3*(1), 25–35.

Hongwei, B., Sung, C., & Steinhoff, M. (2000). ThinPrep pap test promotes detection of glandular lesions of the endocervix. *Diagnostic Cytopathology, 23*(1), 19–22.

Hutti, M., & Hoffman, C. (2000). Cytolytic vaginosis: an overlooked cause of cycle vaginal itching and burning. *Journal of the American Academy of Nurse Practitioners, 12*(2), 55–57.

Keller, C., Fullerton, J., & Mobley, C. (1999). Supplemental and complementary alternatives to hormone replacement therapy. *Journal of the American Academy of Nurse Practitioners, 11*(5), 187–198.

Klingman, L. (1999). Assessing the female reproductive system. *American Journal of Nursing, 99*(8), 37–43.

Magnusson, P., Lichtenstein, P., & Gyllensten, U. (2000). Heritability of cervical tumors. *International Journal of Cancer, 88*(5), 698–701.

Manos, M., Kinney, W., Hurley, L., Sherman, M., Shieh-Ngai, J., Kurman, R., Ransley, J., Fetterman, B., Hartinger, J., McIntosh, K., Pawlick, G., & Hiatt, R. (1999). Identifying women with cervical neoplasia. *JAMA, 281,* 1605–1610.

Martin-Hirsch, P., Lilford, R., Jarvis, G., & Kitchener, H. (1999). Efficacy of cervical-smear collection devices: a systematic review and meta-analysis. *Lancet, 354,* 1763–1770.

Melnikow, J., Chan, B., & Stewart, G. (1999). Do follow-up recommendations for abnormal Papanicolaou smears influence patient adherence? *Archives of Family Medicine, 8,* 510–514.

Montz, F. (1996). Impact of therapy for cervical intraepithelial neoplasia on fertility. *American Journal of Obstetrics and Gynecology, 175,* 1129–1136.

Nguyen, H., & Nordquist, S. (1999). The Bethesda system and evaluation of abnormal pap smears. *Seminars in Surgical Oncology, 16*(3), 217–221.

Rose, P., Bundy, B., Watkins, E., Thigpen, J., Deppe, G., Mainman, M., Clarke-Pearson, D., & Insalaco, S. (1999). Concurrent cisplatin-based radiotherapy and chemotherapy for locally advanced cervical cancer. *New England Journal of Medicine, 340,* 1144–1153.

Selvaggi, S., & Guidos, B. (200). Specimen adequacy and the ThinPrep pap test: the endocervical component. *Diagnostic Cytopathology, 23*(1), 23–26.

Stienstra, K., Brewer, B., & Franklin, L. (1999). A comparison of flat and shallow conical tips for cervical cryotherapy. *Journal of the American Board of Family Practice, 12*(5), 360–366.

U.S. Preventive Services Task Force. (1996). *Guide to clinical preventive services* (2nd ed.). Alexandria, VA: International Medical Publishing.

van Zandt, S. (2000). Pelvic pain in women—Better understanding of an elusive diagnosis. *Clinician Reviews, 10*(9), 51–69.

Wright, T., Denny, L., Kuhn, L., Pollack, A., & Lorincz, A. (2000). HPV DNA testing of self-collected vaginal samples compared with cytologic screening to detect cervical cancer. *JAMA, 283,* 81–86.

Ylitalo, N. (2000). Consistent high viral load of human papillomavirus 16 and risk of cervical carcinoma in situ: a nested case-controlled study. *Lancet, 355,* 2194–2198.

Zenilman, J. (2001). Chlamydia and cervical cancer. *JAMA, 285,* 81–83.

Contraception

Schnare, S. (2000, February). Emergency postcoital contraception. *American Journal for Nurse Practitioners. 4*(2), 15–21.

Robinson, D., Dollins, A., &McConlogue-Shaughnessy. (2000, March). Care of the woman before and after an elective abortion. *American Journal for Nurse Practitioners,* pp. 17–29.

Dysmenorrhea

Wolf, L. (1999, March). Dysmenorrhea. *Journal of the American Academy of Nurse Practitioners,* pp. 126–130.

Endometriosis

Esposito, M., Tureck, R., & Mastroianni, L. (1999, June). Understanding endometriosis. *Female Patient, 24,* 48–55.

Frackiewicz, E. (2000). Endometriosis: an overview of the disease and its treatment. *Journal of the American Pharmaceutical Association, 40*(5), 645–657.

van Zandt, S. (2000). Pelvic pain in women—Better understanding of an elusive diagnosis. *Clinician Reviews, 10*(9), 51–69.

Wellbery, C. (1999). Diagnosis and treatment of endometriosis. *American Family Physician, 60,* 1753–1772.

Wolf, L., & Schumann, L. (1999). Dysmenorrhea. *Journal of the American Academy of Nurse Practitioners, 11*(3), 125–130.

Epididymitis

Centers for Disease Control and Prevention (1998). 1998 Guidelines for treatment of sexually transmitted diseases. *Morbidity and Mortality Weekly Report, 47*(RR-1).

Erectile Dysfunction

Albaugh, J. (1999, April). Erectile dysfunction: Newer treatment options don't reduce need for education, counseling. *Advance for Nurse Practitioners,* pp. 43–44.

Doerfler, E. (1999, March). Male erectile dysfunction: A guide for clinical management. *Journal of the American Academy of Nurse Practitioners, 11*(3), 117–123.

Masters, W., & Johnson, V. (1970). *Human sexual inadequacy.* Boston: Little Brown.

Fibrocystic Breast Disease

Horner, N., & Lampe, J. (2000). Potential mechanisms of diet therapy for fibrocystic breast conditions show inadequate evidence of effectiveness. *Journal of the American Dietetic Association, 100,* 1368–1380.

Klingman, L. (1999). Assessing the female reproductive system. *AJN, 99*(8), 37–43.

Leslie, N., & Leight, S. (1999). Clinical assessment of a breast mass: a case study. *Clinical Excellence for Nurse Practitioners, 3*(3), 149–153.

Morrow, M. (2000). The evaluation of common breast problems. *American Family Physician, 61,* 2371–2390.

Hormone Replacement Therapy

Barclay, L. (July, 2002). Risks of a combination HRT regime outweigh benefits. JAMA288 (3):321–3333, 336–368.

Kaunitz, A. M. (July, 2002). Use of combination hormone replacement therapy in light of recent data from the Women's Health Initiative, Contemporary Issues in Gynecology, Obstetrics and Women's Health, Medscape, Women's Health ejournal (7)4:2002.

Infertility

Lesser, C. (1999, March). Ovarian decline in the later reproductive years: Assessing ovarian reserve. *Advance for Nurse Practitioners,* pp. 36–44.

Menopause

Archer, D., &Utian, W. (2001, May). Decisions in prescribing HRT. *Patient Care for the Nurse Practitioner,* pp. 45–58.

Doughty, S. (2001, July). The postmenopausal woman. *Advance for Nurse Practitioners,* pp. 35–40.

Finkel, M., Cohen, M., & Mahoney, H. (2001). Treatment options for the menopausal woman. *Nurse Practitioner 26*(2), 5–15.

Keller, C., Fullerton, J., & Mobley, C. (1999, May). Supplemental and complementary alternatives to hormone replacement therapy. *Journal of the American Academy of Nurse Practitioners,* pp. 187–198.

Knapp, P. (1999). *Menopause: A look at the transitional changes of midlife.* Reno: University of Nevada, Reno, Orvis School of Nursing.

Nachtigall, L.B., Nachtigall, M.J., & Nachtigall, L.E. (1999, June). Nonprescription alternatives to hormone replacement therapy. *Female Patient, 24,* pp. 39–46.

North American Menopause Society (2000). *Menopause core curriculum study guide.* Cleveland: Author.

Notelovitz, M. (2000, Fall). Tailoring hormone therapy to patients' needs. Menopausal Medicine, 8(3), 28–36.

Ramsey, L.A., Ross, B.S., & Fischer, R.G. (1999, May). Management of menopause: Examining the science behind this alternative approach. Advance for Nurse Practitioners, pp. 27–30.

Reiter, R. (2001, July). One on one with hormone replacement. *Clinical Advisor,* pp. 66–71.

Rousseau, M.E. (1998). Hormone replacement therapy. *Nurse Practitioner Forum, 9*(3), 147–153.

Ovarian Cancer

Cottreau, C., Ness, R., & Kriska, A. (2000). Physical activity and reduced risk of ovarian cancer. *Obstetrics and Gynecology, 96,* 609–614.

Klingman, L. (1999). Assessing the female reproductive system. *American Journal of Nursing, 99*(8), 37–43.

Martin, V. (2000). Listen for the "whispering disease:" Learn the subtle signs and symptoms of ovarian cancer. *Nurse Practitioner, 25*(4), Special section: A guide to women's health, 6–7.

Padilla, L., Radosevich, D., & Milad, M. (2000). Accuracy of the pelvic examination in detecting adnexal masses. *Obstetrics and Gynecology, 96*(4), 593–598.

Shifren, J., Braunstein, G., Simon, J., Casson, P., Buster, J., Redmond, G., Burki, R., Ginsburg, E., Rosen, R., Leiblum, S., Caramelli, K., & Mazer, N. (2000). Transdermal testosterone treatment in women with impaired sexual function after oophorectomy. *New England Journal of Medicine, 343,* 682–688, 730–731.

Pelvic Inflammatory Disease

Grimes, D. (2000). Intrauterine device and upper-genital-tract infection: A review. *Lancet, 356,* 1013–1019.

Hemsel, D., Ledger, W., Martens, M., Monif, G., Osborne, N., & Thomason, J. (2001). Concerns regarding the Centers for Disease Control's published guidelines for pelvic inflammatory disease. *Clinical Infectious Diseases, 32*(1), 103–107.

Jackson, S., & Soper D. (1999). Pelvic inflammatory disease in the postmenopausal woman. *Infectious Diseases in Obstetrics and Gynecology, 7*(5), 248–252.

Keene, G. (1999). Office gynecology—Common reproductive tract disorders. *Clinician Reviews, 9*(1), 58–60.

Merchant, J., Oh, M., & Klerman, L. (1999). Douching: a problem for adolescent girls and young women. *Archives of Pediatric and Adolescent Medicine, 153,* 834–837.

van Zandt, S. (2000). Pelvic pain in women—Better understanding of an elusive diagnosis. *Clinician Reviews, 10*(9), 51–69.

Woodward, C., & Fisher, M. (1999). Drug treatment of common STDs. Part II. Vaginal infections, pelvic inflammatory disease and genital warts. *American Family Physician, 60,* 1716–1726.

Polycystic Ovarian Syndrome

Goodman, A. (2000). Abnormal genital bleeding. *Clinical Cornerstone, 3*(1), 25–35.

Hunter, M., & Sterrett, J. (2000). Polycystic ovary syndrome: It's not just infertility. *American Family Physician, 62,* 1079–1094.

Lewy, V., Danadian, K., Witchel, S., & Arslanian, S. (2001). Early metabolic abnormalities in adolescent girls with polycystic ovarian syndrome. *Journal of Pediatrics, 138*, 38–44.

Tweedy, A. (2000). Polycystic ovary syndrome. *Journal of the American Academy of Nurse Practitioners, 12*(3), 101–105.

Vandermolen, D., Ratts, V., Evans, W., Stovall, D., Kauma, S., & Nestler, J. (2001). Metformin increases the ovulatory rate and pregnancy rate from clomiphene citrate in patients with polycystic ovary syndrome who are resistant to clomiphene citrate alone. *Fertility and Sterility, 75*, 310–315.

Pregnancy

Hobbins-Garbett, D. (1999). Pregnancy. In T.M. Buttaro, Trybulski, J., Polgar-Bailey, P., & Sandberg-Cook, J. (Eds.), *Primary care: A collaborative practice*. St. Louis: Mosby-YearBook.

Premenstrual Syndrome

Hatcher, R., Trussel, J. Stewart, F., Stewart, G., Kowal, D., Guest, F., Cates, W., & Policar, M.S. (1998). *Contraceptive technology* (17th ed.) New York: Irvington.

Ugarriza, D.N., Klinger, S., & O'Brien, S. (September, 1998). Premenstrual syndrome: Diagnosis and intervention. *Nurse Practitioner. 23*(9), 40–56.

Testicular Cancer

Hagan, C.J., & Penrose-White, J. (1999, April). Common but curable: Responding to symptoms of testicular cancer. *Advance for Nurse Practitioners*, pp 25–30.

Uterine/Endometrial Cancer

Bergman, L. Beelen, M. Gallee, M., Hollema, H., Benraadit, J., & van Leeuwen, F. (2000). Risk and prognosis of endometrial cancer after tamoxifen for breast cancer. *Lancet, 356* 868–869, 881–887.

Burns, C.E., Brady, M.A., Dunn, A.M. & Starr, N.B. (2000). Pediatric Primary Care: A Handbook for nurse practitioners (2nd ed.) Philadelphia: W.B. Saunders.

Goodman, A. (2000). Abnormal genital tract bleeding. *Clinical Cornerstone, 3*(1), 25–35.

Hill, D., Weiss, N., Beresford, S., Voigt, L. Daling, J. Stanford, J., & Self, S. (2000). Continuous combined hormone replacement therapy and risk of endometrial cancer. *American Journal of Obstetrics and Gynecology, 183*, 1456–1461.

Jain, M., Howe, G., & Rohan, T. (2000). Nutritional factors and endometrial cancer in Ontario, Canada. *Cancer Control Journal, 7*(3), 288–296.

Keller, C., Fullerton, J., & Mobley, C. (1999). Supplemental and complementary alternatives to hormone replacement therapy. *Journal of the American Academy of Nurse Practitioners, 11*(5), 187–198.

Kerpsack, J., Finan, M., & Kline, R. (1998). Correlation between endometrial cells on Papanicolaou smear and endometrial carcinoma. *Southern Medical Journal, 91*(8), 749–752.

Porth, C.M. (1998). Pathophysiology: Conenpts of Altered Health States (5th ed.) Philadelphia: Lippincott.

Suh-Burgmann, E., & Goodman, A. (1999). Surveillance for endometrial cancer in women receiving tamoxifen. *Annals of Internal Medicine, 131*(2), 127–135.

Vulvodynia

Hutti, M., & Hoffman, C. (2000). Cytolytic vaginosis: an overlooked cause of cyclic vaginal itching and burning. *Journal of the American Academy of Nurse Practitioners, 12*(2), 55–57.

Metts, J. (1999). Vulvodynia and vulvar vestibulitis: Challenges in diagnosis and management. *American Family Physician, 59,* 1547–1565.

Powell, J., & Wojnarowska, F. (1999). Acupuncture for vulvodynia. *Journal of the Royal Society of Medicine, 92,* 579–581.

Rex, J., Walsh, T., Sobel, J., Filler, S., Pappas, P., Dismukes, W., & Edwards, J. (2000). Practice guidelines for the treatment of candidiasis. *Clinical Infectious Disease, 30,* 662–678.

Riley, C. (1998). Vulvodynia: Theory and management. *Dermatologic Clinics, 16*(4), 775–778.

Vulvovaginal Infection

Centers for Disease Control and Prevention (1998). 1998 Guidelines for treatment of sexually transmitted diseases. *Morbidity and Mortality Weekly Report, 47*(RR-1).

Cullins, V., Dominguez, L., Guberski, T., Secor, R., & Wysocki, S. (1999). Treating vaginitis. *Nurse Practitioner, 24*(10), 46–60.

Egan, M., & Lipsky, M. (2000). Diagnosis of vaginitis. *American Family Physician, 62,* 1095–1108.

Hutti, M., & Hoffman, C. (2000). Cytolytic vaginosis: An overlooked cause of cyclic vaginal itching and burning. *Journal of the American Academy of Nurse Practitioners, 12*(2), 55–57.

Woodward, C., & Fisher, M. (1999). Drug treatment of common STDs. Part II. vaginal infections, pelvic inflammatory disease and genital warts. *American Family Physician, 60,* 1716–1726.

RESOURCES

General

American College of Obstetrics and Gynecology
600 Maryland Ave. SW
Suite 300 East
Washington, DC 20024
Telephone: 202-638-5577
www.acog.org

American Foundation for Urological Disease, Incorporated
www.afud.org/

American Society for Reproductive Medicine (formerly the American Fertility Society)
1209 Montgomery Hwy.
Birmingham, AL 35216-2809
Telephone: 205-978-5000
www.asrm.org

American Society of Clinical Gynecology
703-299-0150
www.asco.org/

American Urological Association, Incorporated
www.auanet.org

Association of Reproductive Health Professionals
www.arhp.org

National Center for Homeopathy
www.homeopathic.org

National Center for Complimentary and Alternative Medicine
http://nccam.nih.gov/

National Women's Health Network
514 10th St. NW
Suite 400
Washington, DC 200004
Telephone: 202-628-7814
Women's Health Resources
www.indra.com

Amenorrhea

Society for Menstrual Cycle Research
10559 N. 104th Pl.
Scottsdale, AZ 85258
Telephone: 602-451-9731

Cancer

(Breast, Cervical/Abnormal Pap Smear, Ovarian, Testicular, Uterine/Endometrial)

American Cancer Society
Telephone: 800-ACS-2345
www.cancer.org
www.ca-journal.org

American Society of Colposcopy and Cervical Pathology
www.asccp.orf

Cancer Care, Incorporated
Telephone: 800-813-HOPE (4673)
www.cancercareinc.org

Cancer Survivors Online
www.cancersurvivors.org

College of American Pathologists (CAP)
www.papsmear.org

Gilda's Club
Telephone: 212-647-9700

The Gilda Radner Familial Ovarian Cancer Registry
www.ovariancancer.com

Gynecologic Cancer Foundation
Telephone: 800-444-4441 or 312-644-6610
www.sgo.org

National Action Plan on Breast Cancer
www.napbc.org

National Alliance of Breast Cancer Organizations (NABCO)
9E 37th St., 10th floor
New York, NY 10016-2822
Telephone: 212-719-0154
www.nabco.org

National Breast Cancer Coalition (NBCC)
Telephone: 202-296-7477
www.natlbcc.org

National Cancer Institute
  Telephone: 800-4-CANCER (422-6237)
  TTY: 1-800-332-8615

National Cervical Cancer Coalition
  16501 Sherman Way
  Suite 110
  Van Nuys, CA 91406
  Telephone: 800-685-5531—cervical cancer patients and families
  818-909-3849—office
  818-780-8199—fax
  www.nccc-online.org

National Coalition for Cancer Survivorship (NCCS)
  Telephone: 877-NCCS-YES (622-7937)
  www.cansearch.org

National Comprehensive Cancer Network (NCCN)
  Telephone: 888-909-NCCN (909-6226)
  www.nccn.org

National Lymphedema Network (NLN)
  Telephone: 880-541-3259
  www.lymphnet.org

National Ovarian Cancer Coalition
  www.ovarian.org

OncoLink (University of Pennsylvania)
  www.oncolink.upenn.edu

ONS Online (Oncology Nursing Society)
  Telephone: 412-921-7373
  www.ons.org

Ovarian Cancer National Alliance
  www.ovariancancer.org

Society of Gynecologic Oncologists
  www.sgo.org

Susan G. Komen Foundation
  Telephone: 800-462-9273
  www.breastcancerinfo.com

Testicular Cancer Links, Sites, and Pages
  www.cancerlinks.org

Y-ME National Organization for Breast Cancer Information and Support
  Telephone: 800-221-2141
  www.y-me.org

Women's Cancer Network
  www.wcn.org/

Contraception

Family Planning Council of America
  www.familyplanning.org/

Planned Parenthood Federation of America
  Telephone: 800-230 PLAN
  www.plannedparenthood.org/

Dysmenorrhea/Endometriosis

Endometriosis Association
    8585 North 76th Pl.
    Milwaukee, WI
    Telephone: 800-992 ENDO
    www.endometriosisassn.org

RESOLVE/National Infertility Association
    Telephone: 617-623-0744
    www.resolve.org

The Endometriosis Research Center
    Telephone: 800-239-7280 or 561-274-7442
    www.endocenter.org

Hysterectomy Educational Resources
    Telephone: 610-667-7757

The American Association of Gynecologic Laparoscopists
    (800) 554-2245 (562) 946-8774
    www.aagl.com/

Erectile Dysfunction

Impotence Institute of America
    8201 Corporate Dr.
    Suite 320
    Landover, MD 20785
    Telephone: 301-577-0650

Impotence Resource Center
    P.O. Box 9
    Minneapolis, MN 55440
    Telephone: 800-843-4315
    www.impotence.org/

Sexual Function Health Council
    American Foundation for Urologic Disease
    300 W. Pratt St.
    Suite 401
    Baltimore, MD 21201
    Telephone: 800-242-2383

Infertility

Families of America
    3333 Highway 100 North
    Minneapolis, MN 55422
    Telephone: 612-535-4829

Resolve, Inc. National Office
    P.O. Box 474
    Belmont, MA 02178
    www.resolve.org/international

Menopause

Aeron LifeCycles Laboratory (information about hormone saliva testing)
    1933 Davis St.
    Suite 310
    San Leandro, CA 94577
    Telephone: 800-631-7900

National Resource Center on Osteoporosis
   Telephone: 202-223-0344

North American Menopause Society
   www.menopause.org

Society for Menstrual Cycle Research
   10559 N. 104th Pl.
   Scottsdale, AZ 85258
   Telephone: 602-451-9731

Women's Health America, Madison Pharmacy Associates
   P.O. Box 259690
   Madison, WI 53725
   Telephone: 800-558-7046

Pelvic Inflammatory Disease
   American Social Health Association
   www.ashastd.org

Polycystic Ovarian Syndrome
Polycystic Ovarian Syndrome Association
   Telephone: 877-775-7267
   www.pcosupport.org

Premenstrual Syndrome
National Institute of Mental Health (NIMH)
   6001 Executive Blvd.
   Bethesda, MD 20892-9663
   (301) 443-4513
   nimhinfor@nih.gov
   nimhpubs@nih.gov

Vulvodynia, Vulvovaginal Infections
International Society for the Study of Vulvovaginal Diseases
   20 W. Washington St.
   Suite 1
   Hagerstown MD 21740
   Telephone: 301-733-3640
   Fax: 301-733-5775
   www.issvd.org

National Vulvodynia Association
   P.O. Box 19288
   Sarasota FL 34276-2288
   Telephone: 941-927-8503
   Fax: 941-927-8602
   www.nva.org

Vulvar Pain Foundation
   P.O. Drawer 177
   Graham NC 27253
   Telephone: 336-226-0704
   Fax: 336-226-8518
   www.vulvarpainfoundation.org

ADRENAL INSUFFICIENCY

SIGNAL SYMPTOMS abdominal pain, nausea, salt craving, constipation, recurrent vomiting, weight loss

ICD-9 Codes	255.4	Adrenal insufficiency

Adrenal insufficiency is defined as inadequate adrenocortical function. This may be caused by primary adrenal failure such as adrenal gland destruction from autoimmune disease (Addison's disease) or an infectious process; secondary adrenal failure (abnormal adrenocorticothyroid hormone [ACTH] secretion); or tertiary adrenal failure (abnormal hypothalamic release of ACTH-stimulating hormone). Glucocorticoid and mineralocorticoid secretion are both affected in primary adrenal insufficiency. In secondary and tertiary adrenal insufficiency, mineralocorticoid deficiency is not typically present.

Epidemiology

Primary Adrenal Insufficiency
40–60 cases per 1 million adults

Secondary and Tertiary Adrenal Insufficiency
Much less common

Often due to iatrogenic causes (e.g., administration of exogenous glucocorticoids, surgical or radiation induced ablation of pituitary gland and/or hypothalamus)

Etiology

Primary Adrenal Insufficiency
Destruction of the three layers of the adrenal cortex.

May be caused by autoimmune disease (e.g., Addison's disease) or as part of a polyglandular autoimmune syndrome; granulomatous diseases (histoplasmosis and tuberculosis); metastatic breast and lung carcinoma; infectious (meningococcemia); hemorrhage caused by anticoagulant therapy; and adrenoleukodystrophy, as well as other uncommon infiltrative hereditary diseases.

In infants, causes include congenital adrenal hypoplasia, caused by abnormal in utero development or deficiencies in adrenal enzymes such as cholesterol desmolase deficiency.

Secondary Adrenal Insufficiency

Absent ACTH production

May be caused by congenital absence of the pituitary or secondary to pituitary tumor and its treatments (e.g., radiation, surgery)

Tertiary Adrenal Insufficiency

Hypothalamic disturbance involving the messengers usually sent to the pituitary, which act to stimulate ACTH production.

May be caused by congenital absence, tumor, surgery, or radiation.

Physiology and Pathophysiology

Normally, corticotropin-releasing hormone (CRH) from the hypothalamus stimulates release of ACTH (from the pituitary gland), which in turn stimulates the adrenal gland to release glucocorticoids and mineralocorticoids (the normal hypothalamic–pituitary–adrenal gland axis).

With adrenal insufficiency there is no feedback mechanism to respond to the ever-increasing levels of ACTH. Therefore, very high levels of ACTH may be measured in the face of low cortisol (and other adrenal gland hormones). The physical result of the elevated ACTH level is hyperpigmentation secondary to crossover between ACTH and melanocyte-stimulating hormone (MSH). Therefore, clients with primary adrenal insufficiency will appear deeply tanned or bronzed.

Clinical Manifestations

Subjective

Abdominal pain

Nausea

Salt craving

Constipation

Recurrent vomiting

Weight loss

Unexplained fever

Headache

Muscle weakness and pain

Fatigue

Failure to thrive, signs of adrenal crisis (obtundation, hypotension, hypoglycemia, salt wasting) in the newborn period, or chronic, severe abdominal pain (infants or children with congenital adrenal hypoplasia)

Objective

Amenorrhea (Addison's disease)

Loss of axillary hair in women (Addison's disease)

Signs of dehydration or hypovolemic shock

Hypotension

Hyperpigmentation ("bronzing") or vitiligo (more noticeable on areas not usually tanned; areas of scarring or repeated friction, palmar surfaces, such as the elbows, antecubital areas, waistline; and gums and inner lip areas)

Signs of other autoimmune endocrine deficiencies

Differential Diagnosis

Inflammatory bowel disease (profuse watery diarrhea containing varying amounts of blood, mucus, and pus; tenesmus; severe abdominal pain; fever; chills; anemia and weight loss)

Gastric carcinoma (vague epigastric discomfort, anorexia, weight loss, unexplained iron deficiency anemia)

Diagnostic Tests

Complete blood cell (CBC) count (reveals anemia, eosinophilia).

Serum chemistry profile, including electrolytes (reveals hyponatremia, hyperkalemia, azotemia, hypercalcemia).

Basal plasma cortisol and ACTH levels (basal cortisol level of >20 μg/dl excludes the diagnosis of adrenal insufficiency; basal cortisol level of <10 μg/dl is strongly suggestive but should be confirmed with an ACTH stimulation test).

Once the diagnosis of adrenal insufficiency is made, it should be determined whether it is primary, secondary, or tertiary. If secondary or tertiary adrenal insufficiency (low ACTH, low cortisol) is present brain imaging should be performed to evaluate for the presence of a tumor. If primary adrenal insufficiency is present (high ACTH, low cortisol) additional causes should be pursued (autoimmune, adrenoleukodystrophy, etc.).

Management/Treatment

Pharmacologic Management

Glucocorticoid replacement: Hydrocortisone, prednisone. Initially stress doses of hydrocortisone may be necessary ($50–100$ mg/m^2). Subsequently $10–15$ mg/m^2 hydrocortisone (or equivalent) is given. Dose may be varied depending on symptoms, growth, etc.

Mineralocorticoid replacement: Fludrocortisone, $0.05–0.1$ mg once or twice a day. Typically younger patients require a higher dose.

Nonpharmacologic Management

Fluid replacement to maintain fluid and electrolyte balance

Increased dietary intake of sodium, particularly during hot weather to make up for losses through perspiration

Client Education

Necessity of taking medications regularly and to increase doses in times of stress (fever, illness, surgery, trauma, etc.)

Life-threatening nature, especially during times of increased stress

Medical identification jewelry indicating disease and dependence on steroids

Follow-up

With endocrinologist at quarterly intervals; in children this is of utmost importance for proper growth and development.

Annual laboratory testing.

Referral

Refer to endocrinologist

CUSHING'S SYNDROME

SIGNAL SYMPTOMS new onset diabetes mellitus, rapid weight gain in the absence of other signs, new-onset hypertension, acne and hirsutism in adults. In children the only symptom may be growth failure despite normal or increased weight gain.

ICD-9 Codes	255.0	Cushing's syndrome

Cushing's syndrome results from chronic glucocorticoid excess, resulting in typical clinical signs and symptoms. The glucocorticoid excess can result from endogenous production (ACTH-dependent or ACTH-independent) or from exogenous glucocorticoids. ACTH-dependent disease is referred to as Cushing's disease. Regardless of the etiology, the physical signs and symptoms are similar.

Epidemiology

Cushing's Syndrome

True incidence unknown because of underreporting and underdiagnosis.

A significant portion of cases have been attributed to small-cell lung cancer, which causes ectopic ACTH production and results in glucocorticoid excess; as the number of women smoking has increased this has resulted in women having at least as high an incidence as men.

If due to adrenal tumors (benign and malignant), incidence is 3–8 times higher in women than in men.

Adrenal carcinoma is the cause of half of all cases of childhood Cushing's syndrome, and adenoma accounts for another one sixth; girls are affected slightly more often than boys.

Typically, in children <8 years of age Cushing's syndrome is caused by a primary adrenal disorder and after age 8 years is caused by ACTH-dependent (typically pituitary tumor secreting ACTH).

Cushing's Disease

Occurs mainly in women aged 25–45 years.

Cushing's disease accounts for one third of all childhood cases of Cushing's syndrome; boys and girls are equally affected.

Adrenal tumors have a bimodal age distribution, with small peaks in the

first decade of life for adenomas and carcinomas and major peaks at
about 52 years of age for adenoma and 39 years for carcinomas.
Approximately one fourth of adrenal tumors occur in children.

Etiology

ACTH-Dependent Cushing's Syndrome

Most clients have ACTH-secreting anterior pituitary corticotropic microadeno-
mas; they are rarely malignant. Typically there are slowly progressive symptoms
of glucocorticoid excess, which usually includes hyperpigmentation.

ACTH-Independent Cushing's Syndrome

Exogenous glucocorticoid administration.

Ectopic ACTH secretion: Usually due to small-cell lung cancer; clients may
have sudden onset of symptoms, including acute salt retention,
hypertension, edema, hypokalemia, weakness, and glucose intolerance.
The typical habitus of Cushing's syndrome may be absent.

Adrenocortical tumors: Clients with adenomas typically have gradual onset
of symptoms and lack the hyperpigmentation associated with ACTH
excess. Clients with adrenocortical carcinoma may have a more rapidly
progressive course during which the androgen effects (hirsutism, acne)
may predominate. Abdominal, back, and flank pain may also be present.

Physiology and Pathophysiology

Normally, CRH from the hypothalamus stimulates release of ACTH (from the
pituitary gland), which in turn stimulates the adrenal gland to release glucocorticoids and mineralocorticoids (the normal hypothalamic–pituitary–
adrenal gland axis.)

With Cushing's syndrome/Cushing's disease, increased levels of ACTH continue to further stimulate release of cortisol from the adrenal gland with the end
result being a Cushingoid appearance of the client.

Clinical Manifestations

Many clients early in the course of the disease do not present with the "classic"
signs and symptoms of Cushing's syndrome. Therefore, consider this diagnosis in
adult clients with new-onset diabetes mellitus, rapid weight gain in the absence of
other signs, new-onset hypertension, acne, and hirsutism. In children the only
symptom may be growth failure despite normal or increased weight gain.

Obtain a detailed medication history. Often, clients do not realize their medications may contain steroids (particularly inhaled or topical steroids). In addition, clients may have access to illicit steroids used for increasing muscle mass,
which may have significant glucocorticoid content, resulting in a Cushingoid
appearance.

Subjective

Fatigue, emotional lability, increased irritability, sleep disturbances
Weakness
Weight gain
Easy bruisability

Hirsutism

Acne, oily skin

Impotence, decreased libido

Polydipsia, polyuria

Abdominal pain

Amenorrhea, menstrual irregularities

Headache, anxiety

Backache

Objective

Central obesity, moon face, buffalo hump

Facial plethora

Proximal myopathy

Hypertension,

Striae (red to purple) on abdomen, hips, buttocks, thighs, breasts, and axillae

Ankle edema

Slender extremities, muscle wasting

Vertebral collapse or fracture

Hyperpigmentation

Exophthalmos

Tinea versicolor infection

Renal calculi

Signs of glucose intolerance

Psychological changes

Differential Diagnosis

Exogenous obesity (caused by a caloric intake greater than needed to meet the body's needs)

Exogenous glucocorticoid administration

Diagnostic Tests

Cushing's Syndrome: ACTH-Independent

24-hour urine culture reveals elevated cortisol:creatinine ratio, elevated 17-ketosteroids.

ACTH low.

Salivary cortisol elevated.

Radiologic evaluation may reveal adrenal tumor or other tumor.

Cushing's Syndrome: ACTH-Dependent

24-hour urine culture reveals elevated cortisol:creatinine ratio.

ACTH high.

Salivary cortisol elevated.

Radiologic evaluation may reveal pituitary/hypothalamic tumor.

It is important to keep in mind that cortisol and ACTH release may be episodic even in a client with Cushing's syndrome. Therefore, if the initial laboratory evaluation is negative for Cushing's syndrome, repeat evaluation should be performed in those with a clinical picture consistent with the syndrome.

Cushing's Disease
See "Cushing's Syndrome: ACTH-Dependent."

Management/Treatment
The management of Cushing's syndrome depends on the etiology. The mainstay of treatment is surgical. In some instances some medications are used. Of utmost importance is glucocorticoid replacement perioperatively.

Exogenous Glucocorticoid Administration
Slowly wean drug as tolerated and ultimately discontinue if symptoms allow.

Pituitary Gland Tumor Secreting ACTH (Cushing's Disease)
Transsphenoidal microadenomectomy (cure rate, 80%–90%); macroadenomectomy (cure rate, 50%); or pituitary resection if adenoma cannot be identified (cure rate, 80%–90%).

If the client is not cured with transsphenoidal surgery other options include repeat operation on the pituitary gland, radiation to the pituitary gland, and medical or surgical adrenalectomy.

Ectopic ACTH-Producing Tumor
Surgical resection of the tumor: Unfortunately in the majority of cases the tumor is not resectable, in which case chemotherapy and/or radiation therapy may be helpful. Adrenal enzyme inhibitors are used to decrease the degree of hypercortisolism, which in these cases may be causing more problems than the tumor itself. Ultimately, an adrenalectomy may be necessary to control the symptoms.

Adrenocortical Tumors
Surgical resection of the tumor: In the case of adenomas the cure rate is nearly 100%; however, these patients may have profound suppression of the hypothalamic–pituitary–adrenal axis for several months after surgery. It is therefore imperative that these patients receive steroid replacement therapy. Results for adrenal carcinoma resection are very poor as micrometastases are typically present even when all of the tumor was thought to be removed. In this situation drugs such as mitotane have been used to control the tumor. Ultimately adrenal enzyme inhibitors may be used to control the symptoms of glucocorticoid excess. The long term prognosis for adrenal carcinoma is very poor.

Client Education
Necessity of taking medications regularly (sometimes lifelong need) and to increase their doses in times of stress (fever, illness, surgery, trauma, etc.)

Medical identification jewelry indicating disease and dependence on steroids

Follow-up
Depends on disease state and treatment.

Referral
Refer to endocrinologist.

Refer to surgeon (general or neurosurgeon) as indicated.

Refer to oncologist as indicated.

DIABETES MELLITUS, TYPE 1

SIGNAL SYMPTOMS polydipsia (excessive thirst), polyphasia (excessive hunger), polyuria (excessive urination)

| ICD-9 Codes | 250.1 | Type 1 diabetes mellitus, uncontrolled |

Type 1 diabetes mellitus is a metabolic disorder that results from failure of the pancreas to make the hormone insulin. Insulin helps the body use food by converting sugar or glucose into energy. Without insulin, sugar accumulates in the bloodstream and will cause symptoms. 90% of cases of type 1 diabetes begin in childhood, most between the ages of 10 and 14 years of age, as juvenile onset is the typical pattern.

Epidemiology

Occus in 1 of every 300 children.

Average age of onset is 4 to 11 years old.

Equal incidence between males and females.

Caucasian > African-American > Hispanic.

Incidence increases 3%–5% a year.

15%–30% of people with type 1 diabetes present with diabetic ketoacidosis (DKA).

DKA usually seen in children <5 years of age.

Most have several weeks to months of symptoms.

Etiology

Diabetes mellitus is typically classified into type 1 (insulin-dependent and typically occurring at <30 years of age), type 2 (typically older and overweight), gestational diabetes mellitus, malnutrition-related diabetes, and other. Type 2 diabetes mellitus was previously referred to as non-insulin-dependent diabetes or adult-onset diabetes (see Table 10–1).

Type 2 diabetes implies insulin resistance, and these clients usually have a relative deficiency of insulin as opposed to an absolute deficiency as seen in type 1 diabetes. Obesity (typically seen in type 2) results in some degree of insulin resistance. Over time the pancreas secretes very high insulin levels in an effort to overcome the insulin resistance at the cellular level. Ultimately this may cause a "burnout" of the islet cells, resulting in insulin deficiency.

Type 1 diabetes has two forms. Immune-mediated diabetes mellitus—resulting from autoimmune destruction of the β cells—typically occurs in childhood or adolescence but can arise at any age. Destruction of islet (insulin-producing) cells may be caused by multiple factors, including a genetic tendency, autoimmunity, environmental, and a "trigger," which can be a common viral infection. Islet-cell antibodies are usually present around the time of onset of type 1 diabetes. These patients are rarely obese and are also prone to other autoimmune diseases.

Idiopathic diabetes mellitus has no known cause and no evidence of autoimmunity. This is a rare form, and it is inherited. It is a hereditary disease mani-

Table 10-1   Classification of Diabetes

I. Type 1 diabetes (β-cell destruction)—immune mediated or idiopathic
II. Type 2 diabetes (insulin resistance with relative insulin deficiency or secretory defect with insulin resistance)
III. Other specific types
  -Genetic defects of β-cell function
  -Genetic defects in insulin action
  -Diseases of exocrine pancreas (pancreatitis, trauma/pancreatectomy, neoplasia, cystic fibrosis, hemochromatosis)
  -Endocrinopathies (Acromegaly, Cushing's syndrome, glucagonoma, pheochromocytoma, hyperthyroidism somatostatinoma, aldosteronoma)
  -Drug-or chemical-induced (pentamidine, nicotinic acid, glucocorticoids, thyroid hormone, diazoxide, β-adrenergic agonists, thiazides, dilantin, α-interferon
  -Infections (congenital rubella, cytomegalovirus)
  -Genetic syndromes associated with diabetes (Down's, Klinefelter's, Turner, Wolfram's syndromes and Friedreich's ataxia)

Adapted from Diabetes Care Volume 23 Supplement 1 American Diabetes Association: Clinical Practice Recommendations 2000

fested by glucose intolerance, although the specific genetics of the disease are ambiguous and in most cases of new-onset insulin-dependent diabetes mellitus, there is no family history of type 1 diabetes mellitus.

Physiology and Pathophysiology

The initial destruction of islet cells in the pancreas may begin to occur months prior to presentation of the disease. With destruction of the islet cells there is a decrease in insulin production, and symptoms of diabetes begin to occur. With stress and illness, cellular glucose requirements and insulin needs increase, leading to abnormally high blood sugar levels.

Clinical Manifestations

Subjective

  Polyuria (excessively wet and heavy diapers in children)
  Polydipsia
  Polyphagia
  Nocturia
  Weight loss
  Blurred vision
  Constipation
  Fatigue
  Irritability
  Abdominal pain or tenderness
  Altered mental status

Objective

  Patients often present with DKA.
  Fruity breath.
  Weight loss despite normal or increased appetite.
  Poor skin turgor, reduced muscle mass, dry mucous membranes.
  Kussmaul breathing.

Differential Diagnosis

Glucocorticoid excess (mimics signs of diabetes)

Severe stress (causes diabeteslike symptoms)

Medication use (certain drugs)

Renal glucosuria (genetic condition in which the renal threshold for glucose is abnormally low, causing positive results for urine glucose measurements at normal serum glucose levels)

Transient hyperglycemia

Untreated thyroid disease

Type 2 diabetes (non-insulin-dependent)

Diabetes insipidus (extreme polyuria and polydipsia)

Diagnostic Tests

Fasting blood sugar level >126 mg/dl or casual blood sugar level >200 mg/dl

Presence of ketones in urine and/or blood

Electrolytes, chemistry panel, and venous pH (hyponatremia, hypokalemia/hyperkalemia, (If pH <7.3 or HCO_3 <15 DKA is present)

Hemoglobin A_{1c} test is not typically useful as it is almost always more than 10% by the time a client presents with symptoms of diabetes. If is not clear whether the client has type 1 or type 2 diabetes, testing of autoantibodies may be helpful. The most commonly used are gadolinium-65 (glutamic acid decarboxylase), anti–islet-cell antibody, and anti-insulin antibody. All or some of these are positive in approximately 90% of cases of type 1 diabetes. Therefore, the most useful result is a positive antibody test, which indicates the presence of autoimmune or type 1 diabetes mellitus. (See Table 10–5: American Diabetes Association Criteria for the Diagnosis of Diabetes Mellitus.)

Management/Treatment

Initially, clients who have evidence of DKA or dehydration are very ill and should be admitted to the hospital for stabilization, treatment, and education. The overall goal of diabetes management is to keep blood glucose levels near normal to lower the risk of short- and long term complications. This includes managing the diet with meal planning, helping parents and patients to be comfortable with drawing up insulin and giving injections and storing insulin, sick day and exercise management, treatment of hypoglycemia and hyperglycemia, and who the client should call if help is needed.

Pharmacologic Management

INSULIN (TABLE 10–2)

Recommended doses:

Prepubertal child: 0.5–1.0 U/kg/day

Midpubertal adolescent: 0.75–1.5 U/kg/day

Late pubertal adolescent: 1.0–1.5 U/kg/day

Adult: 0.5–0.8 U/kg/day

Table 10–2 Insulin Action Times

Insulin	Onset	Peak	Duration
Lispro (Humalog)	5–10 minutes	60–90 minutes	2–4 hours
Human Regular	Around 30 minutes	2–3 hours	Around 6 hours
Human NPH	2–3 hours	6–10 hours	12–16 hours
Human Lente	1–4 hours	4–12 hours	12–18 hours
Human Ultralente	6–10 hours	8–12 hours	18–22 hours
Lantis (insulin glargine)	24 hours action without peak (basal insulin)	–	–
70/30 insulin (70% NPH and 30% Regular insulin)	Within 30 minutes	Maximal effect between 2 and approximately 12 hours	Up to 24 hours
75/25 insulin (75% insulin lispro protamine suspension and 25% insulin lispro) (Do not mix Lantis, 70/30 or 75/25 with any other insulin.)	Within 15 minutes	–	May be up to 24 hours

During ketosis, illness, and/or growth increase to 1.0–1.5U/kg/day

Most newly diagnosed children and adults receive three injections of insulin a day. They usually receive humalog insulin and NPH in the morning before breakfast; humalog insulin before dinner, and NPH before bedtime. Consistent timing of checking blood sugar levels and snacks and meals are imperative to being able to see patterns in the blood sugar levels.

Blood sugar levels should be checked at least four times a day; before meals and before bedtime snack. Before, during, and after any vigorous exercise, blood sugar levels should be checked and appropriate food/snacks added.

Goals of glucose management:

Before meals: 80–120 mg/dl

Bedtime: 100–140 mg/dl

Postprandial: <180 mg/dl

SOMOGYI EFFECT

The Somogyi effect is a rebound hyperglycemic reaction that consists of the presence of normoglycemia at bedtime, low blood glucose concentrations at 3 A.M., and symptoms of nocturnal hypoglycemia (nightmares, sweating, hunger, morning headache). It is thought to be related to the waning effects of the evening dose of NPH because insulin is needed to suppress the hepatic glucose output during the fasting state.

Options for counteracting this effect include decreasing the evening NPH dose by 2–3 units and monitoring the blood glucose level at 3 A.M., or shifting the evening injection of NPH from before dinner to bedtime. This effectively shifts the peak action of NPH to the early morning when the client is awake.

DAWN PHENOMENON

A rise in blood glucose concentration (by 30–40 mg/dl) that occurs between 4 and 8 A.M. following a physiologic nadir in the blood glucose concentration that occurs between midnight and 3 A.M. This is inconsistently present from one day to the next.

An increase in the evening NPH dose is indicated. Because this is inconsistent, be sure to monitor the blood glucose concentrations at 3 A.M.

DIABETIC KETOACIDOSIS

See Table 10–3.

Nonpharmacologic Management

Self-monitor blood glucose levels.

Check ketones for blood sugar levels >300 mg/dl.

Exercise.

Possible need for extra snacks before, during, or after exercise.

Do not begin exercise until blood sugar level is under better control.

Depends on intensity and duration

Table 10–3 Treatment of Diabetic Ketoacidosis (DKA) in Children and Adults

Fluid Management	-Normal saline 1 liter per hour for 2–3 hr. -Subsequent fluid replacement: ½ normal saline (NS) or ½ normal saline with 40–80 mEq/L potassium. If peripheral IV is used, no more than 40 meq/L potassium should be in the fluid. Typically the potassium should be divided into potassium acetate and potassium phosphate. IV fluid should run at 1½ maintenance fluids rate. Complete fluid replacement should occur over 24–48 hours. -Fluids should be changed as necessary depending on electrolyte balance. Once blood sugar is around 250 mg/dL, D5 and 0.45% NS is used to meet fluid needs. -Overzealous fluid management has been attributed to an increase risk of cerebral edema.
Insulin Management	-Insulin should only be given IV in a critical care area only. Regular insulin bolus of 0.1 U/kg may be given. -Insulin infusion should be started after rehydration has commenced. Infusion rates for insulin are 0.05–0.1 units/kg/hour. Blood sugar should decline by no more than 100 mg/dL/hour. If there is less than a 10% drop in blood sugar in 2 hr, the rate of insulin infusion should be doubled. When plasma glucose is 250 mg/dl, decrease insulin infusion rate to half. Continue insulin infusion until arterial pH is >7.30, plasma glucose is <250 mg/dl, anion gap is 13–17, and HCO_3 is >15. -The insulin infusion should always be > 0.05 units/kg/hour otherwise the acidosis will worsen. If blood sugar falls too rapidly or too low, increase the dextrose concentration in the IV fluid. This will hasten the resolution of acidosis. The endpoint of therapy is not eyglycemia but resolution of acidosis.

Table continued on following page.

Table 10–3 Treatment of Diabetic Ketoacidosis (DKA) in Children and Adults (Continued)

Electrolyte Management	-Potassium abnormalities—nitially hyperkalemia may be present secondary to intracellular acidosis pushing it out of the cells. Once insulin infusion is started, the potassium is likely to decrease significantly. Many clients will need multiple potassium boluses, typically KCL 1–2 meq/kg IV over several hours. -Sodium abnormalities—initially sodium levels are factitiously low due to hyperglycemia. If initial sodium is high, severe dehydration and/or concurrent diabetes insipidus may be present. -Phosphorous, magnesium abnormalities—with severe diabetic ketoacidosis and prolonged polyuria, phosphorous and magnesium losses may be significant. Both should be replaced as necessary.
Laboratory Evaluation	-EKG every 2 hrs -Hourly blood sugars while on insulin drip -Electrolytes every two hours -Chemistry panel every 4–8 hours -Venous pH -Urine ketones every void -Once the diabetes ketoacidosis has resolved and the patient is on subcutaneous insulin, fingersticks should be checked before each meal, 1½ hours after breakfast and dinner, bedtime and 0400. Electrolytes should be obtained until all potassium, phosphorous, sodium, and magnesium abnormalities are no longer present.
Complications	-Cerebral edema–> 30% of clients have CT scan evidence of cerebral edema, but most do not have clinical evidence. Watch for signs of increased intracranial pressure (Cushing's triad, worsening mentation, worsening headache) -Infection – deep line infection, urinary tract infection, upper respiratory infection, pneumonia, rarely meningitis -Deep venous thrombosis – more common in clients with severe diabetic ketoacidosis with central line placement -Cardiac arrhythmia secondary to electrolyte imbalance.

For short-duration and low to moderate intensity (walking a half mile or leisure bicycling for less than 30 minutes)—If blood sugar level is less than 100 mg/dl, increase food by 10 to 15 g of carbohydrate per hour of exercise. If blood sugar level is 100 mg/dl or greater, it is not necessary to increase food intake.

For moderate exercise (tennis, swimming, jogging for 1 hour)—If blood sugar level is less than 100–170 mg/dl, increase food intake by 25 to 50 g of carbohydrates before exercise, then 10 to 15 g per hour of exercise. If the blood sugar level is 180 to 300 mg/dl, increase food intake by 10 to 15 g of carbohydrates per hour of exercise. If greater than 300 mg/dl, no increase in food intake is necessary.

For strenuous exercise or activity (football, hockey, strenuous swimming)—If the blood sugar level is less than 100 mg/dl increase food intake by 50 g of carbohydrates; monitor blood sugar level closely because hypoglycemia can occur 8–15 hours after strenuous exercise. For a blood sugar level of 100–170 mg/dl, increase food intake by

25–50 g of carbohydrates. For blood sugar levels from 180 to 300 mg/dl, increase food intake by 10–15 g of carbohydrates per hour of exercise. For a blood sugar level >300 mg/dl, the client needs to get blood sugar level under better control before beginning exercise.

Diet

Clients with diabetes are placed on an exchange list/carbohydrate-counting diet plan that is individualized according to their activity pattern and growth requirements. The diet should consist of 50% carbohydrates, 25%–30% protein and 25%–30% fat. For adults, the recommended ADA guidelines are a minimum of 60%–70% carbohydrates, 10%–20% protein, and 10%–20% fats. (If the client has nephropathy, consider protein restriction.)

SICK DAY MANAGEMENT

If the client has an upset stomach (blood sugar level <180 and no ketones) and is unable to tolerate solid foods, use fluids rather than the usual meal plan. These liquids (1–2 oz every 15 minutes) will give the sugar (carbohydrates) of the usual meal plan, but not the fat or protein. Clear liquids such as Jell-O, 7-Up, and apple juice are easily digested and will not cause vomiting as easily as regular food. Cola-flavored soda, orange juice, and Gatorade may prolong vomiting, especially in young children and should be avoided. If the client can tolerate solid foods, extra water and sugar-free drinks should be encouraged. If vomiting persists, a fever of 101°F is present, dehydration occurs, blood sugar levels are continuously >240, and/or ketone levels continue to be moderate to large despite supplemental doses of insulin, the client may need to go to the emergency room for rehydration therapy. Supplemental doses must be individualized, but could be 1–2 U for every 30–50 mg/dl over an agreed-upon target glucose concentration.

Client Education

Pathophysiology, management, risks, and signs, symptoms and management of hyperglycemia and hypoglycemia.

Clients should be instructed on the proper procedure for drawing up insulin, giving injections, and the proper handling of insulin. It is important for clients to also understand each type of insulin, when it peaks, and its duration of action.

Rotation of injection sites to prevent lipohypertrophy and to ensure insulin absorption.

Sick day management.

Exercise and diet.

Need for regular ophthalmologic examinations.

Necessary supplies for treatment and traveling.

Diabetes school protocol. School personnel must be informed of the plan of care and must implement an individualized care plan for the child.

Encourage psychological management and/or support groups to help clients and families cope with the disease.

Follow-up

Quarterly visits with a health-care professional to include evaluation of blood sugar log and/or downloading of blood glucose meter, Hb_{Alc} (should be <7.2), evaluation of injection sites for evidence of lipohypertrophy, height, weight, blood pressure and pubertal status in children.

Annual visit to include the above as well as the following laboratory data: free thyroxine, thyroid-stimulating hormone, fasting chemistry panel and lipid profile, microalbumin in pubertal clients and those who have had diabetes >5 years. In addition, patients should have an annual dilated ophthalmologic examination by a qualified health-care professional who has experience with diabetes.

Clients who present with poor weight gain that cannot be explained by his/her blood sugar control should have laboratory testing for celiac disease. This occurs in approximately 10% of the population with type 1 diabetes. In addition, evaluation for hypothyroidism or hyperthyroidism should be done more often than annually in the presence of symptoms. Approximately 25% of clients with type 1 diabetes ultimately have autoimmune hyperthyroidism and occasionally will have hyperthyroidism.

Referral

Refer to appropriate specialists if there are signs of complications.
Refer to home care or community nurse for patients at risk.

DIABETES MELLITUS, TYPE 2

SIGNAL SYMPTOMS▶ polydipsia, polyuria, polyphasia

| ICD-9 Codes | 250.00 | Type 2 diabetes mellitus, controlled |
| | 250.02 | Type 2 diabetes mellitus, uncontrolled |

Diabetes mellitus is a complex group of metabolic diseases characterized by hyperglycemia resulting from defects in insulin secretion, insulin action, or both. The abnormalities in carbohydrate, fat, and protein metabolism seen in type 2 diabetes are due to deficient action of insulin on target tissues. Deficient action of insulin is due to inadequate secretion of insulin and/or decreased response to insulin at the tissue level. The relative lack of insulin and its action ultimately results in hyperglycemia.

Epidemiology

Affects 16 million in the United States and accounts for approximately 90% of all cases of diabetes; only one third of these individuals are aware that they have diabetes.

The risk of having type 2 diabetes increases with age, obesity, and lack of physical activity; it is more common in subjects with a family history of type 2 diabetes and in individuals with hypertension or dyslipidemia.

The major risk factors for type 2 diabetes include:

Family history of diabetes

Obesity (20% or more over desired body weight or body-mass index >27 kg/m^2)

Race/ethnicity (African-Americans, Hispanic Americans, Native Americans, Asian Americans, Pacific Islanders)

Age ≥45 years

History of impaired glucose tolerance

Hypertension (blood pressure >140/90 mm Hg in adults)

HDL cholesterol level <35 mg/dl and/or triglyceride level >250 mg/dl

History of gestational diabetes mellitus or delivery of babies weighing ≥9 lb

Screening for diabetes may be appropriate in individuals with one or more risk factors; if the results of the first screening are negative, the screening should be repeated every 3 years. It should be stressed that practitioners should be vigilant about questioning patients about risk factors and testing as deemed appropriate.

Etiology

Diabetes mellitus is typically classified into type 1 (insulin-dependent and typically occurring in adults <30 years of age), type 2 (typically older and overweight clients), gestational diabetes mellitus, malnutrition-related diabetes, and other. Type 2 diabetes mellitus was previously referred to as non-insulin-dependent diabetes or adult-onset diabetes. (See Table 10–1.)

Type 2 diabetes implies insulin resistance; these clients usually have a relative deficiency of insulin as opposed to an absolute deficiency as seen in type 1 diabetes. Obesity (typically seen in type 2) results in some degree of insulin resistance. Over time the pancreas secretes very high insulin levels in an effort to overcome the insulin resistance at the cellular level. Ultimately this may cause a "burnout" of the islet cells, resulting in insulin deficiency.

Physiology and Pathophysiology

In the normal (nondiabetic) state there is a finely tuned relationship between insulin production from the islet cells in the pancreas, glucagon release, glycogenolysis, and gluconeogenesis, and this is dependent on the fed or fasting state. In type 2 diabetes, however, this relationship changes. Early on, the changes occur because of insulin resistance at the cellular level. In many clients this is due to obesity, which in turn increases resistance. In others, it may be a genetic defect at the cellular level. As the resistance to insulin increases, the pancreas attempts to compensate by increasing insulin production to ever higher amounts. At this stage the client may still have normal glucose levels on testing but may have very high levels of serum insulin. In addition, on physical examination clients may be noted to have acanthosis nigricans (a dark, velvety appearing skin alteration typically seen on the back of the neck, axillae, and waist). Ultimately, the levels of glucose increase because the pancreas can no longer compensate for the insulin resistance. This leads to hyperglycemia that may be undetected for months to years prior to diagnosis. In many clients the islet cells cease to function properly or even at all, at which point they may become dependent on exogenous insulin to maintain normal blood sugar levels. Prior to losing islet-cell function patients may be treated with oral agents.

Clinical Manifestations

Some clients may present with signs of long-term complications associated with diabetes. These include coronary artery disease, hypertension, retinopathy, blindness, nephropathy, peripheral neuropathy, autonomic neuropathy causing gastrointestinal, genitourinary, and cardiovascular symptoms, and sexual dysfunction. Clients may also present with acute complications such as DKA or nonketotic hyperosmolar syndrome.

In children, behavior problems, declining school performance, delayed puberty, and/or poor growth may also be presenting symptoms.

Subjective

Polyuria, Polydipsia, Polyphagia
Weight loss
Blurred vision
Recurrent infections (e.g., vaginitis or skin infections—especially fungal)
Numbness, tingling

Objective

Abnormal/delayed healing
Signs of dehydration
Weight loss (although the patient is often obese and has a history of hypertension, dyslipidemia, and/or hypertension and coronary artery disease)
Signs of DKA (Kussmaul breathing, dehydration, oral candidiasis) or nonketotic hyperosmolar syndrome
Presence of acanthosis nigricans

Differential Diagnosis

Diabetes mellitus type 1 (Table 10–4)
Diabetes insipidus (extreme polyuria and polydipsia)

Diagnostic Tests

Fasting Plasma Glucose (FPG) Level

FPG is the preferred method of testing for diabetes. This test should be done in a client who has been fasting—no food or drink other than water for at least 8 hours prior to testing. The oral glucose tolerance test [OGTT] (75 g glucose) may also be performed; however, the FPG is easier and faster to perform, is more convenient and acceptable to clients, and is less expensive than the OGTT. The diagnosis of diabetes must be confirmed with a second test on a subsequent day. Other factors, such as medications, fever, and illness, also must be taken into account when interpreting laboratory results. Normoglycemia is defined as a plasma glucose level <110 mg/dl in the FPG and a 2-hour postload value <140 mg/dl in the OGTT (Table 10–5).

Table 10–4   Characteristics of Type 1 and Type 2 Diabetes Mellitus

Characteristic	Type 1 Diabetes Mellitus	Type 2 Diabetes Mellitus
Gender	Females = males	Females>males
Age at diagnosis	Childhood/adolescence (<30 yrs)	>13 yrs; typically >40 yrs
Ethnic group with highest prevalence	Caucasians	African-Americans, Hispanics, and Native Americans
Autoimmunity	Common	Uncommon
Obesity	Uncommon	Common
Acanthosis nigricans	Uncommon	Common
Family history of diabetes	Infrequent	Frequent
Dependence on insulin	Lifelong	Episodic

Hemoglobin A_{1c}

A hemoglobin A_{1c} (a 3-month measurement of the glycosylation of red cells and an indicator of blood sugar control) is not recommended for diagnosing diabetes or glucose intolerance. However, it is useful for providing insight into the mean blood sugar levels over the preceding 2–3 months

Urine Test for Glucose

A urine test is not recommended for diagnosing or screening for diabetes mellitus.

Management/Treatment

The overall goal of the management of diabetes is to lower blood glucose levels to near normal, thereby lowering the risk of short- and long-term complications. Managing type 2 diabetes includes dietary management, exercise, and pharmacologic agents.

The stepped approach to treating type 2 diabetes includes:

Pharmacologic Management

Symptomatic patients and patients with marked hyperglycemia (FPG ≥300 mg/dl) will show marked improvement in both with initiation of an oral agent. Drug therapy should also be an adjunct to diet and exercise, not a substitute. Initiate when diet and exercise have not achieved and maintained FPGs <120 mg/dl and an Hb_{A1c} of

Table 10–5   American Diabetes Association Criteria for the Diagnosis of Diabetes Mellitus

Test	Normo-glycemia	Impaired Fasting Glucose	Impaired Glucose Tolerance	Diabetes Mellitus
Fasting plasma glucose	<110 mg/dl	110–125 mg/dl	–	>126 mg/dl
2-hr postload glucose	<140 mg/dl	–	140–199 mg/dl	>200 mg/dl
Random plasma glucose concentration	–	–	–	>200 mg/dl
Other	–	–	–	Symptoms of diabetes mellitus

Management of Type 2 Diabetes

Diagnosis of type 2 DM: use one of three tests (results should be
confirmed on a subsequent day)
- RPG ≥ 200 mg per dL (11.1 mmol per L) + symptoms
- FPG ≥ 126 mg per dL (7.0 mmol per L)
- OGTT (75 g) with 2 hr PG = 200 mg per dL (11.1 mmol per L)

Patient education/diet and exercise/HBGM
Goals: FPG<126 mg per dL (7.0 mmol per L),
Hba$_{1c}$ < 7 percent: evaluate in three months

Initiate monotherapy if diet and exercise alone are inadequate.

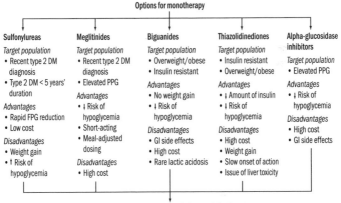

Options for monotherapy

Sulfonylureas

Target population
- Recent type 2 DM diagnosis
- Type 2 DM < 5 years' duration

Advantages
- Rapid FPG reduction
- Low cost

Disadvantages
- Weight gain
- ↑ Risk of hypoglycemia

Meglitinides

Target population
- Recent type 2 DM diagnosis
- Elevated PPG

Advantages
- ↓ Risk of hypoglycemia
- Short-acting
- Meal-adjusted dosing

Disadvantages
- High cost

Biguanides

Target population
- Overweight/obese
- Insulin resistant

Advantages
- No weight gain
- ↓ Risk of hypoglycemia

Disadvantages
- GI side effects
- High cost
- Rare lactic acidosis

Thiazolidinediones

Target population
- Insulin resistant
- Overweight/obese

Advantages
- ↓ Amount of insulin
- ↓ Risk of hypoglycemia

Disadvantages
- High cost
- Weight gain
- Slow onset of action
- Issue of liver toxicity

Alpha-glucosidase inhibitors

Target population
- Elevated PPG

Advantages
- ↓ Risk of hypoglycemia

Disadvantages
- High cost
- GI side effects

Initiate combination therapy if a single agent is inadequate.

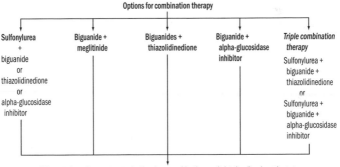

Options for combination therapy

Sulfonylurea +
biguanide
or
thiazolidinedione
or
alpha-glucosidase
inhibitor

Biguanide + meglitinide

Biguanides + thiazolidinedione

Biguanide + alpha-glucosidase inhibitor

Triple combination therapy
Sulfonylurea +
biguanide +
thiazolidinedione
or
Sulfonylurea +
biguanide +
alpha-glucosidase
inhibitor

If therapeutic goals are not met using the above combinations, switch to insulin +/− oral agent.

Stepwise approach for the management of type 2 diabetes in patients inadequately controlled with diet
and exercise. (RPG = random plasma glucose; FPG = fasting plasma glucose; OGTT = oral glucose
tolerance test; PG = plasma glucose; HbA1c = glycosylated hemoglobin A1c; HBGM = home blood
glucose monitoring; DM = diabetes mellitus; GI = gastrointestinal; PPG = postprandial glucose)
Reprinted from *American Family Physician,* Vol 63, No. 9, May 2001.

less than 7 percent after a 3-month trial. There are many types of oral medications for type 2 diabetes mellitus. The most commonly used agents include:

Sulfonylureas: Agents such as glipizide, glyburide, and glimepiride stimulate the β cells in the pancreas to release more insulin. They are typically taken 1–2 times a day. (Not recommended for pregnant women or women who are planning to become.)

Repaglinide (Prandin): Taken three times/day prior to each meal.

Biguanides: Metformin sensitizes the body to insulin already produced and reduces liver production of glucose. Common side effects include diarrhea and the risk of lactic acidosis in acutely ill patients.

Glitazones: Rosiglitazone (Avandia) and pioglitazone (Actose) help endogenous insulin work better in fat and muscle tissues. However, these agents have been associated with liver dysfunction; therefore, liver-function tests should be routinely ordered. Never use if patients have liver disease or if the alanine aminotransferase level is >2.5 times the upper limit of normal.

Acarbose (Precose) and Meglitol: These agents slow or block the breakdown of starches and certain sugars by acting as α-glucosidase inhibitors, causing a slow rise in blood sugar levels after a meal. These agents are taken with the first bite of a meal. Typical side effects include gas and diarrhea.

Nonpharmacologic Management

If fasting plasma glucose measurements are <200 mg/dl and presenting symptoms are not severe, a course of diet and exercise should be initiated first to control the hyperglycemia.

Self-monitoring of blood glucose levels, diet, regular exercise are foundational to the non-pharmacologic management

Complementary/Alternative Therapies

Stress management therapies

Client Education

Diet and exercise—Most patients are overweight, so this is significant because a moderate weight loss will reduce hyperglycemia, dyslipidemia, and hypertension.

Suggest a reduction of 250 to 500 calories per day with 10%–20% of daily intake from protein, 10%–20% from fat (less than 10% saturated), and 60%–70% from carbohydrates.

Pathophysiology, management, risks, and signs and symptoms of complications of diabetes.

Clients should be clearly informed about the medications they are taking, potential side effects, drug interactions, and any changes in the treatment regimen; if they are taking insulin, be sure the client is capable of drawing insulin up in a syringe accurately.

Sick day management.

Need for annual podiatric and ophthalmologic examinations.

If the client is planning a pregnancy, she should be referred for follow-up and switched to insulin if she is on an oral antidiabetic agent before becoming pregnant.

Follow-up

There should be a regularly scheduled follow-up visit each of which should include discussion of a management plan and any changes—e.g., Is the client taking the medications? Monitoring blood sugar levels? Also, blood pressure and weight should be measured and a neurologic and foot examination should be done.

At regular intervals an Hb_{A1c} (keep <7), lipid profile, chemistry panel including blood urea nitrogen and creatinine, and liver-function tests should be performed. Urine should be checked for microalbumin (consider using angiotensin–converting–enzyme inhibitors to slow the progression of microalbuminuria to overt disease in normotensive patients). A dilated retinal examination should be performed by an experienced ophthalmologist or optometrist, and a podiatric examination and electrocardiography should be performed annually.

An annual influenza vaccine should also be administered to all patients with diabetes.

Referral

Refer to endocrinologist, a dietitian/nutritionist, an appropriate specialist if there are signs of complications, at-risk clients to home care nurse.

HYPOGLYCEMIA

SIGNAL SYMPTOMS diaphoresis, blurred vision, headache, weakness, tachycardia

ICD-9 Codes	251.20	Hypoglycemia, unspecified/reactive/spontaneous

Hypoglycemia is a clinical syndrome in which the blood glucose level is <60 mg/100 ml.

Epidemiology

More prevalent in young adults and women
1% of nondiabetic population affected
More common in persons with type 1 diabetes than type 2

Etiology

Endocrine disorders are the most common cause. Inconsistent subcutaneous absorption of insulin, decreased food intake, missed meal, and increased insulin secretion during exercise produce hypoglycemia in diabetics.
Lifestyle patterns also contribute to this condition.
Can be precipitated by stress, pregnancy, intensive control of hyperglycemia, and diabetic gastroparesis.
Pancreatic tumors, severe malnutrition, renal failure, septicemia.
Adrenocortical insufficiency.
Liver disease—hepatitis, cirrhosis, liver congestion.
Propranolol (Inderal), salicylates, quinidine, pentamidine (Pentam 300), disopyramide (Norpace).

Physiology and Pathophysiology

Hypoglycemia causes the brain to receive an inadequate supply of blood glucose to function. In persons with diabetes mellitus, the lack of a glucagon and epinephrine response to low blood sugar levels aggravates the condition. In reactive hypoglycemia, the blood glucose falls 2–5 hours after eating. Very low levels will trigger the release of adrenaline to restore the blood sugar levels. The release of adrenaline produces the symptoms of sweating, trembling and a rapid heart rate.

Clinical Manifestations

Subjective

ADRENERGIC	NEUROGLYCOPENIC
Sweating	Headaches.
Tremulousness	Seizures.
Dizziness	Fatigue.
Confusion	Weakness.
Anxiety	Drowsiness.
Palpitations	Syncope.
	Diplopia and blurred vision.
	Personality changes.

Neurologic manifestations of hemiparesis, convulsions, confusion, and coma are more common in patients with diabetes mellitus.

Objective

Tachycardia (with or without preventricular contractions)
Diaphoresis
Hypothermia or hyperthermia
Coma, seizures
Babinski's sign
Aphasia
Hemiparesis

Differential Diagnosis

Anxiety disorder (palpitations, shortness of breath, dizziness, profuse sweating, pallor of face and extremities)
Panic attacks (tachycardia, anxiousness, dyspnea, trembling, chest pain, palpitations)
Hyperventilation (dizziness, faintness, numbness of fingers and toes, syncope)
Pheochromocytoma (headache, palpitations, sweating, nervousness, nausea, vomiting, hyperglycemia, syncope, weight loss, myocarditis, cardiac dysrhythmia, and heart failure)
Drug/alcohol ingestion
Transient ischemic attacks (disturbance of vision in one or both eyes, dizziness, weakness, dysphasia, numbness or unconsciousness lasting a few minutes)
Cerebrovascular accident (paralysis, weakness, sensory change, speech defect, aphasia, or death)

Diet (meals high in refined carbohydrates, fructose, galactose, and leucine and drugs such as sulfonylureas and salicylates)

Diagnostic Tests

Check blood glucose level while patient is experiencing symptoms. The most reliable method of diagnosing hypoglycemia is with a plasma glucose measurement after a 72-hour fast; this test is performed in the hospital under close observation.

For definitive diagnosis, the patient should have (1) documented occurrences of low blood glucose levels, (2) symptoms that occur while the blood glucose level is low, (3) evidence that symptoms are relieved by sugar or other foods, and (4) identification of the particular type of hypoglycemia.

Measurements of plasma insulin level, insulin antibodies, plasma and urine sulfonylurea levels and C peptide, blood urea nitrogen, creatinine, alcohol levels, liver-function tests during symptoms may also be useful.

To rule out endocrine pathology, obtain cortisol and ACTH levels.

Management/Treatment

Normalize blood glucose levels and treat underlying cause.

Pharmacologic Management

Glucagon, 1.0 mg IM, SC, or IV, which may be repeated if needed and can be given if patient is unresponsive.

Evaluate diabetic medications and change if necessary (e.g., substitute short-acting glipizide for longer-acting glyburide; metformin (glucophage) can be used as monotherapy in patients with type 2 diabetes who have frequent episodes of hypoglycemia).

Nonpharmacologic Management

For acute hypoglycemia—6–12 oz of orange juice or another fruit juice without added sugar.

1 cup of milk.

Diet modifications—high-protein, low-carbohydrate diet divided into six small feedings

Restrict caffeine, refined sugars, and alcohol.

Allergy testing to identify offending foods.

If hypoglycemia is a result of pancreatic or extrapancreatic tumors, surgical excision is recommended.

Client Education

Clients need to monitor blood glucose levels frequently during initiation of lifestyle changes such as diet and exercise.

Monitor blood glucose levels morning, before meals, and at bedtime.

More frequent recording of hypoglycemic events is necessary, especially 12–24 hours after event.

Review need for monitoring blood glucose levels during exercise, and stress need to avoid missing a meal.

Diet modifications—High-protein, low-carbohydrate diet divided into 5–6 small feedings.

Stop smoking; avoid caffeine and alcohol.

Follow-up

Frequent follow-up and evaluation.

On each visit, review record of hypoglycemic events.

Referral

Refer to endocrinologist.

HIRSUTISM

SIGNAL SYMPTOMS ▶ excessive hair growth, amenorrhea

ICD-9 Codes	704.1	Hirsutism

Hirsutism is a condition in women in which excessive growth of hair is present in areas where hair growth is usually minimal or absent. These areas are usually androgen-sensitive areas of the body. Virilization may occur in combination with hirsutism and may include temporal hair loss, loss of female body curvature, deepening of voice, or clitoral enlargement.

Epidemiology

Hirsutism without virilization: Usually benign; sometimes associated with polycystic ovary syndrome.

Hirsutism with virilization: May indicate an adrenal or ovarian tumor or uncontrolled congenital adrenal hyperplasia.

Etiology

Increased secretion of androgens by the ovary or adrenal gland stimulates hair growth, whereas estrogens inhibit hair growth in women.

Most frequent cause is ovarian dysfunction; polycystic ovary syndrome is the most common.

Physiology and Pathophysiology

Under normal circumstances, the circulating testosterone level in women is obtained from direct secretion by the ovary and by extraglandular conversion of androstenedione secreted by the ovary and the adrenal gland. With isolated hirsutism, 25% of the circulating testosterone is from ovarian secretion. When there is an increase in the level of testosterone, it results in an increase of free testosterone and metabolic clearance for testosterone. Mild hirsutism in women may be explained as the presence of an increased number of androgen receptors or increased receptor sensitivity.

Clinical Manifestations

Subjective

Occurring at time of menarche

History of excessive hair growth (may be rapid or gradual)

History of secondary amenorrhea (for at least 6 months)

History of drug usage (phenytoin, danazol, metyrapone, minoxidil, phenothiazines, diazoxide; or drugs used for body-building, or to correct menopause or diminished libido)

Familial occurrence

Objective

Presence of excessive hair growth (face, external genitalia, inner thigh, buttock, areola, linea alba, and chest). Arms are not androgen-sensitive areas.

Differential Diagnosis

Polycystic ovary syndrome (anovulation, amenorrhea, hirsutism, and infertility)

Late-onset adrenal hyperplasia (obesity, hypertension, glucose intolerance)

Ovarian or adrenal-gland tumor (hirsutism with virilization)

Menopause (amenorrhea)

Cushing's syndrome (hirsutism, amenorrhea, polycystic ovaries)

Hyperprolactinemia (one of the more common causes)

Diagnostic Tests

Serum testosterone level (elevated in cases of ovarian causes of virilization and some adrenal tumors)

Dehydroepiandrosterone sulfate (elevated in cases of adrenal causes of virilization)

Basal 17-hydroxyprogesterone (elevated if family history of adrenal hyperplasia)

Prolactin level, luteinizing hormone, follicle-stimulating hormone, estradiol, androstenedione, dehydroepiandrosterone, normal results differ at each laboratory

If no cause is found, perform magnetic resonance scan of the pituitary

Management/Treatment

Treat the cause of the hirsutism.

If caused by medication, discontinue the medication.

Treat hypothyroidism with levothyroxine (Synthroid).

Prolactinoma:

Treat for 6 months to 1 year treatment for partial improvement.

In women with microprolactinomas with amenorrhea who desire contraception, may take oral birth control pills or estrogen replacement safely.

In women with macroprolactinoma, no estrogen should be ordered because it may stimulate the growth of the macroprolactinoma.

Dopamine agonists can be used at bedtime to minimize side effects. Cabergoline dosage is 0.25 mg orally once weekly for 1 week, then 0.25 mg twice weekly for the next week, then 0.5 mg twice weekly until symptoms subside. Also bromocriptine (1.25–20 mg/day PO) or pergolide (0.125–2 mg/day PO) may be used.

Surgical intervention may be necessary for large tumors (transsphenoidal pituitary surgery).

Radiation treatment may be necessary for macroprolactinomas that continue to grow despite various treatments.

Ovarian causes:

Oral contraceptives may stimulate menses, but less effective for hirsutism.

21-Hydroxylase deficiency:

Glucocorticoids: Cortef-hydrocortisone, 15–25 mg PO daily in two divided doses

Increased androgen/testosterone levels:

Antiandrogens: Flutamide, 250–375 mg/day inhibits androgen reception uptake and suppresses serum androgen. It may be used with oral contraceptives. Treatment is applicable only to nonpregnant clients.

Nonpharmacologic Management

Hair-removal therapies (shaving, waxing, depilatories, tweezing, electrolysis)

Client Education

Permanent resolution of hirsutism is uncommon; depends on the cause and treatment

Supportive care

Follow-up

Depends on cause and treatment

Referral

Refer to endocrinologist.

Refer to surgeon for further evaluation of ovarian or adrenal tumor.

HYPERTHYROIDISM/THYROTOXICOSIS

SIGNAL SYMPTOMS ▶ **weight loss despite increased appetite, tremor, nervousness, palpitations**

ICD-9 Codes	242.0	Thyrotoxicosis with or without goiter
	242.1	Toxic uninodular goiter
	242.2	Toxic multinodular goiter
	242.4	Thyrotoxicosis from ectopic thyroid nodule
	242.8	Thyrotoxicosis of other specified origin
	242.9	Thyrotoxicosis without mention of goiter or other cause

Hyperthryoidisim (thyrotoxicosis) is a clinical syndrome involving tissues that are exposed to high level of circulating thyroid hormone. Conditions caused by an increase in thyroid hormone production by the thyroid gland are referred to hyperthyroidism. The most prevalent form of hyperthyroidism is Graves' disease.

Epidemiology

Strong familiar predisposition

Females affected 5 times more often than males

Peak occurrence between the ages of 20 and 40 years

Etiology

Hyperactivity of the thyroid gland

Excessive ingestion of thyroid hormone

Excessive secretion of thyroid hormone from ectopic sites

Physiology and Pathophysiology

Thyrotoxicosis results when tissues are exposed to elevated levels of circulating thyroid hormone. Usually thyrotoxicosis is due to hyperactivity of the thyroid gland, or hyperthyroidism; occasionally it can result from an excessive ingestion of thyroid hormone or excessive secretion of thyroid hormone from ectopic sites. Graves' disease (most commonly seen) is an autoimmune disorder in which T lymphocytes are sensitized to antigens within the thyroid gland and then stimulate the B lymphocytes to produce antibodies to these antigens. While mimicking the action of thyroid-stimulating hormones (TSHs) on the thyroid receptors, the growth and vascularity of the thyroid gland is increased. The antibodies are called thyroid-stimulating immunoglobulins. Hence, the gland itself enlarges (called thyromegaly).

Clinical Manifestations

Subjective

Nervousness, irritability, insomnia
Behavioral problem
Decreased school and work performance
Palpitations
Pedal edema
Amenorrhea or light menses
Diarrhea or frequent bowel movements
Fatigue, muscle weakness, tremors
Weight loss despite increased appetite

Objective

Exophthalmos, decreased visual acuity
Lid lag, lid retraction, stare, loss of extraocular movements
Tremor, nervousness, palpitations
Brisk deep-tendon reflexes
Fine, brittle hair
Atrial fibrillation, congestive heart failure
Bruit over the thyroid gland
Goiter, bruits, thrills
Itchy skin
Heat intolerance; flushed, moist skin
Pretibial myxedema
Plummer's nails (fingernail separates from matrix)

Differential Diagnosis

Acromegaly (gradual marked elongation of the bones of the face, jaw, and extremities)
Anorexia nervosa (prolonged refusal to eat, resulting in emaciation, amenorrhea)

Exogenous thyroid hormone administration

Illicit drug use

Psychiatric disorders

Marine–Lenhart syndrome (toxic multinodular goiter)

Plummer's disease (toxic adenoma)

Hyperthyroid phase of Hashimoto's thyroiditis (asymptomatic goiter; patient may report dysphagia and a feeling of local pressure)

Rare forms of thyrotoxicosis are ovarian struma, metastatic thyroid cancer, hydatidiform mole, TSH-secreting pituitary tumor

Diagnostic Tests

Thyroid-function tests (elevated free thyroxine, rarely elevated triiodothyronine, suppressed TSH, and positive thyroid antibodies)

Thyroid scan

Management/Treatment

Pharmacologic Management

The larger the gland is, the less likely it is for the disease to remit with drug treatment. The size of the gland also dictates amount of medication.

Propylthiouracil and methimazole are the drugs of choice. Propylthiouracil is considered the drug of choice during pregnancy or breast-feeding because it causes fewer problems in the newborn. The dosage is 300–600 mg daily in four divided doses. The dosage of methimazole in children is initially 0.4 mg/kg daily in three divided doses. The maintenance dose is half of the initial dose. For adults, the initial dose is 15–60 mg daily in three divided doses, depending on the severity of the disease. (May have to add antihistamine if rash occurs with medication). Dosage and frequency is generally reduced as symptoms of hyperthyroidism resolve and the free thyroxine level becomes normal.

Propranolol (Inderal) is the treatment of choice for tachycardia. Treatment usually begins with 10 mg PO, and is increased progressively until an adequate response (normal pulse) is achieved—usually 20 mg four times daily.

Radioactive iodine 1131 is used for adults or children in whom medical treatment is not improving the clinical status.

Nonpharmacologic Management

Rest, no vigorous activity or sports until condition improves

Adequate diet and nutrition

Surgery (removal of thyroid gland), if indicated

Complementary/Alternative Therapies

Multivitamin supplements—avoid iodine-enriched supplements

Client Education

Importance of taking medications regularly and consistently

How to check heart rate (pulse), what the normal heart rate is and at what rate to report rapid rate to their health-care provider

How to recognize tremors and report (if tremors, client is suffering from propranolol deficiency)

Decrease activity until symptoms such as increased heart rate, tremors, etc. have normalized

Follow-up

Frequent office visits (monthly) until symptoms normalize

Referral

Refer to endocrinologist.

Refer to surgeon, if indicated.

Refer to ophthalmologist if exophthalamos is present or there is any report of vision difficulty with closing of the eyes (corneal ulceration can occur).

HYPOTHYROIDISM

SIGNAL SYMPTOMS ▶ weight gain, mental/physical lethargy, dry skin, constipation, arthritis, slowing of metabolic process

ICD-9 Codes	243	Hypothyroidism, congenital
	244	Hypothyroidism, postsurgical
	244.1	Hypothyroidism, postablative
	244.3	Hypothyroidism, iatrogenic
	244.8	Hypothyroidism, other acquired/secondary NEC
	244.9	Hypothyroidism, primary NOS

Hypothyroidism is a clinical syndrome of a deficiency of thyroid hormones that results in a generalized decrease in metabolic processes. In infants and young children, this deficiency can result in a marked slowing of growth and development. Mental retardation may be a serious permanent consequence of hypothyroidism if not remedied soon enough. The onset of hypothyroidism in adults results in a generalized slowing down of the organism, which produces the deposition of glycosaminoglycans in the intracellular spaces (especially in the skin and muscle) and produces signs and symptoms of myxedema (loss of mental and physical vigor, dry skin and hair and firm inelastic edema).

Epidemiology

One of every 4000 to 5000 births results in congenital hypothyroidism.

Mental retardation and growth retardation may result in infants who are not treated with supplements; children with Down's and Turner's syndrome have a higher incidence of hypothyroidism.

Symptoms in adults can usually be reversed with therapy.

25% of children with type 1 diabetes mellitus acquire hypothyroidism (also found in adults).

Etiology

May be due to thyroid failure, pituitary TSH deficiency, hypothalamic deficiency of thyroid-releasing hormone (TRH) or an abnormality of the thyroxine (T_4) receptor in the cell. May also be caused by radioactive iodine therapy for Graves' disease, excessive iodide intake (kelp, radiocontrast dyes), iodide deficiency, or hypopituitarism due to pituitary adenoma, pituitary ablative therapy, or pituitary destruction.

Physiology and Pathophysiology

Thyroid agenesis or dysgenesis, enzyme defect in thyroid hormone production, hereditary thyroid hormone resistance, or transfer of thyroid-blocking antibodies across the placenta from the mother can cause congenital hypothyroidism. Ninety percent of these cases are picked up on newborn screening within 3 weeks of age. Long-term issues for children with congenital hypothyroidism include neurologic development and growth. In the absence of good control and compliance or in the event that therapy is not begun until after 6 weeks of age, significant neurologic problems may occur. Impairment of the thyroid gland may be caused by cancer, radiation, surgery, Hashimoto's thyroiditis (autoimmune), decrease in dietary iodine, antithyroid medication, pituitary disorders, or problems with thyroid hormone resistance.

Clinical Manifestations

Subjective

INFANTS AND CHILDREN

Constipation
Prolonged jaundice
Feeding or breathing difficulties

ADULTS

Dyspnea
Myxedema
Hoarseness
Weight gain
Dry and cool skin, cold intolerance
Constipation, decreased appetite
Amenorrhea
Fatigue
Increased menstrual flow
Decreased libido
Severe depression
Confusion, slow speech and thinking, memory loss

Objective

INFANTS AND CHILDREN

Low temperature
Enlarged fontanel
Decreased activity
Hoarse cry
Enlarged, protruding tongue
Umbilical hernia and retarded bone age
Poor growth
Precocious puberty
Short stature
Enlargement of the sella turcica

Delayed puberty

Periorbital swelling
Thick tongue
Thin, brittle hair
Goiter
Weight gain, decreased basal metabolic rate
Dull and apathetic appearance
Myxedema
Severe depression
Anemia
Anovulation, high incidence of spontaneous abortion
Decreased deep tendon reflexes

Differential Diagnosis

Epstein–Barr syndrome (fever of undetermined origin, weight loss, sore throat, tonsillar swelling)
Poor nutrition
Excessive intake of calories
Psychological syndromes
Infertility due to other causes
Growth hormone deficiency

Diagnostic Tests

TSH (will be elevated): TSH may be low if decreased free T_4 is secondary to primary disorder
Free T_4 (will be low)
Anti–thyroid peroxidase antibodies (may be present if mother has had autoimmune thyroid disease)

Management/Treatment

Pharmacologic Management

INFANTS

Replacement dose varies according to age of infant. The initial dose should raise the serum T_4 as rapidly as possible to minimize the consequences of hypothyroidism on cognitive function. A T_4 dosage of 10–15 μg/kg per day is recommended to raise the serum T_4 to >10 μg/dl by 7 days. In a full-term healthy infant, an average initial T_4 dose of 37.5–50 μg/day is appropriate. Mental development and attainment of normal growth are not impaired if adequate thyroxine treatment is initiated before 3 months of age.

Age	Daily μg/kg T_4 (thyroxine)
3–6 months	10–15
6–12 months	5–7
1–10 years	3–6
>10	2–4

Levothyroxine, 50–100 μg QD (Wynne et al., 2002)
Levothyroxine, 25–50 μg QD (Wynne et al., 2002)

Client Education

Compliance with medication; medication must be taken daily.
Soy may affect absorption and effectiveness of medication.
Developmental issues in children; measure heights and weights.

Follow-up

Free T_4 and TSH levels every 1–2 months for newborns for first year of life, then
every 2–3 months for the next 2 years. Every 6 months for clients 3 to 6 years old.
For those over 6 to adult, laboratory tests should be done annually

Referral

Refer to endocrinologist.

METABOLIC ACIDOSIS

SIGNAL SYMPTOMS ▶ wasting, high fever, sepsis, poor skin turgor

ICD-9 Code	276.2	Metabolic acidosis

Metabolic acidosis is a condition due to a loss of bicarbonate (HCO_3^-). This condition is also seen in respiratory alkalosis, but the pH of the blood distinguishes
between the two disorders (pH <7.30 = metabolic acidosis; pH >7.40 = alkalosis). A decrease in the plasma HCO_3^- concentration or an increase in carbon
dioxide decreases the blood pH and leads to acidemia.

Metabolic acidosis may be classified into two categories: acute normochlor-
emic organic acidosis and chronic hyperchloremic acidosis due to diarrhea or
renal acidification defects.

Epidemiology

Clients may produce organic acids as a result of the excess activity of a normal
metabolic pathway. The metabolism of an ingested substance (e.g., methyl alcohol, ethylene glycol) may result in a moderate rate of acid production.

Metabolic acidosis during renal failure is usually accompanied by an increase in the plasma anion gap. During acidemia there is a potent stimulus to
the respiratory center that causes hyperventilation.

Etiology

Overproduction of an organic acid
Renal failure (low glomerular filtration rate)
Infection
Sepsis
Dehydration

Physiology and Pathophysiology

Careful calculation of the anion gap assists in determining the cause of the metabolic acidosis. The anion gap represents the difference between readily measured anions and cations.

In plasma, Na^+ unmeasured cations $= HCO_3^- + CL^- +$ unmeasured anions. Anion gap $= (Na^+) - (HCO_3^- + CL^-)$. Reference ranges for the anion gap depend on differing laboratory methods. (Normal anion gap is $10 - 14$ mEq/L.)

The major unmeasured cations are calcium, magnesium, γ-globulins, and potassium. The major unmeasured anions are negatively charged albumin, phosphate, sulfate, and other organic anions.

A decreased anion gap occurs with a decrease in unmeasured anions or an increase in unmeasured cations. A decrease in unmeasured anions occurs when sodium concentration remains normal, but HCO_3^- and the chloride increase. An increase in unmeasured cations occurs after a fall in the sodium concentration because of an addition of unmeasured cations, but the HCO_3^- and CL^- are not changed. Causes include hypoalbuminemia, bromide intoxication, plasma-cell dyscrasias, and chloride retention.

Increased anion gap acidosis (low HCO_3^-) is associated with normal serum chloride; consequently the anion gap increases. Causes include diabetic ketoacidosis, starvation, renal insufficiency, alcohol ketoacidosis, and lactic acidosis.

A normal anion gap acidosis occurs when the low HCO_3^- of metabolic acidosis is combined with hyperchloremia. Causes include diarrhea, renal tubular acidosis, carbonic anhydrase inhibitors, and loss of HCO_3^-.

A urinary anion gap is used to distinguish between gastrointestinal and renal causes of hyperchloremic acidosis. With a gastrointestinal cause, the HCO_3^- loss is due to diarrhea and the urinary anion gap is negative. In cases in which the cause is distal renal tubular acidosis, the urinary anion gap is positive. With volume depletion, this result is more accurate than the urinary pH.

Clinical Manifestations

Subjective

Depends on the underlying condition; may include:

Diarrhea (primary or laxative-provoked)
Anorexia
History of parental feeding or toxic ingestion
History of diabetes, alcoholism, or renal or liver disease
History of medication use (β-blockers, enzyme inhibitors, spironolactone)

Objective

Depends on the underlying condition; may include:

Hypokalemia or hyperkalemia
Hyperpnea
Wasting
High fever

Sepsis
Poor skin turgor, dry mucous membranes

Differential Diagnosis

Alkalemia (increased bicarbonate or decreased carbon dioxide causes the blood pH to rise)

Diagnostic Tests

Blood pH (easily distinguishes between chronic respiratory alkalosis and metabolic acidosis, if pH <7.4 the primary defect is acidemia (check anion gap next—may be normal in cases of hyperchloremia or increased in cases of normochloremia).

Serum HCO_3^- and partial pressure of carbon dioxide are decreased.

Urinalysis (positive proteinuria, cellular casts found in renal disease; urine ketones show ketoacidosis; urine glucose shows diabetes ketoacidosis; urine oxalate crystals found in ethylene glycol intoxification).

Serum electrolytes and chemistry panel (serum ketones found in ketoacidosis; high blood urea nitrogen and creatinine found in uremic acidosis and distal renal tubular acidosis).

Organic acids, amino acids, lactate, pyruvate, and ammonia toxicology (high serum salicylate level found in salicylate intoxification; high serum lactate concentration found in lactic acidosis).

Management/Treatment

Treatment aimed at the underlying disorder and stabilizing the condition.
Correct fluid and electrolyte balance
Diabetes: Insulin and fluid-replacement therapy.
Hyperkalemia and some forms of normal anion gap acidosis: Supplemental HCO_3^-.
Salicylate intoxication: Alkali therapy (unless blood pH is already alkaline).
Alcoholic ketoacidosis: Thiamine should be given with glucose.
Distal renal tubular acidosis: Supplemental bicarbonate is necessary.
Proximal renal tubular acidosis: Monitor bicarbonate level; if elevated give no supplemental bicarbonate. If extra bicarbonate is necessary, also give potassium if indicated.

Client Education

Proper administration of medications
Side effects of medications
Signs and symptoms of dehydration
Hazards of overmedicating or abuse of salicylate/alcohol

Follow-up

Dependent on client's therapy, response to therapy, and underlying condition.

Referral

Refer to specialist as indicated by underlying condition.
Refer at-risk clients to home care nurse.

METABOLIC ALKALOSIS

SIGNAL SYMPTOMS lethargy, confusion, orthostatic hypotension, obtundation

ICD-9 Codes	276.3	Metabolic alkalosis

Metabolic alkalosis is a hyperbicarbonatemic, alkalemic, hypochloremic disorder (increased extracellular volume depletion). The mark of metabolic alkalosis is an elevated HCO_3^-. (The high HCO_3^- is also seen in chronic respiratory acidosis, but the blood pH distinguishes the two disorders.) This condition can be classified into two groups: saline-responsive and saline-unresponsive alkalosis.

Epidemiology

Most commonly occurs with the loss of gastric contents (hydrochloric acid) with vomiting or diuretic use.

Mineralocorticoid excess is less common; may occur with pyloric stenosis secondary to vomiting.

Etiology

Condition in which there exists an excessive plasma bicarbonate concentration in the body.

If the body does not excrete the excess bicarbonate and it is retained, some mechanism has abolished the kidney's normal bicarbonaturic response, and metabolic alkalosis ensues.

Physiology and Pathophysiology

Bicarbonate comes from exogenous sources or from loss of normally acidic fluid, gastric contents, or urine. Normal response to increased bicarbonate is to quantitatively excrete the excess bicarbonate. If bicarbonate is retained instead of excreted, the kidney's normal bicarbonaturic response is abolished. There are two types of metabolic alkalosis: saline-responsive alkalosis (a sign of extracellular volume contraction) and saline-unresponsive alkalosis (implying volume expansion). Saline-responsive is the most common of the two conditions; it presents with normotensive extracellular volume contraction and hypokalemia and is seen in cases of vomiting, nasogastric suctioning, and diuretic use. In cases of saline-unresponsive alkalosis there is an expansion of extracellular volume with hypertension; this may be seen with mineralocorticoid excess.

Clinical Manifestations

Subjective

History of self-induction of vomiting, diuretic use and abuse, or unusual ingestions

History of seizures, previous kidney dysfunction, gastrointestinal complaints

Muscle cramping/muscle weakness

Decreased cardiac output

Hypoventilation

Objective

Paresthesias (low "free" calcium levels, total normal)

Obtundation

Hypoventilation

Increased or decreased blood pressure

Positive Chvostek's and Trousseau's signs (severe alkalosis)

Signs of hypokalemia/potassium depletion

Lethargy

Confusion

Orthostatic hypotension

Differential Diagnosis

Bartter's syndrome (abnormal physical growth, mental retardation, chronic hypokalemia, alkalosis)

Magnesium depletion (decreased potassium level)

Cushing's syndrome (central obesity, round "moon face," supraclavicular fat pads, striae-covered fat pads on chest and abdomen, oligomenorrhea, edema, muscular atrophy)

Primary hyperaldosteronism (hypertension, alkalosis, muscular weakness, tetany, paresthesias, ventricular arrhythmias, nephropathy)

Malignant hypertension (diastolic pressure greater than 120, severe headaches, blurred vision, and confusion)

Diagnostic Tests

Arterial blood gases (increased HCO_3 level).

Venous pH (pH >7.4 may reveal a primary defect in alkalemia).

Tests to help determine the cause include serum electrolytes, magnesium, chemistry panel, renin, aldosterone, ACTH level.

Management/Treatment

Treatment is aimed at the underlying disorder and stabilizing the condition.

Correct fluid and electrolyte balance.

Severe or symptomatic alkalosis (pH >7.60) requires urgent care.

Saline-responsive alkalosis:

Treatment depends on severity, with possible addition of 0.9% NaCl and KCl.

Diuretics should be discontinued and pH and electrolytes should be stabilized.

Clients who show signs of marked renal insufficiency, may need dialysis.

Administering H_2-blockers in clients with alkalosis due to nasogastric suctioning may be helpful.

Saline-unresponsive alkalosis

Treatment may include removal of mineralocorticoid-producing tumor and treating patient with spironolactone to attempt to block the aldosterone effect.

For clients with primary aldosteronism in metabolic alkalosis, the treatment is potassium repletion.

Client Education
Correct medication administration
Side effects of medications

Follow-up
Dependent on client's therapy and response to therapy.

Referral
Refer to specialist as indicated.
Refer at-risk clients to home care.

REFERENCES

General
Dunphy, L.M., & Winland-Brown, J.E. (2001). *Primary care: The art and science of advanced practice nursing.* Philadelphia: F.A. Davis

Hoekelman, R., Adam, H., Nelson, N., Weitzman, M., & Wilson, M (2001). *Primary pediatric care.* (4th ed.). St. Louis: Mosby

Koda-Kimble, M., Young, L., Kradjan, W., & Guglielmo, B. (2002). *Applied therapeutics: The clinical use of drugs.* Philadelphia: Lippincott Williams & Wilkins

Noble, J., Greene, J. Levinson, W., Modest, G., Mulrow, C., Scherger, J., & Young, M.J. (2001). *Textbook of primary care.* St. Louis: Mosby.

Sperling, M. (1996). *Pediatric endocrinology.* Philadelphia: Saunders

Wilson, J.D. et al. (Eds.) (1998). *Williams textbook of endocrinology* (9th ed.). Philadelphia: Harcourt Health Sciences.

Wynne, A., Woo, T., & Millard, M (2002). *Pharmacotherapeutics for nurse practitioner prescribers.* Philadelphia: FA Davis/.

Diabetes
American Diabetes Association (2000). Clinical practice recommendations. *Diabetes Care, 23* (Supplement 1).

American Diabetes Association (1998): Clinical practice recommendations. Report of the Expert Committee on the Diagnosis and Classification of Diabetes Mellitus. *Diabetes Care, 21* (Supplement 1).

Consensus Guidelines (2000). *ISPAD Consensus guidelines for the management of type I diabetes mellitus in children and adolescents.* Zeist, The Netherlands: Ed. PGF Swift

Kelnar, C. (1995). *Childhood and adolescent diabetes.* New York: Chapman Hall, pp. 9–333.

Rosenbloom A.L., & Hanas R. (1996). Diabetic ketoacidosis (DKA): Treatment guidelines. *Clinical Pediatrics, 35,* 261–266.

Hirsutism
Lifshitz, F. (1996). *Pediatric endocrinology: Hirsutism and polycystic ovary syndrome* (3rd ed.). Brooklyn, NY: Marcel Dekker.

Odom, J.B. (2000) *Andrews' diseases of the skin: Clinical dermatology* (9th ed.). Philadelphia: Saunders, pp. 964–967

Hyperthyroidism and Hypothyroidism
Porterfield, S. (1997). Endocrine physiology (2nd ed.) St. Louis: Mosby, pp. 57–79.

Metabolic Acidosis and Metabolic Alkalosis

Cogan, M. (1991). *Fluid and electrolytes: Physiology and pathophysiology.* Englewood Cliffs, NJ: Appleton and Lange, pp. 203–240.

Finberg, L., Kravath, R.E,. & Hellerstein, S. (1993). *Water and electrolytes in pediatrics: Physiology, pathology, and treatment* (2nd ed.) Philadelphia: Saunders, pp. 179–234.

Tierney, L. (2000). *Current diagnosis and treatment* (39th ed.). New York: Lang Medical/McGraw Hill.

Resources

American Association of Clinical Endocrinologists
www.aace.com

American Association of Diabetes Educators
aade@aadenet.org

American Dietetic Association
www.eatright.org

Barbara Davis Center for Childhood Diabetes at the University of Colorado Health Sciences Center
www.uchsc.edu/misc/diabetes/bdc.html

Juvenile Diabetes Foundation
www.jdfcure.com

Chapter 11

MUSCULOSKELETAL SYSTEM

CARPAL TUNNEL SYNDROME

SIGNAL SYMPTOMS ▶ paresthesia in first three digits

ICD-9 Code	354.0	Carpal tunnel syndrome

Carpal tunnel syndrome is a compressive neuropathy in which the median nerve is constricted by narrowing of the carpal tunnel at the wrist. The resulting entrapment of the median nerve causes motor and sensory deficits in the portion of the hand innervated by the median nerve. Occasionally tendons within the carpal tunnel may also be entrapped, which impairs flexion of the fingers.

Epidemiology

Occurs more often in women than in men.

Occurs at any age, but commonly in adults aged 40–60 years.

Etiology

Most commonly due to repetitive motion or long-term malpositioning.

Other conditions that can cause narrowing of the carpal tunnel include:

Swelling from a Colles fracture of the distal end of the radius

Dislocation of the lunate

Wrist sprains or strains

Pregnancy

Tumor

Hypothyroidism

Diabetes

Congestive heart failure

Renal failure

Systemic conditions such as arthritis or Paget's disease of the bone

Physiology and Pathophysiology

Carpal tunnel syndrome occurs as the carpal tunnel is compressed. The carpal tunnel is formed by the carpal bones and the transverse carpal ligament. Nine tendons and the median nerve run through this fairly rigid structure. Any inflammation, as well as increased exercise or a firm gripping motion, increases pressure within the carpal tunnel. The increased pressure causes mechanical stress that can result in focal demyelination and ischemia of the median nerve.

Clinical Manifestations

Subjective

Paresthesias in the first three and one-half digits (often involves only the first two fingers), may be relieved by shaking the hands.

Night awakening with burning pain or numbness in all or part of median nerve distribution.

Report of pain radiating up the forearm.

Report of weakness.

Objective

Atrophy of thenar muscle in longstanding condition

Tinel's sign (tapping over the median nerve produces tingling)

Phalen's sign (symptoms are reproduced after 1 minute of unforced wrist flexion)

May be weakness in the affected portion of the hand

Differential Diagnosis

Diabetic neuropathy (occurs only with diabetes; most common type occurs in stocking–glove distribution.)

Compression of the median nerve in the proximal or distal forearm (paresthesia in upper and/or lower arm, as well as in the first three and one-half digits)

Tumors (persistent swelling, pain in the bone that impairs sleep, imaging studies revealing the lesion; systemic signs are also present in Ewing's sarcoma or metastatic disease)

Arthritis (pain and swelling rather than paresthesia are the primary symptoms)

Cervical radiculopathy (paresthesia over dermatome supplied by involved nerve)

Vascular occlusion (cool and/or mottled skin)

Reflex sympathetic dystrophy (swelling, burning pain, sensitivity to light touch, dry, glossy skin)

Diagnostic Tests

Wrist x-ray examination (to rule out injury, joint changes, or tumors).

Nerve-conduction studies (to assess for impaired nerve conduction).

Cervical spine and chest x-ray examination (to assess for thoracic-outlet syndromes and pathologic changes in the cervical spine).

If systemic condition is suspected, specific relevant tests should be performed.

Management/Treatment

Pharmacologic Management

Nonsteroidal antiinflammatory drugs (NSAIDs): Opinion differ on the best initial choice. One useful strategy is to begin with a drug from the propionic acid class that has a low rate of side effects. If the initial drug is ineffective, select a drug from another class. Cox II inhibitors have the lowest incidence of adverse gastrointestinal effects. However, they are quite expensive and may offer little advantage over other NSAIDS in persons at low risk for gastrointestinal complications (Table 11–1).

Table 11–1   Treatment: Non-Steroidal Anti-Inflammatory Drugs

Drug Class/ Name	Dosage	Risk Profile	Dosage Forms (mg)
Salicylates			
Aspirin (Ecotrin, ASA, Empirin, Bayer)	325–650 mg PO/PR Q 4–6 H	High risk of GI side effects (gastritis) Low risk of BP elevation	Tablets: 81, 325, 500, 650, 975 Suppository:. 120, 200, 300, 600
Salsalate (Saliflex, Disalcid)	3000 mg/day divided doses Q 8–12 H	*	Tablets: 500, 750
Difunisal (DoloBID)	500–1000 mg initially, then 250–500 mg PO Q 8–12 H	*	Tablets: 250, 500
Propionic Acids			
Flurbiprofen (Ansaid)	200–300 mg/day, divided doses BID/TID/QID	*	Tablets: 50, 100
Ibuprofen (Motrin, Advil, Nuprin, Rufen)	200–800 mg PO TID-QID	Small to moderate risk of BP elevation	Tablets: 100, 200, 300, 400, 600, 800
Ketoprofen (Orudis, Actron)	25–75mg PO TID/QID	*	Tablets: 12.5, 25, 50, 75
Naproxen (Naprosyn)	250–500 mg PO BID	High risk for BP elevation.	Tablets: 200, 250, 375, 500
(Anaprox)	275–550 mg PO BID	High risk for BP elevation	Tablets: 275, 550
(Naprelan)	750–1000 mg PO QD	High risk for BP elevation	Tablets: 375, 500 controlled release
(EC Naprosyn)	375–500 mg PO BID	High risk for BP elevation	Tablets: 375, 500 delayed release
Oxaprozin (Daypro)	1200 mg PO QD	*	Tablets: 600
Acetic Acids			
Diclofenac (Voltaren, Cataflam)	50 mg PO BID/TID	*	Tablets: 50
(Voltaren XR)	100 mg PO QD/BID	*	Tablets: 100
(Voltaren)	75mg PO BID	*	Tablets: 25, 50, 75
Etodolac (Lodine)	200–400 mg PO BID/TID	*	Tablets: 200, 300, 400, 500
(Lodine XL)	400–1200 mg PO QD	*	Tablets: 400, 500, 600 extended release
Indomethacin (Indocin)	25–50 mg PO/PR TID	High risk for BP elevation	Caplets: 25, 50 Suppository: 50

Table continued on following page.

Table 11–1 Treatment: Non-Steroidal Anti-Inflammatory Drugs (Continued)

Drug Class/ Name	Dosage	Risk Profile	Dosage Forms (mg)
Salicylates			
(Indocin SR)	75mg PO QD/BID	High risk for BP elevation	Tablets: 75
Ketorlac (Toradol)	10 mg PO Q 4–6H PRN up to 5 days total duration	High risk for GI side effects.	Tablets: 10
Sulindac (Clinoril)	150–200 mg PO BID	Low risk of BP elevation	Tablets: 150, 200
Nabumatone (Relafen)	1000 mg PO QD/BID	*	Tablets: 500, 750
Tolmetin (Tolectin)	200–600 mg PO TID	*	Tablets: 200, 400, 600
Fenamates			
Meclofenamate (Meclomen)	50–100 mg PO TID/QID	*	Tablets: 50, 100
Oxicams			
Piroxicam (Feldene)	20 mg PO QD	Medium to high risk of BP elevation	Tablets: 10, 20
COX-2 Inhibitors			
Celecoxib (Celebrex)	200 mg PO QD or 100 mg PO BID, RA: 200 mg PO QD or BID	Fewer GI side effects than other NSAIDS Mild to severe effects on BP reported	Tablets: 100, 200
Rofecoxib (Vioxx)	OA: 12.5–25mg PO QD, Acute pain or dysmenorrhea: 50 mg PO QD	Fewer GI side effects than other NSAIDS Mild to severe effects on BP reported	Tablets: 12.5, 25

BP = blood pressure; GI = gastrointestinal.
*All NSAIDS have the potential to cause GI side effects and loss of hypertensive control. For some NSAIDS the magnitude of these effects has not been explored in comparison studies. All NSAIDS should be used with extreme caution in clients who are taking angiotensin-converting–enzyme inhibitors since losss of hypertensive control is common and the potential for hyperkalemia is increased.

Oral prednisolone, 20 mg daily for 2 weeks, followed by 10 mg daily for 2 weeks, may relieve symptoms in some cases.

Consider consultation or referral for injection of methylprednisolone either into the carpal tunnel or proximal to it. Injection proximal to the carpal tunnel is safer, easier to administer, and may have longer efficacy.

Nonpharmacologic Management

Splint wrist in extension. Some sources recommend splinting in neutral position rather than in extension.

Modify work environment or activities involving repetitive motion.

Ultrasound therapy.

Complementary/Alternative Therapies

Hatha Yoga (controversial)

Box 11–1
Hatha Yoga for the Treatment of Carpal Tunnel Syndrome

Hatha Yoga is a practice of controlled breathing and meditation. It is based on a belief that the body contains many channels in which the life-energy current moves. Through breathing and meditation, creative energy is thought to rise up through the lower energy centers or "chakras" to the higher chakras. Hatha Yoga involves practice in purification, "asanas" (postures for strength and flexibility), breathing exercises, "mudras" (postures designed to seal the air within the body), and samadhi, (the state of spiritual bliss and union with God).

Hatha Yoga, particularly the asanas, may be a beneficial adjunct in the treatment of many medical conditions such as arthritis, asthma, backaches, constipation, diabetes, endometriosis, menopause, multiple sclerosis, sciatica, and varicose veins. The breathing and relaxation practices may be a beneficial adjunct in the control of high blood pressure, hypercholesterolemia, migraine headaches, and other stress-related symptoms.

Client Education

Protective measures, including modification of repetitive wrist maneuvers and periodic breaks from work or recreation involving repetitive movement.

Wearing wrist brace during activity requiring repetitive wrist motion.

Follow-up

Every 2–3 weeks during treatment

Referral

Surgery, or orthopedics if client fails to respond to conservative therapy or if symptoms become more severe.

CHRONIC PAIN

ICD-9 Code	780.9	Generalized pain
		Other specific codes depend on the site of the pain.
		Chronic pain is pain that lasts longer than 6 months.

Epidemiology

Distribution within the population varies with the cause of the pain.
May occur at any age.

Etiology

Chronic pain may be caused by ongoing physical damage to tissue, damage to sensory nerves, prolonged activation of the sympathetic nervous system, or psychological factors. Often several of these factors, and possibly others, contribute to the phenomenon of chronic pain.

Pain is interpreted, and a response is generated, in the brain. Multiple factors influence this process, including the extent of physical damage, fatigue, anxiety or depression, past experience with pain, learned responses influenced by culture, age, and gender, and even mental constructs such as the expectation of relief.

Common musculoskeletal causes of chronic pain include:

Repetitive motion disorders
Osteoarthritis
Rheumatoid arthritis
Lumbosacral strain
Cervical strain
Tendinitis/bursitis

Physiology and Pathophysiology

Pain is a complex phenomenon that involves: (a) perception of potentially painful stimuli by pain receptors, (b) conduction of the impulses generated by these receptors to the spinal cord and brain, (c) processing and interpretation of the stimuli at several levels of the spinal cord and brain, and (d) generation of a reaction to the stimuli.

Intense, potentially painful stimuli are received and transmitted to the spinal cord by A-delta and C fibers (the primary afferent nociceptors). A-delta fibers are myelinated, allowing for rapid conduction of painful stimuli, whereas C fibers are unmyelinated and conduct impulses more slowly.

When an impulse reaches the spinal cord, it enters the dorsal horn and is transmitted toward the brain along several pathways (tracts). As the impulse ascends, it passes through the substantia gelatinosa, which is postulated to be the site of the gating process described in the gate control theory. Most pain impulses are transmitted along the spinothalamic tract to the thalamus, the somatosensory cortex, and portions of the cortex associated with emotional responses.

Pain may be modulated (increased or decreased) at several levels. The dorsal horn of the spinal cord, the hypothalamus–midbrain–medula circuit, and the proinflammatory polypeptides produced by nociceptors have all been implicated in pain modulation.

Chronic pain is less well understood than acute pain. Recent animal studies suggest that there may be a central neural plasticity within the dorsal horn, sensory thalamus, and cerebral cortex in response to injury. In some instances a peripheral injury may induce changes in both the structure and function of the central nervous system. These changes result in central nervous system sending messages that produce hyperalgesia, allodynia, and an expanded field of pain long after the original injury has healed. It is not clear why this phenomenon occurs in some situations and not in others.

Clinical Manifestations

Client's report of pain.
May be accompanied by depression or anxiety.
Specific manifestations depend on the cause and site of the pain.

Differential Diagnosis

Depends on the site and characteristics of the pain

Diagnostic Tests

Depends on the cause of the pain

Management/Treatment

Pharmacologic Management

Depends on the cause of the pain. Chronic pain is best managed by an interdisciplinary team and should be individualized based on the site and type of pain as well as on individual pain responses.

Intermittent pain occurring less than 4 days each week may be managed with:

Acetaminophen (Tylenol), 325 mg, two tablets PO Q4H PRN pain
NSAIDs (see Table 11–1)

(Chronic, especially daily, use of acetaminophen or NSAIDs has been associated with renal disease, hepatotoxicity, or coagulopathy. All NSAIDs have the potential to cause ulcers, sometimes very quickly.)

Tramadol (Ultram), 50–100 mg PO Q4–6H PRN pain; maximum of 400 mg/day. **Caution: This drug has many interactions (including with alcohol). It must not be used with cyclobenzaprine (Flexeril) or with antidepressants because it may cause seizures.**

If acetaminophen and NSAIDs are ineffective or contraindicated, short-acting opioids or combination products may be considered (codeine up to 60 mg PO Q4–6H PRN).

Hydrocodone/acetaminophen 5/500 (Lorcet, Vicodin), one to two tablets PO Q4–6H PRN pain; oxycodone/acetaminophen 5/325 or 5/500 (Percocet, Roxicet), one PO Q4–6H PRN pain. (In some states nurse practitioners cannot prescribe controlled substances.)

Frequent or constant pain, especially neuropathic pain may be most effectively treated with:

Amitriptyline (Elavil)—Start with 25 mg PO HS and increase gradually to effective dose, usually between 75 and 200 mg/day.

Sertraline (Zoloft)—Start with 25–50 mg PO daily and increase gradually to effective dose up to 150 mg/day.

Paroxetine (Paxil)—30–70 mg PO daily.

Carbamazepine (Tegretol)—Start with 100 mg PO BID and increase by 100 mg Q12H until pain is controlled. Maximum dose is 1200 mg/day; maintenance dose is 20–400 mg BID. (Must perform CBC and liver-function tests initially and periodically thereafter.)

Gabapentin (Neurontin)—300–1200 mg PO TID. Relief is usually obtained at a daily dosage at or below 1800 mg/day. If no relief is noted at this dosage it is unlikely that higher doses will be effective.

Medications that are less effective for the primary treatment of neuropathic pain may be useful adjuncts to antidepressant and/or antiepileptic therapy. These medications include:

Capsaicin cream (Zostrix), 0.075%—Apply to affected area QID. **Caution: May cause burns, especially in elderly or debilitated persons and persons with neuropathy.**

Mexiletene (Mexitil), 675 mg daily.

Long-acting opioids—Thought to be less likely to build up tolerance than short-acting opioids. Opioids are seldom considered the best option in managing chronic musculoskeletal pain. Nurse practitioners in some states cannot prescribe controlled substances.

Morphine controlled release (MS Contin, Roxanol), 90–120 mg Q12H.

Fentanyl transdermal patches, 25–100 μg/hour. Apply patch Q72H. Do not use above 25 μg/hour in clients who have never taken opiates.

Oxycodone controlled release (OxyContin), 10–40 mg PO Q12H.

Nonpharmacologic Management

Depends on the cause of the pain

Commonly used methods include:

    Transcutaneous electrical nerve stimulation unit (TENS)

    Physical therapy for reconditioning

    Occupational therapy for body mechanics

    Ultrasonography

    Cognitive and behavioral therapy

    Stress management

Complementary/Alternative Therapies

A number of complementary therapies may be useful in the management of chronic pain; selection should be based on the cause and the site of the pain.

Yoga

Massage

Acupuncture

Acupressure

Relaxation therapy

Biofeedback

 CP 11–1 Clinical Pearl: Complementary methods for chronic pain may be paid for by medical insurance.

Client Education

Cause of pain if known

Management strategies

Avoid nicotine (increases pain awareness and decreases plasma levels of antidepressants)

Weight loss strategies, if indicated

Follow-up

Depends on the cause of the pain; In general, clients may initially benefit from follow-up appointments every 1 to 2 weeks. After a degree of pain control is achieved, appointments can be scheduled less frequently.

Referral

Depends on the cause of the pain.
Referral to a pain management center may be beneficial.

DEGENERATIVE JOINT DISEASE (Osteoarthritis)

SIGNAL SYMPTOMS pain with movement, stiffness after rest

ICD-9 Codes	715.0	Osteoarthritis, generalized
	715.1	Osteoarthritis, localized primary
	715.2	Osteoarthritis, localized secondary
	715.9	Osteoarthritis, unspecified whether generalized or localized

Degenerative joint disease (osteoarthritis) is a chronic disease in which there is deterioration of articular cartilage accompanied by bony overgrowth. Although the distinction is often blurred, osteoarthritis is sometimes classified as primary or secondary. In primary disease there is no identifiable underlying cause. In secondary disease there is an identifiable predisposing condition such as trauma, systemic disease, or joint abnormalities.

Epidemiology

At least 2% of the population; although many are asymptomatic, 85%–90% of persons over age 40 show evidence of osteoarthritic changes on autopsy.
More common in women.
Prevalence increases with age.

Etiology

A number of factors seem to influence the development of osteoarthritis including:

Genetic predisposition
Increasing age
Obesity
Previous trauma
Limb deformity or malalignment
Metabolic disorders
Inflammatory or infectious conditions affecting joints

Physiology and Pathophysiology

Articular cartilage is composed of a matrix of proteoglycans, type II collagen fibers, chondrocytes, and water. Over time, proteoglycan levels in the matrix fall and water content increases. This change in composition causes cartilage to stiffen and break down, exposing underlying bone to increased mechanical stress generated by bone-against-bone movement within the joint. Ongoing tissue injury induces a low-level inflammatory response in which cytokines and other inflammatory products cause further breakdown of cartilage. These changes within the joint produce microfractures, pain, and bone hypertrophy.

Clinical Manifestations

Subjective
Pain on movement of involved joint
Joint stiffness after rest that resolves with activity, usually within 1 hour

Objective
Joint tenderness on palpation
Pain and crepitus on passive movement of involved joint
Heberden's nodes: nodular swelling on dorsal aspect of interphalangeal joints
Bouchard's node: nodular swelling on dorsal aspect of proximal interphalangeal joints
Often unilateral joint involvement

Differential Diagnosis
Other arthritides (laboratory studies and analysis of synovial fluid consistent with crystal-induced or immune-mediated arthritis)
Osteoporosis (decreased bone density)
Bone tumors (persistent swelling, bone pain that impairs sleep, imaging studies revealing the lesion, and, in Ewing's sarcoma or metastatic disease, systemic symptoms)
Multiple myeloma (diffuse bone lesions on radiography)
Hemochromatosis (serum ferritin $>200\mu$g/L in menstruating women or 400 μg/L in postmenopausal women and men; gold standard is liver biopsy demonstrating hepatic iron concentration of 200–800 μmol/g dry weight)

Diagnostic Tests
Routine laboratory chemistry panel (to rule out other diagnoses)
CBC and liver- and renal-function tests (obtain prior to long-term analgesic or NSAID therapy to rule out anemia and liver- or renal-function changes)
X-ray examination of affected joints (may show the classic changes in osteoarthritis: narrowing of the joint space, osteophyte formation, subchondral sclerosis, and periarticular bone cysts.

Management/Treatment

Pharmacologic Management
Acetaminophen (Tylenol), 325 mg, two tablets Q4H PRN.
NSAIDs—Begin therapy with an NSAID that has a low side-effect profile, at the lowest effective dose. If initial dose is ineffective, increase dose incrementally until full antiinflammatory dose is reached. If full antiinflammatory dose of

initial NSAID is ineffective, consider changing to NSAID in another group. Check blood pressure and renal function 7–10 days after beginning NSAID therapy. Loss of hypertensive control is common.

Cox II inhibitors (rofecoxib [Vioxx], celecoxib [Celebrex]) or misoprostol (Cytotec) (provides gastric protection)—If client has a high risk for ulcer 100 μg PO BID. **Caution: Do not use misoprostol in pregnancy.**

Capsaicin 0.025% (Capsaicin-P)—Apply to affected areas three to four times daily; can cause burns, especially if a warm pack or heating pad is used concurrently; use with caution for elderly or debilitated clients and for persons with sensory deficits.

Corticosteroid: Intraarticular injection.

Hyaluronate sodium (Hyalgan) or Hylan G-F20 (Synvisc)—Intraarticular injections.

Nonpharmacologic Management

Weight reduction, if weight-bearing joints are involved.

Joint protection with use of cane and/or use of shock-absorbing insoles.

Exercise program to strengthen muscles that support affected joints.

Low-impact aerobic exercise.

Hydrotherapy.

Physical therapy, including application of heat and massage.

Joint aspiration to decrease effusion, if indicated.

Arthroscopic surgery or joint replacement may be beneficial if there is significant disability.

Complementary/Alternative Therapies

Acupuncture.

Acupressure.

Massage.

Glucosamine sulfate and chondroitin sulfate have been widely advertised as a cure for arthritis. While some trials lend support to their possible usefulness in relieving symptoms of osteoarthritis, the results remain controversial.

Client Education

Course of disease, treatment

Follow-up

Return visit 1–2 weeks after initiating NSAID therapy.

Monthly follow-up by telephone may promote good clinical outcome.

Referral

Refer to orthopedist if there is an inadequate response to NSAIDs and conservative nonpharmacologic therapies after 2 months.

 RF 11–1   Red Flag: If there is pain at rest refer client to orthopedist for possible fracture, tumor, or infection.

Refer to surgeon for possible joint replacement if there is significant functional impairment.

FRACTURES

ICD-9 Code	829	Fracture of unspecified bone
		Other specific codes depend on the site and characteristics of fracture.

A fracture is a disruption of the continuity of a bone. Fractures are classified according to:

Location: Bone, part of bone, intraarticular or extraarticlular.

Pattern: Direction and description of the fracture line.

Simple: Broken in two pieces. May be transverse, oblique, spiral or vertical.

Comminuted: Broken into more than two pieces.

Compound: A portion of the fractured bone penetrates the skin or an organ.

Deformity: Displacement of the fracture.

Translation: Front-to-back or side-to-side displacement of fracture surfaces; described as anterior, posterior, lateral, or medial translation.

Angulation: Description of the angle formed by the fracture—e.g., apex posterior

Rotated: Rotary displacement of a fracture fragment.

Impacted: One fracture fragment is wedged into another.

Type: Description of the process leading to fracture—e.g., traumatic, stress, pathologic.

Epidemiology

Common sports injury

More common after bone maturity

Etiology

Commonly caused by trauma.

May also occur with little or no trauma in conditions that produce osteopenia, such as osteoporosis, osteomalacia, or osteogenesis imperfecta.

Physiology and Pathophysiology

Fractures occur when forces applied to the bone exceed the strength of the bone. This is true whether the fracture is traumatic, in which case the force applied to the bone is greater than the normal strength of the bone, or pathologic, in which case the bone is weakened and unable to bear normal forces. Conditions that produce osteopenia, such as osteoporosis, oseomalacia, or osteogenesis imperfecta result in a susceptibility to pathologic fractures.

Clinical Manifestations

Subjective

History of trauma (usually).

Pain.

Client may also report numbness, tingling, and/or loss of function of the involved body part.

Objective

Tenderness

Swelling

Contusion (not always seen)

Deformity (not always seen)

Impaired sensation and/or signs of impaired circulation

Differential Diagnosis

Infection (elevated erythrocyte sedimentation rate [ESR] and white cells [WBCs], fever)

Tumor (persistent swelling, pain in bone that impairs sleep, imaging studies revealing the lesion, and in Ewing's sarcoma or metastatic disease, systemic signs)

Sprain or strain (no bone disruption on x-ray examination)

Tendinitis and/or bursitis (no bone disruption on x-ray examination)

Diagnostic Tests

Laboratory tests are rarely indicated except when there is concern that the fracture is secondary to another condition.

Plain x-ray examination of the affected site; if fracture is strongly suspected but plain x-ray examination fails to demonstrate a defect, consider computed tomography (CT) or magnetic resonance imaging (MRI). (See Box 11–5 for the Ottawa Rules for ankle imaging .)

Management/Treatment

Pharmacologic Management

Narcotic or nonnarcotic analgesic.

Consider NSAIDs after any initial bleeding has subsided (24–36 hours). Ibuprofen, 600 mg Q6H is a rational choice for many clients, but the choice of an NSAID should always be based on the patient's history and the side-effect profile of each NSAID.

Nonpharmacologic Management

Reduction of the fracture.

Immobilization.

Box 11–2
Approach to Diagnosis of Stress Fracture

The typical client with a suspected stress fracture is an athlete or a person who has recently dramatically increased his or her activity level who presents with chronic pain that is worse with activity and is relieved by rest. Often the pain worsens over time. The client has no palpable mass or systemic signs. The first diagnostic strategy should be a plain x-ray examination. Stress fractures are indicated by a horizontal band of sclerosis and a periosteal reaction. If the stress fracture is not evident on plain radiography but clinical suspicion is high, a CT or MRI scan should be done. Although it is more expensive, MRI is the preferred imaging study in this situation because it reveals soft-tissue distortion more clearly.

Elevation for the first 48–72 hours.

Cold packs during first few days—Never use cold packs for more than 20 minutes an hour. Some sources suggest maximum benefit is obtained from 20 minutes Q4–6H.

Sling for upper extremity fracture.

Mobilize joints as soon as possible.

Physical therapy for rehabilitation as needed.

Complementary/Alternative Therapies

Relaxation methods, guided imagery, music therapy, meditation, others as adjunct for pain relief.

Client Education

Cast or splint care: Keep cast clean and dry. Do not put anything in the cast. Protect cast from trauma. Promptly report any foul odor or signs of vascular or nerve compression to health-care provider. Remove splint only as instructed.

Signs of vascular or nerve compression: Numbness, increased pain, cyanosis, increased swelling, coolness of skin distal to cast.

Elevate extremity and use cold packs as directed.

Medications and side effects.

Follow-up.

Follow-up

Depends on the fracture

Referral

Refer to orthopedist for all open (compound), displaced, and unstable fractures and fractures with evidence of nerve, muscle, or vascular damage. Make a referral for fractures in sites that have a high incidence of nonunion (distal tibial diaphysis, carpal navicular [scaphoid], and proximal diaphysis of fifth metatarsal.

GOUT

SIGNAL SYMPTOMS ▶ red, swollen, tender joint

ICD-9 Codes	274.0	Gouty arthropathy
	274.9	Gout unspecified

Gout is a crystal-induced arthritis in which monosodium urate crystals accumulate in tissues, including bones, joints, and subcutaneous tissue. Hyperuricemia precedes gout, but gout does not develop in all persons with hyperuricemia. Gout may be classified as primary (idiopathic) or secondary (related to an identified cause).

Epidemiology

The incidence in men is greater than that in women (5.0–6.6/1000 men; 1.0–3.0/1000 women).

Most commonly begins in middle age (30–50 years); uncommon under age 30.

Etiology

Develops because of an overproduction of uric acid, a reduction in the excretion of uric acid, or both.

Physiology and Pathophysiology

Uric acid is a by-product of purine metabolism. When uric acid accumulates, from overproduction or from impaired excretion, a supersaturated level (>0.42 mmol/L) of sodium urate in body fluids may lead to precipitation of crystals. Because urate crystals form very slowly and are coated with apolipoprotein, they may not initially induce the inflammatory response. Ultimately, however, the interaction of immunoglobulin G with urate crystals activates neutrophils and monocytes. These leukocytes phagocytose the urate crystals and release inflammatory mediators that produce pain, erythema, and swelling. Secondary gout may arise in connection with diabetes, hypertension, renal insufficiency, alcohol abuse, or the use of diuretics, salicylate, or cyclosporine.

Clinical Manifestations

Subjective

Painful joint.

Attacks may be precipitated by stress, illness, surgery.

Objective

Red, swollen, very tender joint.

Usually affects only one joint; often the initial attack involves the metatarsophalangeal joint of the great toe.

May be accompanied by fever.

Tophi: Deposits of urate crystals in subcutaneous tissue (deposits form in men with longstanding disease, but tophi may develop early in women with the disease).

Differential Diagnosis

Pseudogout (calcium pyrophosphate dihydrate crystals in aspirated synovial fluid)

Cellulitis (increased WBCs; elevation to 15,000/ml may occasionally be seen in gout; no crystals in joint aspirate)

Bursitis (no crystals in joint aspirate, pain with direct pressure on bursa)

Other arthritides (laboratory studies, radiographs, and analysis of synovial fluid consistent with osteoarthritis or immune-mediated arthritis)

Hyperparathyroidism (hypercalcemia)

Diagnostic Tests

Synovial fluid aspirate for urate crystals (gold standard for diagnosis of gout)

Serum uric acid (elevated in gout)

ESR (elevation indicates an inflammatory process; elevation seen during episodes of acute gout)

24-hour urinary uric acid excretion (elevated in gout associated with overproduction of uric acid)

CBC (to rule out infection)

Rheumatoid factor titers (to rule out other arthritides)

X-ray examination (may be done to rule out other possible diagnoses)

Management/Treatment

Pharmacologic Management

ACUTE ATTACK

NSAIDs; avoid aspirin. Traditionally, indomethacin, 150 mg PO initially, then 50 mg PO Q8H until pain is relieved, but a lower dose of indomethacin or another NSAID (e.g., ibuprofen) may be better tolerated.

Colchicine, 1.0–1.2 mg PO initially, then 0.5–1.2 mg PO Q12H until pain is relieved or unacceptable side effects occur.

Corticosteroid therapy: Either triamcinolone, 60 mg IM, or prednisone, starting with 20–50 mg PO daily and tapering.

CHRONIC DISEASE

Wait at least 2 weeks after resolution of the acute attack before beginning therapy for chronic disease.

Allopurinol (Zyloprim): Use for overproduction of uric acid—24-hour uric acid output of >900 mg/day; with 100 mg/day PO; may titrate up to 300 mg/day. Also use NSAID or colchicine, 0.6 mg PO BID, for first few months of allopurinol therapy. Allopurinol has many undesirable side effects. It should be avoided in clients with renal insufficiency and used only for persons who have frequent acute episodes or have chronic tophi and associated symptomatic episodes.

Probenecid (Benemid): Use for impaired renal clearance of uric acid; 250 mg PO BID for 1 week, then 500 mg PO BID.

Nonpharmacologic Management

Rest joint.

Elevation.

Avoid high-purine foods (liver and other organ meats, spinach, mushrooms, cocoa, asparagus, oatmeal).

Limit alcohol consumption.

Increase fluids.

Complementary/Alternative Therapies

Relaxation modalities (guided imagery, music therapy, meditation, etc.) as adjunct for pain relief.

Client Education

Disease process

Diet modifications

Medications and side effects

Follow-up

See client in 24 hours to assess pain relief.

Return appointment in 1 month to evaluate need for prophylactic therapy.

Referral

Refer to orthopedist if there is evidence of joint destruction.

LUMBOSACRAL STRAIN (Low Back Pain)

ICD-9 Codes	724.5	Back pain (postural)
	724.2	Low back pain
	724.8	Stiff back
	847.9	Back strain

Lumbosacral strain (low back pain) is trauma to the muscles and tendons of the lower back. Many conditions may cause low back pain, including disk herniation, infection, malignancies, arthritides, fractures, and neurologic conditions.

Epidemiology

Extremely common; as many as 90% of American adults experience low back pain at some point.

Low back pain is the fifth most common symptom among persons who seek medical care.

Incidence greater in men than in women.

Occurs primarily in adults but can occur at any age.

Prevalence varies from 7.6%–37%.

Etiology

Generally occurs with unaccustomed physical effort, often involving lifting, pulling, or pushing.

Physiology and Pathophysiology

Excessive stress on the musculotendinous units in the lower back results in overstretching or tearing the involved muscles and/or tendons.

Clinical Manifestations

Subjective

Aching pain in the back, buttocks, and sometimes thighs.

Occurs after overexertion.

Pain is relieved by lying still and worsened with movement.

Objective

There may be paravertebral tenderness and tightness of muscles in the lower back

Positive straight-leg raising—Radicular pain extending below the knee when leg is raised between 30 and 70 degrees is found in herniated nucleus pulposus.

Decreased spinal range of motion, possibly with pain.

Pain with heel and toe walking may be present.

Differential Diagnosis

Herniated intervertebral disk (herniated nucleus pulposus) (paresthesia in leg, sciatica—pain that radiates below the knee along the back of the leg, pain increased with sitting and decreased with standing, positive straight leg test, pain may be increased with sitting or cough) (See Box 11–3.)

Fracture (usually a history of trauma, tenderness over spinous process)

Malignancy (progressive aching pain at rest, pain increased with supine position or cough, history of prior malignancy)

Abdominal aortic aneurysm (pulsatile abdominal mass)

Referred abdominal pain (primarily abdominal symptoms)

Infection (fever, abnormal laboratory results—e.g., elevated ESR and/or WBCs, pain with percussion of vertebral bodies)

Osteoarthritis (ache or shooting pain that increases when walking up an incline, pain decreased with sitting)

Spinal stenosis (pseudoclaudication, pain increases during the day)

Ankylosing spondylitis (tenderness over sacroiliac joints, progressive, morning stiffness)

Diagnostic Tests

Generally none are indicated. May consider ESR, CBC, purified protein derivative if malignancy or infection is suspected.

Plain x-ray examination is usually not useful.

MRI best for soft-tissue findings; indicated if infection or neoplasm is suspected or if considering referral for surgery.

Box 11–3
Differentiating between Lumbar Strain and Herniated Nucleus Pulposus

Lumbosacral strain is characterized by dull pain that may be referred to the buttock and posterior thigh. Muscle tenderness and stiffness are the primary findings on physical examination.

Herniated nucleus pulposus (HNP) classically occurs in young adults. It is rare after age 50 because the nucleus pulposus becomes less gelatinous with increasing age. Typically the client with HNP will report sharp pain that may have begun suddenly after unaccustomed activity or may have worsened gradually or occurred intermittently for some time. Patients who have a sudden onset sometimes will report a tearing sensation at the time of injury. Eventually, sciatica, a shooting or shocklike pain that radiates down the posterior leg to below the knee, develops. The physical examination demonstrates decreased range of motion with forward bending and motor, sensory, or reflex changes along a specific nerve root. The straight-leg raise, in which the client rests in the supine position with legs straight and the examiner elevates the leg to 70 degrees, is positive, eliciting radicular pain extending down the back of the leg to below the knee. The sensitivity of a positive straight-leg test for HNP is around 80%. A crossed straight-leg test, in which there is radicular pain extending down the back of the affected leg to below the knee when the unaffected leg is raised, may also be positive. The crossed straight-leg test has poor sensitivity but high specificity for HNP.

CT best for viewing cortical bone; less expensive than MRI.
May consider bone scan.

Management/Treatment

Pharmacologic Management
NSAIDs (see Table 11–1)

Muscle relaxants:

    Cyclobenzaprine (Flexeril), 10 mg PO Q8H or at night only. Do not use with tramadol (Ultram).

    Metaxalone (Skelaxin), 800 mg PO Q8H or at night only

    Carisopradol (Soma), 350 mg PO TID or QID with meals and HS (controlled substance)

Narcotics may be helpful initially for acute pain, but are not a mainstay for treatment of low back pain.

Nonpharmacologic Management
Bedrest for up to 2 days may be beneficial if there is acute radiculopathy.

Modify activities to prevent re-injury.

Warm and cold packs.

Exercise program to promote weight loss, if overweight.

Strengthening and stretching exercises for the lower back. Many excellent brochures describing exercises to increase the flexibility and strength of the lower back are available commercially. One good resource is *Griffith's Instructions for Patients* (Moore, 1998). The copyright page includes a statement that material from this book may be copied and distributed to patients for instructional purposes.

Some exercises that the nurse practitioner may wish to recommend include:

    Pelvic tilt: Lie on back with knees bent. Feet should be flat against the floor or mat and arms should be relaxed at sides. Use abdominal muscles to push the small of the back flat against the floor. Hold for 10–60 seconds and release. Repeat several times as tolerated.

    Belly breathing: Lie on back with lower legs supported on a chair or pillows. Exhale, pushing abdomen toward spine. Hold for several seconds and relax abdomen while inhaling. Repeat several times as tolerated.

    Knee to chest: Lie on back with knees bent. Tighten abdomen and pull right knee toward chest while exhaling. Hold for several seconds then return leg to starting position while inhaling. Repeat several times as tolerated. Repeat exercise with left knee.

Complementary/Alternative Therapies
Acupuncture.

Massage.

Relaxation methods.

Chiropractic manipulation; consider only for lumbar strain. If other pathology is suspected, do not recommend chiropractic until other causes of low back pain have been ruled out.

Client Education

Usual course of recovery

Medications and side effects

Nonpharmacologic treatment methods

Back exercises

Ergonomics

Encourage maintenance of normal weight

Follow-up

Reevaluate in 24 hours if pain is severe or unrelieved or if new symptoms develop.

Reevaluate in 1 week if pain is mild to moderate and there are no symptoms suggesting serious neurologic, infectious, vascular, or systemic condition.

Referral

 RF 11–2 Red Flag: Surgical emergency: Refer to neurosurgeon or to emergency department any client with saddle anesthesia, bladder dysfunction, and sensorimotor symptoms. These suggest cauda equina syndrome.

Refer to neurosurgeon any client with neurologic deficit that is severe and progressive.

Refer to oncologist or orthopedist any client with a history of cancer, recent infection that may have extended into spinal structures, IV drug abuse, immunodeficiency, major trauma, minor trauma in the elderly, systemic symptoms, or pain that increases when supine.

Refer to orthopedist if pain lasts longer than 6 weeks, or if client is <18 or >50 years of age.

NECK (Cervical) STRAIN

SIGNAL SYMPTOM ▶ neck pain

ICD-9 Codes	847.0	Sprains and strains of neck
	847.1	Sprains and strains of thoracic part of the back

Cervical strain is characterized by neck pain resulting from trauma to the musculotendinous structures of the neck and upper back. Pain may also involve the upper shoulder close to the neck.

Epidemiology

Can occur at any age; more common in adults.

Etiology

In many cases the etiology of cervical strain is unknown. Hyperflexion and/or hyperextension (e.g., whiplash injuries) are responsible for some cases. In other cases there may be a report of lifting a heavy object above shoulder level. Osteoarthritis of the cervical spine may also be a predisposing factor.

Physiology and Pathophysiology

Excessive stress on the musculotendinous units in the neck results in over-stretching or tearing the involved muscles and/or tendons.

Clinical Manifestations

Subjective

Neck pain
Upper back and or trapezius pain
Headaches are common

Objective

Muscle spasm and/or tenderness

Differential Diagnosis

Cervical disk herniation (radiculopathy commonly seen)
Tumor (pain at night, systemic symptoms)
Infection (fever, systemic symptoms, pain on percussion of the vertebral body)
Arthritis (diagnostic tests consistent with arthritis)
Fracture, dislocation, or subluxation (x-ray examination indicates the structural abnormality)

Diagnostic Tests

Generally none are indicated. May consider ESR, CBC, purified protein derivative if malignancy or infection is suspected.
Plain x-ray examination may be useful if there is a history of trauma or neurologic deficit, if pain persists, if the client has rheumatoid arthritis, or if there are risk factors for osteoporosis.
MRI is indicated for radiculopathy lasting more than 3–4 weeks, for persistent pain, or for myelopathy.

Management/Treatment

Pharmacologic Management

NSAIDs (see Table 11–1)
Muscle relaxants:
Cyclobenzaprine (Flexeril), 10 mg PO q8h or at nighttime only
Metaxalone (Skelaxin), 800 mg PO Q8H or at night only
Carisopradol (Soma), 350 mg PO TID or QID with meals and HS (controlled substance)

Nonpharmacologic Management

Modify activities to prevent re-injury.
Warm and cold packs.
Physical therapy: Ultrasonography and traction therapies may be beneficial.
Exercises to increase strength and flexibility; examples include:
Neck releases: Begin with head in neutral position, looking straight ahead. Turn head to the right while exhaling. Hold for several seconds. Return to

neutral position while inhaling. Turn head to the left while exhaling. Hold for several seconds. Return to neutral position while inhaling. Repeat this sequence several times. Next, slowly tilt head toward the right shoulder while exhaling. Hold for several seconds. Return to neutral position while inhaling. Slowly tilt head toward the left shoulder while exhaling. Hold for several seconds. Return to neutral position while inhaling. Repeat this sequence several times. Finish this exercise by tilting head backward while inhaling. Hold for several seconds, then lower head toward chest while exhaling. Repeat this sequence several times.

Chin circles: Extend chin forward and draw an imaginary circle with your chin. At the end of the circle, tuck chin toward chest. Repeat several times.

Isometric exercises: Use the hand to resist movement as effort is made to tilt head side to side, bow head, and tilt head backward. The head should not actually move. Repeat each maneuver several times.

Complementary/Alternative Therapies
Relaxation methods
Massage

Client Education
Usual course of recovery
Medications and side effects
Nonpharmacologic treatment methods
Stretching and range-of-motion exercises
Ergonomics

Follow-up
Reevaluate in 24 hours if pain is severe or unrelieved, or if new symptoms develop.

Reevaluate in 1 to 2 weeks if pain is mild to moderate and there are no symptoms suggesting a serious neurologic, infectious, vascular, or systemic condition.

Referral

RF 11–3   Red Flag: Refer to orthopedist any client with a neurologic deficit that is severe and progressive, if the client has myelopathy, or if the client has radicular pain that persists after 1 to 2 weeks of conservative therapy.

Refer to orthopedist, or appropriate specialist, any client with a history of cancer, recent infection that may have extended into spinal structures, IV drug abuse, immunodeficiency, major trauma, or systemic symptoms.

OSTEOPOROSIS

ICD-9 Code	733	Osteoporosis

Osteoporosis is a group of disorders of bone metabolism that result in loss of bone mass sufficient to increase the likelihood of fractures. Three types of primary osteoporosis are generally recognized. Idiopathic osteoporosis occurs in young people, including children, who have normal estrogen and androgen levels. Type I osteoporosis occurs in postmenopausal women who have increased bone resorption leading to abnormal losses of trabecular bone. Type II osteoporosis occurs in elders of both genders who have abnormal loss of both trabecular and cortical bone. Parathyroid hormone levels in this type of osteoporosis are generally high. Secondary osteoporosis may be found in any age group and is attributable to an identified cause.

Epidemiology

The incidence in women is greater than that in men.

Affects more than 25 million Americans (mostly women).

Most common in Caucasian and Asian women.

Responsible for 1.5 million fractures annually, exceeding $10 billion per year.

Etiology

Although the underlying causes of osteoporosis are often unclear, predisposing factors include:

Hormonal disturbances (excess parathyroid, thyroid, and adrenal corticosteroid hormones; deficiency in insulin or gonadal hormones)

Chronic illnesses, especially rheumatoid arthritis

Nutritional factors (inadequate consumption of calcium, vitamin D, or vitamin C; intestinal or liver disorders)

Inadequate weight-bearing

Medications, including corticosteroids, anticonvulsants, tetracyclines, heparin, chemotherapy, and radiation therapy

Smoking

Excessive alcohol consumption

Malignancies (multiple myeloma, metastases, hormonally active neoplasms)

Genetic factors

Physiology and Pathophysiology

Although the pathogenesis of primary osteoporosis is not fully understood, excessive bone loss is the defining characteristic. Bone remodeling (resorption by osteoclasts and formation by osteoblasts) is a lifelong process. While at any given time most bone surfaces are quiescent and are not involved in the remodeling process, a balance of bone formation and resorption at active sites is necessary to maintain skeletal mass. Bone mass peaks at about age 30 in women and at about age 35–40 in men. After this peak bone resorption exceeds bone formation. Men lose about 3% of their bone mass per decade. Women lose about 3%–8% of their bone mass each decade until menopause, at which time bone loss accelerates. Factors that are known to have an impact on bone mass and the rate of bone loss include:

Peak bone mass

Nutrition

Life style

Hormone levels

Clinical Manifestations

Subjective

Back pain caused by vertebral compression fractures

 RF 11–4 **Red Flag:** Limp or knee pain with weight-bearing may indicate a possible impending fracture; refer to orthopedist if suspected.

Objective

Kyphosis

Loss of height caused by vertebral compression fractures

Radiographic evidence of fracture with minimal or no trauma

Differential Diagnosis

Osteoarthritis (x-ray film showing changes consistent with osteoarthritis)

Multiple myeloma or other malignant neoplasm (diffuse bone lesions on x-ray examination; may have systemic symptoms)

Malabsorption disorders (laboratory studies showing low levels of involved nutrients)

Vitamin D deficiency (laboratory studies showing low level of vitamin D)

Endocrine disorders (laboratory studies showing endocrine abnormality)

Collagen disorders (i.e., polyarteritis, systemic lupus erythematosus, rheumatic fever)

Renal disease (i.e., decreased creatinine clearance, hemoglobin, hematocrit; increased magnesium, amylase, uric acid)

Effects of medications (history of medications that can alter bone metabolism—i.e., corticosteroids)

Diagnostic Tests

Laboratory tests are usually normal in primary osteoporosis, although alkaline phosphatase may be elevated after a fracture. Laboratory tests useful in determining a cause in secondary osteoporosis include:

Thyroid-function tests

Serum calcium level

Parathyroid hormone level

Glucose level

Estrogen level

Urinary free cortisol level

Serum 25-hydroxyvitamin D level

CBC

Serum protein electrophoresis

Serum osteocalcin level

X-ray examination (plain films)

Before vertebra collapse: Vertical striations on the vertebra, prominence of vertebral end plates, and biconcavity of the vertebra

After fracture and vertebra collapse: Decreased anterior height of the vertebra and, if fractures are old, osteophytes

CP 11–2   Clinical Pearl: A decrease in bone density is not a sensitive measure because bone mass may be reduced up to 30% before it is detectable on x-ray examination.

Bone mass measures (decreased bone density)
Single-photon absorptiometry
Dual-photon absorptiometry
Quantitative CT
Dual energy x-ray absorptiometry

Management/Treatment

Pharmacologic Management

HORMONE-REPLACEMENT THERAPY

Conjugated estrogen (Premarin), 0.625 mg PO daily for women who have had a hysterectomy, or medroxyprogesterone (Provera), 2.5–10 mg daily either continuously or cyclically with 0.625 mg conjugated estrogen for women who have their uterus.

Prempro combines 0.625 mg conjugated estrogen and either 2.5 or 5 mg of medroxyprogesterone and can be taken either continuously or cyclically.

Recent evidence suggests that a lower dose of 0.45 mg of conjugated estrogens and 1.5 mg medroxyprogesterone acetate may be as effective for 80%–85% of women in early menopause.

Elderly women who start on hormone-replacement therapy can be started on 0.3 mg conjugated estrogens and the dose may not have to be raised if they show increased lumbar spine density and no loss at femoral neck. If no change in density may have to increase dose.

For women who cannot take hormone-replacement therapy, consider:

Raloxifene (Evista), 60 mg PO daily.

Alendronate sodium (Fosamax), 5–10 mg PO daily; may be taken 70 mg PO weekly. Take with 8 oz of water first thing in the morning. Must remain upright and have no other oral intake for at least 30 minutes. Hypocalcemia must be corrected before beginning alendronate therapy.

Risendronate sodium (Actonel), 5mg PO daily.

Calcium intake of 1000–1500 mg daily with adequate vitamin D. If client has little exposure to sunlight daily, vitamin D intake should total 400–800 IU daily. Calcium supplementation may be contraindicated for clients who have a history of calcium-containing urinary stones.

Synthetic salmon calcitonin (Miacalcin), 200 IU (1 puff) intranasally daily. Alternate nostrils. Use calcium supplement and vitamin D with this medication.

Synthetic salmon calcitonin (Calcimar), 100 IU subcutaneous injection daily. Use calcium supplement and vitamin D with this medication.

Nonpharmacologic Management

Encourage measures to promote maximum bone mass in children and young adults and for middle-aged and older adults to minimize bone loss:

Adequate calcium and vitamin D intake
Weight-bearing exercise regularly
Refrain from smoking, heavy use of alcohol
Minimize caffeine intake

Complementary/Alternative Therapies

None recommended. Herbal products containing estrogen have varying amounts of estrogen

Client Education

Disease process
Adequate intake of calcium, and exposure to sunlight >10 minutes daily
  or intake of adequate vitamin D
Moderate exercise (weight-bearing)
Discourage high-protein diet
Negative effects on bone health of cigarette smoking and heavy alcohol use

Follow-up

1–2 months initially; then every 3–6 months.
If taking calcium supplements, check urinary calcium excretion every 6
  months.
Consider annual bone density test to evaluate treatment effectiveness.
Annual well-woman examination, Pap smear, and mammography as
  indicated.

Referral

Refer to orthopedist if fracture occurs.

RHEUMATOID ARTHRITIS

SIGNAL SYMPTOM ▷ morning stiffness

ICD-9 Code	714.0	Rheumatoid arthritis

Rheumatoid arthritis (RA) is a systemic, progressive, inflammatory disease of connective tissue, involving primarily the joints.

Epidemiology

Affects about 1% of the population.
Great variation in age at first symptoms and in the severity of the disease.
About 90% of clients with severe disease are disabled within 20 years.
Presence of extraarticular symptoms or severe disease is associated with
  increased mortality.
Female:male ratio, 3:1.
Most common age of onset is between 20 and 50 years (see Box 11–4.)

Etiology

Immune-mediated disorder.
Possible triggers include genetic, infectious, and autoimmune factors.

Box 11–4
Juvenile Rheumatoid Arthritis

Possibly 250,000 children in the United States are affected by juvenile rheumatoid arthritis (JRA). It is difficult to delineate the exact prevalence of this disease because not all childhood arthritis is JRA, and differentiating between causes of arthritis in children is often very difficult.

Criteria for the diagnosis of JRA set by the American College of Rheumatology include:

1. Peripheral articular marginal and subchondral erosions
2. Axial joint erosions
3. Fusion of axial or peripheral joints
4. Ballooned and/or premature epiphyseal closure
5. Underdeveloped long bones resulting in growth retardation
6. Micrognathia
7. Osteopenia

Although these criteria are somewhat useful in diagnosing JRA, many difficulties remain. In some children all criteria may not be evident. In others, joint symptoms may not be present at all. Conversely, children with juvenile spondyloarthopathy may meet all of these criteria but do not have JRA. Rheumatoid factor is rarely found in JRA. Antinuclear antibody is sometimes found, and perhaps 35% of affected children have antineutrophil cytoplasmic antibody.

Three major categories of JRA are recognized:

Pauciarticular disease in which four or fewer joints are affected

Polyarticular disease in which more than four joints are affected

Systemic disease in which systemic symptoms predominate and there may be little or no joint involvement

Pauciarticular disease is the most common. Fever and malaise are not seen, and although few joints are affected, ocular disease is common. Iridocyclitis, band keratopathy, and cataract formation may permanently damage vision if not detected and treated. Polyarticular disease affects 30%–40% of children with JRA. In addition to more extensive joint involvement, these children often have low-grade fever, malaise, and in about one third of the cases, pericarditis. Systemic JRA (also called Still's disease) is the least common form. Systemic symptoms including fever spikes to 103°F twice each day, lymphadenopathy, hepatosplenomegaly, pleuritis, and pericarditis are often seen. A salmon-colored macular rash that occurs when pressure or heat is applied to the skin is common. Articular symptoms are variable, and most children recover from this form during adolescence.

A large number of inflammatory products are thought to play a role in producing the pathologic effects commonly seen.

Physiology and Pathophysiology

Whatever the trigger (e.g., autoimmune response, infectious agents such as human parvovirus 19, and Epstein–Barr virus), a multitude of inflammatory cells including T lymphocytes, B lymphocytes, synoviocytes (members of the monocyte–macrophage family), mast cells, and neutrophils are found in joints and surrounding tissue. A variety of cytokines produced and/or induced by these inflammatory cells are thought to participate in the pathologic process of RA. Current evidence suggests that tumor necrosis factor and interleukin-1 play a dominant role.

There are two major pathogenic processes in RA—joint inflammation (synovitis) and cartilage and bone destruction. It is uncertain whether these processes are mediated by the same or by different pathologic pathways.

Clinical Manifestations

Subjective
Prodromal weakness and fatigue
Morning stiffness that lasts more than 1 hour

Objective
Anemia, lymphadenopathy, anorexia
Bilateral, symmetric joint symptoms, usually involving several joints
Commonly affects hands, wrists, elbows, shoulders, feet, ankles, and knees
Tender, swollen joints
Subcutaneous nodules over joints
Joint deformities in more advanced disease, including contractures, subluxations, and dislocations

 RF 11–5   Red Flag: Refer to rheumatologist for intractable joint pain at rest or for severe joint deformity.

Extraarticular findings may include inflammation of tendon sheaths and bursae, splenomegaly, scleritis and episcleritis, vasculitis, pericarditis, pneumonitis, pulmonary fibrosis, skin nodules.

American College of Rheumatology criteria (five of the seven criteria must be evident).
1. Morning stiffness >1 hour for more than 6 weeks
2. Arthritis of at least three joint groups with soft tissue swelling or fluid for more than 6 weeks
3. Swelling of at least one of the following joints for more than 6 weeks: proximal interphalangeal, metacarpophalangeal, or wrists
4. Symmetrical joint swelling for more than 6 weeks
5. Subcutaneous nodules
6. Positive rheumatoid factor
7. Radiographic changes consistent with RA

Differential Diagnosis
Osteoarthritis (often unilateral, radiographic findings consistent with osteoarthritis)
Systemic lupus erythematosus (malar rash, laboratory studies consistent with systemic lupus erythematosus—i.e., thrombocytopenia, positive for antinuclear antibodies, positive Coombs test, increased creatinine level, leukopenia)
Lyme disease (rash, history of tick bite)
Polymyositis (muscle weakness, painless)
Sclerodema (skin thickening)
Crystal-induced arthritides (hyperuricemia, crystals in joint aspirate)

Diagnostic Tests

Rheumatoid factor (positive [>1:80 titer] in about 80% of persons with RA; also occurs in other diseases and in a small percentage of the general population)

Antinuclear antibodies (high titers are found in about one third of persons with RA)

ESR (usually elevated in RA but is typically elevated with any inflammatory process)

CBC (anemia of chronic disease often seen; WBC count elevated)

Synovial fluid analysis (decreased viscosity, WBCs may be elevated)

X-ray examination of involved joints (typical findings include narrowing of joint space, soft-tissue swelling, juxtoarticular osteoporosis, loss of articular cartilage and bone erosions)

Management/Treatment

Pharmacologic Management

NSAIDs.

Corticosteroids (controversial).

Prednisone, 5–15mg PO daily until symptoms are relieved.

Disease-modifying antirheumatic drugs alone or in combination therapy. (Adult dosages given; refer children to rheumatologist.)

Gold salts:

Auranofin (Ridaura), 6–9mg PO daily or BID.

Injectable gold: Refer to rheumatologist.

D-penicillamine, 250 mg PO daily, may increase slowly to 750–1000 mg/day; no more than 8–12 weeks at maximum dose.

Methotrexate (Folex, Rheumatrex): Adults: 5–15 mg/week PO in one dose or divided doses.

Hydroxychloroquine (Plaquenil): Adults: 400 mg PO HS for 2–3 months, then 200 mg PO HS.

Sulfasalazine (SSZ, Azulfidine): Adults: 500 mg PO daily. May increase up to 2000 mg/day.

Infliximab (Remicade): Refer to rheumatologist.

Etanercept: Refer to rheumatologist.

Nonpharmacologic Management

Balance of rest and activity

Physical therapy, including exercise, splinting, assistive devices, and heat or cold applications

Immunoadsorption column for apheresis

Complementary/Alternative Therapies

Relaxation therapy

Keeping a journal for the purpose of chronicling pain and response to medications

Social support
Imagery

Client Education
Disease process
Medications and side effects
Moderate exercise balanced with rest
Nutrition

Follow-up
At 2 weeks, then every 2 weeks to 3 months depending on client's condition and treatments

Referral
Refer to rheumatologist if a 3-month trial of NSAIDs is ineffective or if there is significant disability, extraarticular manifestations, or evidence of cartilage or bone changes on x-ray examination. Also refer any ambiguous case for diagnosis.

STRAINS AND SPRAINS

ICD-9 Codes	848.9	Unspecified site of sprain and strain
		Other specific codes depend on site of sprain/strain

A sprain is an injury in which a ligament is overstretched or torn. Sprains may be graded to indicate severity:

Grade I results in pain and tenderness at the joint with minimal or no swelling and no ligament laxity.

Grade II is characterized by joint pain and tenderness, greater swelling, ecchymosis, and ligament laxity.

Grade III has all the characteristics of grade II, along with marked joint instability.

A strain is an injury to the musculotendinous unit.

Epidemiology
Very common in physically active persons

Etiology
Sprains usually result from trauma
Strains usually result from overuse

Physiology and Pathophysiology
Injury to ligaments, tendons, or muscles induces the inflammatory response. The release of inflammatory mediators produces pain, swelling, erythema, and decreased range of motion.

Clinical Manifestations

Subjective
Pain.
Client may report a tearing sensation or may hear a pop.

Objective
Swelling
Inability to bear weight (grade II or III lower-extremity sprain)
Decreased range of motion
Increased laxity of ligaments (grade II or III sprain)
Ecchymosis (grade II or III sprain)

 CP 11–3   Clinical Pearl: Always palpate the Achilles tendon when examining a client with an ankle injury. Rupture of the Achilles tendon is sometimes painless.

Differential Diagnosis
Fracture (x-ray film showing fracture)
Tendinitis (minimal swelling)
Arthritides (laboratory tests and x-ray films consistent with arthritis)
Bursitis (pain with direct pressure on bursa)

Diagnostic Tests
X-ray examination (no evidence of fracture) (see Box 11–5).

Management/Treatment
It is often not possible to determine whether a given injury is a sprain, a strain, or both. Treatment is guided more by the degree of pain, swelling, laxity, and instability rather than by the diagnosis of strain, sprain, or both.

Pharmacologic Management
NSAIDs on a regular schedule for the first several days
Muscle relaxant for muscle spasms that can occur with strains:
   Cyclobenzaprine (Flexeril), 10 mg one PO TID PRN (*Note:* Do not give with Ultram.)
   Metaxalone (Skelaxin), 400 mg two PO TID PRN
   Orphenadrine (Norflex), 100 mg one PO BID PRN
May wish to consider narcotic analgesics for grade II–III sprains and severe strains.

Box 11–5
Evaluation of a Foot or Ankle Injury: Is X-ray Examination Necessary?

Ottawa ankle rules (rules used to determine the appropriateness of x-ray examination of ankle or foot) may be useful in determining the necessity of radiography for foot and ankle injuries. Pain or tenderness in any of the areas listed below or inability to bear weight immediately after the injury and at the time of medical evaluation suggests a need for radiography.

Pain at the posterior edge or tip of either the lateral or medial malleolus
Navicular pain
Pain at the base of the fifth metatarsal

Nonpharmacologic Management

Immobilization:

Grade I sprain: Elastic bandage (Ace) wrap applied snugly around affected hand or foot then more loosely as wrapped up the lower leg or forearm.

Grade II sprain: Air cast, splint, or unna boot.

Grade III sprain: Cast

Some sources suggest that because there is a high rate of poor healing and recurrence with ligament injuries, a more rigid form of immobilization is preferable.

Rest.

Elevate affected area if possible.

Crutches for grade II–III ankle sprains.

Cold packs for 15–20 minutes Q4–6H for the first 24–72 hours.

Rehabilitation after pain and swelling subside:

Start isometric exercises and gentle stretching exercises at 1–3 weeks.

Wear ankle brace when weight bearing is resumed.

Progress slowly with activities.

Complementary/Alternative Therapies

Cold therapy

Relaxation exercises as an adjunct for pain control

Client Education

Sprains heal slowly; complete healing may take months after a grade III sprain.

Body mechanics for prevention of recurrent strains.

Medications and side effects.

Rest, ice, compression, elevation.

Use of crutches if indicated

Follow-up

Follow-up depends on the severity of the injury and type of treatment.

Referral

Refer to orthopedist if suspected grade III sprain or fracture.

SYSTEMIC LUPUS ERYTHEMATOSUS

SIGNAL SYMPTOMS malaise, joint pain, butterfly rash, weight loss, anorexia

ICD-9 Code	710.0	Systemic lupus erythematosus

Systemic lupus erythematosus (SLE) is a multisystem, inflammatory, autoimmune disease. Its manifestations vary from mild to severe, and its course is marked by exacerbations and remissions.

Epidemiology

Prevalence approximately 1 in 2500.

Occurs predominantly in women (incidence in women 7–10 times that in men).

Can occur at any age but most commonly develops between ages 20 and 50.

Etiology

Underlying cause is unknown.

Genetic, hormonal, and infectious components have been implicated as etiologic factors.

Malfunction of suppressor T cells is thought to initiate the autoimmune events leading to clinical manifestations of SLE.

Physiology and Pathophysiology

It is commonly believed that defective functioning of suppressor T cells in SLE permits uncontrolled activation of B cells. Mature plasma cells arising from this polyclonal activation of B cells produce antibodies that lack the usual specificity for foreign antigens. These antibodies may interact with autoantigens in the host's tissues or with products produced by damaged host cells, forming antigen–antibody complexes. Complement is activated by the antigen–antibody complexes, initiating an inflammatory reaction that damages tissue at the sites of deposition. Deposition of circulating antigen–antibody complexes can occur widely, most often in semipermeable membranes.

Clinical Manifestations

Subjective

Fatigue
Joint pain
Abdominal pain
Headache
Pleuritic pain

Objective

Joint tenderness and swelling
Skin lesions (molar or discoid rash)
Alopecia
Raynaud's phenomenon
Fever
Weight loss
Oral ulcers
Photophobia
Neurologic signs
Lymphadenopathy
Pleural effusion
Thrombocytopenia
Proteinuria and cellular casts

Criteria of the American Rheumatism Association (four or more criteria must be present to diagnose SLE):

Butterfly rash

Discoid rash

Photosensitivity

Oral ulcers

Arthritis

Serositis (pleuritis or pericarditis)

Renal disease

Neurologic disorder

Hematologic disorder (hemolytic anemia, leukopenia, lymphopenia, thrombocytopenia)

Immunologic disorder

Positive lupus erythematosus(LE)–cell preparation

Anti-DNA

False positive serologic test for syphilis

Positive antinuclear antibody test

Differential Diagnosis

RA (joint destruction present)

Scleroderma (skin thickening; prominent gastrointestinal symptoms; dry eyes and mouth)

Polyarteritis nodosa (hypertension; gastrointestinal symptoms in most clients; triad of fever, weight loss, and mononeuritis multiplex with foot drop often seen)

Drug reactions (medication history; rash resolves when drug is discontinued)

Malignancy (progressive aching pain at rest; pain increased with supine position or cough; history of prior malignancy)

Diagnostic Tests

CBC with differential (anemia, leukopenia, lymphopenia, thrombocytopenia often present in SLE; also helps to rule out infectious process)

Antinuclear antibody tests (positive in almost all clients with SLE; however, test not specific for SLE)

LE-cell preparation (positive in SLE; neutrophils show reddish-purple inclusion)

Anti-DNA antibody test (positive in 65%–80% of clients with SLE)

Anti-Sm (Smith nuclear antigen) (positive in SLE)

Urinalysis (proteinuria and red-cell casts may be present in SLE; may indicate deteriorating renal function)

Blood urea nitrogen and creatinine (evaluates renal function)

Partial thromboplastin time (may be prolonged in SLE)

Chest x-ray examination (pulmonary infiltrates and/or pleural effusion may be present in SLE)

Echocardiography (valvular heart disease may be present in SLE)

Management/Treatment

Pharmacologic Management

NSAIDs for joint pain (avoid ibuprofen, sulindac, and tolmetin—possibility of aseptic meningitis).

Hydrochloroquine (Plaquenil), 400 mg, one PO HS for 2–3 months, then 200 mg one PO HS for 2–3 months for arthritis not controlled by NSAIDs or for dermal manifestations of SLE.

Prednisone, 10–20mg/day for short-term treatment of joint symptoms not controlled with NSAIDs.

Higher-dose prednisone, 1 mg/kg/day may be required for nephritis, myocarditis, pericarditis, neurologic, and hematologic (hemolytic anemia or thrombocytopenia) manifestations.

Topical steroids for dermal lesions

Immunosuppressants (e.g., cyclosporine, methotrexate), danazol, and immunoglobulins may be considered for severe renal, neurologic, or hematologic involvement. Refer clients to rheumatologist if consideration of these treatments seems warranted.

Nonpharmacologic Management

Recommend support group or other stress-management techniques.

Sun protection: Sunscreen, avoiding prolonged exposure to sun or other ultraviolet light.

Warm or cold packs for joint pain.

Low-salt, low-fat diet.

Contraception counseling.

Complementary/Alternative Therapies

Relaxation therapy

Recommend support group or other stress-management techniques

Client Education

Treatment and side effects of medications

Importance of regular follow-up

Protection from sun exposure and use of sun screen

Prompt treatment of infections

Birth control options (oral contraception may be associated with exacerbation of SLE)

Follow-up

Initially: Every 1–2 weeks

During remissions: Every 3 months

During exacerbations: More frequent follow-up

Referral

Refer to appropriate specialists (rheumatology, nephrology, perinatology) for all newly diagnosed clients and those with exacerbation of disease or deterioration of renal, cardiac, hematologic, pulmonary, or neurologic function.

TENDINITIS/BURSITIS

SIGNAL SYMPTOMS ▶ tendinitis: pain with movement of involved area; bursitis: pain with pressure on affected bursa

ICD-9 Codes	726.9	Tendinitis
	727.3	Bursitis
		Other codes for specific locations

Tendinitis is injury and subsequent inflammation of a tendon—a fibrous band that attaches muscle to bone.

Bursitis is inflammation of a bursa, a cushioning sac between tendons and bones in areas prone to frequent pressure or friction.

Epidemiology

Occurs commonly

Most common in adults but can occur at any age

Occurs slightly more frequently in men than in women

Common sites include:

Shoulder: Frequently seen in football, baseball, and tennis players

Elbow (tennis elbow): Frequently seen in tennis players and golfers

Hips

Knee (housemaid's knee)

Heel: In association with Achilles tendinitis

Etiology

Most cases caused by chronic overuse, resulting in repetitive trauma to the tendons and bursae.

Other causes: Acute trauma, gout, immune-mediated disorders, or infection.

Physiology and Pathophysiology

In the most common type of tendinitis/bursitis, overuse causes microtears in a tendon. Over time, repetitive trauma induces an inflammatory response involving the tendon and adjacent structures, including bursae. Bursae, sacs lined with a synovial membrane, form in sites where muscles and tendons move over bony protuberances. They cushion stress and reduce friction at these vulnerable sites. When inflamed, bursae become swollen with fluid and are painful.

Clinical Manifestations

Subjective

Pain at site of musculotendinous unit or bursa

Stiffness

Objective

May be swelling at the site

Tendinitis: Pain with movement of involved area

Bursitis: Pain with pressure on affected bursa

May be mild erythema and warmth over involved area

Differential Diagnosis

Tendinitis (history of overuse, no findings consistent with fracture or arthitides on radiography)

Bursitis (pain with direct pressure on the bursa)

Arthritides (laboratory studies or x-ray examinations consistent with an arthritis)

Sprain (history of trauma, pain, and possibly laxity at the joint)

Stress fracture (horizontal band of sclerosis and a periosteal reaction on radiography)

Diagnostic Tests

X-ray examinations (not routinely ordered, but if done, no fracture shown)

MRI (may be ordered if tendon tear if suspected; no tendon tear is shown)

Management/Treatment

Pharmacologic Management

NSAIDs

Corticosteroid and/or local anesthetic injection

Nonpharmacologic Management

R—rest

I—ice

C—compression

E—elevation

Splint if appropriate.

Strengthening exercises after site is pain-free.

May need to aspirate swollen bursa to rule out infection.

Complementary/Alternative Therapies

Acupuncture

Relaxation methods as adjunct for pain relief

Client Education

Cause of disorder

Treatment

Strengthening exercises and when they may be started

Medications and side effects

Follow-up

1 to 2 weeks

Referral

Refer to orthopedist if:

Septic bursitis is suspected.

Symptoms continue after 2 months of conservative therapy.

Bursitis not relieved with rest, ice and NSAIDs; consider referral for aspiration or injection with corticosteroid and/or local anesthetic.

REFERENCES

General

Anderson, B.C. & Kersey, R. (1998). *Office orthopedics for primary care: Diagnosis and treatment.* Philadelphia: Saunders.

Cash, J.C., & Glass, C.A. (Eds.) (1999). *Family practice guidelines.* Philadelphia: Lippincott.

Damjanov, I. (2000) *Pathology for the health-related professions* (2nd ed.). Philadelphia: Saunders.

Dunn, S.A. (1998). *Mosby's primary care consultant.* St. Louis: Mosby.

Dunphy, L.M. (Ed.) (1999). *Management guidelines for adult nurse practitioners.* Philadelphia: F.A. Davis

Fauci, A.S., Braunwald, E., Issebacher, K.J., Wilson, J.D., Martin, J.B., Kasper, D.L., Hauser, S., L., & Longo, D. L. (Eds.) (1998). *Harrison's principles of internal medicine* (14th ed.). New York: McGraw-Hill.

Ferri, F.F. (Ed.) (2000). *Ferri's clinical advisor.* St. Louis: Mosby.

Kaufman, C.E., & McKee, P. A. (1996). *Essentials of pathophysiology.* Philadelphia: Lippincott Williams and Wilkins

Luskin, F.M., Newell, K.A., Griffith, M., Holmes, M., Telles, S., DiNucci, E., Marvasti, F.F., Hill, M., Pelletier, K.R., & Haskell, W.L. (2000). A review of mind/body therapies in the treatment of musculoskeletal disorders with implications for the elderly. *Alternative Therapies, 6* (2), 46–56.

Moore, S.W. (1998). *Griffith's instructions for patients* (6th ed.). Philadelphia: Saunders.

Wilson, J.L., & Cohen, M.D. (1998). Making sense of musculoskeletal disorders. *Comprehensive Therapy, 24* (2), 64–70.

Carpal Tunnel Syndrome

Ebenbichler, G.R., Resch, K.L., Nicolakis, P., Wiesinger, G.F., Url, F., Ghanem, A.H., & Fialka, V. (1998). Ultrasound treatment for treating the carpal tunnel syndrome: Randomized "sham" controlled trial. *British Medical Journal, 316,* 731–735.

Garfinkel, M.S., Singhal, A., Katz, W.A., Allan, D.A., Reshetar, R., & Schumacher, H.R., Jr. (1998). Yoga-based intervention for carpal tunnel syndrome. *JAMA, 280,* 1601–1603.

Chronic Pain

Marcus, D.A. (2000). Treatment of nonmalignant chronic pain. *American Family Physician, 61,* 1331–1338, 1345–1346.

Degenerative Joint Disease

Klahr, P.D., Caplan, P.S., Levy, M.S., & Starz, T.W. (1999). New treatments for osteoarthritis and rheumatoid arthritis. *Emergency Medicine, 31*(5), 28–44.

Fractures

Pope, T.L. (1998). Cost-effective strategies for radiologic referral. *Emergency Medicine, 30*(5), 45–46.

Ritchie, J.V., & Munter, D.W. (1999). Emergency department evaluation and treatment of wrist injuries. *Emergency Medicine Clinics of North America, 17*(4) 823–842.

Roberts, D.M., & Stallard, T.C. (2000). Emergency department evaluation and treatment of knee and leg injuries. *Emergency Medicine Clinics of North America, 18* 1), 67–83.

Wedmore, I.S. & Charette, J. (2000). Emergency evaluation and treatment of ankle & foot injuries. *Emergency Clinics of North America, 18*(1), 85–109.

Gout

Harris, M.D., Siegel, L.B., & Alloway, J.A. (1999). Gout and hyperuricemia. *American Family Physician, 59*(4), 925–934.

McGill, N.W.(1997, January 6). Gout and other crystal arthropathies. *MJA Practice Essentials—Rheumatology, 166*, pp. 33–38.

Lumbosacral Strain

Bratton, R.L. (1999). Assessment and management of acute low back pain. *American Family Physician, 60*, 2299–2306.

Connelly, C. (2000). A rational approach to low back pain. *Patient Care, 34*(6) 23–48.

Della-Giustina. (1999). Emergency department evaluation and treatment of back pain. *Emergency Medicine Clinics of North America, 17*(4), 877–893.

Ghoname, E.A., Craig, W.F., White, P.F., et al. (1999). Percutaneous electrical nerve stimulation for low back pain: A randomized crossover study. *JAMA, 281*, 818–823.

Goldsmith, M.E., & Wiesel, J. W. (1998). Clinical evaluation of low back pain. *Comprehensive Therapy, 24*, 370–377.

Patel, A.T., & Ogle, A.A. (2000). Diagnosis and management of acute low back pain. *American Family Physician, 61*(6), 1779.

Rose-Innes, A.P., & Engstrom, J.W. (1998). Low back pain: An algorithmic approach to diagnosis and management. *Geriatrics, 53*(10), 26.

Sarrdhu, F.A., & McGrail, K.M. (1999). The evaluation and management of low back pain. *Emergency Medicine, 31*(10), 20–46.

Neck (Cervical) Strain

Pawl, R.P. (1999). Chronic neck syndromes: an update. *Comprehensive Therapy, 25*(5), 278–282.

Osteoporosis

Schapira, D. (1999). Prevention and treatment of osteoporosis. *Comprehensive Therapy, 25*(11/12), 467–478.

Staley, C.A. (2000). Oral bisphosphonates: Alendronate and risendronate. Prevention and treatment of osteoporosis. *Women's Health in Primary Care, 3*, 662–680.

Rheumatoid Arthritis

Alexiades, M.M. (1999). Determining surgical priorities in rheumatoid arthritis. *Comprehensive Therapy, 25*(2), 101–108.

Klahr, P.D., Caplan, P.S., Levy, M.S. & Starz, T.W. (1999). New treatments for osteoarthritis and rheumatoid arthritis. *Emergency Medicine, 31*(5), 28–44.

Medsger, T.A., Jr. (1999). Laboratory tests in the diagnosis of rheumatic diseases. *Emergency Medicine, 31*(5), 12–28.

Rothschild, B.M. (1999). Recognition and treatment of arthritis in children. *Comprehensive Therapy, 25* (6/7), 347–359.

Speroff, L., Gallagher, V.M., Penkerton, J.V., & Raisz, L.G. (2001, July supplement). Menopause management: The impact of low dose HRT. *Contemporary OB/GYN for the Nurse Practitioner.*

Strains and Sprains

Bassewitz, H.L. & Shapiro, M.S. (1997). After ankle sprain: Targeting the causes. *Physician and Sportsmedicine 25*(12), 58–67.

Garrick J.G., & Schelkun, P.H. (1997). Managing ankle sprains: Keys to preserving motion and strength. *Physician and Sportsmedicine 25*(3), 57–68.

Safran, M.R., Benedetti R.S., Bartolozzi A.R. III, & Mandelbaum B.R. (1999). Lateral ankle sprains: A comprehensive review. Part 1: Etiology, pathoanatomy, histopathogenesis, and diagnosis. *Medicine & Science in Sports and Exercise 31*(7 Suppl.), S429–S437.

RESOURCES

General

American Academy of Orthopedic Surgeons
6300 N. River Rd.
Rosemont, IL 60018
Telephone: 847-823-7186 or 800-346-AAOS
Fax: 847-823-8125
www.aaos.org

American College of Rheumatology
1800 Century Pl.
Suite 250
Atlanta, GA 30345
Telephone: 404-633-3777
Fax: 404-633-1870
E-mail: acr@rheumatology.org
www.rheumatology.org

Arthritis Foundation
Western Missouri/Greater Kansas City Chapter
3420 Broadway
Suite 105
Kansas City, MO 64111
Telephone: 816-753-2220 or 888-719-5670
E-mail: info.wmo@arthritis.org
www.arthritis.org

Arthritis National Research Foundation
200 Oceangate
Suite 400
Long Beach, CA 90802
Telephone: 800-588-CURE (2873)
www.curearthritis.org

National Institute of Arthritis and Musculoskeletal and Skin Diseases
Information Clearinghouse
National Institutes of Health
1 AMS Circle
Bethesda, MD 20892
Telephone: 301-495-4484 or 877-22-NIAMS (toll-free)

National Institute of Arthritis and Musculoskeletal and Skin Diseases
Office of Communications and Public Liaison
National Institutes of Health
Bldg. 31
Rm. 4C05
31 Center Drive, MSC 2350
Bethesda, MD 20892
Telephone: 301-496-8190
Fax: 301-480-2814
www.nih.gov/niams

Chronic Pain

American Academy of Pain Management
13947 Mono Way, #A
Sonora CA 95370
Telephone: 209-533-9744
E-mail: aapm@aapainmanage.org
www.aapainmanage.org

American Chronic Pain Association
P.O. Box 850
Rocklin, CA 95677
Telephone: 916-632-0922,
Fax: 916-632-3208
E-mail: acpa@pacbell.net
http://members.tripod.com

American Society of Anesthesiologists
520 N. Northwest Hwy.
Park Ridge, IL 60068
Telephone: 847-825-5586
Fax: 847-825-1692
E-mail: mail@asahq.org
www.asahq.org

Osteoporosis
National Institutes of Health
Osteoporosis and Related Bone Diseases
National Resource Center
1232 22nd St. NW
Washington, DC 20037
Telephone: 202-223-0344 or 800-624-BONE
E-mail: orbdnrc@nof.org
www.osteo.org

National Osteoporosis Foundation
1232 22nd St. NW
Washington, DC 20037
Telephone: 202-223-2226
E-mail: communications@nof.org
www.nof.org

Systemic Lupus Erythematosus
Lupus Foundation of America
1300 Piccard Dr.
Suite 200
Rockville, MD 20850
Telephone. 301-670-9292 or 800-558-0121
www.lupus.org

BELL'S PALSY

SIGNAL SYMPTOMS ▶ facial numbness, drooping

ICD-9 Code	351.0	Bell's palsy

Bell's palsy is a paralysis or weakness of cranial nerve VII (facial nerve; it is usually unilateral.

Epidemiology

Usually affects individuals over age 30 years.

Incidence is 25 per 100,000 persons in the United States.

Equal male:female predominance.

Recurrence occurs in 7%–9% of population, and it is more likely in those with a positive family history.

Etiology

Idiopathic

Other possible causes:

Viral infection (including reactivated herpes simples virus)

Vascular entrapment

Autoimmune reactions

Infectious diseases

Physiology and Pathophysiology

Swelling and an acute inflammatory reaction of cranial nerve VII (facial nerve) results in weakness and/or paralysis of the mouth, cheek, and eyes; it is usually limited to one side of the face.

Clinical Manifestations

Subjective

Onset of symptoms is usually sudden (<48 hours).

One-sided weakness or paralysis of face.

Drooling may be present.

Unable to close one eye.

May have excessive tearing.
May have dry eye.
May experience some loss of taste.
Earache/pain possible.

Objective

Peripheral paralysis of cranial nerve VII (facial nerve) (Table 12–1)
Parotid gland and neck normal
Possible widened palpebral fissure
Possible decrease in corneal reflex

Differential Diagnosis

Malignant neoplasm (tumors of head/neck) (diagnosed via magnetic
resonance imaging [MRI] or computed tomographic [CT] scan)
Ramsay Hunt syndrome (Bell's palsy associated with herpes zoster) (usually
within or behind the ear)
Infectious processes:
Otitis media (ear pain with abnormal otologic examination; see "Otitis
Media" sections in Chapter 4)
Meningitis (stiff neck, fever, headache, photophobia, skin rash;
diagnosed via positive spinal tap)

Table 12–1   Grading Facial Nerve Dysfunction

Grade	
I: Normal	Normal function
II: Mild dysfunction	Slight weakness noticeable on close inspection; may have very slight synkinesis Normal symmetry and tone at rest Forehead: Moderate to good movement Eye: Complete closure with minimum effort Mouth: Slight asymmetry
III: Moderate dysfunction	Obvious weakness, but not disfiguring difference between two sides Noticeable, but not severe synkinesis, contracture, and/or hemifacial spasm Normal symmetry and tone at rest Forehead: Slight to moderate movement Eye: Complete closure with effort Mouth: Slightly weak with maximum effort
IV: Moderately severe dysfunction	Obvious weakness and/or disfiguring asymmetry Normal symmetry and tone at rest Forehead: No movement Eye: Incomplete closure Mouth: Asymmetry with maximum effort
V: Severe dysfunction	Barely perceptible movement Asymmetry at rest Forehead: No movement Eye: Incomplete closure Mouth: Slight movement
VI: Total paralysis	No movement

Adapted from: House JW, Brackmann DE. (1985). *Otolaryngol Head Neck Surg.*

Osteomyelitis (bone inflammation diagnosed via positive culture)

Measles, mumps, rubella, varicella (skin rashes)

Guillain–Barré syndrome (an acute febrile polyneuritis; refer to section on "Guillain–Barré Syndrome" below)

Head injury (review patient history; diagnosed via MRI or CT scan)

Brainstem stroke (unilateral numbness, loss of function, diagnosed via MRI or CT scan; refer to section on "Cerebrovascular Accident/Transient Ischemic Attack" below)

Diagnostic Tests

Audiometric testing is indicated for all clients (to rule out hearing loss) (findings should be normal, except for possible absent ipsilateral acoustic reflex)

Electrodiagnostic testing (reveals extent of paralysis)

MRI or CT scan (to rule out other pathology, if suspected)

Management/Treatment

Prognosis is generally good in all clients, with the majority (85%) regaining full function of facial nerve by 3 weeks:

~5% will have severe facial deformity.

10%–15% will be bothered by some asymmetrical movement.

Pharmacologic Management

Corticosteroids are the mainstay of treatment: Prednisone (Deltasone), 1 mg/kg/day; usually 60 mg/day for 7–10 days, then taper to 50, 40, 30, 20, 10.

If concurrent herpes simplex virus (HSV) infection is present, treat with acyclovir (Zovirax), 400 mg five times a day for 10 days.

If patient is unable to blink, saline eye drops should be used, and ophthalmic ointment should be used at bedtime.

Nonpharmacologic Management

Usually none.

Can tape eye lids shut if they do not cover the cornea.

Surgical decompression of the facial nerve is an option, but it remains controversial.

Client Education

Proper dosing of medications

Course of disease

Side effects of medications

Follow-up

Usually 48–72 hours to see if treatment is working.

Referral

Refer to neurologist if paralysis does not disappear (usually within 10 days).

Refer to ophthalmologist if eyes fail to improve.

CEREBROVASCULAR ACCIDENT/TRANSIENT ISCHEMIC ATTACK

SIGNAL SYMPTOMS unilateral numbness, loss of function

| ICD-9 Codes | 436 | Stroke (brain attack) |
| | 435.9 | Transient ischemic attack |

A cerebrovascular accident (CVA), or stroke, is the complete interruption of blood flow to the brain, resulting in irreversible injury.

A transient ischemic attack (TIA) is a brief interruption of blood flow to the brain, resulting in temporary focal neurologic deficit.

Epidemiology

Prevalence of TIAs ranges from 1.5%–4%.

Strokes occur in 30% of persons who have had a TIA.

Approximately 500,000 persons experience a stroke each year.

There are 150,000 stroke-related deaths each year.

Stroke is the leading cause of disability in the United States.

Only 10% of stroke victims experience a near-complete recovery.

Medical and lost employment costs are approximately $40 billion annually.

Risk increases with age.

An estimated 50% of stroke survivors will have concurrent depression.

Etiology

80% of strokes are due to ischemic cerebrovascular disease.

Other causes:

Cardioemboli secondary to valvular or mural pathology

Hemorrhagic

Hypercoagulable states

Posttraumatic

Risk factors:

Age

High blood pressure

Family history

Cardiac disease

Atrial fibrillation

Smoking

Diabetes

Elevated cholesterol level

Previous history of TIA

Physiology and Pathophysiology

Strokes may be ischemic or hemorrhagic.

Ischemic stroke: a clot forms, usually somewhere else in the body, breaks off and travels through the cerebrovascular system until it lodges in a vessel that is too small to permit its passage. Ischemia to that particular area of the brain results, and ultimately causes permanent damage, depending on the severity of blood flow reduction and length of time.

Hemorrhagic stroke: Bleeding occurs within the brain, usually as the result of ruptured blood vessels or aneurysms.

Clinical Manifestations

Subjective

Imperative to include in your assessment:

Complete symptom analysis

History of previous events

Current medications

Chronic risk factors

CVA:

Sudden weakness or tingling in extremities

Sensory loss and/or paralysis

Aphasia

Vision problems

Vertigo, dizziness

Severe headache

Nausea and vomiting

Ataxia

Loss of consciousness

TIA:

Symptoms similar to CVA, but come and go suddenly, usually <5 minutes.

Objective

Neurological assessment should include the following:

Level of consciousness

Cognition

Motor abilities (including strength)

Cranial-nerve testing

Sensation

Proprioception

Cerebellar testing

Deep tendon reflexes

Differential Diagnosis

Complex migraine headache (normal diagnostic tests; thorough patient history; refer to sections on "Headache" below)

Brain tumor (diagnosed with MRI or CT scan)

Bell's palsy (facial drooping, numbness; see section on "Bell's Palsy" above)

Drug overdose (review patient history)

Hypoglycemia (fatigue, irritability, weakness, and possible delirium diagnosed via decreased serum glucose)

Malingering (consider after above have been ruled out)

Diagnostic Tests

Complete blood cell (CBC) count (to rule out infectious process).

Chemistry profile (include cholesterol and glucose) (to rule out cardiac disease and/or abnormal glucose levels).

Prothrombin time and partial thromboplastin time (to determine any coagulation problems).

Sedimentation rate (to rule out any general inflammation).

Pulse oximetry (to determine oxygen saturation).

Electrocardiography (ECG) (to rule out cardiac problems).

Cranial CT scan without contrast (preferred test for acute stroke).

MRI scan may be warranted.

Management/Treatment

 RF 12–1 Red Flag: A CVA is a medical emergency; client needs immediate referral and treatment.

Emergency care includes:

Maintaining the airway

Maintaining oxygenation

Monitoring vital signs

Performing a physical examination, with special attention to the neurologic examination

Evaluating for use of thrombolytic therapy (Table 12–2)

Pharmacologic Management

Once client is stable, management includes:

Aggressive treatment of hypertension (<140/90 mm Hg)

Aggressive management of diabetes (if applicable)

Table 12–2 Guidelines for Use of Thrombolytic Therapy in Acute Ischemic Stroke

Client age 18 or older

Clinical diagnosis of ischemic stroke causing a measureable neurologic deficit

Time of symptom onset <180 min before treatment would begin

No contraindications; contraindications include:

    Intracranial or subarachnoid hemorrhage

    Active internal bleeding

    Known bleeding diathesis

    History of intracranial surgery, head trauma, or previous stroke within 3 mo

    Systolic blood pressure 185 mm Hg or diastolic blood pressure ≥110 mm Hg or higher at time treatment begins

    History of intracranial hemorrhage

    Known arteriovenous malformation or aneurysm

    Client observed to have had seizure at same time as onset of stroke symptoms

    History of gastrointestinal or urinary tract hemorrhage within 21 days

    Recent arterial puncture at a noncompressible site

    Recent lumbar puncture

    Abnormal blood glucose level (<50 or >400 mg/dl)

    Only minor or rapidly improving stroke symptoms

    Postmyocardial infarction pericarditis

Aggressive management of hypercholesterolemia (with use of "statins")
Use of coumadin or aspirin therapy, or other antiplatelet medications, especially in clients with atrial fibrillation

Nonpharmacologic Management
Once client is stable, management includes:

Surgical management of carotid stenosis (if applicable)
Stroke rehabilitation
Smoking cessation program
Limiting alcohol intake
Weight loss, if necessary
Encouraging physical activity
Encouraging a balanced, low-fat, low-cholesterol diet
Stress management
Cognitive therapy, if depression is present

Client Education
Course of disease and prognosis
Side effects of medications
Client empowerment and responsibility

Follow-up
Continual assessment of the following should be done:

Neurologic function
Dysphagia
Bladder/bowel function
Skin breakdown
Nutrition status
Physical activity
Sleep patterns
Psychological assessments

Referral
Refer to neurologist for initial evaluation and management plan and/or if worsening symptoms occur.

DEMENTIA

SIGNAL SYMPTOMS ▶ cognitive function impairment

ICD-9 Codes	345	Senile dementia
	290.10	Presenile dementia, uncomplicated
	290.40	Arteriosclerotic dementia, uncomplicated
	331.0	Alzheimer's disease

Dementia is the broad, global impairment of intellectual function (cognition). It is usually progressive, and it interferes with social and occupational activities. Dementia may have numerous etiologies. Dementia of Alzheimer's type is the most common form of dementia; it is marked by continual, yet variable deterioration of higher cortical functioning.

Dementia is differentiated from delirium, which is a state of mental confusion and excitement characterized by disorientation for time and place, usually with illusions and hallucinations. Causes include fever, shock, exhaustion, anxiety, or drug overdose. Delirium, unlike dementia, is reversible.

Epidemiology

Some type of cognitive dementia will develop in an estimated 80% of elders (people >85 years of age).

Prevalence in the United States is 1500/100,000.

The incidence in men and women is equal.

Over 4 million people in the United States currently have dementia.

Alzheimer's dementia incidence increases with increasing age:

0.5% in ages 60–64
3% in ages 65–74
18.7% in age 75–84
47.2% in ages ≥85

Etiology

Primary: Alzheimer's disease (50%–60% of all cases of dementia); genetic predisposition (at least 15% of patients report a positive family history).

Secondary: Brain tumors, several medical or surgical diseases.

Physiology and Pathophysiology

Multiple pathways of physiology based on the different etiologies.

Clinical Manifestations

Subjective

CP 12–1 Clinical Pearl: Usually it is helpful, or imperative, to illicit history from a spouse and/or family members.

Behaviors often seen in dementia include:

Anger, agitation, screaming
Wandering
Resistance
Difficulties with eating
Inappropriate actions
Repetitive actions
Sleep disturbances
Paranoia, delusions, hallucinations
Impaired short- and long-term memory
Impaired judgment
Personality changes
Restlessness, hyperactivity
Tremor

Seizures

Include in your history taking:

Onset of disease (gradual vs. sudden; intermittent vs. continual symptoms)
Medication history
History of acute illness
Dehydration
Constipation
Depression/fatigue
Use of any alcohol or street drugs
Activities of daily living (ADL) assessment
Environmental assessment
Family assessment

Objective

Include in your examination:

Complete physical examination
Neurologic examination and mental status
Mini–Mental State examination
Geriatric Depression Scale

Diagnostic Criteria

The diagnostic criteria from the *Diagnostic and Statistical Manual of Mental Disorders,* 4th ed. (DSM-IV) include:

Development of multiple cognitive deficits, including memory impairment and inability to recall or learn new information
Gradual onset and continued cognitive decline over time
Significant impairments in social, occupational, and daily functions
And at least one of the following:

Aphasia
Agnosia
Apraxia
Disturbances in executive functioning

Differential Diagnosis

Delirium (a state of mental confusion, which can be reversed)
Vascular dementia (dementia secondary to vascular disease)
Infectious etiologies (fever, elevated white-cell count)
Normal-pressure hydrocephalus (increased accumulation of cerebrospinal fluid [CSF] in the ventricles of the brain)
Depression (mental depression characterized by altered mood; use DSM-IV criteria to diagnose; refer to section on "Depression" in Chapter 13)
Mental disorder (review patient history; refer to Chapter 13)
Age-associated dementia (cognitive impairment associated with age)
Chronic subdural hematoma (review patient history for trauma/injuries)
Hypothyroidism (fatigue, weight gain, dry skin; diagnosed via elevated levels of thyroid-stimulating hormone [TSH])

Vitamin B_{12} deficiency (fatigue, weakness, confusion; diagnosed using CBC)

Diagnostic Tests

Urinalysis (to rule out urinary tract infection)
Chest x-ray examination (to rule out lung infection)
ECG (to rule out cardiac problems)
CT or MRI scan of head (to rule out brain disorders, tumors, masses)
Electroencephalography (to rule out seizures)
CSF analysis—possible decreased amyloid b protein and increased tau
   protein
Blood studies may include
   CBC count with differential (to rule out systemic infection)
   Serum folate
   Vitamin B_{12} (to rule out vitamin B_{12} deficiency)
   Rapid plasma reagin test (to rule out syphilis)
   Chemistry panel (to rule out electrolyte imbalances)
   Blood urea nitrogen and creatinine (to rule out renal impairment)
   TSH (to rule out hyper/hypothyroidism)
   Human immunodeficiency virus (HIV) studies (to rule out HIV infection)

Management/Treatment

Pharmacologic Management

Effective in only ~30% of clients.
Tracine (Cognex), 10 mg PO QID, with 10-mg QID increments every
   4 weeks, up to 40 mg QID.
Donepezil (Aricept), 5 mg PO QHS; increased to 10 mg QHS after 1 month
Antidepressants may be helpful in patients with depression; serotonin
   selective reuptake inhibitors work best.
Antipsychotics for sundowning, aggressive behaviors (haloperidol [Haldol],
   thioridazine HCl [Mellaril]).
Hypnotics (tamazepam [Restoril], zolpidem tartrate [Ambien]) for sleep
   disturbances; use with caution.

Nonpharmacologic Management

Daily schedules, routines
Behavioral strategies
Support and education for caregivers (provide information on support
   groups)
Adult day care

Complementary/Alternative Therapies

Gingko biloba extract, 40 mg PO TID, may help with performance.

Client (Caregiver) Education

Disease process and prognosis
Importance of utilizing support groups
Use of hospice care, especially with disease worsening

Follow-up

Regularly and in conjunction with medical management team, assess:

Mental status
Nutritional status
Environment safety
Status of caregiver(s)

Referral

Refer to neurologist and/or specialist in Alzheimer's disease for initial diagnosis and management plan.
Refer family members and caregivers to support groups.
Refer client to a hospice.

FIBROMYALGIA

SIGNAL SYMPTOMS ▸ chronic muscle/solt tissue pain

ICD-9 Codes	345.90	Neurasthenia
	729.1	Fibromyalgia

Fibromyalgia (fibromyalgia syndrome [FMS]) is a rheumatic syndrome that is characterized by pain (especially specific tender points), generalized muscle aches, stiffness, fatigue, and nonrestorative sleep. Fibromyalgia is often associated with chronic fatigue syndrome (CFS); 75% of clients with CFS also meet the criteria for FMS.

There are two types of FMS:

Primary FMS: No secondary diagnosis is present.
Secondary FMS: Syndrome has an underlying cause, such as trauma or skeletal malalignment.

Epidemiology

Approximately 6 million people have been diagnosed with FMS.
Overall prevalence is 2% (3.4% for women; 0.5% for men).
There is a 3:1 predominance for women as compared with men.
Common in women aged 50 years and older.
Depression is present in 20% of patients with FMS.

Etiology

Cause is unknown; CFS and FMS have been thought to be linked to the Epstein–Barr virus.

Physiology and Pathophysiology

The current theory is that of central sensitization, or the increased excitability of second-order spinal cord neurons. This results in pain, more specifically, the perception of that pain is greater than what is to be expected (hyperalgesia). FMS is thought to be a combination of neuroendocrine abnormalities, muscle-tissue abnormalities, neurotransmitter changes, and sleep disturbances.

Clinical Manifestations

Subjective

Obtain a complete history, including social, family, stress, and work history.

Stiffness, usually in the morning (75%–90% of clients).

Nonrestorative sleep.

Overfatigue.

Headaches (45%–60% of clients).

Feeling of "puffiness" in joints.

Chemical hypersensitivity (adverse reactions to strong odors, such as pollution, fumes, perfume).

Irritable bowel and bladder symptoms may also be present (40%–60% of clients).

Depression may be present.

Objective

Perform a thorough review of systems (include musculoskeletal, sleep, gastrointestinal, genitourinary, pain).

May need to observe patient over time to confirm diagnosis.

Diagnostic Criteria

Defined by the American College of Rheumatology. See Table 12–3.

Differential Diagnosis

Chronic Epstein–Barr virus infection (diagnosed via Epstein–Barr antibody test)

Chronic fatigue syndrome (severe, prolonged fatigue)

HIV infection (diagnosed with positive enzyme-linked immunoassay/Western blot tests)

Hypothyroidism (fatigue, weight gain, dry skin; diagnosed by elevated TSH level)

Lymphoma (consider if signs and symptoms persist despite treatment)

Multiple sclerosis (weakness/numbness in one or more limbs; visual disturbances; diagnosed via MRI; refer to section on "Multiple Sclerosis" below)

Neuropathies (numbness in extremities; refer to section on "Peripheral Neuropathies" below)

Rheumatoid arthritis (diagnosed via positive rheumatoid factor, elevated erythrocyte sedimentation rate and antinuclear antibody [ANA] test)

Sleep apnea (constant fatigue, waking in the middle of the night gasping for air; diagnosed via sleep studies)

Depression/anxiety (mental depression characterized by altered mood; use DSM-IV criteria to diagnose; refer to section on "Depression" in Chapter 13)

Diagnostic Tests

CBC, electrolytes, sedimentation rate, ANA, and rheumatoid factor (to rule out immune system diseases)

TSH and thyroid profile (to rule out thyroid disease)

Table 12–3 Diagnostic Criteria for Fibromyalgia*

History Criteria	Pain is considered widespread when ALL of the following are present: Pain in the left side of the body Pain in the right side of the body Pain above the waist Pain below the waist Axial skeletal pain (cervical spine, anterior chest, thoracic spine, or low back)
Pain Criteria	Pain exists in 11 of 18 tender points (trigger points) on digital palpation (at a force of at least 4 kg): Occiput: bilateral, at the suboccipital muscle insertions Low cervical: bilateral, at the anterior aspects of the intertransverse spaces at C5–C7 Trapazius: bilateral, at the midpoint of the upper border Supraspinatus: bilateral, at origins above the scapula spine near the medial border Second rib: bilateral, at the second costochondral junctions, just lateral to the junctions on upper surfaces Lateral epicondyle: bilateral, 2 cm distal to the epicondyles Gluteal: bilateral, in upper quadrants of buttocks in anterior fold of muscle Greater trocanter: bilateral, posterior to the trocanteric prominence Knee, bilateral, at the medial fat pad proximal to the joint line For a tender point to be "positive," the client must state that the palpation was painful. A statement of "tender" is not considered "painful."

*Client must have a history of widespread pain (present for at least 3 months) in specific anatomic areas and must exhibit this pain during an examination of tender points.

X-ray examination (to rule out suspected orthopedic problems, if indicated)
MRI, nerve-conduction studies (to rule out neurologic pathologies, if indicated)

Management/Treatment

Pharmacologic Management

 CP 12–2 Clinical Pearl: It is important to start LOW and go SLOW.

ANALGESICS

Acetaminophen (Tylenol), 650 mg Q4–6H

Tramadol HCl (Ultram), 50 mg Q4–6H

Nonsteroidal antiinflammatory drugs (NSAIDs) generally are not necessary, because FMS is not an inflammatory process. However, if concurrent musculoskeletal pain and/or arthritis is present, NSAIDs may be on option.

MUSCLE RELAXANTS

Cyclobenzaprine (Flexeril), 10 mg Q8H, is helpful (may cause drowsiness). Do not use with Ultram.

ANTIDEPRESSANTS

Serotonin selective reuptake inhibitors (Prozac, Zoloft, and Paxil) are especially helpful, and should be given in the morning.

Tricyclic antidepressants (amitriptyline, nortriptyline) and other antidepressants (trazadone) can be helpful with nonrestorative sleep.

Low-dose anesthetic injections at tender points (2–3 ml of 1% lidocaine can provide relief, but should not be given routinely).

Nonpharmacologic Management

Exercise, especially walking and water exercise, is strongly encouraged (advise patients to start slowly and gradually increase time and endurance).

Massage.

Stretching.

Healthy, balanced diet.

Behavioral modification for physical and emotional stress.

Transcutaneous electrical nerve stimulation.

Complementary/Alternative Therapies

Acupuncture

Chiropractic medicine

Tai chi

Biofeedback

Hypnosis

Client Education

It is imperative to discuss the course of the disease, and that time and patience are necessary in the treatment course. FMS is a documented disorder with real symptoms; however, it does not have to be crippling or life-threatening.

Encourage functional improvement, not total pain eradication.

Encourage empowerment of clients in the course of their treatment.

Advise patients about the side effects of medications.

Educate patients on local and national resources.

Follow-up

At initial diagnosis, follow-up should be quite regular, to establish most effective treatment plan.

Once treatment plan is effective and stabilized, clients do not need to be seen as often.

Referral

Refer to rheumatologist, especially for initial diagnosis and treatment failures.

GUILLAIN–BARRÉ SYNDROME

SIGNAL SYMPTOM limb weakness

ICD-9 Code	357.0	Guillain–Barré Syndrome

Guillain–Barré syndrome is a disorder of sudden onset of progressive weakness, often beginning distally, and progressing to sensory loss.

Epidemiology

0.5–2.0 cases per 100,000 U.S. population annually.
Occurs in all ages.
Equal male:female predominance.
Usually affects individuals 50–75 years of age.
Mortality rate is 3%–10%.

Etiology

Thought to be autoimmune.
Can follow infectious process.
1976–77 swine flu vaccine triggered 1/100,000 cases.

Physiology and Pathophysiology

Destruction of the myelin sheath that covers peripheral nerves, usually via an autoimmune inflammatory pathway, causes paralysis and loss of motor function. Guillain–Barré syndrome is usually triggered by surgery, pregnancy, or vaccinations.

Clinical Manifestations

Subjective

Gradual onset of:

Weakness, usually in lower limbs, and progresses to upper limbs
"Glove and stocking" numbness sensation
Back pain
Double vision
Possible urinary difficulties

Objective

Do a complete physical examination, including neurologic and respiratory assessment. Findings may include facial diplegia, ophthalmoplegia, blood pressure fluctuations, cardiac arrhythmias, and decreased ankle reflexes progressing proximally.

Differential Diagnosis

Any of the following diagnoses can present with weakness or numbness

Paralysis (complete loss of sensation)
Spinal cord lesions (review patient history; diagnosed via MRI)
Polio (review patient history, including immunizations)
Myasthenia gravis (muscular weakness with fatigue)
Vitamin B_{12} deficiency (fatigue, weakness, confusion; diagnosed via CBC)
Metals/toxins exposure (review patient history)

Diagnostic Tests

CBC (to rule out systemic infection)
Chemistry panel (to rule out electrolyte disorders)
TSH level (to rule out thyroid disorders)
Urinalysis (to rule out urinary disorders)

Management/Treatment

There is no cure for Guillain–Barré syndrome; however, most clients recover. Treatment includes IV fluids, nutritional support, and prevention of complications.

Client Education

Explain disease process and prognosis.
Encourage physical rehabilitation.

Follow-up

After hospitalization and regularly for 6–12 months afterward.

Referral

Refer to physician (neurologist) for hospitalization.
Referral for psychological counseling may be necessary to help patients adjust.

HEADACHE: CLUSTER

SIGNAL SYMPTOMS ▶ headache, eye pain, tearing

ICD-9 Codes	345	Headache
	346.2	Variants of migraine (includes cluster/histamine)

Cluster headaches are attacks of severe, unilateral pain around the eye and temple area, with ipsilateral lacrimation, rhinorrhea, ptosis, miosis, and nasal stuffiness. They may occur 1–3 times per day, for up to 12 weeks, followed by 1–24 months without an attack. They seem to occur during characteristic times of the year, particularly vernal and autumnal equinoxes, hence the name "clusters."

See Table 12–4 for general information about headaches.

Epidemiology

Very rare
69 per 100,000 population
Occur more commonly in men (6:1 ratio)
Mean age of onset—30 years in men, later in women
Sufferers are more likely to abuse nicotine and/or alcohol
Often misdiagnosed
Average primary-care provider will see 1–2 cases in entire career

Etiology

Cause unknown
Possibilities:
Disorder of arterial tone in cerebral arteries
Disturbance in circadian rhythms based in hypothalamus
Disorder of serotonin metabolism or transmission in the central nervous system (CNS)
Disorder of histamine concentrations or receptors

Table 12–4 Headaches

Headaches can indicate myriad diagnostic possibilities, but fortunately, they usually are not caused by underlying disease. Fewer than 1% of cases of headache represent a serious disease process.

In 1988, the International Headache Society (IHS) published a hierarchical classification system and operational diagnosis criteria for all headaches.

1 Migraine
2 Tension-type headache
3 Cluster headache and chronic paroxysmal hemicrania
4 Miscellaneous headaches not associated with a structural lesion
5 Headache associated with head trauma
6 Headache associated with vascular disorders
7 Headache associated with nonvascular intracranial disorder
8 Headache associated with substances or their withdrawal
9 Headache associated with noncephalic infections
10 Headache associated with metabolic disorder
11 Headache or facial pain associated with disorder of cranium, neck, eyes, ears, nose, sinuses, teeth, mouth, or other facial or cranial structures
12 Cranial neuralgias, nerve trunk pain, and deafferentation pain
13 Headache not classifiable

Headache is the second most common chronic symptom presented to health-care providers.
Headaches affect up to 90% of the population annually.
Over 75% of females and over 50% of males report at least one significant headache per month.
Only 5%–7% of the population will seek medical assistance for their headache symptoms.
45 million Americans suffer from chronic severe headache pain.
Usual age of onset is 15–35 years; prevalence is highest in the 35–45 age group.
Incidence tends to decrease in those >45 years of age.
Headache is three times more common in women than in men.
   There is a correlation between headache and the reproductive phase.
   Headaches usually begin during adolescence and taper off after menopause.
   There are some women who have headaches only premenstrually, related to prostaglandin synthesis at that time.
   Migraine in pregnancy may improve after the first trimester; however, failure of migraine to improve during pregnancy implies greater likelihood of pre-eclampsia.
Cost of headaches
   >150 million work days lost annually
   >$50 billion lost each year (absenteeism, reduced employee productivity, and medical expenses)
Primary headaches:
   Includes migraine, cluster, and common tension-type/muscle contraction headaches
   Comprise 90%–98% of headaches
   "Rules of Thumb":
      Linked to hormonal cycles
      Worse with sensory stimuli (sight, sound, smell)
      Improved with sleep
      Change location
   Almost all clients have one of three benign (primary) headache disorders:
      Cluster headache
      Migraine headache
      Tension-type/muscle contraction headache
Secondary headaches:
   A result of an identifiable structural or physiologic pathology (cerebrovascular lesions; meningeal irritation; intracranial pressure changes; and facial, cervical, systemic, or traumatic causes)
   Red flags:
      First headache
      Worst headache patient has ever had
      Different headache
      No response to treatment

Table continued on following page.

Table 12–4   Headaches (*Continued*)

Abnormal neurologic examination
History of trauma
Abnormal vital signs
Altered level of consciousness
Stiff neck
Papilledema
Pupils unreactive
Visual-field deficit

Only 1 in 250,000 clients who present with a chief symptom of headache will have a secondary cause of headache.

Physiology and Pathophysiology

A cluster headache is thought be due to a neuronal component, with implication of the trigeminal nerves and the trigeminal vascular system. There may also be involvement of the hypothalamus, with the biologic clock mechanism.

Clinical Manifestations

Subjective

Episodes of constant, severe, unilateral orbital pain with rapid onset (within 15 minutes) and rapid resolution (within 2 hours).

Episodes occur in clusters lasting weeks to months.

Severe, piercing, or boring pain.

Objective

Ipsilateral lacrimation (84%)
Infected conjunctiva (58%)
Ptosis (57%)
Nasal stuffiness (48%)
Rhinorrhea (43%)
Bradycardia (43%)
Nausea (40%)
Perspiration (26%)

Differential Diagnosis

Headache secondary to other pathology (positive findings on diagnostic tests)

Migraine headache (usually not behind eye; may have concurrent neurologic symptoms)

Trigeminal neuralgias (tender facial points, can have violent muscle spasms)

Temporal arteritis (headache, facial pain, visual loss)

Pheochromocytoma (elevated blood pressure)

Diagnostic Tests

Generally not done, unless to rule out differential diagnosis; MRI scan may be done for atypical presentations.

Management/Treatment

Pharmacologic Management

ABORTIVE TREATMENT

Because these headaches develop rapidly and are short and often severe, treatment must work rapidly and be highly effective; daily administration of medication may be necessary.

Sumatriptan (Imitrex), 6 mg SC, may repeat dose in 1 hour.

100% oxygen at 10–12 L per minute via non-rebreather mask for 10–15 minutes provides relief for 70%–80% of clients.

PROPHYLACTIC TREATMENT

Ergotamine (Cafergot) (timed to provide peak dose at anticipated time of attack), 2 mg PR 1 hour before; 1–2 mg PO 2 hours before

Prednisone (Deltasone), 80 mg /day, followed by rapid tapering over 6 days OR 40 mg/day for 5 days, tapering over 3 weeks

Lithium carbonate (Eskalith), 300 mg 2–4 times daily

Nonpharmacologic Management

Rest.

Avoid bright lights or glare.

Avoid nicotine and alcohol.

Client Education

Educate about nature of headaches.

Assist patients in learning self-treatment methods.

Discuss side effects of medications.

Follow-up

If treatment does not work or headaches become more frequent.

Referral

Refer to neurologist, especially if treatment fails.

HEADACHE: MIGRAINE

SIGNAL SYMPTOMS ▶ headache, neurologic symptoms

ICD-9 Codes	345	Classical migraine
	345.90	Variants of migraine
	346.9	Migraine, unspecified
	345	Headache, unspecified

The word *migraine* comes from the Latin roots *hemi* and *cranium,* meaning "one side of the head." A migraine headache, commonly referred to just as a "migraine," generally is a throbbing, unilateral headache, often preceded by neurologic manifestations. Migraine headaches are one of the more common reasons patients visit their primary-care providers.

Table 12–5 Migraine Headaches

Criteria	Migraine without Aura
A Headache frequency	At least 5 attacks fulfilling criteria B–D
B Duration	Headache lasting 4 to 72 h (untreated or unsuccessfully treated)
C Headache characteristics (headache has at least two of the characteristics listed)	Unilateral location Pulsating quality Moderate or severe intensity (inhibits or prohibits daily activities) Aggravation by walking stairs or similar routine physical activity
D Concurrent symptoms (during headache, at least one of the criteria listed is present)	Nausea and/or vomiting Photophobia and phonophobia
E Physical examination (at least one of the criteria listed)	History, physical, and neurological examinations do not suggest one of the disorders listed in groups 5–11 in Table 12–5. History and/or physical and/or neurologic examinations do suggest such a disorder, but it is ruled out by appropriate investigations. Such a disorder is present, but migraine attacks do not occur for the first time in close temporal relation to the disorder

Criteria	Migraine with Aura
A Headache frequency	At least two attacks fulfilling B
B Headache characteristics (at least three of the four characteristics listed)	One or more fully reversible aural symptoms indicating focal cerebral cortical and/or brainstem dysfunction. At least one aural symptom develops gradually over more than 4 minutes or two or more symptoms occur in succession. No aural symptom lasts more than 60 min. If more than one aural symptom is present, accepted duration is proportionally increased. Headache follows aura with a free interval of less than 60 min. (It may also begin before or simultaneously with the aura.)
C Physical examination (at least one of the criteria listed)	History, physical, and neurologic examinations do not suggest one of the disorders listed in groups 5–11 (in Table 12–4). History and/or physical and/or neurologic examinations do suggest such a disorder, but it is ruled out by appropriate investigations. Such a disorder is present, but migraine attacks do not occur for the first time in close temporal relation to the disorder.

Adapted from: New International Headache Society Definition of Migraine without Aura and Migraine with Aura Headache Classification Committee of the International Headache Society (1988). Classification and diagnostic criteria for headache disorders, cranial neuralgias and facial pain. *Cephalalgia.* 8(Suppl. 7), 1–96.

The International Headache Society (IHS) (see Table 12–5) classifies migraine headaches into three categories:

Migraine with aura (formerly called "classic")

Migraine without aura (formerly called "common")

Aura without headache

Epidemiology

More than 23 million Americans suffer from migraine headaches; over 10 million of these people experience moderate to severe disability.

3:1 predominance in females.

80% of patients with migraines have a family history of migraine headache.

Onset is usually during adolescence. Age of first onset usually between ages 10 and 30.

Etiology

Unknown; however, there is evidence that supports a strong genetic influence.

Can be "triggered" by stimuli in a susceptible individual. Common triggers include:

Certain foods (nitrites, chocolate)

Stress

Changes in temperature/weather

Fluctuating hormone levels/menstrual cycles

Disruption of sleep patterns (too much or too little)

Depression or anxiety

Too much or too little exercise

Smoking

Missed medication

Caffeine withdrawal, especially sudden withdrawal

Bright lights

Strong odors

Fasting

Head trauma

Loud noises

Physiology and Pathophysiology

Previous thoughts regarding the pathophysiology for migraine headaches included a rather simplistic vasoconstriction/vasodilatation theory. However, it is now believed that migraine headaches involve a complex interaction of vascular, biochemical, and neurologic factors.

Release of vasoactive substances (substance P, peptides, and neurokinin A) from the trigeminal nerves causes an inflammatory reaction around the blood vessels at the base of the brain and in the blood vessels of the dura and pia. This "neurogenic inflammation" may be accompanied by vasodilation (causing headache pain) and is triggered by nerve impulses in the caudal trigeminal nucleus. Because specific serotonin receptors (5-hydroxytryptamine) mediate this process, the newer "triptan" medications (which are 5-hydroxytryptamine blockers) work effectively to abort migraine headache pain.

Clinical Manifestations

Subjective

PREHEADACHE PHASE:

Prodrome: Up to 50% of clients with migraines suffer from a prodrome—symptoms that begin insidiously and develop slowly over the 24 hours preceding a migraine attack. Symptoms include mood fluctuations, gastrointestinal disturbances, food cravings, excessive yawning, and speech disturbances.

Aura: 10%–20% of clients with migraines experience an aura—distinct visual or other neurologic symptoms that last about 20–40 minutes then disappear before the pain of a headache begins. Symptoms include:

Flashing/shimmering lights (photopsia)

Zig-zag lines (fortification spectra)—Usually begin in the periphery of the visual field and spread toward the midline

Peripheral numbness/tingling

HEADACHE PHASE

Headache is usually unilateral, but not always.

Throbbing pain, that gradually increases in intensity, peaking in about 1 hour; may last for a few hours to several days (4–72 hours).

Nausea and/or vomiting may be present.

Increased sensitivity to light, sound, smells, and motion.

POSTHEADACHE PHASE

Once the pain has faded, client may be left with some or all of the following: diminished appetite, mood swings, fatigue, sore muscles.

Important subjective items to include in history are:

Onset

Duration

Frequency

Pain location

Pain quality

Associated symptoms

Triggers

Relieving factors

Objective

General appearance (note photophobia)

Vital signs (especially blood pressure, temperature)

Mental status (done throughout examination)

Neurologic examination:

Cranial nerves

Motor (gait, heel/toe walk, Romberg, deep knee bend, pronator drift)

Sensory (pain, vibration, stereognosis)
Reflexes
Scalp tenderness (cranial artery inflammation)
Eyes (pupils for light reflex, size, reactivity)
Corneas (clouding—glaucoma)
Neck (nuchal rigidity)

Differential Diagnosis

Tension headache (pain in head and neck; usually no neurologic symptoms; refer to section on "Headache: Tension" below)

Sinus headache/sinusitis (concurrent nasal drainage, possible fever, congestion)

Cluster headache (sharp pain behind eye, constant tearing; refer to section on "Headache: Cluster" above)

Temporal/cranial arteritis

Hypertension (elevated blood pressure)

Meningitis (nuchal rigidity, fever, hyperphotosensitivity, rash; diagnosed via spinal tap)

Temporomandibular joint dysfunction (jaw and/or ear pain, "clicking")

Trigeminal neuralgia (tender facial points, can have violent muscle spasms)

Ischemic events (review patient history; confirmed via diagnostic testing)

Subdural hematoma (review patient history for trauma/injuries; confirmed via diagnostic testing)

Mass lesions/brain abscess (confirmed via diagnostic testing)

Diagnostic Tests

Generally speaking, the client with a normal physical and neurologic examination and a history consistent with one of the patterns of a benign headache, should NOT be subjected to further diagnostic testing.

Keep in mind that sometimes diagnostic testing is used only for purposes of reassurance.

In clients who meet the criteria for migraine and have a normal neurologic examination, only 0.4% of imaging studies are positive for any abnormality.

Management/Treatment

Pharmacologic Management

<u>ABORTIVE TREATMENT</u>

NSAIDs:

Salicylic acid (ASA), 1 g Q6H, up to 4 g daily

Acetaminophen (Tylenol), 1 g Q6H, up to 4 g daily

Ibuprofen (Advil, Motrin), 800 mg Q6H, up to 2.4 g daily

Naproxen sodium (Anaprox), 825 mg initially; 220–550 mg Q3–4H, up to 1.5 g daily

Excedrin Migraine (aspirin, 250 mg ; acetaminophen, 250 mg; and caffeine, 65 mg)

Midrin (isometheptene dichlorophenazone acetaminophen), two capsules at onset of headache; can repeat one capsule Q1H up to five total (in 12 hours)

Butalbital-containing medications:

Fiorinal (aspirin, 325 mg; butalbital, 50 mg; and caffeine, 40 mg)

Fioricet/Esgic (acetaminophen, 325 mg; butalbital, 50 mg; and caffeine 40 mg)

Semispecific agents with ergotamine:

Cafergot (ergotamine tartrate, 2 mg; and caffeine, 100mg), one rectally at onset; one after 1 hour if needed (up to two total)

Wigraine (ergotamine tartrate, 1 mg; and caffeine, 100 mg): two PO at onset; one every 30 minutes PRN, up to six total

"Triptans:"

Naratriptan (Amerge), 1 or 2.5 mg PO with fluid;, repeat once after 4 hours when necessary

Rizatriptan (Maxalt), 5 or 10 mg PO; repeat once after at least 2 hours when necessary

Sumatriptan (Imitrex), 6 mg SC; repeat once after at least 1 hour when necessary; 5, 10, or 20 mg intranasally; repeat once after 2 hour when necessary; 50 mg PO with fluid,; repeat at intervals of at least 2 hours when necessary

Zolmitriptan (Zomig), 2.5 or 5 mg; dose can be repeated after 2 hours

Other

DHE-45 (dihydroergotamine), 1 mg IM or IV at onset; can give another 1 mg after 1 hour (up to 2 mg maximum)

Dihydroergotamine mesylate (Migranal) nasal spray, one spray each nostril (0.5 mg/spray), repeat 15 minutes later, up to six sprays maximum in 24 hours

SYMPTOMATIC TREATMENT

Nausea and vomiting

Prochlorperazine (Compazine), 5–10 mg IM

Promethazine (Phenergan), 25–50 mg IM or PR Q4–6H

Improve gastric motility and efficacy of oral agents

Metoclopramide (Reglan), 10 mg

PROPHYLACTIC TREATMENT

Use if:

Attacks occur more than two times per month.

Client has attacks with sufficient severity or disability.

Abortive agents do not work.

Client has a concurrent medical condition that is a relative indication for preventive therapy (e.g., hypertension and β-blocker use).

There is a question about quality of life.

β-blockers
  Atenolol (Tenormin), 50–100 mg QD
  Metoprolol (Lopressor), 50–300 mg QD
  Propranolol (Inderal), 40–320 mg QD
  Timolol (Blocadren), 20–60 mg QD

Tricyclic antidepressants
  Amitriptyline (Elavil), 10–300 mg QD
  Nortriptyline (Pamelor), 10–150 mg QD
  Doxepin (Sinequan), 10–200 mg QD
  Particularly useful with concurrent depression

Calcium Channel Blockers
  Verapamil (Calan, Isoptin), 120–720 mg QD

Anticonvulsants (clients with anxiety, bipolar disorder, or seizure disorder)
  Valproic acid (Depakene), 250–1500 mg QD

Nonpharmacologic Management

Eat regular meals; do not skip meals.
Try to avoid food triggers; limit caffeine intake.
Try to keep same sleep schedule.
Practice stress reduction/relaxation techniques.
Take hot baths.

Complementary/Alternative Therapies

Massage.
Biofeedback.
Acupuncture.
White willow bark can be helpful for headaches (dose unknown).
Feverfew (*Tanacetum parthenium*), 125 mg QD (25 mg of dried leaves BID or 82 mg of dried powdered leaves QD; however, higher doses may be needed) of standardized extract can be taken for migraine prophylaxis.
  Not recommended in pregnancy.
  Induces menstruation.
  Caution with anticoagulants.

Client Education

Explain diagnosis (in simple terms).
Educate about false beliefs.
Supply information about triggers.
Give information about all medications, including dosage, frequency, contraindications, and side effects.
Encourage patient to keep a headache diary:
  Date of attack
  Location, quality of pain
  Precipitating/relieving factors
  Associated symptoms

Follow-up

2–4 weeks after initial diagnosis to evaluate treatment plan

Once stabilized, in 6—12 months, depending on severity and frequency of headaches

Follow-up immediately if symptoms change or worsen

Referral

Refer to neurologist if all treatments fails.

Refer to pain specialist.

HEADACHE: TENSION

SIGNAL SYMPTOMS head, neck pain

ICD-9 Codes	345.90	Tension headache
	784.0	Headache, unspecified

A tension headache is described as an ache or sensation of tightness, pressure, or constriction that is widely varied in intensity, frequency, and duration. It is steady and dull, and it worsens as the day progresses. A tension headache can also be described as a bandlike pressure across the forehead and occiput. The headache may be accompanied by occipital and nuchal soreness. It is often associated with stress. The IHS differentiates tension headaches into episodic and chronic (Table 12–6).

Epidemiology

Approximately 90% of headaches are tension headaches.

40% of tension headaches sufferers have a positive family history.

Can occur at any age; rare in childhood and common in adulthood.

75% of sufferers are female.

Etiology

No single factor responsible

Commonly associated with psychological stress

Precipitants may include anxiety, depression, and situational stress, of which patients may be unaware

May occur secondary to muscle strain from cervical spondylosis or temporomandibular joint disease

Physiology and Pathophysiology

The pathophysiology is poorly understood. Experts suggest that the mechanism of tension headaches lies in the tender spots within the affected muscles, which transmit signals to the central nervous system through the A and C fibers of the trigeminal nerve and the upper three cervical roots. Once these signals are in the dorsal columns of the cord, the fibers ascend and ultimately reach the thalamus, which results in the perception of pain.

Table 12–6   Tension Headaches

Criteria	Episodic Tension-Type Headache	Chronic Tension-Type Headache
A Headache frequency	At least 10 previous headache episodes fulfilling criteria B-D. Number of days with such headache <180/year (<15/month). Headache lasting from 30 min to 7 days.	Average headache frequency 15 days/month (180 days/year) for 6 months fulfilling criteria B-D.
B Pain (at least 2 of the pain characteristics listed)	Pressing/tightening (nonpulsating) quality. Mild or moderate intensity (may inhibit but does not prohibit activities). Bilateral location. No aggravation by walking stairs or similar routine physical activity.	Pressing/tightening quality. Mild or moderate severity (may inhibit but does not prohibit activities). Bilateral location. No aggravation by walking stairs or similar routine physical activity
C Other (both of the criteria listed)	No nausea or vomiting (anorexia may occur). Photophobia and phonophobia are absent, or one but not the other is present.	No vomiting. No more than one of the following: nausea, photophobia, or phonophobia.
D Physical examination (at least one of the criteria listed)	History, physical, and neurologic examinations do not suggest one of the disorders listed in groups 5–11 in Table 12-4. History and/or physical and/or neurologic examinations do suggest such a disorder, but it is ruled out by appropriate investigations. Such a disorder is present, but tension-type headache does not occur for the first time in close temporal relation to the disorder.	History, physical, and neurologic examinations do not suggest one of the disorders listed in groups 5–11 in Table 12-4. History and/or physical and/or neurologic examinations do not suggest such a disorder, but it is ruled out by appropriate investigations. Such a disorder is present, but tension-type headache does not occur for the first time in close temporal relation to the disorder.

Adapted from: New International Headache Society Definition of Tension-Type Headache Headache Classification Committee of the International Headache Society (1988). Classification and diagnostic criteria for headache disorders, cranial neuralgias and facial pain. *Cephalalgia. 8* (Suppl. 7): 1–96.

Clinical Manifestations

Subjective

Mild or moderate dull ache or feeling of pressure.

Often reported as *bandlike* tightness around the head, or a *tight-cap* on top of the head.

Usually occurs bilaterally.

Can extend into the neck and shoulders.

May last an hour, all day, or longer.

Acute attacks often occur in the late afternoon or evening, when stress builds up.

Usually no nausea or vomiting.

Objective

Client may appear fatigued or stressed.

Results of examination are usually normal.

Results of cranial-nerve examination are normal.

Some muscles tightness may be palpated in the neck and shoulders.

Differential Diagnosis

Migraine headache (headache, often with neurologic symptoms; refer to section on "Headache: Migraine" above)

Cervical (musculoskeletal) spasm (cervical muscle tightness, decreased range of motion)

Diagnostic Tests

Usually not done, unless to rule out other pathology.

Management/Treatment

Pharmacologic Management

Analgesics are the standard line of treatment.

NSAIDs:

Ibuprofen (Advil, Motrin), 400–2400 mg/day

Naproxen (Aleve), 500 mg BID or TID

Naproxen sodium (Anaprox), 275 mg BID or TID

Ketoprofen (Orudis, Actron), 75 mg BID or TID

Muscle relaxants:

Cyclobenzaprine (Flexeril), 10 mg Q8H

Metaxalone (Skelaxin), 800 mg 3–4 times a day

Orphenadrine citrate (Norflex), 100 mg BID

Diazepam (Valium), 2–10 mg Q6–8H; most effective muscle relaxant, but use with caution because of addictive tendencies

Other:

Indomethacin (Indocin), 25–200 mg/day

Diclofenac sodium (Voltaren), 100–150 mg/day

Sulindac (Clinoril), 150–200 mg BID

Nonpharmacologic Management

Psychological therapy:

Stress management.

Formal psychotherapy may also be useful for patients who have associated anxiety and/or depression.

Physical therapy:

Ultrasound treatment

Electrical stimulation

Hot/cold packs

Stretching exercises
Aerobic exercise
Massage therapy

Complementary/Alternative Therapies
Biofeedback
Relaxation therapy
Hypnosis
Massage therapy

Client Education
Reassure.
Teach about medications and side effects.
Encourage clients to keep headache diary.
Stress reduction:
Help identify stressors.
Teach prioritizing.
Prescribe exercise and physical activity.

Follow-up
2–4 weeks after initial diagnosis to evaluate treatment plan, then 6–12 months after treatment stabilization.

Referral
Refer to neurologist or pain specialist if treatment fails.
Refer to physical therapist to assist in treatment.
Refer to psychotherapist to assist in stress reduction.

MENINGITIS (Bacterial and Viral)

SIGNAL SYMPTOMS ▶ stiff neck, fever, photophobia

ICD-9 Codes	320	Bacterial meningitis
	47.9	Unspecified viral meningitis

Meningitis is an inflammation of the meninges, in response to either bacteria or viruses.

Epidemiology
Incidence of bacterial meningitis is 20–100 per 100,000 newborns.
Infection with *Neisseria meningitidis* is 4.5 per 100,000 in children
3 months to 5 years of age.
Infection with *Streptococcus pneumoniae* is 2.5 per 100,000 children.
70% of meningitis cases occur in children under age 5 years.

Etiology
Bacterial:
Group B streptococcus (most common in first month of life)
Escherichia coli

Listeria monocytogenes
Streptococcus pneumoniae
Neisseria meningitidis
Haemophilus influenzae type b (rare because there is a vaccine)
Viral:
Coxsackievirus
Enteroviruses
Poliovirus
Mumps
Herpes (simplex and zoster)
Epstein–Barr virus
Cytomegalovirus
Previous upper respiratory infection

Physiology and Pathophysiology

Meningitis usually begins via nasopharyngeal colonization of bacteria or viruses. Pathogens enter the bloodstream via phagocytosis. It is then believed that continual exposure of the pathogens to the central nervous system results in an inadequate defense mechanism and, thus, replication within the cerebral spinal fluid.

Clinical Manifestations

The signs and symptoms listed below are for adults; for signs and symptoms in infants, see Age-Related Considerations 12–1.

Subjective
Fever/chills
Headache
Stiff neck
Nausea and vomiting
Light sensitivity

 Signs and Symptoms of Meningitis in Infants

Fever
Poor feeding
Lethargy
Irritability
Seizures
Rash
Jaundice
Vomiting/diarrhea
Altered sleep patterns
Bulging fontanelle (rare, and often late sign)

Skin rash, can be pruritic

Rhinitis, cough

Anorexia

Myalgias

Objective

Elevated temperature

Possible tachypnea

Irritability

Positive Kernig's sign (flexion of hip and knee, followed by straightening elicits resistance or pain)

Positive Brudzinski's sign (flexion of the neck produces hip and knee flexion)

Erythematous, macular, or vesicular rash

Differential Diagnosis

Seizures (convulsions; confirmed by electroencephalography)

Brain abscess (confirmed by CT or MRI scan)

Encephalitis (nuchal rigidity, changes in level of consciousness)

Migraine headache (headache, often with neurologic changes; refer to section on "Headache: Migraine" above)

Viral syndrome (symptoms can vary; negative diagnostic tests)

Trauma/injury (review patient history)

Child abuse (review patient history; refer to section on "Abuse: Physical" in Chapter 13)

Subdural hematoma (review patient history for trauma/injuries)

Diagnostic Tests

CBC with differential (to rule out infectious process)

CSF analysis (via lumbar puncture)—protein, glucose, cellular differential, Gram's stain (to confirm meningitis)

CSF, blood, and urine for bacterial culture (to determine specific pathogen)

Management/Treatment

Management of meningitis often involves hospitalization.

Pharmacologic Management

If bacterial, IV antibiotics are needed:

Ampicillin (Principen), 300–400 mg/kg

Cefotaxime (Claforan), 200 mg/kg/day Q4–6H

Ceftriaxone (Rocephin), 100 mg/kg/day Q12–24H

Aminoglycoside (tobramycin), 7.5 mg/kg/day Q6–8H

Vancomycin (Vancocin), 10 mg/kg IV Q6H or 500–2000 mg PO

If viral, antibiotics are not indicated, but are often given until diagnosis is firmly established:

If HSV is suspected, acyclovir (Zovirax), 10–15 mg/kg Q8H for 10 days.

If HIV is suspected, multidrug retroviral drug treatment is warranted.

Analgesics for pain:

Meperidine (Demerol), 25–50 mg IM Q4–6H

Morphine sulfate, 2–5 mg IM or IVQ4–6H

Antiemetics:

Promethazine (Phenergan), 25 mg IM Q4–6H

Proclorperazine (Compazine), 10 mg IM Q4–6H

Antipyretics:

Acetaminophen (Tylenol), 650 mg PO or PR Q4H (children: 10–15 mg/kg/dose)

Nonpharmacologic Management

Provide supportive care for patient and family.

Low lighting may be helpful for photophobia.

Client Education

Educate about course of disease and prognosis.

Stress importance of hospitalization.

May need to discuss possible complications for anticipatory guidance.

Follow-up

Monitor for complications such as deafness, seizure disorders (20%–30% of clients), motor deficits, language deficits, behavior disorders, and mental retardation.

Referral

Admit to hospital.

Refer to neurologist.

MULTIPLE SCLEROSIS

SIGNAL SYMPTOMS muscle weakness, visual changes

ICD-9 Code	340.0	Multiple sclerosis

Multiple sclerosis (MS) is a chronic disease of autoimmunity; it affects the myelin sheaths of the central nervous system (CNS), and usually affects people in the prime of lives. MS has a highly variable course, ranging from very mild to very severe.

Types of MS include:

Relapsing-remitting (the most common): Characterized by acute worsening of symptoms followed by stable periods, usually within 24 hours to weeks to months

Primary progressive: Characterized by slow progression of the disease, with or without improvements

Secondary progressive: Usually develops within 10 years in clients with relapsing MS; characterized by incomplete resolution of disability

Progressive relapsing (the least common): Clients with primary progression with one or more relapses

Epidemiology

Prevalence: 350,000 in the United States.

Incidence: 5/100,000 in the United States.

Seems to occur more commonly in the northern United States.

Scandinavians have a high occurrence of MS.

Typically occurs between ages 15 and 50, with peak onset around age 30.

The ratio of cases in women:men is 2:1.

95% of cases occur in Caucasians.

Etiology

The etiology is unknown, but current hypotheses include:

Viral etiology: Viral infection is the initial cause of MS.

Autoimmune etiology: The immune system is unable to respond and regulate myelin self-antigens.

Physiology and Pathophysiology

CNS lesions called plaques form in the white matter, and occasionally in the gray matter, of the brain and are characterized by inflammation and demyelination.

Clinical Manifestations

Subjective

Symptoms usually present very obscurely and can be highly varied.

Sensory changes—numbness, paresthesias

Weakness

Spasticity

Pain

Visual changes or difficulties

Peripheral facial weakness

Difficulty maintaining balance

Impaired mobility

Dizziness

Fatigue

Depression

Cognitive deficits

Genitourinary symptoms—bladder dysfunction

Objective

Unilateral or bilateral weakness

Hyperreflexia or loss of reflexes

Increased tone

Atrophy of muscles

Loss of peripheral sensation

Gait unsteadiness, uncoordination

Nystagmus

Decreased visual acuity and visual fields

Optic neuritis

Depressed affect

A neurologist will make the diagnosis. See Table 12–7 for the criteria for the diagnosis of MS.

Differential Diagnosis

Amyotrophic lateral sclerosis (muscle weakness and atrophy with spasticity and hyperreflexia)

Brainstem/cerebellar/spinal cord tumors (symptoms can vary from mild to complete paralysis; diagnosed with MRI)

Systemic lupus erythematosus (a chronic connective-tissue disease that can affect the skin, joints, and nervous system; can present with fever, joint pain, and malaise)

Lyme disease (red annular lesion ["target rash"] with associated fever, fatigue, headache, and malaise)

Sarcoidosis (a disease of widespread granulomatous lesions)

Cerebrovascular disease/vasculitis (unilateral weakness, numbness; refer to section on "Cerebrovascular Accident/Transient Ischemic Attack" above)

CNS infections (fever, changes in level of consciousness, headache)

Pernicious anemia (fatigue, weakness, possible confusion; diagnosed via CBC)

Leukodystrophies (a group of diseases of abnormal myelin formation)

Optic neuropathies (visual changes secondary to neurologic changes)

Diagnostic Tests

No single test can diagnose MS.

MRI (to identify lesions of the white matter).

CSF (to reveal increased mononuclear cells and protein and immunoglobulin levels).

Table 12–7   Criteria for the Diagnosis of MS

Definite MS	Clinical diagnosis: Two symptomatic attacks and clinical evidence of two separate lesions OR Two attacks, clinical evidence of 1 lesion, and paraclinical evidence of second lesion (e.g., MRI or evoked potential testing)
	Laboratory-supported diagnosis: Oligoclonal bands of increased immunoglobulin G synthesis in CSF AND Two attacks and clinical or paraclinical evidence of one lesion OR One attack and clinical evidence of two lesions OR One attack, clinical evidence of one lesion and paraclinical evidence of second lesion
Probable MS	Two attacks and clinical evidence of one lesion OR One attack and clinical evidence of two lesions OR One attack, clinical evidence of one lesion, and paraclinical evidence of second lesion

Evoked potential testing, including visual, brainstem/auditory, and somatosensory (to help detect the effects of demyelination).

Management/Treatment

All initial treatment will be decided by a neurologist.

Pharmacologic Management

Immunomodulators:

Betaseron (interferon beta-1b), 8 million IU SQ injections QOD

Avonex (recombinant human interferon beta-1a), 30 μg IM weekly

Noninterferon, nonsteroidal agents:

Copaxone (Glatiramer acetate), 20 mg SC injections daily

Acute relapse symptom management:

Methylprednisolone (Medrol), 1 g in 250 ml 5% dextrose in water, infused over 2–4 hours for 3–5 days

Followed by oral prednisone (Deltasone)

Fatigue:

Pemoline (Cylert), 37.5 mg PO QD (may increase 18.75 mg/day at weekly intervals up to 112.5 mg daily maximum)

Methylphenidate (Ritalin), 10–60 mg PO divided BID–TID

Amantadine, 100 mg PO BID–TID

Depression:

Fluoxetine (Prozac), 10–80 mg QD

Amitriptyline (Elavil), 75–150 mg PO BID–TID

Muscle spasticity:

Baclofen (Lioresal), 5 mg PO TID and titrate up to 100 mg/day TID–QID

Diazepam (Valium), 10–40 mg/day

Clonazepam (Klonopin), 0.5 mg PO TID

Nonpharmacologic Management

Energy conservation—naps

Moderate exercise

Occupational therapy

Client Education

Educate about disease process and progression.

Educate about systemic involvement and appropriate medications.

Explain high concurrence of depression.

Encourage healthy behaviors:

Not smoking.

Good nutrition—high fiber to prevent constipation.

Exercise in moderation.

Limited alcohol intake.

Client self-monitoring.

Pregnancy may cause relapse.

Follow-up

Regular client follow-up with neurologist is recommended.

Referral

Refer to neurologist for initial diagnosis and management plan.
Refer to urologist if bladder dysfunction persists,
Refer for counseling/therapy for persistent depression.
Refer to physical therapist for mobility problems.

PARKINSON'S DISEASE

SIGNAL SYMPTOMS rigidity, tremor, slow movement

ICD-9 Code	331.0	Parkinson's disease

Parkinson's disease is a progressive movement disorder of the CNS, of unknown etiology, with four characteristic features: slowness of movement, muscular rigidity, resting tremor, and postural instability.

Categories of Parkinson's disease include:

Idiopathic
Symptomatic
Parkinson-plus syndrome
Other heredodegenerative diseases
"Drug-induced" parkinsonism (seen in heroin addicts)

Epidemiology

Affects over 1 million Americans.
Fourth most common neurodegenerative disease.
Affects 1% of the population over age 65 years; 0.4% of population over age 40 years.
Mean onset is 57 years.
Incidence is greater in men, with a 3:2 ratio.

Etiology

Unknown
Possible factors include:
    Arteriosclerosis (blood supply to basal ganglia is compromised).
    Viral infections (encephalitis).
    Environmental toxins (pesticides) have been suspected.
    Drugs such as the phenothiazines and reserpine (reversible when discontinued)

Physiology and Pathophysiology

There is widespread destruction of neural cells in the zona compacta of the substantia nigra, the locus ceruleus, and the autonomic ganglia, due to a variety of causes. Thus, dopamine (DA), which is normally secreted in the caudate nucleus and putamen is no longer available to refine motor movements. There is also a loss of DA receptors in the caudate nucleus and putamen, further contributing to loss of refinement of motor movements. Acetylcholine-secreting neurons (excitatory signals) remain active.

Clinical Manifestations

Subjective

In initial stages, many clients do not have movement problems. They may report anxiety and difficulty sleeping.

Primary symptoms include:

Resting tremor (about two thirds of clients)
Bradykinesia (slowness of movement)
Postural instability (propulsion vs. retropulsion)
Rigidity

Other motor symptoms may include:

Dysarthria (reduced volume and/or raspy/hoarse quality)
Dysphagia
Flexed posture
"Freezing" at initiation of movement
Hypomimia (diminution of facial expression)
Hypophonia
Micrographia (very small handwriting)
Reduced frequency of blinking and swallowing
Decreased arm swing and slight food drag

See Table 12–8.

Objective

Assess autonomic system for:

Bladder and anal sphincter disturbance
Constipation
Diaphoresis
Orthostatic blood pressure changes
Paroxysmal flushing
Sexual disturbances

Assess mental status changes, including:

Confusional state
Dementia
Psychosis (paranoia, hallucinations)
Sleep disturbances

Assess for other changes, including:

Fatigue
Oily skin
Pedal edema
Seborrhea
Weight loss

Inclusion criteria

Presence of 1 year or more of two of the three cardinal motor signs:
    Resting/postural tremor
    Bradykinesia

Table 12–8   Rating Rigidity, Tremor, and Akinesia in Parkinson's Disease

Rating	Rigidity	Tremor	Akinesia (body bradykinesia and hypokinesia)
0	Absent	None	None
1	Slight or detectable only when activated by mirror or other movements	Slight Present infrequently	Minimal slowness Movement has a deliberate character (could be normal for some) Possibly reduced amplitude
2	Mild to moderate	Mild in amplitude Persistent OR Moderate in amplitude but only intermittently present	Mild slowness Poverty of movement (abnormal movement) Some reduced amplitude
3	Marked Full range of motion (ROM) easily achieved	Moderate in amplitude Present most of the time	Moderate slowness Poverty of movement OR Small amplitude
4	Severe ROM achieved with difficulty	Marked in amplitude Present most of the time	Marked sloweness Poverty of movement OR Small amplitude

Adapted from: Duvoisin, R.C. (1990). The differential diagnosis of Parkinson's disease. In G.M. Stern (ed.), *Parkinson's disease (pp. 431–491).* London: Chapman & Hall.

Rigidity

Positive response to levodopa therapy with moderate to marked improvement and duration of improvement for 1 year or more.

Differential Diagnosis

Essential tremor (a benign tremor made worse with action or movement)

Drug-induced parkinsonism (review patient history and medications)

Multisystem atrophy (loss of general muscle tissue)

Progressive supranuclear palsy (neck dystonia, rigidity, ocular changes)

Huntington's disease (progressive dementia with bizarre involuntary movements)

Normal-pressure hydrocephalus (increased accumulation of CSF in the ventricles of the brain)

Multiple lacunar strokes (review patient history; refer to section on "Cerebrovascular Accident/Transient Ischemic Attack" above)

Posttraumatic parkinsonism (review patient history)

Depression (mental depression characterized by altered mood; refer to section on "depression" in Chapter 13)

Diagnostic Tests

No laboratory test can confirm the diagnosis.

MRI or CT scan (to rule out mass lesion, silent infarcts, or pressure hydrocephalus).

Management/Treatment

Explain to clients and family that there is no cure for Parkinson's disease. The goals of therapy are to delay disease progression, relieve symptoms, and preserve functional capacity; with the primary goal to maintain the client at *maximum function* with *minimal medication.*

Pharmacologic Management

MEDICATIONS THAT INCREASE DOPAMINE LEVELS

Sinemet (levodopa/carbidopa), 25/100 mg TID
  Combination helps cross the blood-brain barrier; helps prevent nausea and vomiting associated with dopamine.
  Most efficacious treatment.
  Helps confirm diagnosis
  Short duration of action requires frequent dosing.
  Can have a "wearing off" phenomenon.
Symmetrel (amantadine), 100 mg BID
  Works synergistically with levodopa.

MEDICATIONS THAT STIMULATE DOPAMINE RECEPTORS

Parlodel (bromocriptine), 5–40 mg/day
Permax (Pergolide), 1–5 mg/day
Mirapex (Pramipexole), 0.125–4.5 mg/day in divided doses
Requip (Ropinirole), up to 24 mg/day TID
Adjuncts to levodopa therapy to help control motor fluctuations

MEDICATIONS THAT INHIBIT DOPAMINE METABOLISM

Eldepryl (Selegiline), 5 mg BID (monoamine oxidase B inhibitor)
Tasmar (Tolcapone), 100–200 mg TID
Adjunct therapy to levodopa to help improve psychomotor function

MEDICATIONS THAT RESTORE BALANCE BETWEEN CHOLINERGIC
AND DOPAMINERGIC INFLUENCES

Anticholinergics (may be helpful in reducing incidence of akinesia, rigidity, and tremor)
  Trihexyphenidyl (Artane), 2–5 mg BID/TID
  Benztropine (Cogentin), 1–2mg BID
  Diphenhydramine (Benadryl), 25 mg QHS

Nonpharmacologic Management

SURGERY

Thalamotomy
  Electrode is burrowed to thalamus.
  Intermedius region is usual target.
  Improves tremors and rigidity.
Pallidotomy
  Part of the basal ganglia is destroyed.
  Performed with local anesthetic, so client may participate in demonstrating mobility and cognition.

Adrenal medullary grafting.

Implantation of adrenal medulla tissue into nigra-striatal region

Mixed results.

Symptoms often return within 6 months.

SUPPORTIVE MEASURES

Physical therapy

Psychological support/therapy

Nutritional counseling/supplements

Techniques to manage sleep disturbances

Client Education

Be honest.

Give anticipatory guidance regarding the course of the disease.

Discuss the need for trial and error to obtain maximum medication benefit and minimal side effects.

Explain the need for frequent visits during initiation period.

Follow-up

Initially, follow up with neurologist to confirm diagnosis and initiate treatment.

May need occasional visits to neurologist.

Follow-up depends on response to pharmacological management.

Referral

Refer to neurologist.

PERIPHERAL NEUROPATHIES

SIGNAL SYMPTOMS peripheral pain, numbness

ICD-9 Codes	345.90	Peripheral neuropathy NOS
	345	Numbness, burning, or tingling
	782.0	Paresthesia NOS

Peripheral neuropathy is the sensation of numbness and occasionally pain, often associated with type 1 or type 2 diabetes mellitus.

Types of neuropathy include:

Diffuse

Peripheral

Autonomic (cardiovascular, gastrointestinal, genitourinary)

Focal (uncommon)

Epidemiology

Prevalence ranges from 10%–100% in clients with diabetes.

Seen in approximately 20% of clients with type 2 diabetes at times of diagnosis.

Foot ulcers will develop in 15% of clients with peripheral neuropathy; 25% of those clients will require amputation.

Etiology

Etiology is unknown; current theory holds that hyperglycemia coupled with insulin deficiency results in functional and structural defects, causing nerve damage and symptoms.

Physiology and Pathophysiology

Sensory neurons are damaged, resulting in loss of sensation and possibly ultimately pain.

Clinical Manifestations

Subjective

"Stocking and glove" (feet and hands) loss of sensation
Numbness, tingling in lower extremities and hands
Burning sensation
Pain

Objective

 CP 12–3   Clinical Pearl: It is important to do a thorough neurologic examination, focusing on the sensory portion, using a monofilament.

Decreased sensation
Diminished vibratory sensation
Decreased fine motor movement
Loss of ankle reflexes
Muscle weakness, atrophy
Charcot's joint (midfoot muscular collapse)

Also important to assess:
    Pulses
    Skin integrity, including between the toes

Differential Diagnosis

Pernicious anemia (fatigue, weakness, possible confusion; diagnosed via CBC)
Autoimmune diseases (wide variety of symptoms; diagnosed via elevated sedimentation rate and antinuclear antibodies)
Lyme disease (red annular lesion ["target rash"] with associated fever, fatigue, headache and malaise)
Toxic neuropathies (review patient history)

Diagnostic Tests

Nerve conduction studies may be useful (to confirm neuropathies)

Management/Treatment

 CP 12–4   Clinical Pearl: Strict glucose control may help prevent peripheral neuropathies.

Pharmacologic Management

Amitriptyline (Elavil), 150–200 mg/day PO

Carbamazepine (Tegretol), 100 mg PO BID, increased to 1000 mg/day

Ibuprofen (Advil, Motrin), 600 mg PO QID

Naproxen (Aleve), 250 mg PO Q6–8H

Capsaicin (Zostrix) cream (0.075%) applied topically TID–QID

Nonpharmacologic Management

Discuss and demonstrate strict foot care.

Use transcutaneous electrical nerve stimulation unit.

Physical therapy may be useful.

Client Education

Discuss and encourage meticulous foot care.

Discuss medication and side effects.

Encourage strict glucose control.

Follow-up

2–4 weeks after treatment plan initiated; sooner if symptoms worsen and/or change

Referral

Refer to neurologist if treatment fails.

Refer to physical therapist for additional treatment.

SEIZURES

SIGNAL SYMPTOM ▶ convulsions

ICD-9 Codes		
	345.90	Convulsions
	780.31	Fever convulsions
	345.0	Epilepsy, nonconvulsive
	345	Petit mal seizures
	345.90	Epilepsy, convulsive NOS
	345.10	Grand mal seizures

A seizure is a sudden alteration of behavior that may be characterized by changes in sensory or motor activities, or both. Epilepsy is a disease state characterized by recurrent seizures. Seizures are classified as:

Partial (focal) seizures (70% of seizures)—begin in a localized section of the brain

Simple partial

Complex partial

Partial seizures with secondary generalization

Generalized seizures

Absence seizures

Myoclonic seizures

Clonic seizures

Tonic seizures

Tonic–clonic seizures

Atonic seizures

Unclassified epileptic seizures

Epidemiology

2 million Americans have epilepsy.

10% of clients with epilepsy have a positive family history.

Isolated seizures can occur in 10% of population.

Etiology

Risk factors for epilepsy include:

Head trauma

CNS infection

Stroke

Brain surgery

Risk factors for nonepileptic seizures include:

Medications

Hypoglycemia

Migraines

Hypertension

Metabolic disorders

Physiology and Pathophysiology

Ionic imbalances, both intracellularly and extracellularly, cause depolarization and hyperpolarization. These changes in ionic gradients, along with activated neurotransmitters can cause seizures.

Clinical Manifestations

Subjective

May include but not limited to:

Fever

Headache

Loss of consciousness

Repetitive muscle contractions

Sustained muscle contractions

Include in history:

Location, onset, duration of seizure

Events preceding and following seizure

Sensory changes

Motor symptoms

Mood/affect changes

Pain/discomfort

Medical history

Prenatal history, labor, and delivery

Family history

Exposure to metals/toxins

Objective

Perform a complete physical examination, including a thorough neurologic assessment.

Differential Diagnosis

Any of the following diagnoses can cause seizures; it is imperative to take a thorough patient history.

Hypoxia
Injury
Infection
Fever
Metabolic disorder
Drug/alcohol withdrawal
Tumor
Vascular disease

Diagnostic Tests

Electroencephalogram (to confirm brain-wave abnormalities)
CBC with differential (to rule out infection)
Urinalysis (to rule out urinary infection)
Drug/alcohol screening (to rule out drug/alcohol withdrawal)
Lead/metal screening (to rule out exposure to toxins)
ECG (to rule out cardiac disorders)
Chemistry panel (to rule out electrolyte disorder)
CT scan (to rule out cerebral abnormalities such as tumor or mass)
Lumbar puncture (to rule out neurologic infectious process, such as meningitis)

Management/Treatment

Pharmacologic Management

 CP 12–5   Clinical Pearl: It is important to start LOW and go SLOW.

Carbamazepine (Tegretol), 200–300 mg PO BID
Phenytoin (Dilantin), 300–500 mg PO QD
Valproate (Depakote), 500–4000 mg QD
Phenobarbital (Donnatal), 60–240 mg PO QD
Neurontin (Gabapentin), 300 mg PO TID

Newer drugs include:

Lamotrigine (Lamictal), 25 mg PO QOD
Topiramate (Topamax), 25 mg PO BID
Tiagabine (Gabitril), 4 mg PO QD
Fosphenytoin (Cerebyx), 10–20 phenytoin-equivalents/kg IV or IM (not approved for pediatric patients)
Diazepam rectal gel (Diastat), 15–20 mg PR (infants and children: 2.5–5.0 mg PR)

Nonpharmacologic Management
Possible ketogenic diet
Medication compliance

Client Education
Type of seizure.
Monitoring of symptoms.
Medications used and side effects.
Clients who are seizure-free for 2 years, may be considered for medication withdrawal.

Follow-up
Blood work may be necessary to determine serum levels, depending on the medication used.

Referral

Refer to neurologist for initial diagnosis and management plan, and/or if control is not achieved.

REFERENCES

Bell's Palsy
Billue, J.S. (1997). Bell's palsy: An update on idiopathic facial paralysis. *Nurse Practitioner, 22*(8), 88–105.

Zalvan, C.H., Huo, J., & Selesnick, S.H. (1999). Bell's palsy: An update on causes, recognition, therapy. *Consultant 39*(1), 39–48.

Cerebrovascular Accident/Transient Ischemic Attack
Boderick, J.P. (1998). Practical considerations in the early treatment of ischemic stroke. American Family Physician, 57(1), 73–80.

Hart, R.G. & Benavente, O. (1999). Stroke: Part I. A clinical update on prevention. *American Family Physician, 59,* 2475–2482.

Kelley, R.E. (1999). CT versus MRI: Which is better for diagnosing stroke? *Patient Care, 33*(6), 175–182.

Ozer, M.N., Roth, E., & Young, M.A. (1999). New approaches, improved outcomes in stroke rehabilitation. *Patient Care, 33*(7), 162–180.

Ryan, M., Combs, G., & Penix, L.P. (1999). Preventing stroke in patients with transient ischemic attacks. *American Family Physician, 60,* 2329–2336.

Selman, W.R., Tarr, R., & Landis, D. (1997). Brain attack: emergency treatment of ischemic stroke. *American Family Physician, 55,* 2655–2662.

Schretzman, D. (1999). Acute ischemic stroke. *Nurse Practitioner, 24*(2), 71–88.

Dementia
Bryant, H. (1998). Dementia in the primary care setting. *Advance for Nurse Practitioners, 6*(7), 29–33.

Delagarza, V.W. (1998). New drugs for Alzheimer's disease. *American Family Physician, 58,* 1175–1182.

Fletcher, K., & Damgaard, P. (1998). A glimmer of hope. *Advance for Nurse Practitioners, 6*(5), 49–84.

Kelley, R.E. (1999). Keeping current on Alzheimer's disease. *Patient Care, 33*(10), 127–146.

Mangino, M., & Middlemiss, C. (1997). Alzheimer's disease: Preventing and recognizing a misdiagnosis. *Nurse Practitioner, 22,* 58–75.

Oiler, C., & Vernon, G.M. (1998). Primary care of the older adult with end-stage Alzheimer's disease. *Nurse Practitioner, 23*(4), 63–83.

Sloane, P.D. (1998). Advances in the treatment of Alzheimer's disease. *American Family Physician, 58,* 1577–1586.

Fibromyalgia

Alarcon, G.S. (1999). Fibromyalgia: Dispelling diagnostic and treatment myths. *Women's Health in Primary Care, 2,* 775–784.

Clark, S., & Odell, L. (2000). Fibromyalgia syndrome: Common, real and treatable. *Clinician Reviews, 10*(5), 57–83.

Marlowe, S.M. (1998). Calming the fire of fibromyalgia: Examining symptoms and strategies. *Advance for Nurse Practitioners, 6*(1), 51–55.

Millea, P.J., & Holloway, R.L. (2000). Treating fibromyalgia. *American Family Physician, 62,* 1575–1582.

Headache

Barrett, E. (1996). Primary care for women: Assessment and management of headache. *Journal of Nurse Midwifery, 41,* 117–124.

Bartleson, J.D. (1999). Treatment of migraine headaches. *Mayo Foundation for Medical Education and Research, 74,* 702–708.

Biondi, D.M., Elkind, A.H., & Silberstein, S.D. (1998). Emerging migraine treatments. *Patient Care Nurse Practitioner, 1*(7), 10–26.

Coutin, I.B., & Glass, S.F. (1996). Recognizing uncommon headache syndromes. *American Family Physician, 54,* 2247–2252.

DeRaps, P.K. (1999). Migraine management: New approaches focus on serotonin receptors. *Advance for Nurse Practitioners, 7*(5), 51–55.

Diamond, S., Lipton, R.B., Cady, R.K., Diamond, M.L., & Kaniecki, R.G. (2000). Migraine: New perspectives on diagnosis and therapy. *Consultant, 40*(11), S1–S32.

Kumar, K.L., Ninan, T.M., & Silberstein, S.D. (1995). Migraine: Finding the road to relief. *Patient Care, 29*(14), 1–18.

Headache Classification Committee of the International Headache Society (1988). Classification and diagnostic criteria for headache disorders, cranial neuralgias and facial pain. *Cephalalgia, 8*(Suppl. 7), 1–96.

Login, I.S. (2000). New approaches to diagnosing and managing migraine in women. *Women's Health in Primary Care, 3*(8), 569–580.

Mendizal, J.E. (1998). The clinical challenge of chronic daily headaches. *Patient Care Nurse Practitioner, 1*(5), 41–46.

Moloney, M.F., Matthews, K.B., Scharbo-Dehaan, M., & Strickland, O.L. (2000). Caring for the woman with migraine headaches. *Nurse Practitioner 25*(2), 17–39.

Moore, K.L,. & Noble, S.L. (1997). Drug treatment of migraine, Part I. Acute therapy and drug-rebound headache. *American Family Physician XX,* 2039–2051.

Noble, S.L., & Moore, K.L. (1997). Drug treatment of migraine, Part II. Preventive therapy. *American Family Physician, XX,* 2270–2286.

Pfeiffer, G.M. (1997). Tension headaches: A systematic approach. *Advance for Nurse Practitioners, 8,* 25–31.

Weiss, J. (1999). Assessing and managing the patient with headaches. *Nurse Practitioner, 24*(7), 18–35.

Meningitis

Norris, C.M., Danis, P.G., & Gardner, T.D. (1999). Aseptic meningitis in the newborn and young infant. *American Family Physician, 59,* 2761–2770.

Willoughby, R.E., & Polack, F.S. (1999). What's new in meningitis management. *Patient Care, 33*(11), 237–254.

Tunkel, A.R., & Scheld, W.M (1997). Issues in the management of bacterial meningitis. *American Family Physician, 56,* 1355–1362.

Multiple Sclerosis

Giesser, B.S. (1998). Managing multiple sclerosis. *Clinical Advisor, 1*(5), 61–65.

Greenstein, J.I. (2000). A family physician's guide to multiple sclerosis: Diagnostic and treatment considerations. New York: National Multiple Sclerosis Society.

Holland, N., & Halper, J. (1999). Management of multiple sclerosis. *Advance for Nurse Practitioners, 7*(3), 27–32.

Hess, G.C. (2000). Multiple sclerosis: New help, new hope. *Consultant, 40*(5), 1085–1100

Smiroldo, J., & Coyle, P.K. (1999). Advances in the treatment of multiple sclerosis. *Patient Care, 33*(11), 88–106.

Stuibergen, A., Becker, H., Rogers, S., Timmerman, G., & Kullberg, V. (1999). Promoting wellness for women with multiple sclerosis. *Journal of Neuroscience Nursing, 31*(2), 73–79.

Parkinson's Disease

Duvoisin, R.C. (1990). The differential diagnosis of Parkinson's disease. In G.M. Stern (Ed.), *Parkinson's disease* (pp. 431–491). London Chapman & Hall.

Goetz, C. (1999). Augmentation therapies for advanced Parkinson's disease. *Patient Care, 33*(2), 108–121.

Imke, S. (1998). Parkinson's disease: A medical management update. *Advance for Nurse Practitioners, 6*(1), 24–28.

Lucey, G. (1998). *Parkinson's disease.* Prepared for Pharmacist's Letter and Prescriber's Letter. Document no. 140511. Stockton, Therapeutic Research Center.

Lustis, S. (1997). Pathophysiology and management of idiopathic Parkinson's disease. *Journal of Neuroscience Nursing, 29*(1), 24–31.

Tapper, V. (1997). Pathophysiology, assessment and treatment of Parkinson's disease. *Nurse Practitioner, 22*(7), 76–95.

Young, R. (1999). Update on Parkinson's disease. *American Family Physician, 59,* 2155–2170.

Peripheral Neuropathies

Apfel, S.C., Comi, R.J., & White, P.F. (2000). Diabetic neuropathy: Update your management. *Patient Care, 34*(17), 47–58.

Mangan, M.M. (1999). Diabetic neuropathy: Clinical evaluation and pain management. *Clinician Reviews, 9*(9), 61–78.

Seizures

Allen, T.G. (1997). Seizure disorders: A primary care guide. *Advance for Nurse Practitioners, 5*(10), 32–66.

Champi, C., & Gaffney-Yocum, P.A. (1999). Managing febrile seizures in children. *Nurse Practitioner, 24*(10), 28–43.

Hilton, G. (1997). Seizure disorders in adults: Evaluation and management of new onset seizures. *Nurse Practitioner, 22*(9), 42–59.

Hwang, J.Y., & Morrell, M.J. (1998). Coping with epilepsy in women. *Women's Health in Primary Care, 1*(6), 520–527.

Marks, W.J., & Garcia, P.A. (1998). Management of seizures and epilepsy. *American Family Physician, 57*(7), 1589–1600.

McAbee, G.N., & Wark, J.E. (2000). A practical approach to uncomplicated seizures in children. *American Family Physician, 62,* 1109–1115.

Smith, M. (1998). Epilepsy in the 90s. *Clinical Advisor, 1*(4), 60–65.

Thomson, L.R. (1998). Nonepileptic seizures. *Clinician Reviews, 8*(3), 81–96.

Valente, L.R. (2000). Seizures and epilepsy: Optimizing patient management. *Clinical Reviews, 10*(3), 79–103.

Valente, M.B., & Valente, S.M. (1998). Pediatric epilepsy : Primary care treatment and health care management. *Nurse Practitioner, 23*(11), 38–57.

RESOURCES

General

American Medical Association
    Telephone: 312-464-5000
    www.ama-assn.org/migraine

American Neurological Association
    Telephone: 612-545-6284
    www.aneuroa.org

Cerebrovascular Accident/Transient Ischemic Attack

National Stroke Foundation
    96 Inverness Dr., E.
    Suite I
    Englewood, CO 08112-5112
    Telephone: (800) STROKES (800-787-6537)
    www.stroke.org

National Aphasia Association
    156 Fifth Ave.
    Suite 707
    New York, NY 10010
    Telephone: (800) 922-4622
    www.aphasia.org

Stroke Connection of the American Stroke Association (part of American Heart Association)
    7272 Greenville Ave.
    Dallas, TX 75231-4596
    Telephone: (800) 553-6321
    www.americanheart.org/Stroke/index.html

National Association of Area Agencies on Aging
    927 15th St., NW
    6th Floor
    Washington, DC 20005
    Telephone: (202) 296-8130
    www.n4a.org

Dementia

The Alzheimers Association
    Telephone: (800) 272-3900
    www.alzheimers.com
    www.alz.org

National Hospice Organization
    1901 N. Moore St.
    Suite 901
    Arlington, VA 22209
    Telephone: (703) 243-5900

Alzheimer's Disease and Related Disorders Association Information
        and Referral Center
    Telephone: (800) 272-3900

National Alliance for the Mentally Ill
    Telephone: (800) 950-6264

National Institute of Aging Information Center
    Telephone: (800) 222-4225

Fibromyalgia

The Fibromyalgia Network
    P.O. Box 31750
    Tucson, AZ 85751
    Telephone: (800) 853-2929
    www.fmnetnews.com

Fibromyalgia Alliance of America
    P.O. Box 21990
    Columbus, OH 43221-0990
    Telephone: (888) 717-6711
    www.fmaa.org

National Fibromyalgia Awareness Campaign
    2415 N. River Trail Rd., #200
    Orange, CA 92865
    Telephone: (714) 921-0150
    www.fmaware.org

Oregon Fibromyalgia Foundation
    1221 Southwest Yamhill
    Suite 303
    Portland, OR 97221
    www.myalgia.com

The Arthritis Foundation (can assist with local support groups)
    1330 W. Peachtree St.
    Atlanta, GA 30309
    Telephone: (800) 283-7800
    www.arthritis.org

Guillain–Barré Syndrome

Guillain–Barré Syndrome Foundation International
    P.O. Box 262
    Wynnewood, PA 19096
    Telephone: (215) 667-0131

Headache

National Headache Foundation
    Telephone: (800) 843-2256
    www.headaches.org

American Academy of Neurology
Telephone: (800) 879-1960
www.aan.com

American Council for Headache Education
Telephone: (609) 423-0258
www.achenet.org

Migraine Information Center (Cerenex/Glaxo Wellcome)
Telephone: 800-716-5499

American Association for the Study of Headache:
Telephone: 609-423-0043
www.aash.org

Migraine Awareness Group—A National Understanding for Migraineurs (MAGNUM)
Telephone: 703-739-9384
www.migraines.org

Meningitis

American Academy of Pediatrics
141 Northwest Blvd.
P.O. 927
Elk Grove Village, IL 60009-0927
Telephone: (800) 433-9016
www.aap.org

Multiple Sclerosis

Multiple Sclerosis Foundation, Inc (MSF)
6350 N. Andrews Ave.
Fort Lauderdale, FL 33309
Telephone: (954) 776-6805 or (800) 441-7055
www.msfacts.org
E-mail: msfact@icanect.net

National Multiple Sclerosis Society
733 Third Ave.
New York, NY 10017
Telephone: (800) FIGHT MS (800-344-4867)
www.nmss.org
E-mail: info@nmss.org

Parkinson's Disease

American Parkinson's Disease Foundation.
Telephone: (800) 223-2732
www.apdaparkinson.com

National Parkinson's Foundation
Telephone: (800) 327-4545

Parkinson's Disease Foundation
Telephone: (800) 457-6676

United Parkinson Foundation
Telephone: (312) 733-1893

International Tremor Foundation
Telephone: (913) 341-3880

Peripheral Neuropathies

American Diabetes Association
    Telephone: (800) DIABETES
    www.diabetes.org

Learning about Foot Care
    www.diabetesresource.com

Seizures

Epilepsy Foundation of America
    4351 Garden City Dr.
    Landover, MD 20785
    Telephone: (800) EFA-1000
    www.efa.org

Chapter 13

MENTAL HEALTH

ABUSE: PHYSICAL

SIGNAL SYMPTOMS ▶ physical and/or mental mistreatment

ICD-9 Codes	995.5	Physical Abuse of a Child
	995.5	Sexual Abuse of a Child
	995.5	Neglect of a Child
	995.81	Physical Abuse of Adult (inclusive of older adults)
	995.81	Sexual Abuse of Adult

Abuse is the severe mistreatment of one individual by another through, physical abuse, psychological abuse, sexual abuse, or adult/child neglect. Anyone can be a victim of abuse: men, women, children, elderly adults, and teenagers. Anyone can also be an abuser: men, women, children, elderly adults, and teenagers.

Epidemiology

Child Physical/Sexual Abuse

In 1994, 1 million cases of child abuse were substantiated.

2000–4000 children die each year because of abuse and neglect.

150,000–200,000 cases of child sexual abuse are reported each year.

Perpetrators of child abuse are parents (75%), other relatives (15%), or unrelated caretakers (10%).

The perpetrator of physical abuse is more likely the mother than the father.

Sexual abuse perpetrators: father/stepfather (7%–8%), uncles or older siblings (16%–42%), friends (32%–60%), strangers (1%).

Adult Physical/Sexual Abuse

1.8 million battered wives in the United States (estimated).

15%–25% of pregnant women are abused.

In 2000, the incidence of reported rape was 0.6/1000, a decrease from 1999 of 0.9/1000.

Only 4 or 5 of 10 rapes are reported.

Older Adult Abuse

10% of adults >65 years old are abused.

Etiology

Factors for high risk of physical abuse: stressful living conditions, social isolation, parental history of physical and/or sexual abuse

Factors for high risk of sexual abuse: child living with single parent, marital conflict, parental history of physical and/or sexual abuse

Factors for high risk of elder abuse: history of family conflict, person is very old and frail, victim lives with assailants who may be financially dependent on the victim

Factors for high risk of spousal abuse: history of substance abuse in the family; husband raised in violent home; husband is immature, dependent, and nonassertive and lacks self-esteem. Predominance of spousal abuse involves husband abusing wife. Battered wives/partners frequently show signs of somatization, including chronic headaches, hypertension, diabetes out of control, eating disorders, and depression.

Rapist characteristics: white (51%), black, (47%), other races (2%); tend to rape victim of same race; often accompanied by another crime (e.g., robbery)

Physiology and Pathophysiology

Perpetrators of Child Abuse

Long-term exposure as a child to violent home life, pain, and torment.

Thinking and judgement impaired by substance abuse.

Mental disorder that impairs judgement or thought process (e.g., psychosis).

Clinical Manifestations

Subjective

Chart review: A thorough reading of the client's chart may reveal data related to abuse; this may require obtaining information from other providers if the client has not been seen consistently by a single provider or facility.

Objective

CHILD PHYSICAL ABUSE

Suspicious bruises or marks with a symmetrical pattern or outline of a specific shape (belt buckle, open hand, cord)

Symmetrical round burns (cigarettes)

Sock-, glove-, or doughnut-shaped burns (immersion in boiling water)

Retinal hemorrhage (shaking of an infant)

Unexplained abdominal trauma

Multiple and spiral fractures

Metaphyseal fragmentation, periosteal hemorrhage, periosteal calcification, layer of calcification around long bones, epiphyseal separation, and periosteal shearing

CHILD SEXUAL ABUSE

Detailed knowledge about sex inappropriate for developmental level

Sexual play and behaviors alone and with peers

Extreme fear of adults

Difficulty in walking and sitting
Genital or rectal bleeding
Genital bruising, pain, itching
Recurrent urinary tract infections or vaginal discharges
Sexually transmitted diseases

ADULT SEXUAL ABUSE/RAPE

Feelings of shame, humiliation, fear
Posttraumatic stress disorder (PTSD) symptoms: anxiety, insomnia,
    flashbacks, hypervigilance, recurrent recollections of the event, avoidance
    of anything associated with the trauma
Vaginismus

OLDER ADULT ABUSE

Physical/sexual abuse: bruises; welts; fractures; burns; physical restraint;
    lack of personal care; difficulty walking or sitting; pain, bruising, or
    bleeding of genitalia or rectum
Psychological abuse: threats, assault, harassment, withholding of security
    and affection
Exploitation: misuse of victim's income or financial assistance
Medical abuse: withholding or improper administration of medications,
    treatments, or medically necessary aids (e.g., false teeth, hearing aids)

Differential Diagnosis

In the psychiatric assessment of abuse clients, the differential diagnosis focuses
on identifying the psychiatric illnesses that are often the sequelae of abuse.
Clients can present with myriad signs and symptoms. Usually this indicates a
one-time accident. Other times it is part of a pattern of abuse. Characteristic
symptoms of the more common comorbid illnesses are as follows:

Major depression (related to impact of abuse on self-esteem, interruptions
    in social, occupational functioning, or other important areas of
    functioning)
PTSD (hypervigilance, flashbacks, distressing recollections of the event,
    acting or feeling as though the trauma were recurring, avoidance of
    things associated with the traumatic event
Substance abuse or dependence (consumption of substance to decrease or
    stop distressing recollections or flashbacks of the event, decrease anxiety,
    decrease insomnia, decrease hypervigilance
Dissociative identity disorder (formerly multiple personality disorder)
    (extremely rare; occurs most often in persons sexually abused repeatedly
    over time; inability to recall important information beyond ordinary
    forgetfulness; presence of two or more distinct identities or personality states

Diagnostic Tests

Diagnostic tests as indicated, such as x-ray examination, computed tomographic or magnetic resonance imaging (MRI) scan as indicated by physical
and neurologic examination (to identify client's immediate needs as well as to

identify historical and/or unreported injuries that may establish a pattern of injury/abuse).

Management/Treatment

Crisis counseling
Therapy
Individual therapy
Group therapy

Referral

Reporting

<u>MANDATORY CHILD SEXUAL ABUSE REPORTING REQUIREMENTS</u>

All states and the District of Columbia have statutes identifying mandatory reporters (nurses are included) of child maltreatment and under what circumstances they are to report.

Mandatory Elder Abuse Reporting Requirements

All states and the District of Columbia except Colorado, Illinois, Iowa, Kentucky, New York, North Dakota, Pennsylvania, South Dakota, and Wisconsin have elder abuse reporting requirements. Reporting requirements vary widely by state, as do the penalties for failure to report elder abuse.

Refer to psychotherapist (M.S.N., Ph.D., M.S.W., M.D., M.A.)
Refer to psychopharmacologist (M.S.N., M.D.)
Refer to infectious disease specialist (M.D.)
Refer to social worker (if available)
Refer to local rape and sexual abuse center

ABUSE: SUBSTANCE

SIGNAL SYMPTOM ▶ overuse of a substance

ICD-9 Codes		(Alcohol codes provided as an example.)
	303.90	Alcohol Dependence
	305.00	Alcohol Abuse
	303.00	Alcohol Intoxication
	291.8	Alcohol Withdrawal

Similar categories and ICD codes exist for amphetamines, caffeine, cannabis (marijuana), cocaine, hallucinogens (LSD), inhalants (huffing), nicotine, opioids (heroin), phencyclidine (PCP), sedatives, hypnotics, and anxiolytics, as well as unknown or other substances.

Intoxication

Development of a substance-specific syndrome due to recent
ingestion/exposure to a substance
Clinically maladaptive behavioral or psychological changes due to the effect
of the substance on the central nervous system

Withdrawal

Development of a substance-specific syndrome due to the cessation of or reduction in substance use that has been heavy and prolonged.

Substance-specific syndrome causes clinically significant distress or impairment in social, occupational, or other important areas of functioning.

Dependence

Use of a substance causing significant impairment or distress as manifested by three or more of the following within the past year

TOLERANCE (DEFINED BY EITHER OR BOTH OF THE FOLLOWING)

Need of increased amounts of the substance to achieve intoxication or desired effect

Markedly diminished effect with continued use of the same quantity of the substance

WITHDRAWAL (DEFINED BY EITHER OR BOTH OF THE FOLLOWING)

Characteristic withdrawal syndrome for the substance or another substance taken to relieve or avoid withdrawal symptoms.

Substance is taken in larger amounts or over a longer period of time than was intended.

Persistent desire or unsuccessful efforts to cut down or control substance use.

Great deal of time spent in activities to obtain the substance, use the substance, or recover from its effects.

Important social, occupational, or recreational activities are given up or reduced because of substance use.

Use is continued despite knowledge of having a persistent or recurrent physical or psychological problem likely to have been caused by the substance.

Abuse

Maladaptive pattern of substance use leading up to clinically significant impairment or distress as evidenced by one or more of the following in a 13-month period (the person cannot have met the criteria for substance dependence for this class of substance):

Recurrent substance use resulting in failure to fulfill major obligations at work, school, or home (e.g., absences from work/school; neglect of child)

Recurrent substance use in situations in which it is physically hazardous (e.g., driving a car)

Recurrent substance-related legal problems

Continued use despite having persistent or recurrent social or interpersonal problems caused or exacerbated by the effects of the substance (e.g., arguments, fights with spouse)

Epidemiology

10% with substance dependence may commit suicide

Ratio of men:women—5:1

200,000 deaths each year directly related to alcohol

Etiology

Psychological, behavioral, genetic, neurotransmitter, and co-addiction theories provide the base from which new theories propose that varying contributions and combinations of theories promote the development of a substance-abuse problem.

Physiology and Pathophysiology

Opioid, dopamine, norepinephrine, and γ-aminobutyric acid neurotransmitters have all been implicated in substance abuse.

Dopamine neurons projecting to the nucleus accumbens in the limbic system are probably involved in the sensation of reward of amphetamine and cocaine use.

Adrenergic neurons in the locus ceruleus may mediate opiate and opioid use.

SELECTED COMPLICATIONS OF SUBSTANCE ABUSE/DEPENDENCE

Alcohol: Seizures, delirium tremens, cerebellar degeneration, cardiomyopathy

Amphetamines: Cerebrovascular accidents, cardiac incidents, psychosis

Cannabis: Delirium, psychosis, flashbacks, amotivational syndrome

Cocaine: Cerebral infarctions, spinal cord hemorrhages, myocardial infarction, arrhythmias

Hallucinogens: Flashbacks, delirium, psychosis, mania, anxiety

Inhalants: Psychosis, depression, panic disorder, generalized anxiety disorder

Nitrate inhalants: May negatively affect the immune system

Nitrous oxide: Exposure has been associated with reduced fertility

Opioids: Human immunodeficiency virus, hepatitis

Phencyclidine: Convulsions, coma, death, hyperthermia, seizures

Sedatives/hypnotics/anxiolytics: Paranoia, nystagmus, delirium, psychosis

Clinical Manifestations

See Table 13–1.

Differential Diagnosis

The differential diagnosis in substance abuse/dependence addresses three variables: Is this a substance issue, a nonsubstance mental illness, or a combination of these? The clinician must consider the high comorbidity of substance issues and nonsubstance mental illnesses. The clinician also must consider the possibility of multiple nonsubstance mental illnesses being comorbid with the abuse of multiple substances. Depending on presentation, the psychiatric differential diagnosis should include:

Bipolar disorder (with and without psychosis; patient exhibits both manic and depressive episodes; refer to section on "Mood Disorders" below)

Eating disorders (includes anorexia and/or bulimia; refer to section on "Eating Disorders" below)

Generalized anxiety disorder (patient exhibits anxious behavior; refer to section on "Anxiety Disorders" below)

Table 13–1 Clinical Manifestations of Intoxication and Withdrawal: Selected Substances

Substance	Intoxication	Withdrawal
Alcohol	Slurred speech, incoordination, unsteady gait, nystagmus, memory impairment, stupor, coma	Autonomic hyperactivity, hand tremor, insomnia, nausea/vomiting, transient hallucinations or illusions, psychomotor agitation, anxiety, seizure
Amphetamines	Tachycardia or bradycardia, pupillary dilation, elevated or lowered blood pressure, perspiration or chills, nausea/vomiting weight loss, psychomotor agitation or retardation, arrhythmias, respiratory depression, confusion, seizures, dyskinesias, dystonias, coma	Fatigue, vivid unpleasant dreams, insomnia or hypersomnia, increased appetite, psychomotor agitation or retardation
Cannabis	Conjunctival injection, increased appetite, dry mouth, tachycardia	Psychological dependence; irritability, restlessness, insomnia, anorexia, mild nausea (only after abruptly stopping high doses)
Cocaine	Tachycardia or bradycardia, pupillary dilation, elevated or lowered blood pressure, perspiration or chills, nausea/vomiting, weight loss, psychomotor agitation or retardation, arrhythmias, respiratory depression, confusion, seizures, dyskinesias, dystonias, coma	Fatigue, vivid unpleasant dreams, insomnia or hypersomnia, increased appetite, psychomotor agitation or retardation
Hallucinogens	Pupillary injection, tachycardia, sweating, palpitations, blurring of vision, tremors, incoordination	Psychological dependence; no physical dependence nor withdrawal symptoms
Inhalants	Dizziness, nystagmus, incoordination, slurred speech, unsteady gait, lethargy, depressed reflexes, psychomotor retardation, tremor, generalized muscle weakness, blurred vision or diplopia, stupor, coma, death	Tolerance; withdrawal symptoms fairly mild
Opioids	Drowsiness, coma, slurred speech, impairment in attention or memory	Dysphoria, nausea/vomiting, muscle aches, lacrimation or rhinorrhea, pupillary dilation, piloerection, sweating, diarrhea, yawning, fever, insomnia
Phencyclidine	Vertical or horizontal nystagmus, hypertension or tachycardia, numbness or diminished response to pain, ataxia, dysarthria, muscle rigidity, seizures, coma, hyperacusis	Rare; a function or dose and duration of use
Sedatives/ Hypnotics/ Anxiolytics	Slurred speech, incoordination, unsteady gait, nystagmus, memory impairment, stupor, coma	Autonomic hyperactivity, hand tremor, insomnia, nausea/vomiting, transient hallucinations or illusions, psychomotor agitation, anxiety, seizure

Major depressive disorder (with and without psychosis; patient exhibits mental depression characterized by altered mood; refer to section on "Mood Disorders" below)

Panic disorder (with and without agoraphobia; patient exhibits acute anxiety, terror or fright; refer to section on "Mood Disorders" below)

PTSD (patient exhibits characteristic symptoms after a psychologically traumatic experience; refer to section on "Anxiety Disorders" below)

Schizophrenia (patient exhibits unique type of disorder thinking, affect, and behavior; may include delusions and hallucinations; refer to section on "Mood Disorders" below)

Social phobia (patient exhibits persistent irrational fears and the need to avoid any situation in which he/she might be exposed and/or potentially embarrassed; refer to section on "Anxiety Disorders" below)

Diagnostic Tests

Tests performed will depend on suspected substance and may include:

Blood alcohol level (to rule out alcohol intoxication)

Urine drug screen (to rule out drug use; preferred test, because it is noninvasive; drug levels are higher in urine or are not detectable in blood, and drug metabolites are excreted for a longer time through urine)

Other, for example, complete blood count (CBC) with differential, chemistry profile, electrolytes, liver-function studies, creatinine, creatine kinase MB isoenzyme (CK-MB)/CK, electrocardiography (ECG), electroencephalography (EEG) (to rule out infection, hypoglycemia or hyperglycemia, electrolyte imbalance, liver and/or kidney dysfunction, cardiac problems and neurologic problems, respectively)

Management/Treatment

Treatment will depend on which substance is abused.

Pharmacologic Management

Anticonvulsants (for seizures)

Diazepam (Valium), 2–10 mg BID–QID; infants and children: 1–2.5 mg TID–QID (for agitation, seizures)

Haloperidol (Haldol), 0.5–2 mg BID–TID; infants and children: 0.05–0.15 mg/kg/day (for assaultive/aggressive behavior)

Lidocaine (for ventricular arrhythmias), 1 mg/kg IV bolus followed by IV infusion at 1–4 mg/min

Naloxone (Narcan), 0.4–2 mg IV, IM, or SC, repeat 2–3 minutes for desired response; infants and children: 0.01 mg/kg initially (for opiate overdose)

Nitroprusside (for hypertensive crisis), 0.3–5 mcg/kg/min IV infusion

Propranolol (Inderal), 10–30 mg TID–QID; not recommended for children (for tachycardia)

Activated charcoal (for alcohol, amphetamines, cocaine, hallucinogens, phencyclidine)

Nonpharmacologic Management

Gastric lavage (for alcohol, amphetamines, cocaine, hallucinogens, phencyclidine)

Dialysis (for alcohol)

Supportive care:
  Quiet room
  Supplemental oxygen

Client Education

Negative sequelae of substance abuse/dependence on physical and mental health and on work, family, and social functioning

Multitude of services available to those with substance abuse/dependence issues

Support groups, such as Al-Anon, Alcoholics Anonymous, Cocaine Anonymous, Codependents Anonymous, Narcotics Anonymous

Referral

Refer to psychiatrist.

Refer to psychologist.

Refer to psychopharmacologist (M.S.N, M.D.).

Refer to psychotherapist (M.S.N., Ph.D., M.S.W., M.D., M.A.).

Refer to in- or out-client substance abuse/dependence treatment.

Refer to specialty programs that address dual diagnosis for presence of both a substance disorder and a nonsubstance mental illness.

ANXIETY DISORDERS

SIGNAL SYMPTOM▶ anxious behavior; may vary in intensity

ICD-9 Codes	293.89	Anxiety disorder due to (indicate general medical condition)
	300.0	Anxiety disorder NOS
	308.81	Panic disorder without agoraphobia
	300.2	Generalized anxiety disorder
	300.01	Panic attack
	300.23	Social phobia
	308.81	Specific phobia
	300.3	Obsessive-compulsive disorder (OCD)
	308.3	Acute stress disorder
	309.81	Posttraumatic stress disorder (PTSD)

Anxiety is differentiated from fear in that anxiety is a response to an unknown, internal, vague, or conflictual threat. On the other hand, fear is a response to a known, external, definite, or nonconflictual threat. However, anxiety has many positive qualities in that it helps to alert us to the threat of bodily harm, pain, punishment, and threats to our success or wholeness. It is when anxiety escalates beyond these adaptive functions and begins to interfere with occupational, social, and other important functioning that assessment for an anxiety disorder is indicated.

Table 13–2 Anxiety Disorders: Epidemiology

Disorder	Lifetime Prevalence; Gender Differences
Acute Stress Disorder	Depends on the severity and pattern of the stressor and degree of exposure to the stressor
Generalized Anxiety Disorder	5%; 2/3 female, 1/3 male
Obsessive-Compulsive Disorder (OCD)	2.5%; Equally common in males and females
Panic Disorder (with and without Agoraphobia)	1.5%–3.5%; 1/3 to 1/2 have agoraphobia; With agoraphobia diagnosed twice as often in women; Without agoraphobia diagnosed three times as often in women
Post Traumatic Stress Disorder (PTSD)	1%–14% (General Population); 3%–58% (At risk populations: combat veterans, victims of disaster or violence); men's trauma is typically combat related; women's trauma is typically an assault or rape
Social Phobia	3%–13%; Unclear as whether more women or men are affected
Specific Phobia	10%–11.3%; Animal/natural environment type and situational type 75%–90% female

Epidemiology

See Table 13–2.

Etiology

See Table 13–3.

Table 13–3 Anxiety Disorders: Etiology

Disorder	Etiology
Acute Stress Disorder	Biological (increased autonomic nervous system activity; hyperactive noradrenergic, endogenous opiate, and hypothalamic-pituitary-adrenal axis), psychodynamic, stressor
Generalized Anxiety Disorder	Biological (GABA and serotonin dysfunction; abnormalities in basal ganglia, limbic system and the frontal cortex), genetic, psychosocial
Obsessive-Compulsive Disorder (OCD)	Behavioral (conditioned response to stimulus, learned avoidance), genetic, neurotransmitter dysfunction (serotonin in particular)
Panic Disorder (with and without Agoraphobia)	Biological (Neurotransmitter dysfunction in the brainstem, limbic system, and prefrontal cortex), genetic, psychosocial
Post Traumatic Stress Disorder (PTSD)	Biological (increased autonomic nervous system activity; hyperactive noradrenergic, endogenous opiate, and hypothalamic-pituitary-adrenal axis), psychodynamic, stressor
Specific and Social Phobia	Behavioral (conditioned response to stimulus), neurochemical (adrenergic dysfunction, possibly dopaminergic dysfunction), genetic, psychosocial

Physiology and Pathophysiology

Similar to substance abuse, no one hypothesis on the origin of anxiety disorders can account for all anxiety and its variable presentations. Some of the stronger hypotheses thought to explain anxiety individually or in various combinations include adrenergic, serotonergic, autonomic, and neuroendocrine dysfunction.

Clinical Manifestations

See Table 13–4.

Differential Diagnosis

See Table 13–4.

Table 13–4   Anxiety Disorders: Clinical Manifestations and Differential Diagnosis

Anxiety Disorder	Clinical Manifestations	Differential Diagnosis
Acute Stress Disorder	Similar symptoms as seen in PTSD but they have occurred and resolved within 1 month or less of the traumatic event.	Head injury, epilepsy, alcohol use disorders, acute substance intoxication or withdrawal, borderline personality disorder
Generalized Anxiety Disorder	Excessive anxiety and worry; client has difficulty controlling the worry; restlessness or feeling keyed up or on edge, easily fatigued; difficulty concentrating, irritability, muscle tension, sleep disturbance	Substance abuse or dependence, panic disorder, OCD, major depressive disorders, vitamin deficiency, endocrine dysfunction, neurological disorders, toxic poisoning
Obsessive-Compulsive Disorder (OCD)	Obsessions (recurrent and persistent thoughts, impulses or images that are intrusive and inappropriate; not just worry about real life problems; a thought or action is used to neutralize the thoughts, images or impulses) Compulsions (repetitive behaviors or mental acts aimed at preventing distress, a dreaded event or situation	Tourette's disorder, other tic disorders, temporal lobe epilepsy, schizophrenia, phobias, major depressive disorders
Panic Attack (not a disorder itself)	Palpitations, sweating, trembling, chest pain or discomfort, shortness of breath, nausea, paresthesias, feeling of choking, feelings of unreality; chills or hot flashes; fear of losing control, going crazy, or dying	See Panic Disorder
Panic Disorder (with and without Agoraphobia)	Recurrent panic attacks; concern about further attacks, and/or implications of the attacks; significant behavior change related to the attacks	Myocardial infarction, asthma, anemia, vitamin deficiency, endocrine dysfunction; substance abuse, epilepsy, brain lesion, heavy mental poisoning; social and specific phobias, depressive disorders, schizophrenia

Table continued on following page.

Table 13–4 Anxiety Disorders: Clinical Manifestations and Differential Diagnosis (*Continued*)

Anxiety Disorder	Clinical Manifestations	Differential Diagnosis
Post Traumatic Stress Disorder (PTSD)	Person confronted, experienced or witnessed an event(s) that involved threatened death or serious injury to self or others; response involved intense fear, helplessness or horror; traumatic event is persistently reexperienced; persistent avoidance of stimuli associated with the trauma; persistent symptoms of increased arousal (e.g., hypervigilance, insomnia); persists greater than 1 month	Head injury, epilepsy, alcohol use disorders, acute substance intoxication or withdrawal, borderline personality disorder
Social Phobia	Marked and persistent fear of social situations that include unfamiliar people or possible scrutiny by others; Client is concerned that he or she will do something embarrassing or humiliating	Substance abuse, CNS tumors, cerebrovascular disease, schizophrenia, panic disorder, agoraphobia, avoidant personality disorder
Specific Phobia	Excessive or unreasonable fear of a specific object or situation; exposure to object or situation invariably provokes an anxiety response	See Social Phobia

Diagnostic Tests

Tests performed will depend on presentation and differential diagnosis and may include tests such as blood toxicology (e.g., lead) screen, CBC with differential, creatinine, electrolytes, liver-function studies, endocrine/vitamin levels, urine drug screen, MRI, EEG (to rule out toxic substances, infection, kidney dysfunction, electrolyte imbalance, liver dysfunction, vitamin deficiency, drug abuse, and neurologic problems, respectively)

Management/Treatment

Pharmacologic Management

ACUTE STRESS DISORDER

Benzodiazepines

Selective serotonin reuptake inhibitors (SSRIs):

    Citalopram (Celexa), 20–60 mg/day (not recommended for children)

    Fluvoxamine (Luvox), 50–300 mg/day, infants and children: 25–200 mg/day

    Fluoxetine (Prozac), 20–80 mg/day (not recommended for children)

    Paroxetine (Paxil), 10–60 mg/day (not recommended for children)

    Sertraline (Zoloft), 50–200 mg/day; infants and children: 25–200 mg/day

GENERALIZED ANXIETY DISORDER

Benzodiazepines

SSRIs

Tricyclic antidepressants

Venlafaxine (Effexor XR), 75–375 mg/day divided TID (not recommended for children)

OBSESSIVE–COMPULSIVE DISORDER

Clomipramine (Anafranil), 25–250 mg in divided doses; infants and children: 25–100 mg/day in divided doses (or up to 3 mg/kg/day)

SSRIs

PANIC DISORDER (WITH AND WITHOUT AGORAPHOBIA)

Clomipramine (Anafranil), 25–250 mg in divided doses; infants and children: 25–100 mg/day in divided doses (or up to 3 mg/kg/day)

Imipramine (Tofranil), 75–200 mg/day ; adolescents: 30–100 mg/day (not recommended for children)

SSRIs

PTSD

Amitriptyline (Elavil), 75–150 mg/day in divided doses (not recommended for children)

Imipramine (Tofranil), 75–200 mg/day ; adolescents: 30–100 mg/day (not recommended for children)

SSRIs

SPECIFIC AND SOCIAL PHOBIA

SSRIs

Nonpharmacologic Management

Behavioral therapy (individual, group)

Cognitive behavioral therapy (individual, group)

Therapy using other theoretical frameworks (individual, group)

Complementary/Alternative Therapies

Biofeedback

Relaxation therapy, including deep breathing, muscle relaxation

Massage

Meditation

Yoga

Client Education

Support groups

Referral

Refer to psychiatrist.

Refer to psychologist.

Refer to psychopharmacologist (M.S.N., M.D.).

Refer to psychotherapist (M.S.N., Ph.D., M.S.W., M.D., M.A.)

EATING DISORDERS

ICD-9 Codes	307.1	Anorexia Nervosa
	307.50	Eating Disorder NOS
	307.51	Bulimia Nervosa

Anorexia

Anorexia nervosa is an illness in which clients refuse to maintain a minimum weight (at least 85% of normal weight), fear gaining weight, and intentionally lose weight due to misinterpretations of their body image and shape.

Types include:

Restricting type: No binge eating or purging behavior

Binge-eating/purging type: Regularly binge eats and/or purges

Bulimia

With bulimia nervosa, clients are preoccupied with food, weight, and body shape. Clients with bulimia have complications related to repeated bingeing and purging (vomiting or abuse of laxatives) rather than to complications related to minimal calorie intake and significant weight loss.

Types include:

Purging type: Uses self-induced vomiting or misuses laxatives, diuretics, or enemas

Nonpurging type: Compensates for eating through fasting or excessive exercise

Epidemiology

Anorexia

0.5%–1% of adolescent girls

Onset usually in adolescence

10 to 20 times more frequent in females

Bulimia

1%–3% of young women

Onset usually later than that for anorexia nervosa

Significantly more frequent in females

Up to 40% of female college students may have engaged in occasional binge eating and/or purging

Often occurs in normal-weight clients

Etiology

Anorexia

BIOLOGIC

Endogenous opioids may be involved in denial of hunger that leads to decreased appetite, which progresses to starvation. Some studies have shown significant weight gain in clients administered opiate antagonists. Starvation causes biochemical and neuroanatomical changes. Hypercortisolemia, depressed thyroid function, lowered hormonal levels (leading to amenorrhea), and enlarged sulci and ventricles in the brain are all reversed with realimentation.

SOCIAL

May come from homes with high levels of hostility, chaos, and isolation, as well as low levels of nurturance and empathy.

PSYCHOLOGICAL

Some young women may perceive their bodies to be under the control of their parents. Through starvation they hope to gain validation as an autonomous individual.

Bulimia

BIOLOGIC

The neurotransmitters serotonin and norepinephrine have been implicated in bulimia through the success of antidepressants in some clients. Because of the increased endorphin levels after vomiting, the well-being associated with the endorphins may reinforce the vomiting behavior.

SOCIAL

These clients tend to be high achievers and more responsive to societal pressures to be thin. The families of bulimic clients tend to be less close and more conflictual than the families of anorexic clients. Parents can be described as rejecting and neglectful.

PSYCHOLOGICAL

Clients with bulimia tend to be outgoing, angry, and impulsive. Their overeating is seen as ego dystonic, and as such, tend to seek help more often than their anorexic counterparts. The impulsivity is expressed through bingeing and purging, as well as through shoplifting, substance abuse, self-destructive sexual relationships, and emotional lability.

Physiology and Pathophysiology

Starvation causes biochemical and neuroanatomical changes. Hypercortisolemia, depressed thyroid function, lowered hormonal levels (leading to amenorrhea), and enlarged sulci and ventricles in the brain are all reversed with realimentation.

The bingeing and purging behavior seen in bulimia nervosa has been associated with hypotension, bradycardia, dehydration, electrolyte disturbances (e.g., hypokalemia), and metabolic disturbances (hypochloremic alkalosis).

Clinical Manifestations

Anorexia

Refusal to maintain body weight at or above normal weight for age and height

Intense fear of gaining weight or becoming fat, even though underweight

Undue influence of body weight or shape on self-evaluation

Denial of seriousness of the current low body weight

Disturbance in how one experiences one's body weight or shape

Amenorrhea for three consecutive cycles in postmenarcheal females

Bulimia

Eating within 2 hours an amount of food definitely larger than most people would under similar circumstances

Sense of a lack of control over eating

Recurrent inappropriate compensatory behavior to prevent weight gain: self-induced vomiting; misuse of laxatives, diuretics, enemas, or other medications; fasting; or excessive exercise

Behavior occurs at least twice a week for 3 months

Self-evaluation unduly influenced by body shape and weight

Differential Diagnosis

Anorexia

Body dysmorphic disorder (patient exhibits preoccupation with a defect in appearance)

Major depressive disorder (patient exhibits mental depression characterized by altered mood; refer to section on "Mood Disorders" below)

Obsessive–compulsive disorder (patient exhibits recurrent obsessions or compulsions severe enough to cause distress because of the time involved or the interference it may cause in normal life)

Schizophrenia (patient exhibits unique type of disorder thinking, affect, and behavior; may include delusions and hallucinations; refer to section on "Mood Disorders" below)

Social phobia (patient exhibits persistent irrational fears and the need to avoid any situation in which he/she might be exposed and/or potentially embarrassed; refer to section on "Anxiety Disorders" below)

Bulimia

Anorexia nervosa, binge eating/purging type (patient exhibits signs and symptoms of anorexia, but also engages in binge eating and purging)

Borderline personality disorder (patient exhibits difficulty maintaining a consistent stable mood and self-image; refer to section on "Mood Disorders")

Major depressive disorder (patient exhibits mental depression characterized by altered mood; refer to section on "Mood Disorders" below)

Diagnostic Tests

Tests performed will depend on presentation and differential diagnosis and may include tests such as CBC with differential, chemistry profile, creatinine, electrolytes, liver-function studies, ECG, MRI, EEG (to rule out infection, hypoglycemia or hyperglycemia, electrolyte imbalances, liver dysfunction, cardiac disorders, and neurologic disorders, respectively)

Management/Treatment

Nonpharmacologic Management

Behavioral therapy (individual, group)
Cognitive therapy (individual, group)
Interpersonal therapy (individual, group)
Family therapy

Client Education

Teach don't preach!
Encourage client to talk with clinician, therapist, parent, school counselor, or other adult whom the client trusts.
Teach about healthy eating (balanced diet using food pyramid).
Teach about healthy exercising.
Provide factual information on possible sequelae of the eating disorder.

Referral

Hospitalization may be necessary in some cases.
Refer to an eating-disorder specialist and/or program (in- or out-client).
Refer to psychotherapist who specializes in working with individual family members, couples (for parents), and families.

MOOD DISORDERS

SIGNAL SYMPTOMS ▶ **altered mood and behavior**

ICD-9 Codes	296.XX	Depressive disorders
	296.2X	Single episode
	296.3X	Recurrent
	296.XX	Bipolar disorders (formerly manic–depressive disorders)
	296.40	Hypomanic
	296.4X	Most recent episode hypomanic
	296.5X	Recent episode depressed
	296.6X	Most recent episode mixed
	300.4	Dysthymic disorder
	311	Depressive disorder not otherwise specified

The fifth digit in the ICD code for mood disorders specifies the severity of illness: 1 = mild, 2 = moderate, 3 = severe without psychotic features, 4 = severe with psychotic features, 5 = in partial remission, 6 = in full remission.

Mood disorders encompass a range of severity and intensity. Differential diagnosis can be difficult because of the tendency of mood disorder characteristics to fluctuate over time without following a particular pattern.

Mood disorders include:

Depression (periods of low energy, sadness, poor concentration, etc.).
Mania (periods of inflated self-esteem, flights of ideas, poor judgment, decreased sleep, etc.).
Hypomania (similar to mania but does not cause the impairment seen in mania).
Bipolar I disorder includes mania and usually a depressive episode.

Bipolar II disorder includes hypomania and usually a depressive episode.
Dysthymia (persistent low level of depressive symptoms).
Cyclothymia (dips and elevations in mood that are much less severe than
the bipolar disorders but causes significant distress nonetheless).

Epidemiology

Lifetime Prevalence

Major depression: 10%–25% women; 5%–12% men
Dysthymic disorder: 6%
Bipolar I disorder: 0.4%–1.6%
Bipolar II disorder: 0.5%
Bipolar I or II disorder with rapid cycling: 5%–15% of clients with bipolar
illness
Cyclothymic disorder: 0.4%–1.0%

Etiology

Biological

Neurotransmitter dysregulation of neurotransmitters, in particular,
decreased levels of serotonin and norepinephrine have been implicated in
depression. Decreased levels of dopamine in depression and increased
dopamine in mania have been hypothesized.
Neuroendocrine dysregulation has also been implicated in mood disorders.
For example, cortisol, thyroid function, and growth hormone
abnormalities have been observed in depression.
Kindling has been proposed as an explanation for bipolar disorder. Kindling
is the electrophysiologic process by which repeated stimulation of a
neuron eventually causes an action potential. When this occurs in
enough neurons, a seizure results. Because of the success of
anticonvulsants in bipolar disorder, it has been hypothesized that
kindling is a process shared by epilepsy and bipolar disorder.

Genetic

First-degree relatives of clients with bipolar disorder are 8–18 times more
likely than controls to have bipolar disorder and 2–10 times more likely
to have major depression.
First-degree relatives of clients with major depression are 1.5–2.5 times
more likely than controls to have bipolar I disorder and 2–3 times more
likely to have major depression.
50% of all clients with bipolar I have at least one parent with a mood
disorder.
25% chance of a child having a mood disorder if one parent has bipolar
disorder.
50%–75% chance of a child having a mood disorder if both parents have
bipolar disorder.
Concordance rates in monozygotic twins: 50% in major depression;
33%–90% in bipolar I disorder.

Other Theories

Life events and environmental stress, family functioning, individual premorbid personality factors, learned helplessness, and cognitive theory have all proposed theories of mood disorders from their respective viewpoints.

Physiology and Pathophysiology

Dysregulation of neurotransmitters, in particular, decreased levels of serotonin and norepinephrine has been implicated in depression. This is because of the relative success of tricyclic antidepressants, SSRIs, and a serotonin–norepinephrine reuptake inhibitor in improving the symptoms of depression by increasing levels of serotonin and/or norepinephrine.

Clinical Manifestations

See Table 13–5.

Differential Diagnosis

See Table 13–6.

Diagnostic Tests

Tests performed will depend on presentation and differential diagnosis and may include tests such as blood toxicology (e.g., lead) screen, CBC with differential, creatinine, electrolytes, liver-function studies, endocrine/vitamin levels, urine

Table 13–5   Mood Disorders: Clinical Manifestations

Major Depressive Episode	Manic Episode	Mixed Episode	Hypomanic Episode
Depressed mood	Inflated self-esteem or grandiosity	Criteria are met for both a major depressive episode and a manic episode concurrently	Inflated self-esteem or grandiosity
Anhedonia	Decreased need for sleep		Decreased need for sleep
Weight loss or gain	More talkative than usual or pressured speech		More talkative than usual or pressured speech
Insomnia or hypersomnia	Flight of ideas or racing thoughts		Flight of ideas or racing thoughts
Psychomotor agitation or retardation	Too distractible		Too distractible
Fatigue or loss of energy	Increased goal directed activity: socially, at work or school, or sexually		Increased goal directed activity: socially, at work or school, or sexually
Feelings of worthlessness, severe guilt	Poor judgement in activities with a high potential for painful consequences: sexual indiscretions, unrestrained buying sprees		Poor judgement in activities with a high potential for painful consequences: sexual indiscretions, unrestrained buying sprees
Poor concentration			Does not cause marked impairment in functioning nor hospitalization as seen in mania
Thoughts of death			

Table 13–6   Mood Disorders: Differential Diagnosis

Disorder	Psychiatric Differential	Medical Differential
Bipolar I	Bipolar II Disorder Cyclothymic Disorder Dysthymic Disorder Major Depressive Disorder Psychotic Disorders Substance induced mood disorder	Cerebral neoplasms/trauma CNS infections Huntington's disease Hyperthyroidism Pharmacological agents Postpartum mania Temporal lobe epilepsy Vitamin B12 deficiency
Bipolar II	Bipolar I Disorder Cyclothymic Disorder Dysthymia Disorder Major Depressive Disorder Psychotic Disorders Substance induced mood disorder	Essentially the same as for Bipolar I Disorder
Cyclothymic Disorder	Bipolar I with rapid cycling Bipolar II with rapid cycling Borderline Personality Disorder Substance induced mood disorder	Amphetamines Attention deficit disorder Cocaine Personality disorders Seizures Steroids See Bipolar and Depressive Disorders rule outs as well
Dysthymic Disorder	Major Depressive Disorder Personality disorder Feature of chronic psychosis Substance induced mood disorder	Essentially the same as for major depressive disorder
Major Depressive Disorder	Bipolar disorder Cyclothymic Disorder Dementia Dysthymic Disorder Schizoaffective disorder Substance induced mood disorder Schizoaffective disorder	AIDS Cancer Cerebral neoplasms/trauma CNS Infections Endocrine Disorders Inflammatory disorders Neurological Disorders Pharmacological agents Postpartum mood disorders Systemic Infections Vitamin deficiencies

drug screen, MRI, EEG (to rule out toxic substances, infection, kidney dysfunction, electrolyte imbalance, liver dysfunction, vitamin deficiency, drug abuse, and neurologic disorders, respectively)

Management/Treatment

Pharmacological Management

DEPRESSION

First-Line Agents

Citalopram (Celexa), 20–60 mg/day (not recommended for children)

Venlafaxine XR (Effexor XR), 75–375 mg/day divided TID (not recommended for children)

Paroxetine (Paxil), 10–60 mg/day (not recommended for children)

Fluoxetine (Prozac), 20–80 mg/day (not recommended for children)

Bupropion SR (Wellbutrin SR), 100–450 mg/day divided BID–TID (not recommended for children)

Sertraline (Zoloft), 50–200 mg/day; infants and children: 25–200 mg/day

Second-Line Agents

Tricyclic antidepressants (generally more side effects)

MANIA

First-Line Agents

Carbamazepine (Tegretol) 200–1000 mg/day divided BID–QID; infants and children: 10–35 mg/kg divided TID–QID

Lithium carbonate (Lithobid/Lithonate), 900–1800 mg/day divided BID–TID (not recommended for children)

Olanzapine (Zyprexa), 10–20 mg/day (not recommended for children)

Valproate (Depakote), 10–60 mg/kg/day

 CP 13–1 Clinical Pearl: Carbamazepine is not officially approved for the treatment of mania by the Food and Drug Administration. However, because of widespread and long-term use, carbamazepine is generally accepted as primary consideration for its treatment.

Second-Line Agents

Gabapentin (Neurontin), 300–3600 mg/day divided TID (not recommended for children)

Lamotrigine (Lamictal), 25–500 mg/day divided BID; infants and children: 0.15–5 mg/kg/day divided BID

Risperidone (Risperdal), 2–16 mg/day divided BID (not recommended for children)

Topiramate (Topamax), 25–1600 mg/day divided BID; infants and children: 1–9 mg/kg/day divided BID

 CP 13–2 Clinical Pearl: These second-line agents are not officially approved for the treatment of mania by the Food and Drug Administration. However, anecdotal reports in the psychiatric literature indicate positive benefits in some cases and warrant consideration on failure of the first-line agents to achieve a good outcome. Ongoing, double-blind, placebo-controlled studies are under way to study the efficacy in mania/bipolar disorder for most of these agents.

Nonpharmacologic Management

Cognitive behavioral therapy (individual, group)

Therapy using other theoretical frameworks (individual, groups)

Support groups for clients, families, and significant others

Client Education

Mood disorders are illnesses like any other.

The client did not contract this illness because they did anything wrong or because he or she is too weak to handle life's problems.

Mood disorders are generally chronic illnesses and require long-term follow-up.

Mood disorder medications are available and must be taken on a consistent basis.

A great number of people lead very "normal" lives and unless the client told you, you would never know that a mood disorder is part of his or her life.

Referral

Refer to psychiatrist.

Refer to psychologist.

Refer to psychopharmacologist (M.S.N., M.D.).

Refer to psychotherapist (M.S.N., Ph.D., M.S.W., M.D., M.A.).

STRESS

SIGNAL SYMPTOM ▶ disrupted equilibrium

ICD-9 Codes	300.00	Anxiety NOS
	308.81	Nervousness
	309	Grief reaction
	309.81	Posttraumatic stress, acute
	309.82	Posttraumatic stress, chronic
	780.50	Sleep disturbance NOS

Stress is a response to an experience, a memory, or a subconscious thought that provokes a sense of danger. Stress, similar to anxiety, is helpful initially. However, in the long run stress can become chronic and contribute to a variety of illnesses. It is often difficult to differentiate between these illnesses, which are both physical and mental, in practice.

Epidemiology

43% of all adults suffer adverse health effects attributable to stress.

75%–90% of all visits to primary care physicians are for stress-related symptoms.

Etiology

Many agree that stress is a factor in many illnesses; however, no one theory, such as pathophysiologic, genetic, emotional conflict, organ vulnerability, or conflict interactions, has emerged as primary in this controversial discussion.

Physiology and Pathophysiology

Stress is the response of nearly all systems to a perceived threat. The hypothalamic–pituitary–adrenal axis releases cortisol and neurotransmitters such as dopamine, norepinephrine, and epinephrine, which affect systems throughout the body. The amygdala initiates an emotional response to a stressful event and signals the hippocampus to store the experience in long-term memory.

The systems are responding to input from the autonomic nervous system. In particular, the sympathetic nervous system prepares one to deal with normal events as well as to act quickly, as in a fight-or-flight situation. The parasympathetic nervous system serves to control the activity of the sympathetic nervous system by countering the changes brought on previously.

A summary of autonomic nervous system activity is presented in Table 13–7.

Clinical Manifestations

See Table 13–8.

Differential Diagnosis

See Table 13–8.

Diagnostic Tests

Tests performed will depend on presentation and differential diagnosis and may include tests such as CBC with differential, chemistry profile, creatinine, electrolytes, liver-function studies, CK-MB/CK, ECG, MRI, EEG (to rule out infection, hypoglycemia or hyperglycemia, kidney dysfunction, electrolyte imbalance, liver dysfunction, cardiac problems, and neurologic problems, respectively)

Management/Treatment

Depending on the presentation and differential diagnosis, treatment should focus on the most potentially life-threatening issue first, including that of suicide (see Table 13–9).

Secondarily, the clinician can address issues of stress reduction through exercise, diet, and medication to decrease the impact of stress on the presenting physical illness(es). Other therapies that may be used include biofeedback, relaxation

Table 13–7   Summary of Autonomic Nervous System Activity

System	Sympathetic Response	Parasympathetic Response
Adrenal medulla	Stimulates secretion of epinephrine and norepinephrine	
Airways	Relaxes bronchial muscles	Constricts bronchial muscles
Blood vessels: generally	Constricts	
Blood vessels: gastrointestinal tract		Dilates
Gallbladder		Stimulates bile release
Heart rate and force	Increases	Decreases
Intestine: large	Inhibits motility	Increases secretions and motility
Intestine: small	Inhibits motility	Increases digestion
Kidneys	Inhibits urine secretion	Stimulates urine secretion
Liver	Stimulates glucose production and release	
Oral/nasal mucosa	Inhibits mucus production	Stimulates mucus production
Pupils	Dilates	Constricts
Salivation	Inhibits	Stimulates
Stomach	Inhibits digestion	Stimulates digestion
Sweat glands	Stimulates secretion	
Urinary bladder	Relaxes	Contracts

Table 13–8 Stress: Clinical Manifestations and Differential Diagnosis

Cardiovascular System	Respiratory System	Gastrointestinal System
Cardiac arrhythmias	Bronchial asthma	Anorexia nervosa
Congestive heart failure	Hay fever	Peptic ulcer
Coronary artery disease	Hyperventilation	Obesity
Essential hypertension	Tuberculosis	Ulcerative colitis
Raynaud's phenomenon		
Vasomotor syncope		

Neurologic System	Musculoskeletal System	Endocrine
Brain disease	Fibromyalgia	Diabetes mellitus
Brain tumor	Low back pain	Hyperthyroidism
Epilepsy	Rheumatoid arthritis	Idiopathic amenorrhea
Multiple sclerosis		Infertility
Stroke		Menopausal distress
		Premenstrual dysphoria

Headaches	Other Considerations	Skin Disorders
Migraine headaches	Allergic disorders	Generalized pruritus
Tension headaches	Anxiety disorders	Localized pruritus
	Cancer	Hyperhidrosis
	Chronic pain	
	Immune disorders	
	Infectious diseases	

Table 13–9 Suicide

Epidemiology

In 1997, more teenagers and young adults died from suicide than from cancer, heart disease, AIDS, birth defects, stroke, pneumonia and influenza and chronic lung disease combined

Persons under age 25 accounted for 15% of all suicides in 1997

From 1952–1995, the incidence of suicide among adolescents and young adults nearly tripled

More people die annually from suicide than from homicide

Suicide is the eighth leading cause of death for all Americans

Suicide is the third leading cause of death for young people aged 15–24

Nearly 3 of every 5 suicides in 1997 (58%) were committed with a firearm

Etiology

Sociological (social, familial, financial, and cultural reasons for suicide), psychological (repressed desire to harm someone else or the acting out of fantasies of revenge, power and control), and physiological factors (genetics, neurotransmitter dysregulation) have all been proposed. The etiology is probably a combination of these, which is highly variable between individuals.

High Risk Factors Associated with Suicide

Consumes alcohol

Depression

Male

Older adult

Poor physical/mental health

Poor social support

Prior suicidal behavior

Recent loss or separation

Single

Unemployed or retired

Table continued on following page.

Table 13–9   Suicide (*Continued*)

Crisis Intervention for the Suicidal Client

Ask direct, non-blaming questions

Encourage client to share feelings

Normalize client's feelings: discuss that others have had similar thoughts

Help is available and you plan to help them presently

Work with client to achieve positive outcome: appointment with a mental health professional, hospitalization, medication trial, ensure patient has safe environment to return to with people who will be with patient continuously in the short run

Provide local crisis information: emergency room locations, phone numbers

Schedule follow-up: shows the client you are interested in the client in the future

Table 13–10   Teaching Clients About Grief

Normal

Kübler-Ross' Stages of Grief

Denial and Isolation:	"It's not true." "No one here can help me."
Anger:	"It isn't fair. I don't deserve this."
Bargaining:	"If I do these good things maybe the cancer will remit."
Depression:	"I am going to die. I'm sad and depressed."
Acceptance:	"It is true that I am going to die. I cannot change this. I plan to make the best of the time I have left as I have been fortunate to do many things and know so many kind people."

Kübler-Ross' model is not linear. A client may skip over a stage or regress a stage or two. The important information to convey to your clients is that grief is normal and grief involves many emotions. Encourage them to talk about their loss (e.g., the client's own declining health, or the death of a family member or friend).

Pathological: Can present as delayed or absent grief; extremely intense or prolonged grief (keep culture under consideration); grief with psychosis or suicidal ideation; believing the deceased is still alive despite the evidence.

training, deep breathing, group therapy, massage, meditation, muscle relaxation, and yoga.

If the client's stress is related to a loss, teach the client about grief (see Table 13–10).

Referral

Arrange for direct admission to psychiatric hospital as needed.

Employee Assistance Program (if available at client's worksite).

Local Crisis Intervention or Suicide Hotline.

Refer to psychiatrist.

Refer to psychologist.

Refer to psychopharmacologist (M.S.N., M.D.).

Refer to psychotherapist (M.S.N, Ph.D., M.S.W., M.D., M.A.)

REFERENCES

General

American Bar Association. (1998). *Facts about law and the elderly.* Available online at www.abanet.org/media/factbooks/.

American Institute of Stress. (2000). *Stress—America's #1 health problem.* Available online at www.stress.org/problem.htm.

American Psychiatric Association (1994). *Diagnostic and statistical manual of mental disorders (4th ed.)*. (*DSM-IV*). Washington, D.C.: American Psychiatric Press.

Centers for Disease Control and Prevention. (2000). *Suicide in the United States*. Available online at www.cdc.gov/ncipc/factsheets/suifacts.htm.

Center for Mental Health Services. (2000). *Knowledge exchange network (KEN)*. Available online at www.mentalhealth.org/.

Fischbach, F. (1999). *A manual of laboratory & diagnostic tests* (6th ed.). Philadelphia: Lippincott.

Kaplan, H. I., & Sadock, B. J. (1997). *Kaplan and Sadock's synopsis of psychiatry: Behavioral science, clinical psychiatry* (8th ed.). Philadelphia: William & Wilkins.

Kübler-Ross, E. (1969). *On death and dying*. New York: Macmillan.

Purves, D., Augustine, G.J., Fitzpatrick, D., Katz, C., LaMantia, A.S., & McNamara, J.O. (1997). *Neuroscience*. Sunderland, MA: Sinauer.

Schatzberg, A.P., & Nemeroff, C.B. (1995). *Textbook of psychiatry*. Washington, D.C.: American Psychiatric Press.

Springhouse Corporation (2001). *Professional guide to diseases* (7th ed.). Springhouse, PA: Springhouse.

U.S. Department of Health and Human Services & National Clearinghouse on Child Abuse and Neglect Information. (1999). *Child abuse and neglect: State statutes elements, reporting laws number 2: Mandatory reporters of child abuse and neglect*. Available online at www.calib.com/nccanch/.

WebMD, Inc. (2000). *Health: Stress*. Available online at http://my.webmd.com/

RESOURCES

General

National Alliance for the Mentally Ill
Telephone: (800) 950-6264
www.nami.org/

National Institute of Mental Health
Telephone: (301) 443-4513
www.nimh.nih.gov/

National Mental Health Association
Telephone: 703/684-7722
www.nmha.org/

Abuse: Physical

National Center on Elder Abuse
Telephone: (202) 898-2586
www.gwjapan.com/NCEA/

National Domestic Violence/Abuse Hotline
Telephone: (800) 799-7233 or (800)787-3224 (TDD)

Rape, Abuse and Incest National Network (RAINN)
Telephone: (800) 656-4673
http://feminist.com/rainn.htm

Rape Recovery and Information Page
http://raperecovery.terrashare.com/

Sexual Assault Information Page
www.cs.utk.edu/~bartley/saInfoPage.html

Abuse: Substance

Al-Anon
Telephone: (800) 356-9996

Alcoholics Anonymous—Check Local White Pages

Alcohol & Drug Help Line
Telephone: (800) 821-4357

Healthy Nations Initiative: Reducing Substance Abuse Among Native Americans
Telephone: (303) 315-9272
www.hsc.colorado.edu/sm/hnp/

National Clearinghouse for Alcohol Information and Drug Information
Telephone: (800) 729-6680
www.health.org

National Council on Alcoholism and Drug Dependency
Telephone: (800) 622-2255
www.ncadd.org/

National Rehabilitation Information Clearinghouse
Telephone: (800) 346-2742

Anxiety Disorders

Anxiety Disorders Association of America
Telephone: (301) 231-9350
www.adaa.org/

the Anxiety Panic Internet Resource (tAPir)
www.algy.com/anxiety/

Generalized Anxiety Home Page
www.anxietynetwork.com/gahome.html

National Center for Post Traumatic Stress Disorder
Telephone: (802) 296-5132
www.ncptsd.org/

Obsessive Compulsive Foundation
Telephone: (203) 315-2190
www.ocfoundation.org/

Social Phobia/Social Anxiety Association
www.socialphobia.org/

Eating Disorders

American Anorexia Bulimia Association
Telephone: (213) 575-6200
www.aabainc.org/home.html

National Association of Anorexia Nervosa and Associated Disorders
[ANAD] (847) 831-3438
www.anad.org/

Mood Disorders

Bipolar Disorder Sanctuary
www.mhsanctuary.com/bipolar/

Depression and Related Affective Disorders Association (DRADA)
Telephone: (410) 955-4647
www.med.jhu.edu/drada/

National Depressive and Manic–Depressive Association (DMDA)
Telephone: (800) 826-3632
www.ndmda.org/

Stress

American Association of Suicidology
Telephone: (202) 237-2280
www.suicidology.org/

NAMI: Suicide—Learn More, Learn to Help
www.nami.org/helpline/suicide.htm

StopStress.Com
www.stopstress.com/

Stress Management and Emotional Wellness Links
http://imt.net/~7Erandolfi/StressLinks.html

Suicide Prevention Advocacy Network (SPAN)
Telephone: (888) 649-1366
www.spanusa.org/

Chapter 14

INFECTIOUS DISEASES

AIRBORNE TRANSMITTED INFECTION

TUBERCULOSIS

SIGNAL SYMPTOMS ▶ night sweats, anorexia, fatigue, pleuritic chest pain

ICD-9 Code	011.9	Pulmonary tuberculosis, unspecified

Tuberculosis (TB) is a common infection of the lung caused by an airborne bacillus. *Tuberculosis infection* is the presence of a positive tuberculin skin test in an individual with no physical findings of disease and a normal chest x-ray examination or a chest x-ray examination that shows only granulomas or calcifications. An individual with *tuberculosis disease* has signs, symptoms, and chest x-ray findings that indicate colonization with *Mycobacterium tuberculosis*.

Epidemiology

Incubation period is 2–12 weeks.

An estimated 10–15 million persons in United States are infected with *M. tuberculosis*.

85% cases involve lung; TB disease develops in 10% of persons who are exposed.

In 2000, a total of 16,377 cases of tuberculosis were reported, for a rate of 3.5 per 100,000 population.

See Risk Factors 14–1.

Etiology

Aerobic, non–spore-forming, nonmotile bacillus, *M. tuberculosis* (MTb).

Physiology and Pathophysiology

The *M. tuberculosis* organism lodges in the lung periphery, usually the upper lobe, and multiplies, causing nonspecific pneumonitis. Some bacilli migrate to the lymphatic system and lodge in the lymph nodes. The inflammatory process in the lungs causes neutrophils and macrophages to invade areas, with the macrophages engulfing and isolating bacilli. The neutrophils and macrophages

RF 14–1 Risk Factors: *Tuberculosis*

- HIV infection
- Substance Abuse
- Recent infection with M. tuberculosis (within past 2 years)
- Chest x-ray with findings suggestive of previous TB–no evidence of treatment
- Diabetes mellitus
- Silicosis
- Prolonged steroid therapy
- Other immunosuppressive therapy
- Cancer
- Hematologic or reticuloendothelial disease
- End stage renal disease
- Intestinal bypass or gastrectomy
- Chronic malabsorption syndrome
- Low body weight (10% or more below ideal)

wall off bacilli, forming a granulomatous lesion known as a tubercle. The infected tissue in the tubercle dies, forming a caseous necrosis. This collagenous scar tissue forms around the tubercle, further isolating the bacilli. The isolation of the bacilli and a good immune response cause bacilli to be dormant for life.

Clinical Manifestations

Subjective
Anorexia.
Fever.
Night sweats.
Productive cough.
Hemoptysis.
Fatigue.
Pleuritic chest pain.
Children have less obvious symptoms.

Objective
Lung examination (apical crackles, dull percussion, increased tactile fremitus over consolidated area, positive whispered pectoriloquy)
Weight loss
Adenopathy
Hepatospenomegaly

Differential Diagnosis
Human immunodeficiency virus (HIV) infection (positive HIV test)
Pneumonia (cough, fever; pleuritic chest pain; chill; dark, thick, rusty sputum)
Silicosis (cough, dyspnea)

Melioidosis (fulminant, characterized by pneumonia, empyema, lung abscess, septicemia, acquired by direct contact with infected animals)

Neoplasm

Chronic bronchitis (early morning cough for 3 months or more)

Pulmonary embolus (history of sedentary lifestyle or deep vein thrombus, acute onset)

Lymphomas

Atypical mycobacteria infection (*Mycobacterium* organism other than *M. tuberculosis*)

Diagnostic Tests

Tuberculin skin test (purified protein derivative [PPD] skin test) (to detect exposure; positive PPD skin test appears 2–10 weeks after exposure)

Test is positive if:

Induration >5 mm: Clients with HIV infection, immunosuppression, clinical evidence of disease, close contact with client with TB, recent exposure

Induration >10 mm: Clients with diabetes; cancer; end-stage renal disease; immigrants from Asia, Africa, Latin America; medically underserved clients; low-income clients; high-risk minorities; residents of nursing homes or other institutional settings (e.g., prisons); health-care workers

Induration >15 mm: Clients >4 years of age and all other clients not listed above

Sputum specimen for acid-fast bacillus stain (to isolate organism; stain/smear is positive)

Culture and sensitivity (to isolate organism and detect drug resistance; positive MTb culture)

Chest x-ray examination (to evaluate pulmonary infiltration and extent of involvement; shows infiltrates or granulomas)

Gastric aspiration for acid-fast bacilli and culture (to isolate organism)

Bone marrow biopsy (to isolate organism and detect disseminated infection)

Management/Treatment

See Table 14–1 for the classification of TB.

Pharmacologic Management

For treatment of HIV-infected clients, see Table 14–2.

For treatment of TB disease, see Table 14–3.

For disease-treatment regimens, see Table 14–4.

For disease-treatment regimens of HIV-related TB, see Table 14–5.

For first- and second-line anti-TB medications, see Table 14–4.

Nonpharmacologic Management

Airborne isolation

High-calorie, high-protein diet

Table 14–1   Tuberculosis Classification System

Class	Type	Description
0	No TB exposure Not infected	No history of exposure Negative PPD reaction
1	TB exposure No evidence of infection	History of exposure Negative PPD reaction
2	TB infection No disease	Positive PPD skin test Negative bacteriologic test No clinical, bacteriological or radiographic evidence of active TB
3	TB disease Clinically active disease	*M. tuberculosis* cultured Clinical, bacteriologic, or radiographic evidence of current disease
4	TB disease Not clinically active	History of TB or Abnormal with no radiographic findings, Positive PPD reaction, Negative bacteriologic studies and No clinical or radiographic evidence of current disease
5	TB suspected	Diagnosis pending

Source: Centers for Disease Control and Prevention. (2000). Core curriculum on Tuberculosis (4th ed.). Atlanta, Georgia: CDC.

Complementary/Alternative Therapies

Supplementation with pyridoxine, 10–50 mg/day.

Client Education

Emphasize importance of medication compliance
Medication side effects

Follow-up

Monthly follow-up during treatment.
Confirm chest x-ray regression in 2–3 months.
Sputum culture after 2–3 months treatment.
Notify local health department.
Notify contacts of persons with active disease.

Table 14–2   Latent TB Infection for HIV Infected Clients Regimen

Drug	Duration: Adult	Duration: Children
INH	Daily: 9 months Twice Weekly: 9 months	Daily: 9 months Twice Weekly: 9 months
RIF and PZA	Daily: 2 months Twice Weekly: 2–3 months	Not recommended
RFB and PZA	Daily: 2 months Twice Weekly: 2–3 months	Not recommended

EMB—ethambutol, INH—isoniazid, PZA—pyrazinamide, RFB—rifabutin, RIF—rifampin
Adapted Centers for Disease Control & Prevention Division of Tuberculosis Elimination Core Curriculum on Tuberculosis 4th edition, Atlanta, GA,. 2000.

Table 14–3 TB Disease Treatment Regimen

Indication	Induction Phase Drugs	Induction Phase Interval/ Duration	Continuation Phase Drugs	Continuation Phase Interval/ Duration
Option 1 Pulmonary and extrapulmonary TB in adults and children *Total Duration:* 24 weeks	INH, RIF, PZA, EMB or SM	Daily for 8 weeks	INH, RIF	Daily or 2 or 3 times/week for 16 weeks
Option 2 Pulmonary and extrapulmonary TB in adults and children *Total Duration:* 24 weeks	INH, RIF, PZA, EMB or SM	Daily for 2 weeks and then 2 times/week for 6 weeks	INH, RIF	2 times/week for 16 weeks
Option 3 Pulmonary and extrapulmonary TB in adults and children *Total Duration:* 24 weeks	INH, RIF, PZA, EMB or SM	3 times/week for 24 weeks	INH, RIF, PZA, EMB or SM	3 times/week for 24 weeks
Option 4 Smear- and culture negative pulmonary TB in adults *Total Duration:* 16 weeks	INH, RIF, PZA, EMB or SM	Follow option 1, 2, or 3 for 8 weeks	INH, RIF, PZA, EMB or SM	Daily or 2 or 3 times/week for 8 weeks
Option 5 Pulmonary and extrapulmonary TB in adults and children when PZA is contraindicated *Total Duration:* 36 weeks	INH, RIF, EMB or SM	Daily for 4–8 weeks	INH, RIF	Daily or 2 times/ week for 28–32 weeks

EMB–ethambutol, INH–isoniazid, PZA–pyrazinamide, RIF–rifampin, SM–streptomycin
Adapted Centers for Disease Control & Prevention Division of Tuberculosis Elimination Core Curriculum on Tuberculosis 4th edition, Atlanta, GA,. 2000

Direct observed therapy for clients who have multidrug-resistant TB or potential for noncompliance.

Referral

Refer to infectious disease specialist to treat clients with HIV, multidrug-resistant TB, or extrapulmonary TB.
Refer to pulmonologist for bronchoscopy.

Table 14–4 First and Second Line Anti-TB Medications

First-Line Drugs	Route	Adult Daily Dose in mg/kg (maximum dose)	Child Daily Dose in mg/kg (maximum dose)
Isoniazid (INH)	PO or IM	Daily: 5 (300 mg) 2 Times/Week: 15 (900 mg) 3 Times/Week: 15 (900 mg)	Daily: 10–20 (300 mg) 2 Times/Week: 20–40 (900 mg) 3 Times/Week: 20–40 (900 mg)
Rifampin (RIF)	PO or IV	Daily: 10 (600 mg) 2 Times/Week: 10 (600 mg) 3 Times/Week: 10 (600 mg)	Daily: 10–20 (600 mg) 2 Times/Week: 10–20 (600 mg) 3 Times/Week: 10–20 (600 mg)
Rifabutin (RFB)	PO or IV	Daily: 5 (300 mg, or 150 mg, or 450 mg) 2 Times/Week: 5 (300 mg, or 450 mg) 3 Times/Week: Not known	Daily: 10–20 (300 mg or 150 mg or 450 mg) 2 Times/Week: 10–20 (300 mg or 450 mg) 3 Times/Week: Not known
Pyrazinamide (PZA)	PO	Daily: 15–30 (2g) 2 Times/Week: 50–70 (4g) 3 Times/Week: 50–70 (3g)	Daily: 15–20 (2g) 2 Times/Week: 50–70 (4g) 3 Times/Week: 50–70 (3g)
Ethambutol (EMB)	PO	Daily: 15–25 2 Times/Week: 50 3 Times/Week: 25–30	Daily: 15–25 2 Times/Week: 50 3 Times/Week: 25–30
Streptomycin (SM)	IM or IV	Daily: 15 (1g) 2 Times/Week: 25–30 (1.5g) 3 Times/Week: 25–30 (1.5g)	Daily: 20–40 (1g) 2 Times/Week: 25–30 (1.5g) 3 Times/Week: 25–30 (1.5g)
Second-Line Drugs			
Capreomycin	IM or IV	15–30 (1g)	Safety and effectiveness in children has not been established
Kanamycin	IM or IV	15–30 (1g) Not approved by FDA for TB treatment	15–30 (1g)
Amikacin	IM or IV	15–30 (1g) Not approved by FDA for TB treatment	15–30 (1g)
Ethionamide	PO	15–20 (1g)	15–20 (1g)
Para-amino salicylic acid (PAS)	PO	150 (16g)	150 (16g)
Cycloserine	PO	15–20 (1 g)	15–20 (1g)
Ciprofloxacin (cipro)	PO	750–1500 Not approved by FDA for TB treatment	Not used in children
Ofloxacin (floxin)	PO	600–800 Not approved by FDA for TB treatment	Not used in children

Table continued on following page.

Table 14–4 First and Second Line Anti-TB Medications (*Continued*)

Second-Line Drugs	Route	*Adult Daily Dose in mg/kg (maximum dose)*	*Child Daily Dose in mg/kg (maximum dose*
Levofloxacin (levaquin)	PO	500 Not approved by FDA for TB treatment	Not used in children
Clofazimine	PO	100–300 Not approved by FDA for TB treatment	100–300 Not approved by FDA for TB treatment

Adapted from: Centers for Disease Control & Prevention Division of Tuberculosis Elimination Core Curriculum on Tuberculosis 4th edition, Atlanta, GA, 2000

Table 14–5 HIV Related TB Disease Treatment Regimen

Total Duration (months)	Induction Phase Drugs	Induction Phase Interval/ Duration	Continuation Phase Drugs	Continuation Phase Interval/Duration
6	INH, RFB, PZA, EMB	Daily for 2 months (8 weeks)	INH, RFB	Daily or 2 times/ week for 4 months (18 weeks)
	OR INH, RFB, PZA, EMB	Daily for 2 weeks and then 2 times/week for 6 weeks	INH, RFB	2 times/week for 4 months (18 weeks)
9	INH, SM, PZA, EMB	Daily for 2 months (8 weeks)	INH, SM, PZA	2-3 times/week for 7 months (30 weeks)
	OR INH, SM, PZA, EMB	Daily for 2 weeks and then 2 times/week for 6 weeks	OR INH, SM, PZA	2-3 times/week for 7 months (30 weeks)
6	INH, RIF, PZA, EMB or SM	Daily for 2 months (8 weeks)	INH, RIF	Daily or 2-3 times/week for 4 months (18 weeks)
	OR INH, RIF, PZA, EMB or SM	Daily for 2 weeks and then 2-3 times/week for 6 weeks	INH, RIF	Daily or 2-3 times/ week for 4 months (18 weeks)
	OR INH, RIF, PZA, EMB or SM	3 times/week for 2 months (8 weeks)	INH, RIF, PZA, EMB or SM	3 times/week for 4 months (18 weeks)

EMB—ethambutol, INH—isoniazid, PZA—pyrazinamide, RFB—rifabutin, RIF—rifampin, SM—streptomycin
Adapted Centers for Disease Control & Prevention Division of Tuberculosis Elimination Core Curriculum on Tuberculosis 4th edition, Atlanta, GA,. 2000.

Table 14–6 Latent TB Infection in HIV Negative Persons Regimen

Drug	Duration: Adult	Duration: Children
INH	Daily: 9 months Twice Weekly: 9 months	Daily: 9 months Twice Weekly: 9 months
INH	Daily: 6 months Twice Weekly: 6 months	Not recommended
RIF and PZA	Daily: 2 months Twice Weekly: 2–3 months	Not recommended
RIF	Daily: 4 months Twice Weekly: Not recommended	Daily: 4 months Twice Weekly: Not recommended

EMB—ethambutol, INH—isoniazid, PZA—pyrazinamide, RIF—rifampin,
Adapted Centers for Disease Control & Prevention Division of Tuberculosis Elimination Core Curriculum on Tuberculosis 4th edition, Atlanta, GA,. 2000

BLOODBORNE VIRUS INFECTION

HEPATITIS (Viral)

SIGNAL SYMPTOMS▷ jaundice, tender hepatomegaly, malaise and nausea, vomiting and diarrhea.

ICD-9 Codes	070.1	Hepatitis A
	070.3	Hepatitis B
	070.44	Chronic hepatitis C with hepatic coma
	070.54	Chronic hepatitis C without mention of hepatic coma

Viral hepatitis is an acute or chronic inflammation of the liver resulting from a viral infection.

Epidemiology

Hepatitis A

Incubation period is 15–50 days.
Outbreaks due to food and water contamination.
In 1998 there were 23,229 cases of hepatitis A reported.

Hepatitis B

Incubation period is 45–160 days.
Acute cases of hepatitis B decreased by 50%.
In 1998 a total of 10,258 cases of hepatitis B were reported.
Hepatitis B accounts for approximately 50% of cases of hepatitis.
Currently, worldwide over 350 million carriers exist, but less than 2% of
  the US population is HbsAg positive. Portions of South America, Africa,
  Indonesia and Canada have over 8% of the population with positive HbsAg.

Hepatitis C

Incubation period is 2 weeks to 6 months.

It is estimated that approximately 242,000 new cases of hepatitis C infection occur each year.

Hepatitis D

Incubation period is 45–160 days.
Exists as a coinfection with hepatitis B.

Hepatitis E

Incubation period is 15–60 days.

Hepatitis G

Percutaneously transmitted.
Chronic viremia for about 10 years.
Identified in 50% of long-term drug users, 30% of clients who undergo hemodialysis, 20% of clients with hemophilia, and 15% of clients with hepatitis B or C.

Etiology

Hepatitis A (HAV): a picornavirus, RNA virus
Hepatitis B (HBV): a hepadnavirus, DNA virus
Hepatitis C (HCV): a flavivirus, RNA virus
Hepatitis D (HDV): a viruslike particle consisting of a hepatitis B surface antigen (HBsAg) and a unique delta antigen, a defective RNA virus
Hepatitis E (HEV): a calicivirus, RNA virus
Hepatitis G: Flavivirus.

Physiology and Pathophysiology

Hepatitis viruses cause hepatic-cell necrosis, scarring, Kupffer-cell hyperplasia, and infiltration of mononuclear phagocytes. This cellular injury is promoted by cell-mediated immunity. The inflammatory process damages and obstructs bile canaliculi, leading to jaundice.

Hepatitis A: Transmitted through the fecal–oral route.
Hepatitis B: Transmitted through blood and blood products, needle sharing, and sexual contact.
Hepatitis C: Transmitted through blood and blood products, needle sharing, and sexual contact.
Hepatitis D: Transmitted through blood or blood products, needle sharing, or sexual contact.
Hepatitis E: Transmitted through the fecal–oral route.
Hepatitis G: Transmission appears to be through blood and blood products, needle sharing, and sexual contact.

Clinical Manifestations

Subjective

Anorexia
Nausea
Vomiting

Fever

Right-upper-quadrant pain

Pruritus

Changes in color of urine (dark color)

Changes in color of stool (light or clay colored)

Objective

General symptoms

Hepatic enlargement (liver palpable)

Jaundice (yellow sclera, dark-colored urine, skin discoloration, clay-colored stool)

Weight loss

Prodromal or Preicteric Phase

Fatigue, malaise

Anorexia, nausea, vomiting

Headache

Hyperalgia

Cough, pharyngitis

Coryza

Changes in taste, or taste aversion

Right-upper-quadrant pain

Weight loss

Active or icteric phase

Jaundice

Clay colored stool

Hepatic enlargement

Pruritus

Posticteric phase

Jaundice resolves (liver enzymes decrease)

Decreased symptoms

Differential Diagnosis

Alcoholic hepatitis (history of alcoholism)

Drug-induced hepatitis

Autoimmune hepatitis

Infectious mononucleosis (severe fatigue, pharyngeal exudate)

Hepatic malignancy

Epstein–Bar virus infection (increased number of atypical lymphocytes, fever, petechiae at border of hard and soft palate, gelatinous grayish-white exudative tonsillitis for 7–10 days, diffuse hyperemia and hyperplasia of oropharyngeal lymphoid tissue)

Chronic fatigue syndrome (history of chronic fatigue)

Depression

Hypothyroidism (low triiodothyronine and/or thyroxine level)

Anemia (low hemoglobin)

Diagnostic Tests

Hepatitis antibody panel (to detect type of viral infection and stage of viral infection; positive in hepatitis) (see Table 14–7)

Liver-function tests (to determine extent of liver damage; liver enzymes elevated in acute phase, decrease in posticteric phase)

CBC (to rule out infection)

Liver biopsy (to determine extent of liver damage)

Monospot test (to rule out mononucleosis)

Thyroid-function tests (to rule out hyperthyroidism or hypothyroidism)

HIV antibody test (to rule out HIV infection)

Management/Treatment

Pharmacologic Management

Phenothiazine (Compazine): adults, 5–10 mg PO 3–4 times a day; children <2 years, not recommended; 20 to 29 lb, 2.5 mg once or twice daily; 30 to 39 lb, 2.5 mg 2–3 times a day; 40 to 85 lb, 2.5 mg three times a day or 5 mg twice daily.

AquaMephyton (vitamin K): infant, 2 mg PO/IM; child, 5–10 mg PO/IM, adult, 2–25 mg PO/IM based on prothrombin-time results.

For prophylaxis and treatment, see Table 14–8.

Nonpharmacologic Management

Activity as tolerated.

Bedrest recommended during initial acute phase.

Adequate hydration.

High-calorie, low-fat diet.

Complementary/Alternative Therapies

Baths to relieve itching

Table 14–7 Hepatitis Antibody Panel: Interpreting Results

Positive Test Result	Interpretation
IgM HAV	Acute Hepatitis A infection
IgG HAV	Convalescence Hepatitis A infection
HBsAg	Active Hepatitis B infection; early acute Hepatitis B infection
HBsAg, Anti-HBc; IgM	Acute Hepatitis B infection
HBsAg, Anti-HBc	Chronic Hepatitis B carrier
Anti-HBs	Immunity to Hepatitis B (vaccination)
Anti-HBs; Anti-HBc	Immunity to Hepatitis B; recovery from Hepatitis B infection
HBeAg	Hepatitis B infection that is highly infectious
Anti-HBe	Less infectious Hepatitis B status
Anti-HCV	Hepatitis C infection
Anti-HDV	Co-infection with Hepatitis D
IgM HEV	Acute Hepatitis E infection
IgG HEV	Convalescence Hepatitis E infection

Table 14–8 Viral Hepatitis Prophylaxis and Treatment

Hepatitis Virus	Prophylaxis/Vaccination	Treatment
Hepatitis A	IgG 0.02 ml/kg once before exposure or during incubation period (best within 2 weeks) HAV vaccine 1 ml IM 2 doses separated by 6–12 months	Appropriate prophylaxis within 2 weeks
Hepatitis B	HB IgG 0.06 ml/kg IM within 24–48 hours of exposure HBV vaccine 1 ml IM given in 3 doses–first dose, 2nd dose 1 month after 1st dose, 3rd dose 6 months after 1st dose	Appropriate prophylaxis with HBIg and HBV vaccine Pharmacologic intervention minimally beneficial
Hepatitis C	No vaccine	Interferon alpha 2b 3 million units SQ TIW plus oral ribavrin 1,000 or 1,200 mg daily–therapy may be required for 6 months
Hepatitis D	Hepatitis B vaccination	Supportive; IV fluids as needed
Hepatitis E	No vaccine	Supportive; IV fluids as needed

Client Education

Instruct about proper hygiene, good handwashing.
Instruct about modes of transmission.
Encourage safe-sex practices, including condom use.
Avoid alcohol or drugs metabolized by the liver.
Avoid birth control pills.
Avoid strenuous exercise.

Follow-up

Weekly for first month then monthly follow-up to monitor disease progression.
Liver-function tests may be performed every 2 months to monitor disease progression.

Referral

Refer to gastroenterologist to evaluate severity and potential for treatment. Referral is necessary for persistently elevated liver enzymes or for further diagnostic studies (liver biopsy).

HUMAN IMMUNODEFICIENCY VIRUS (HIV) INFECTION AND ACQUIRED IMMUNODEFICIENCY SYNDROME (AIDS)

SIGNAL SYMPTOMS frequently asymptomatic initially, but some patients exhibit flu like symptoms or a mononucleosis-like illness.

ICD-9 Codes	042	HIV infection with specified conditions
	043	HIV infection causing other specified conditions
	044	Other HIV infection
	V08	Asymptomatic HIV
	042.9	AIDS, unspecified

Human immunodeficiency virus (HIV) infection is a chronic infection that results in acquired immunodeficiency. The end stage of this chronic infection caused by a retrovirus is a collection of symptoms known as the acquired immunodeficiency syndrome (AIDS).

Epidemiology

Incubation period 10–14 years.

Epidemic and pandemic.

Disproportionately affects African American and Hispanic populations.

Disproportionately affects minority women.

Perinatal (vertical) infection rates decreasing.

Pediatric cases primarily a result of vertical transmission.

HIV transmitted through exchange of blood and bodily fluids—sexual transmission, exchange of blood or contact with blood on needles and syringes, perinatal transmission.

As of June 2000, there were 130,352 reported cases of HIV infection from 36 states and/or territories.

As of June 2000, there were 745,103 adult/adolescent cases of AIDS; 47% were men who have sex with men; 25% were injection-drug users; 6% were men who have sex with men and inject drugs; 10% were heterosexual contacts; 1% had hemophilia; 1% had had a blood transfusion; and 9% had no risk reported or identified.

As of June 2000, there were 8804 pediatric (<13 years of age) cases of AIDS; 91% came from a mother at risk for HIV infection; 4% were from blood transfusions; 3% were attributable to hemophilia; and 2% had no risk reported or identified.

Etiology

Retrovirus, HIV type 1 (HIV-1)

Physiology and Pathophysiology

HIV-1 attaches to CD4+ cells and replicates inside the host cell. Strands of HIV RNA are injected into the host cytoplasm on entry into the host cell and the HIV enzyme reverse transcriptase makes a template of host-cell DNA for further replication. The HIV enzyme polymerase assists in duplication and cleavage of viral particles into double-stranded DNA virus. The HIV enzyme integrase promotes the insertion of HIV-1 viral DNA into host-cell DNA. This continual viral replication and budding kills CD4+ cells.

Clinical Manifestations

Subjective

Mononucleosislike syndrome (fever, rash, myalgia, and malaise occurring after initial infection)

Chronic fatigue

Anorexia

Objective

Acute Infection

Mononucleosislike syndrome

May have HIV antibody

Asymptomtic Infection

Presence of HIV antibodies

No symptoms or opportunistic infections

Persistent Generalized Lymphadenopathy

Lymph-node enlargement ≥ 1 cm in two or more extrainguinal sites persisting for longer than 3 months

AIDS

Presence of AIDS-defining opportunistic infections or secondary cancers (see Table 14–9)

Differential Diagnosis

Malignancy

Tuberculosis (history of recent exposure, foreign travel)

Depression

Malnutrition

Enterocolitis

Vaccination

Hepatitis B vaccination(recombivax): < 19 years: 5(0.5) μg (ml) IM in deltoid then repeat at 1 and 6 months; 20 years and above: 10(1.0) μg(ml) Im in deltoid then repeat at 1 and 6 months.

Table 14–9   AIDS Defining/Indicator Conditions

Candidiasis of bronchi, trachea or lungs
Candidiasis, esophageal
Cervical cancer, invasive
Coccidoidomycosis, disseminated or extrapulmonary
Cryptococcosis, extrapulmonary
Cryptosporidiosis, chronic intestinal (> 1 month duration)
Cytomegalovirus disease, other than liver, spleen or lymph nodes
HIV encephalopathy
Herpes simplex: chronic ulcers of > 1 month duration or bronchitis, pneumonitis, or esophagitis
Histoplasmosis, disseminated or extrapulmonary
Isosporiasis, chronic intestinal of > 1 month duration
Kaposi's sarcoma
Lymphoma, Burkitts
Lymphoma, immunoblastic
Lymphoma, brain
Mycobacterium avium complex or M. kansasii, disseminated or extrapulmonary
Mycobacterium tuberculosis, pulmonary or extrapulmonary
Mycobacterium, other unidentified species, disseminated or extrapulmonary
Pneumocystis carinii pneumonia
Progressive multifocal leukoencephalopathy (PGL)
Salmonella septicemia, recurrent
Toxoplasmosis, brain
Wasting syndrome

MMR vaccination: adults and children 25mcg/ml SC; not recommended for children <15 months

Diagnostic Tests

Enzyme-linked immunosorbent assay (ELISA) (screening test to detect HIV infection)

Western blot (confirmatory test for HIV infection)

Polymerase chain reaction (PCR) (to detect HIV infection early, especially with children)

Viral culture (to isolate HIV organism)

CD4+ cell count (to detect amount of immunosuppression) (see Table 14–10)

T-lymphocyte subset analysis (to detect amount of immunosuppression)

Viral load assay (to detect amount of viral replication)

Serology for syphilis (to detect syphilis infection)

Viral hepatitis panel (to detect viral hepatitis)

Toxoplasmosis titer (to detect toxoplasmosis infection)

Management/Treatment

The Department of Health and Human Services guidelines for the use of anti-retroviral agents in HIV-infected adults and adolescents are found in Table 14–11, while the International AIDS Society guidelines are found in Table 14–12.

Table 14–10 AIDS Definition for Adolescents and Adults*

	Clinical Categories		
CD4+ T cells (cells/mm³)	(A) Asymptomatic, Acute or Primary HIV or PGL	(B) Symptomatic, not conditions in (A) or (C)	(C) AIDS Defining/ Indicator Conditions
> 500	A1	B1	C1
200–499	A2	B2	C2
< 200	A3	B3	C3

*Shaded areas classify client with an AIDS diagnosis.
Source: Centers for Disease Control and Prevention (1992). 1993 Revised classification system for HIV infection and expanded surveillance case definition for AIDS among adolescents and adults. Morbidity and Mortality Weekly Report, 44(RR-17):1–19.

Table 14–11 Initiation of Therapy (DHHS Guidelines)

Clinical Category	CD4+ T cell count and HIV RNA	Recommendation
Symptomatic (AIDS, thrush, unexplained fever)	Any value	Treat
Asymptomatic	CD4+ count < 500 cells/mm³ or HIV RNA > 10,000 (bDNA) or > 20,000 (RT-PCR) copies/ml	Treatment should be offered to client
Asymptomatic	CD4+ count > 500 cells/mm³ and HIV RNA < 10,000 (bDNA) or < 20,000 (RT-PCR) copies/ml	Experts recommend observing and delaying treatment; some experts treat.

Source: DHHS Panel on Clinical Practices for Treatment of HIV Infection. (2000). Guidelines for use of antiretroviral agents in HIV-infected adults and adolescents. [on-line]: Available at: http://hivatis.org or http://hiv.medscape.com/guidelines/adults.

Table 14-12 International AIDS Society Guidelines for Initiation of Therapy

Initiation of Therapy	CD4+ Count (Cells/mm³)	Plasma HIV RNA (Copies/ml)
Defer	>500	<5,000
Consider	350–500	<5,000
	>500	5,000–30,000
Recommend	<350	<5,000 5,000–30,000 >30,000
	350–500	5,000–30,000 >30,000
	>500	>30,000

Adapted from: Carpenter, C., Cooper, D., Fischl, M. et al. (2000). Antiretroviral therapy in adults: Updated recommendations of the International AIDS Society-USA Panel. Journal of the American Medical Association, 283:381–390.

Pharmacologic Management

See Table 14–13 for initial antiretroviral pharmacologic therapy.

Vaccinations

Annual trivalent influenza (Fluzone) vaccination: Persons > 12 years old: 0.5 mg IM in deltoid. Children 3–12 years old may get 1 or 2 doses given 1 month apart of 0.5ml IM. Children 6 months–35 months may receive 0.25 ml Im in anterolateral thigh. The vaccine is not recommended for children less than 6 months old. Two doses are administered to children less than 9 years old who are being vaccinated for the first time. Trivalent may be given concurrently with other vaccines. It is optimally given from October to mid November. (Pneumovax)—adults and children >2 years, 0.5 ml IM or SC; not recommended <2 years

Table 14–13 Initial Antiretroviral Pharmacologic Combinations

Recommended Combinations by Medication

Zidovudine (AZT) and Lamivudine (3TC) plus a protease inhibitor (PI)
Lamivudine (3TC) and stavudine (d4T) plus a PI
Zidovudine (AZT) and didanosine (ddI) plus a PI
Didanosine (ddI) and stavudine (d4T) plus a PI
Zidovudine (AZT) and zalcitabine (ddC) plus a PI
Saquinavir (fortovase, invirase) and ritonavir (norvir) plus a nucleoside reverse transcriptase inhibitor

Recommendation by Drug Classification

2 nucleoside reverse transcriptase inhibitors (NRTIs) plus PI
2PI
non-nucleoside reverse transcriptase inhibitior (NNRTI) plus 2 NRTI
PI plus NNRTI plus NRTI

Source: DHHS Panel on Clinical Practices for Treatment of HIV Infection. (2000). Guidelines for use of antiretroviral agents in HIV-infected adults and adolescents. [on-line]: Available at: http://hivatis.org or http://hiv.medscape.com/guidelines/adults.

Hepatitis B vaccination: 11–19 years, 10 μg IM in deltoid then repeat at 1 and 6 months; >19 years, 20 μg IM in deltoid then repeat at 1 and 6 months

MMR vaccination: adults and children, 25 μg SC; not recommended for children <15 months.

Polio vaccination must be inactivated; adults, 0.5 ml IM or SC; **do not administer live polio, varicella zoster, bacille Calmette–Guérin, or any live attenuated vaccine except measles–mumps–rubella;** prophylactic medications and treatment medications for opportunistic infections; testosterone replacement therapy for males

Fever-Reduction

Ibuprofen (children's Advil), 6 months–2 years, 5 mg/kg for temperature <102.5°F AND 10 mg/kg for temperature >102.5°F Q6–8H; adults, ibuprofen (Motrin), 400–800 mg 3–4 times a day

Nonpharmacologic Management

Balanced diet
Exercise—aerobic and muscle-mass-building exercises
Hydration

Complementary/Alternative Therapies

Vitamin supplementation
Protein supplementation

Client Education

Safe-sex practices, condom use
Food preparation to avoid contamination
Household cleaning to eliminate molds and spores
Daily oral care
Signs and symptoms of opportunistic infections and disease progression

Follow-up

Notification of sexual partners
Monitor viral load and monitor CD4+ cell count; for asymptomatic with no antiretroviral therapy, monitor every 3–6 months; for patients receiving initial antiretroviral therapy, monitor in 4 weeks; for patients with medication change, monitor in 4 weeks; for stable clients on antiretroviral therapy, monitor every 1–3 months
Dental examination at least yearly
Ophthalmology examination at least yearly

Referral

 CP 14–1 Clinical Pearl: HIV/AIDS reporting: HIV infection is not a reportable disease in every state. The clinician should be familiar with the state law requirement for reporting HIV infection. AIDS is a reportable disease in the United States. Clinicians are required to report clients with an AIDS diagnosis to the appropriate public health professional as required by their state's law.

Table 14–14 HIV Testing and Counseling

The following clients should be referred for HIV testing and counseling:
    Clients with positive PPD skin test
    Clients practicing unprotected sex
    Clients sharing needles, syringes or drug paraphernalia
    Clients with other diagnosed STDs
Pre-test HIV counseling should include a minimum of the following content:
    HIV test method, procedure and follow-up
    Meaning of HIV test
    Overview of HIV/AIDS
    Modes of transmission
    Risk behaviors
    Preparation for test results
    Personal risk reduction plan
    Confidentiality
Post-test Positive HIV counseling should include a minimum of the following content:
    Meaning of Positive test result
    Personal risk reduction plan
    Partner notification
    Referral for early intervention, support group, and other resources
    Assess for suicidal ideation
    Healthy lifestyle behaviors
    Confidentiality
Post-test Negative HIV counseling should include a minimum of the following content:
    Meaning of Negative test result
    Personal risk reduction plan
    Referral for HIV prevention case management
    Confidentiality

Refer to infectious-disease specialist for evaluation and determination of treatment regimen (see Table 14–14).
Support group for emotional counseling
Sexual partner notification for contact tracing
Dentist to evaluate for periodontal disease
Ophthalmologist to evaluate for ocular cytomegalovirus infection

CHILDHOOD ILLNESSES

FIFTH DISEASE (Erythema Infectiosum)

SIGNAL SYMPTOMS ▶ fever, erythematous rash beginning on cheeks—slapped cheeks

ICD-9 Code	057.0	Fifth Disease

Fifth disease is a viral exanthem that affects primarily school-aged children.

Epidemiology

Commonly acquired in winter and spring.
Infection common in childhood.
50% of adult population has evidence of prior exposure.
Incubation period of 4–14 days.

Period of infectivity prior to onset of symptoms.

Etiology

Human parvovirus B19

Physiology and Pathophysiology

Fifth disease is transmitted through direct contact with infected respiratory secretions or blood. It presents as a mild flulike illness during initial viremia at 7–10 days. The characteristic rash represents the immune response that occurs at 10–17 days. Infection during pregnancy can cause fetal hydrops and death. Adults may have complications of arthritis and arthralgias.

Clinical Manifestations

Subjective

Mild systemic symptoms (sore throat, cough, malaise)
Small-joint arthritis in adults (less common in children)

Objective

Begins with a lacy erythematous maculopapular rash on both cheeks (slapped-check appearance)
Rash spreads to upper arms, legs, trunk, hands, and feet; palms and soles are not affected; rash may worsen with heat or sunlight and last from 2 to 39 days (average 11 days)
Mild fever

Differential Diagnosis

Rubella (Forschheimer's sign—small rose-colored to reddish spots located on soft palate that appear before the general rash)
Lyme disease (history of recent tick bite, camping, hiking, hunting)
Rheumatoid arthritis (symmetric joint involvement, pain, swelling, erythema, warmth)
Drug reaction (history of recent medication)
Infectious mononucleosis

Diagnostic Tests

Typically none
Parvovirus B19 antibody panel (test for immunoglobulin [Ig] M confirms current infection; parvovirus B19 IgG indicates previous infection and immunity)
CBC (to rule out infection)
Lyme titers (to rule out Lyme disease)
Monospot test (to rule out mononucleosis)

Management/Treatment

Pharmacologic Management

Ibuprofen (children's Advil): 6 months–2 years, 5 mg/kg for temperature <102.5°F AND 10 mg/kg for temperature >102.5°F Q6–8H; adults: ibuprofen (Motrin), 400–800 mg 3–4 times a day

Intravenous immunoglobulins for clients with red-cell aplasia: children, immunoglobulin 20–40 ml IM every month; adults, immunoglobulin 30–50 ml IM every month or IV 100 mg/kg every month

Nonpharmacologic Management
Supportive
Fever management with fluids and light clothing

Complementary/Alternative Therapies
Multivitaminas once a day

Client Education
Reassure about benign nature
Avoid excessive play, rest (avoid overheating)

Follow-up
Not necessary unless signs and symptoms do not resolve or become worse

Referral
Refer to rheumatologist for further evaluation of signs of severe or erosive arthritis.

RUBEOLA (Measles)

SIGNAL SYMPTOMS ▶ 3 Cs of measles = cough, coryza, and conjunctivitis

ICD-9 Code	055.9	Rubeola

Rubeola is an acute viral epidemic childhood exanthem disease that presents with fever, rash, cough, coryza, or conjunctivitis.

Epidemiology
Infectious 1–2 days before symptoms, 3–5 days prior to onset of rash to 4 days after rash disappears, person becomes infective about the 9th day and is contagious for 1 week.
Incubation period 10–14 days (adults up to 3 weeks).
Rubeola is no longer indigenous to the US. In 1998, a total of 100 cases of rubeola were reported. 71 of those cases were importation related.

Etiology
Measles virus genus *Morbillivirus,* in the Paramyxovirus family

Physiology and Pathophysiology
Rubeola is transmitted by direct contact with infectious droplets. The prodrome consists of fever, cough, conjunctivitis, coryza, and leukopenia. Complications are otitis media, pneumonia, croup, and encephalitis.

Clinical Manifestations
Subjective
Fever (up to 106°F)
Malaise

Photophobia
Cough
Anorexia
Sore throat
Irritability

Objective

Classic triad (brassy cough, coryza, conjunctivitis)
Confluent, erythematous, maculopapular rash begins behind ears,
   progresses to forehead and neck, to trunk, upper extremities, buttocks and
   lower extremities; rash fades in 3 days in same sequence of appearance
   then desquamates
Koplik spots (white papules of 1–2 mm on erythematous base) on buccal
   mucosa, fades after 3 days

Diagnosis/Initial Impression

History
Physical examination

Differential Diagnosis

Drug reaction (history of recent medication)
Infectious mononucleosis (severe fatigue, pharyngeal exudate)
Rubella (Forschheimer's sign)
Erythema infectiosum (erythematous cheeks—slapped appearance)
Roseola infantum
Scarlet fever (rash occurs after sore throat)
Kawasaki disease (fever, conjunctival injection without exudates, rash,
   inflammatory changes in lips and oral cavity, "strawberry tongue")

Diagnostic Tests

None are necessary
CBC (to rule out infection)
ELISA for measles antibodies (to detect presence of infection)
Viral culture can be obtained of exfoliative tissue (to grow organism and
   confirm infection)

Management/Treatment

Pharmacologic Management

Ibuprofen (children's Advil): 6 months–2 years, 5 mg/kg for temperature
   $<102.5°F$ AND 10 mg/kg for temperature $>102.5°F$ Q6–8H; adults,
   ibuprofen (Motrin) 400–800 mg 3–4 times a day
Passive immunization of IgG, 0.25 mg/kg IM within 6 days of exposure
   (double dose for immunocompromised clients)

Nonpharmacologic Management

Humidification
Fluids
Supportive

Complementary/Alternative Therapies

Vitamin A, 200,000 IU per day for 2 days for children >1 year; 100,000 IU for ages 6–12 months

Client Education

Respiratory isolation until 4 days after onset of rash.

Avoid exposure to other children.

Avoid bright lights.

Instruct on vaccination schedule.

Follow-up

Monitor for complications.

Follow-up usually not necessary unless complications develop.

Referral

Refer to neurologist to evaluate for central nervous system complications.

Refer to pulmonologist to evaluate for pneumonia complications.

RUBELLA (German Measles)

SIGNAL SYMPTOMS ▶ prodrome, lymphadenopathy, rash

ICD-9 Codes	056.9	Rubella
	771.0	Congenital
	V04.3	Vaccination

Rubella is a mild contagious viral exanthem illness that causes severe congenital defects to fetuses.

Epidemiology

Peaks in late winter and early spring.

Contagious 1–2 days before symptoms and until 5–7 days after rash clears.

Incubation period is 14–21 days.

No longer indigenous to the US, most cases are imported. In 1998, a total of 364 cases of rubella were reported.

Etiology

Rubella virus, genus *Rubivirus,* in the Togaviridae family

Physiology and Pathophysiology

Rubella is spread by direct contact with infected secretions of the nose or throat. The prodrome consists of nonspecific respiratory symptoms and postauricular and occipital adenopathy. Infants with congenital rubella may shed virus for months after birth. Congenital rubella can result in cataracts, retinopathy, heart defects such as patent ductus arteriosus and pulmonary artery stenosis, sensorineural deafness, and neurologic disorders and developmental delay.

Clinical Manifestations

Subjective

Prodrome 1–5 days (low-grade fever, headache, malaise, anorexia, cough, sore throat, arthralgia)

Objective

Soft-palate petechiae (Forschheimer's sign)

Posterior auricular, posterior cervical, and suboccipital adenopathy

Blotchy, erythematous maculopapular rash beginning on face and neck descending to trunk and limbs (pediatric exanthem)

Differential Diagnosis

Drug reaction (history of recent medication)

Rubeola (Koplik spots)

Scarlet fever (rash occurs after sore throat)

Infectious mononucleosis (severe fatigue, pharyngeal exudates)

Roseola infantum (erythematous cheeks)

Kawasaki disease (fever, conjunctival injection without exudates, rash, inflammatory changes in lips and oral cavity, "strawberry tongue")

Diagnostic Tests

None necessary

CBC (to rule out infection)

Rubella-specific antibody panel (IgM, IgG) (to detect stage of infection)

Management/Treatment

Pharmacologic Management

Ibuprofen (children's Advil): 6 months–2 years, 5 mg/kg for temperature <102.5°F AND 10 mg/kg for temperature >102.5°F Q6–8H; adults, ibuprofen (Motrin) 400–800 mg 3–4 times a day

Nonpharmacologic Management

Supportive

Rest

Hydration

Complementary/Alternative Therapies

Multivitamins

Client Education

Educate about birth control methods.

Limit contact with susceptible persons.

Women should not attempt to become pregnant within 3 months of rubella vaccination.

Avoid pregnancy during infection.

Instruct about vaccinations.

Follow-up

Not necessary unless complications develop.

Pregnant women require frequent monitoring.

Referral

Refer children to pediatrician to evaluate for congenital rubella syndrome.

VARICELLA (Chickenpox)

SIGNAL SYMPTOMS ▶ centripetal rash beginning on trunk—teardrop lesions

ICD-9 Code	052.9	Varicella

Varicella is an acute contagious viral illness characterized by diffuse papulo-vesicular rash.

Epidemiology

Common in late winter and early spring.

Incubation period 10–21 days.

Contagious 24–48 hours prior to vesicle outbreak and until lesions have crusted.

Incidence increased in immunocompromised clients.

In 1998 a total of 82,455 cases of chicken pox were reported.

Varicella causes 4 million cases each year in the US. 90% of those cases are children. Approximately 1000 patients are hospitalized and about 100 patients die. Varicella is the leading cause of vaccine-preventable deaths. (CDC).

Etiology

Human (alpha) herpesvirus 3, a member of the *Herpesvirus* group.

Physiology and Pathophysiology

Varicella is spread by direct contact with airborne respiratory secretions or contact with vesicular fluid. The virus remains latent in sensory ganglia. A prodrome of fever, respiratory symptoms, and headache occurs about 1–3 days prior to rash. Preeruptive pain may last several days.

Clinical Manifestations

Subjective

Fever

Pruritus

Malaise

Anorexia

Arthralgia

Chills (from fever)

Headache

Objective

Initial 3- to 4-mm papules erupt on trunk.

Papules progress to clear vesicles that erupt and crust in 5–14 days (vesicular exanthem).

Rash spreads to face and extremities in a centripetal distribution.

Fever greatest with vesicle eruption.

Differential Diagnosis

Contact dermatitis (rash only on area of exposure)

Herpes simplex virus (vesicular lesion)

Coxsackievirus (type A—upper respiratory infection, febrile, herpangina, acute pharyngitis, hand–foot–mouth disease; type B—pleurodynia (sudden severe chest pain) orchitis, myocarditis/pericarditis)

Scabies (white to gray burrows on skin)

Impetigo (honey-colored, crusted lesion)

Insect bites

Urticaria

Diagnostic Tests

None necessary

CBC (to rule out infection)

Serum varicella titers (to detect level of infection)

Tzanck smear (to isolate organism)

Management/Treatment

Pharmacologic Management

Ibuprofen (children's Advil): 6 months–2 years, 5 mg/kg for temperature <102.5°F AND 10 mg/kg for temperature >102.5°F Q6–8H; adults, ibuprofen (Motrin) 400–800 mg 3–4 times a day

Acetaminophen (children's Tylenol): 10–15 mg/kg every 4–6 hours not to exceed 5 doses in 24 hours for children under 12 years of age. Children over 12 and adults: 650–1000 mg every 6 hours

Do not use aspirin

Oral acyclovir (Zovirax). 20 mg/kg QID for 5 days, preferably within 24 hours of onset; intravenous acyclovir, 500 mg/m^2 or 10 mg/kg Q8H for 7–10 days for immunocompromised clients

Varicella–zoster immunoglobulin, 125 U/10 kg IM to prevent infection in susceptible clients; may repeat 3 weeks later

Nonpharmacologic Management

Use antipruritic lotions (calamine lotion)

Take tepid baths

Use .mild soaps

Drink fluids

Rest

Cut nails

Complementary/Alternative Therapies

Oatmeal baths

Baths with baking soda or colloidal oatmeal (Aveeno)

Client Education

Emphasize importance of handwashing.

Instruct to avoid picking lesions.

Instruct about vaccination.

Instruct not to take aspirin.

Follow-up

Not necessary unless complications develop.

Immunocompromised client should receive follow-up and possible hospitalization.

Referral

Refer immunocompromised clients to infectious-disease specialist.

SEXUALLY TRANSMITTED DISEASES

CHLAMYDIAL INFECTION

ICD-9 Codes	.1	Urethritis
	615.0	Inflammatory disease of uterus
	616.0	Cervicitis

Chlamydial infection is a common sexually transmitted disease that results in urethritis, cervicitis, and epididymitis; it is frequently asymptomatic.

Epidemiology

Over 4 million infections annually.

Majority of cases in women are asymptomatic.

3%–5% of general population infected.

In 1999, a total of 659,441 cases of chlamydia infection reported, for a rate of 254.1 per 100,000 population; a 8.5% increase from 1998.

Etiology

Prokaryotic, obligate intracellular organism, *Chlamydia trachomatis.*

Physiology and Pathophysiology

Chlamydial infection requires squamous-columnar and columnar epithelial cells for infection. These organisms attach to a host cell and enter by endocytosis. The active parasite reproduces within the cell until it is destroyed and ruptures, disseminating infectious organisms that produce a polymorphonuclear inflammatory reaction.

Clinical Manifestations

Subjective
Purulent discharge (thick, cloudy)
Dysuria
Vaginal or abdominal pain
Postcoital bleeding
Women often asymptomatic

Objective
Mucopurulent discharge (thick, cloudy)
Edema and erythema of mucosa
Easily induced cervical bleeding

Differential Diagnosis
Gonorrhea (yellow to green discharge)
Urinary-tract infection (frequency, urgency, dysuria)
Pelvic inflammatory disease (cervical-motion tenderness)
Proctitis (pain with defecation, feeling of rectal fullness)
Urethritis (involvement of urethra only)
Cervicitis
Cystitis (suprapubic tenderness)
Appendicitis (right-lower-quadrant pain)

Diagnostic Tests
Culture (to isolate organism)
PCR (to detect presence of infection)
DNA probes (to detect presence of infection)
Monoclonal antibody immunofluorescence (to detect presence of infection)

Management/Treatment

PHARMACOLOGIC MANAGEMENT

Azithromycin (Zithromax), 1 g PO in a single dose or doxycycline (Vibramycin), 100 mg PO BID for 7 days

Nonpharmacologic Management
Supportive

Complementary/Alternative Therapies
Multivitamin once a day

Client Education
Encourage safe-sex practices, including condom use.
Abstain from sexual intercourse until treatment completed for both partners.
Wear clean cotton undergarments.

Follow-up

Notify all sexual partners.

Retesting after treatment is not required unless symptoms persist or reinfection is suspected.

Testing for cure not required.

Referral

Refer for HIV and syphilis testing and counseling at private, public, or community-based agency.

GENITAL HERPES SIMPLEX VIRUS INFECTION

SIGNAL SYMPTOMS ▶ itching, fever, dysuria, dyspareunia, tingling sensation 24 hours before eruption of lesion

| ICD-9 Code | 054.10 | Genital herpes simplex virus infection |

Genital herpes simplex virus (HSV) infection is a sexually transmitted herpes simplex double-stranded DNA virus infection involving the genital organs.

Epidemiology

Incubation period is 2–20 days.

Reactivation of HSV-2 is twice as common as HSV-1.

In 1999, a total of 10,149 cases of genital herpes were reported.

Etiology

Double stranded DNA virus, HSV-2.

HSV-1 can infect the genital organs.

Physiology and Pathophysiology

HSV enters mucosa or abraded skin and replicates in dermis or epidermis. HSV replication results in cell destruction, transudation, and vesicle formation. It spreads to contiguous cells and sensory-nerve tissue and remains latent in dorsal-root ganglion; reactivation results in increased replication of HSV, with resulting vesicular lesions.

Clinical Manifestations

Subjective

Genital lesion first episode

Itching

Painful genital ulcer

Fever

Headache

Malaise

Myalgia

Burning sensation

Dysuria (female)

Dyspareunia

Prodromal symptoms with recurrent lesions

Burning

Numbness

Tingling

Paresthesia of genital site about 24 hours before vesicle eruption

Objective

Primary Genital Lesion, First Episode

Vesicle on an edematous erythematous base that ulcerates, crusts over and resolves in about 21 days.

Nonprimary Genital Lesion, First Episode

Vesicle on nonedematous erythematous base that ulcerates, crusts over, and resolves in about 2 weeks.

Recurrent Genital Lesion

Prodromal symptoms, vesicle on a nonedematous erythematous base that ulcerates, crusts over, and resolves in about 7–10 days.

Differential Diagnosis

Pemphigus (thin-walled bullae, arising from normal skin or mucous membrane, that rupture and leave raw patches)

Erythema multiforme (polymorphous eruption of skin and mucous membrane, "target" lesions, macules, papules, nodules)

Syphilis (see section on "Syphilis" below)

Chancroid (highly contagious sexually transmitted disease; begins as papule that grows, ulcerates, and forms vesicles or bullae)

Follicular abscess (surrounds hair follicle)

Folliculitis (surrounds hair follicle)

Herpes zoster (vesicular lesion)

Lymphogranuloma venereum (sexually transmitted disease characterized by ulcerative genital lesions, marked swelling of lymph nodes in groin, headache, fever, and malaise)

Diagnostic Tests

Viral tissue culture (to grow and isolate organisms)

Tzanck smear (to isolate organisms)

ELISA monoclonal antibody (to detect presence of antibodies and infection)

Management/Treatment

Pharmacologic Management

First Episode

Acyclovir (Zovirax), 400 mg PO TID for 7–10 days

Acyclovir, 200 mg PO five times a day for 7–10 days

Famciclovir (Famvir), 250 mg PO TID for 7–10 days
Valacyclovir (Valtrex), 1 g PO BID for 7–10 days

Episodic Recurrence

Acyclovir (Zovirax), 400 mg PO TID for 5 days
Acyclovir, 200 mg PO five times a day for 5 days
Acyclovir, 800 mg PO BID for 5 days
Famciclovir (Famvir), 125 mg PO BID for 5 days
Valacyclovir (Valtrex), 500 mg PO BID for 5 days
Burrow's solution 4–6 times a day

Suppressive Therapy

Acyclovir (Zovirax), 400 mg PO BID
Acyclovir, 200 mg TID to five times daily (indicated only for patients with
frequent or severe recurrences; can be continued for up to 5 years, but it is
recommended that therapy be stopped after 1 year of continuous therapy
to assess patient's rate of recurrent episodes)

Severe

Acyclovir (Zovirax), 5–10 mg/kg IV Q8H for 5–7 days or until resolution
Acetaminophen: 10–15 mg/kg every 4–6 hours not to exceed 5 doses in 24
hours for children under 12 years old. For adults and children over 12
years old give 650–1000 mg every 6 hours.,
Burrow's solution 4–6 times a day

Nonpharmacologic Management

Supportive
Cool compresses

Complementary/Alternative Therapies

Multivitamin once a day
Oatmeal baths

Client Education

Safe-sex practices; avoid sexual contact during lesion outbreak or with
prodromal symptoms.
Viral shedding can occur at any time.

Follow-up

Notify sexual partners.
Follow-up required if complications develop.

Referral

Refer to obstetrician or infectious-disease specialist for evaluation and
management of pregnant women.
Refer for HIV and syphilis testing and counseling at private, public or
community-based agency.

GONORRHEA

SIGNAL SYMPTOMS ▶ purulent discharge, dysuria, lower abdominal pain, dysmenorrhea

ICD-9 Code	098.20	Gonorrhea

Gonorrhea is a purulent inflammation of the mucous membranes caused by a sexually transmitted organism.

Epidemiology

Approximately 1 million new cases a year.

Transmitted through unprotected sex.

Incubation period is 2–7 days.

Cases in women are frequently asymptomatic.

In 1999, a total of 369,076 cases of gonorrhea were reported, for a rate of 133.2 per 100,000 population, a 1.2% increase from 1998.

Etiology

Gram-negative diplococcus, *Neisseria gonorrhoeae.*

Physiology and Pathophysiology

Gonorrhea is transmitted by intimate sexual contact. Humans are the natural host for gonorrhea. Pili of the organism attach to epithelial cells of the host's mucous membranes, most likely infecting the columnar, transitional, and stratified squamous epithelial cells. The organism invades cells and changes cellular mucosa, resulting in a leukocytic inflammatory response and exudate production.

Clinical Manifestations

Subjective

Dysuria

Testicular pain

Dysmenorrhea

Lower abdominal pain

Fever

Tenesmus

Rectal burning or itching

Rectal bleeding

Purulent discharge (yellow to green)

Sore throat (pharyngeal)

Eyelid edema (eye infection)

Fever, chills

Arthralgias (disseminated syndromes)

Change in urination pattern: frequency, urgency, nocturia (prostate infection)

Objective

Purulent urethral discharge (history of stained undergarments)
Cervical-motion tenderness (progressing to pelvic inflammatory disease)
Meatal edema

Differential Diagnosis

Chlamydia (thick, cloudy discharge, postcoital bleeding in women, dyspareunia)
Urinary-tract infection (costovertebral and/or pelvic tenderness, frequency, urgency, dysuria)
Nongonococcal urethritis (mild dysuria, scanty penile discharge—white, clear, thin, or purulent; hypertrophic erosion of cervix and purulent cervical mucus develops in women)
Trichomonas (malodorous, frothy discharge and trichomonads on wet mount)
Bacterial vaginosis (grayish color, a fishy musty odor, clue cells on wet mount)

Diagnostic Tests

Culture (Thayer–Martin or Martin–Lewis medium) (to isolate *N. gonorrhoeae*)
Gram stain (to isolate organism—positive Gram stain for diplococci)

Management/Treatment

Pharmacologic Management

Uncomplicated Cervical, Urethral, or Rectal Infection

Cefixime (Suprax), 400 mg PO single dose
Ceftriaxone (Rocephin), 125 mg IM single dose
Ciprofloxacin (Cipro), 500 mg PO single dose
Ofloxacin (Floxin), 400 mg PO PLUS azithromycin (Zithromax), 1 g PO, or doxycycline (Vibramycin), 100 mg PO BID for 7 days

Pharyngeal

Ceftriaxone (Rocephin), 125 mg IM
Ciprofloxacin (Cipro), 500 mg PO
Ofloxacin (Floxin), 400 mg PO PLUS azithromycin (Zithromax), 1 g PO or doxycycline (Vibramycin), 100 mg PO BID for 7 days

Conjunctival

Ceftriaxone (Rocephin), 1 g IM and lavage eye with saline solution

Disseminated

Ceftriaxone (Rocephin), 1g IM or IV Q24H

Meningitis and Endocarditis

Ceftriaxone (Rocephin), 1–2 g IV Q12H

Nonpharmacologic Management
Education

Complementary/Alternative Therapies
Multivitamins

Client Education

Encourage safe-sex practices, including condom use.
Avoid sexual contact until therapy is complete.
Wear cotton undergarments.

Follow-up

Retesting not necessary unless symptoms persist.
Notify sexual partners.

Referral

Refer for HIV and syphilis testing and counseling at private, public or community-based agency.

HUMAN PAPILLOMAVIRUS INFECTION (Genital Warts, Condyloma Acuminatum)

SIGNAL SYMPTOMS pruritus, presence of growth

ICD-9 Code	078.1	Condyloma acuminatum

Human papillomavirus (HPV) infection is soft, skin-colored, fleshy contagious sexually transmitted warts.

Epidemiology

About 40 million Americans infected.
1 million persons infected yearly.
Over 60 types of HPV.
HPV may precede neoplasia.

Etiology

Human papillomavirus
HPV types 6, 11, 16, 18, 31, and 33 are associated with condyloma acuminatum.

Physiology and Pathophysiology

The initial HPV infection follows trauma to epithelium. HPV infects basal cells of the epithelium, which supports viral replication. The infected epithelial cells undergo transformation and proliferate into warty growths.

Clinical Manifestations

Subjective
Irritation
Pruritus
Presence of growth on genitals

Objective

Skin-colored, pink, or red soft-tissue growth (surface smooth to very rough, tumor presentation ranges from pinhead papules to cauliflowerlike masses)

Soft growth usually in clusters but may be solitary

Differential Diagnosis

Condyloma latum (fleshy wart)

Intraepithelial neoplasia

Molluscum contagiosum (umbilicated firm papule)

Mole

Skin tag

Folliculitis (involves hair follicle)

Lichen planus (small, flat, purplish papules or plaques with fine gray lines on flexor surface of wrist, abdomen, ankles, and sacrum)

Seborrheic keratosis (slightly raised tan to black warty lesions on skin, macules loosely covered with greasy crust)

Diagnostic Tests

Biopsy (to detect tissue infection)

Colposcopy (to detect tissue infection)

Pap smear (to detect cervical-tissue changes)

Acetowhitening (to visualize infected cervical tissue)

Management/Treatment

Pharmacologic Management

External Warts (Administered by Client)

Podofilox 0.5% solution or gel

Imiquimod 5% cream

External Warts (Provider Administered)

Cryotherapy with liquid nitrogen or cryoprobe

Podophyllin resin 10%–25 %

Trichloroacetic acid or bichloroacetic acid 80%–90%

Surgical removal by tangential scissors excision, tangential shave excision, or electrosurgery

Vaginal Warts

Cryotherapy with liquid nitrogen or trichloroacetic acid or bichloroacetic acid 80%–90%

Podophyllin 10%–25% in tincture of benzoin

Urethral Warts

Cryotherapy with liquid nitrogen

Podophyllin 10%–25% in tincture of benzoin

Anal Warts

Cryotherapy with liquid nitrogen or trichloroacetic acid or bichloroacetic acid 80%–90%

Surgical removal

Oral Warts

Cryotherapy with liquid nitrogen

Surgical removal

Nonpharmacologic Management

Supportive

Complementary/Alternative Therapies

Multivitamin once a day

Client Education

Encourage safe-sex practices, including condom use.

Need for regular Pap smear—may need proctoscopy if rectal warts are severe.

Assess self for recurrence.

Avoid sexual intercourse until warts are gone.

Follow-up

Annual Pap smear.

Notify sexual partners.

Referral

Refer for HIV and syphilis testing and counseling at private, public or community-based agency.

SYPHILIS

SIGNAL SYMPTOMS painless indurated chancre, fever, malaise, sore throat

ICD-9 Code	097.9	Syphilis

Syphilis is an acute and chronic sexually transmitted treponemal disease that affects multiple systems.

Epidemiology

Incubation period is 10 days–3 months, usually 3 weeks.

Period of contagion is variable.

Contagious during primary, secondary mucocutaneous lesions, and up to 4 years latent.

In 1999, a total of 556 cases of congenital syphilis were reported.

In 1999, a total of 6657 primary and secondary cases of syphilis were reported.

Etiology

Spirochete *Treponema pallidum*

Physiology and Pathophysiology

The syphilis bacterium is transmitted through skin abrasions during intercourse. Primary syphilis begins at the site of bacterial invasion and multiplication in epithelium, producing granulomatous tissue known as a chancre. Some microorganisms may drain into the lymphatic system and bloodstream, causing the systemic symptoms of secondary syphilis. Hypersensitivity reactions to organisms result in the destruction of skin, bone, and soft tissue into the gummas that indicate tertiary syphilis. Neurosyphilis is the invasion of the central nervous system and cerebrospinal fluid.

Clinical Manifestations

Subjective

Primary

Painless sore (indurated lesion)

Secondary

Sore throat
Fever
Malaise

Latent

Asymptomatic
Ulcerative lesions (gummas)

Objective

Primary

Painless, indurated lesion appears 3 weeks after exposure.

Secondary

Generalized, hyperpigmented erythematous rash that involves the palmar and plantar surfaces; rash develops within 6 weeks of painless papule (palmar and plantar rash is characteristic)
Indurated lesion

Early Latent

Asymptomatic
<1 year after infection

Late Latent

>1 year after infection
Gummas (nodular, ulcerative lesions) involving the skin or mucous membranes, cardiovascular symptoms such as aneurysm, aortic regurgitation

Neurosyphilis
  Asymptomatic or symptomatic
  Paralysis
  Tabes dorsalis
  Iritis
  Leukoplakia

Differential Diagnosis

Primary syphilis (lesion)
Secondary syphilis (rash)
Tertiary or late syphilis (>1 year after infection)
Congenital syphilis (mother has active syphilis at time of delivery)
Yaws (chronic ulcerating sores anywhere on the body with eventual tissue
  and bone destruction)

Diagnostic Tests

Dark-field microscopy of lesion fluid (to visualize organism)
Nontreponemal serology (Venereal Disease Research Laboratory [VDRL] test
  or rapid plasma reagin test) (to detect presence of antibody)
Treponemal serology (fluorescent treponemal antibody test or
  microhemagglutination assay) (to detect presence of antibody)
Cerebrospinal fluid analysis via lumbar puncture for VDRL (to detect
  neurologic involvement)
Lumbar puncture (to detect neurologic involvement)

Management/Treatment

Pharmacologic Management

Primary and Secondary

Penicillin G benzathine, 2.4 million units IM

Penicillin Allergy

Doxycycline (Vibramycin), 100 mg PO BID for 2 weeks
Tetracycline (Achromycin V), 500 mg PO QID for 2 weeks

Early Latent

Penicillin G benzathine, 2.4 million units IM

Late Latent or Latent of Unknown Duration

Penicillin G benzathine, 7.2 million units IM total divided into three doses
  of 2.4 million units IM each at 1-week intervals

Tertiary

Penicillin G benzathine, 7.2 million units IM total divided into three doses
  of 2.4 million units IM each at 1-week intervals

Neurosyphilis

Aqueous crystalline penicillin G, 18–24 million units a day divided into 3–4
  million units IV Q4H for 10–14 days

Nonpharmacologic Management
Supportive

Complementary/Alternative Therapies
Multivitamin once a day

Client Education

Encourage safe-sex practices, including condom use.

Avoid intercourse until treatment is complete.

Encourage compliance with medication regimen.

Human immunodeficiency virus (HIV) testing and counseling.

Follow-up

Notify sexual partners.

Repeat quantitative nontreponemal test at 1, 3, 6, and 12 months.

Pregnant women need monthly test until delivery.

Referral

Refer clients with HIV infection, pregnant clients, or clients who need penicillin desensitization to infectious-disease specialist.

Refer for HIV testing and counseling at private, public or community-based agency.

REFERENCES

General

Centers for Disease Control and Prevention (1998). 1998 Guidelines for treatment of sexually transmitted diseases. *Morbidity and Mortality Weekly Report, 47*(RR-1):1–116.

Centers for Disease Control and Prevention (1999). Summary of notifiable diseases, United States 1998. *Morbidity and Mortality Weekly Report, 47*(53):1–92.

Centers for Disease Control and Prevention (1999). *1999 STD Surveillance.* Available online at www.cdc.gov/nchstp/dstd/Stats_Trends/1999SurvRpt.htm.

Hay, W., Hayward, A., & Sondheimer, J. (2000). *Current: Pediatric diagnosis and treatment.* Stamford, CT: Appleton & Lange.

McCance, K., & Huether, S. (1997). *Pathophysiology: The biologic basis for disease in adults and children* (3rd ed.). St. Louis: Mosby-Yearbook.

Prescribing Reference Inc. (2000, Spring). *Nurse practitioners' prescribing reference.* New York: Author.

Tierney, L., McPhee, S., & Papadakis, M. (2000). *Current: Medical diagnosis and treatment* (39th ed.). Stamford, CT: Appleton & Lange.

Woodward, C., & Fisher, M. (1999). Drug treatment of common STDs: Part I. Herpes, syphilis, urethritis, chlamydia, and gonorrhea. *American Family Physician, 60,* 1387–1394.

Airborne Transmitted Infection: Tuberculosis

Centers for Disease Control and Prevention (2000). *Core curriculum on tuberculosis* (4th ed.). Atlanta: CDC.

Centers for Disease Control and Prevention (1999). Reported TB in US, 1999. Available online at www.cdc.gov/nchstp/tb/surv/surv99/surv99.htm.

Centers for Disease Control and Prevention (2000). Targeted tuberculin testing and treatment of latent tuberculosis infection. *Morbidity and Mortality Weekly Report, 49*(RR-6): 1–51.

Bloodborne Virus Infection: Hepatitis (Viral)

Achara, G., & Sadovsky, R. (2000). Hepatitis C virus: An overview of epidemiologic factors and natural history. *Family Practice Recertification, 22*(8):3–7.

Bockhold, K. (2000). Who's afraid of hepatitis C? *American Journal of Nursing, 100*(5):26–31.

Centers for Disease Control and Prevention (1999). Prevention of hepatitis A through active or passive immunization: Recommendations of the advisory committee on immunization practices (ACIP). *Morbidity and Mortality Weekly Report, 44*(RR-12): 1–37.

Centers for Disease Control and Prevention (1998). Recommendations for prevention and control of hepatitis C virus (HCV) infection and HCV-related chronic disease. *Morbidity and Mortality Weekly Report, 47*(RR-19):1–39.

Emmert, D. (2000). Treatment of common cutaneous herpes simplex virus infections. *American Family Physician, 61,*1697–1704.

Gish, R. (2000). Hepatitis C virus: Evaluation and management. *Family Practice Recertification, 22*(8):8–12.

Pawlotsky, J. (2000). Virologic tools for the diagnosis and management of hepatitis C. *Family Practice Recertification, 22*(8):13–16.

Sulkowski, M. (2000). Treatment and outcomes of hepatitis C infection. *Family Practice Recertification, 22*(8): 17–25.

Bloodborne Virus Infection: Human Immunodeficiency Virus (HIV) Infection and Acquired Immunodeficiency Syndrome (AIDS)

Brennan, C., & Porche, D. (1997). HIV immunopathogenesis. *Journal of the Association of Nurses in AIDS Care, 8*(4):7–25.

Carpenter, C., Cooper, D., Fischl, M. et al. (2000). Antiretroviral therapy in adults: Updated recommendations of the International AIDS Society—USA Panel. *Journal of the American Medical Association, 283,* 381–390.

Centers for Disease Control and Prevention (2000). *HIV/AIDS Surveillance Report. 12*(1):1–41.

Centers for Disease Control and Prevention (1999). 1999 USPHS/IDSA guidelines for the prevention of opportunistic infections in persons infected with human immunodeficiency virus. *Morbidity and Mortality Weekly Report, 48*(RR-10): 1–66.

Centers for Disease Control and Prevention (1992). 1993 Revised classification system for HIV infection and expanded surveillance case definition for AIDS among adolescents and adults. *Morbidity and Mortality Weekly Report, 44*(RR-17):1–19.

DHHS Panel on Clinical Practices for Treatment of HIV Infection (2000). Guidelines for use of antiretroviral agents in HIV-infected adults and adolescents. Available online at: http://hivatis.org or http://hiv.medscape.com/guidelines/adults

Sexually Transmitted Diseases: Human Papillomavirus Infection

Carson, S. (1997). Human papillomatous virus infection update: Impact on women's health. *Nurse Practitioner, 22*(4):24–37.

RESOURCES

General

Centers for Disease Control and Prevention
1600 Clifton Rd., NE
Atlanta, GA 30333
www.cdc.gov

The National Foundation of Infectious Diseases
    4733 Bethesda Ave.
    Suite 750
    Bethesda, MD 20814
    www.nfid.org/

Hepatitis

American Hepatitis Association
    30 E. 40th St.
    Room 305
    New York, NY 10016

Human Immunodeficiency Virus (HIV) Infection and Acquired Immunodeficiency Syndrome (AIDS)

Gay Men's Health Crisis
    129 W. 20th St.
    New York, NY 10011
    http://noah.cuny.edu/providers/gmhc.html

National AIDS Hotline (24 hours a day)
    Telephone: 1-800-342-2437 or 1-800-344-7432 (Spanish)

National Association of People with AIDS
    2025 I St. NW
    Suite 415
    Washington, DC 20006
    www.napwa.org

Tuberculosis

American Lung Association
    1740 Broadway
    New York, NY 10019
    www.lungusa.org/

INDEX

Page numbers in *italics* denote figures; those followed by "t" denote tables.